4/2017

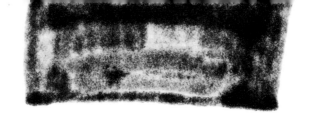

SEDENTARY BEHAVIOR AND HEALTH

CONCEPTS, ASSESSMENTS, AND INTERVENTIONS

WEIMO ZHU, PhD
University of Illinois at Urbana-Champaign

NEVILLE OWEN, PhD
Baker IDI Heart & Diabetes Institute
and Swinburne University of Technology

EDITORS

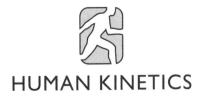

HUMAN KINETICS

Library of Congress Info

Names: Zhu, Weimo, 1955- editor. | Owen, Neville, editor.
Title: Sedentary behavior and health: concepts, assessments, and interventions / Weimo Zhu, Neville Owen, editors.
Description: Champaign, IL: Human Kinetics, [2017] | Includes bibliographical references and index.
Identifiers: LCCN 2016015868| ISBN 9781450471282 (print) | ISBN 9781492538080 (ebook)
Subjects: | MESH: Sedentary Lifestyle | Health Behavior | Risk Reduction Behavior | Motor Activity | Exercise
Classification: LCC RA776.95 | NLM W 85 | DDC 613--dc23 LC record available at https://lccn.loc.gov/2016015868

ISBN: 978-1-4504-7128-2 (print)

The web addresses cited in this text were current as of October 2016, unless otherwise noted.

Acquisitions Editor: Amy N. Tocco; **Developmental Editor:** Judy Park; **Managing Editor:** Stephanie M. Ebersohl and Anne Cole; **Copyeditor:** Joy Hoppenot; **Indexer:** Dan Connolly; **Permissions Manager:** Dalene Reeder; **Graphic Designer:** Whitney Milburn; **Cover Designer:** Keith Blomberg; **Photo Asset Manager:** Laura Fitch; **Photo Production Manager:** Jason Allen; **Senior Art Manager:** Kelly Hendren; **Illustrations:** © Human Kinetics, unless otherwise noted; **Printer:** Sheridan Books

Printed in the United States of America   10 9 8 7 6 5 4 3 2 1

The paper in this book is certified under a sustainable forestry program.

Human Kinetics
Website: www.HumanKinetics.com

United States: Human Kinetics
P.O. Box 5076
Champaign, IL 61825-5076
800-747-4457
e-mail: info@hkusa.com

Canada: Human Kinetics
475 Devonshire Road Unit 100
Windsor, ON N8Y 2L5
800-465-7301 (in Canada only)
e-mail: info@hkcanada.com

Europe: Human Kinetics
107 Bradford Road
Stanningley
Leeds LS28 6AT, United Kingdom
+44 (0) 113 255 5665
e-mail: hk@hkeurope.com

Australia: Human Kinetics
57A Price Avenue
Lower Mitcham, South Australia 5062
08 8372 0999
e-mail: info@hkaustralia.com

New Zealand: Human Kinetics
P.O. Box 80
Mitcham Shopping Centre, South Australia 5062
0800 222 062
e-mail: info@hknewzealand.com

E6212

To the three mentors who significantly influenced my life: Baolin Zhang 张宝林 at the Nanjing Normal University, China; Xinming Tao 陶心铭 at the Shanghai University of Sport, China; and Margaret J. Safrit at the University of Wisconsin-Madison, United States.

Weimo Zhu

To my late brother, Professor Alan Owen.
Neville Owen

CONTENTS

PREFACE

Our genetic makeup and the conditions of our lives have become incongruent. As the human genome developed through the process of natural selection, daily physical exertion was obligatory. Our biochemistry and physiology evolved to function optimally under such circumstances. However, today's mechanized, technologically oriented conditions promote and sometimes force us to have an unprecedentedly sedentary lifestyle: Most people now spend the majority of their waking hours *sitting*.

It is now understood and accepted among scientists, health practitioners, and the lay public that a *lack of physical activity* (too little exercise) has major adverse health consequences and that adopting physical activity has significant preventive benefits. However, recent evidence suggests strongly that *too much sitting* poses an additional and widespread health risk.

Prolonged periods of time spent sitting are now ubiquitous in the workplace, in automobile commuting, and at home, whether viewing television or using computers and electronic entertainment technologies. In this context, the newly emerging science of sedentary behavior has made impressive initial progress in identifying prolonged sitting as a health risk that appears to be distinct from a lack of physical activity or exercise and points to novel opportunities for innovative initiatives in public health, occupational health, and clinical and social policies.

Many important health problems are likely to be exacerbated by sedentary behaviors—*too much sitting*—including obesity, atherosclerosis, age-related fractures, and diabetes. The consequences of sedentary behavior on society (e.g., the high cost of health care) are also likely to be significant. Furthermore, with rapid technological changes, opportunities for passive work, passive recreation, and passive transport are only likely to increase. Thus, the influence of sedentary behavior on health and society is likely to be of ongoing and potentially growing concern.

Many new scientific, public health, and broader social questions about sedentary behavior now need to be addressed. Why does sedentary behavior appear to be such a mismatch with our born-to-move genes? What roles have ergonomics, design, and the industrial and information revolutions played concerning sedentary behavior? What is the effect of environmental changes on people's sedentary behavior and health outcomes?

Written by a group of the finest scientists and experts in their areas, the chapters in *Sedentary Behavior and Health* address these and a plethora of other questions. The collection of 27 chapters in this book provides the latest and most comprehensive coverage on the topic of sedentary behavior and health. This book is unique because it draws on perspectives that go beyond the more conventional physiological, behavioral, and epidemiological perspectives that have shaped the recent development of this field. It provides depth and breadth of perspective, in ways that will be informative for researchers, practitioners, and students in kinesiology, public health, preventive medicine, physical activity, health behavior, health promotion, sociology, and human engineering or industry.

The development of this book has been one arm of a project. The other arm was the conference Sedentary Behavior and Health: Measurement Issues and Research Challenges at the University of Illinois at Urbana-Champaign in October 2015. The majority of the chapter contributors of this book were speakers at the conference. Following the conference, all authors were given the opportunity to review their chapters in the light of what they learned from preparing their own presentations, feedback from other presenters, and new perspectives that arose at the meeting. Through these synergies of the conference and the set of chapters in this book, the new research field on sedentary behavior and health has been further consolidated and new research opportunities and practical and policy implications are emerging. Early indications exist that new research programs and other initiatives for better understanding why and how to reduce sedentary behavior will be fostered.

Broad Readership Interest

This book has several purposes: It serves as a key reference for a rapidly emerging research area, as a textbook for courses and workshops on physical activity and inactivity or sedentary behavior and health, and as key reading for courses and workshops on public health and health promotion.

The primary audience for this book is traditional kinesiology and exercise science professionals and students including those with a focus on physical activity and health, physical fitness, and physical education, as well as professionals and students in public health, physical therapy, occupational therapy, and ergonomics. The secondary audience is professionals and students in public health and medicine, including those with a focus on community health, obesity, worksite wellness, health disparity, and disability. The tertiary audience is professionals and students in broader areas of applied behavioral science, such as transport and urban planning, environmental health, and many other areas that address behavior changes based on thorough environment and policy interventions, computers, and technology.

Because sedentary behavior is quickly becoming a global issue and burden, this book touches on many different aspects and effects of sedentary behavior. Professionals in a diverse range of fields will also be interested in reading it. Industrial engineering, environment design, social science, radiology and anthropology, and measurement and statistical data analysis are just a few examples of interested fields.

Organization of the Book

Each chapter provides learning objectives, a summary of key concepts, and a set of study questions to direct the reader to key studies and commentaries in the specific area under consideration.

To address its goals, the book is organized into five parts:

▶ Part I—Sedentary Behavior Concepts and Context—has six chapters providing a perspective on contemporary developments in the sedentary behavior research field, a thorough review of the physiology of sedentary behavior and the relationship between modern technologies and sedentary behavior, and evolutionary and industrial engineering and design perspectives on sitting.

▶ Part II—Sedentary Behavior and Health—has six chapters providing the most up-to-date review on the relationship between sedentary behavior and several major chronic diseases, specifically obesity, cardiovascular disease, cancer, diabetes, and lower back pain.

▶ Part III—Measuring and Analyzing Sedentary Behavior—has five chapters addressing this topic comprehensively. To properly understand sedentary behavior, we must be able to measure it accurately and analyze the relevant data appropriately. Both conventional approaches in measuring sedentary behavior and future possibilities are covered by leading researchers in the field.

▶ Part IV—Sedentary Behavior and Subpopulations—has four chapters on issues specific to sedentary behavior in children, in working adults, in older adults, and in minorities. To design effective interventions for reducing or eliminating sedentary behavior, a good understanding of characteristics of subpopulations' sedentary behavior is an absolute must.

▶ Part V—Changing Sedentary Behavior—has six chapters covering mainstream intervention methods based on both behavioral theories and psychological models, plus broader perspectives in which environmental, social, community, worksite, and technology-based interventions are considered.

Finally, in the Epilogue, the editors provide their overall conclusions about the state of this new field, identifying promising key research topics, strategies, and future directions and suggesting future public health and broader social implications.

A Consolidated, Broadly Based Overview

Now is an ideal time for a consolidated and broadly based scientific and critical overview of what is known from the rapidly emerging body of research about sedentary behavior and health, where important new opportunities are emerging for reducing the health risks associated with too much sitting. This book contains the evidence required for pursuing well-informed, wide-reaching initiatives.

Sedentary behavior, although presently mismatched with many aspects of our genetic makeup, is quickly emerging as a primary human behavior as well as a likely new public health threat. Studying sedentary behavior and health to design effective interventions will be a hot field in the coming decades. We are confident that *Sedentary Behavior and Health: Concepts, Assessments, and Interventions* will serve as a rich learning resource and reference for this emerging field.

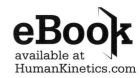

ACKNOWLEDGMENTS

This book is a by-product of the successful Sedentary Behavior and Health conference (www.sedentaryconference.com) held at the University of Illinois at Urbana-Champaign (UIUC) October 15 to 17, 2015. After organizing two previous successful conferences, Aging and Measurement and Walking for Health, at UIUC in 2003 and 2005, respectively (as well as jointly with the Cooper Institute on Diversity in Physical Activity and Health in 2007), I started wondering several years ago what would be the next hot topic for kinesmetrics (i.e., measurement and evaluation in kinesiology) to address. It did not take me too long to identify a coming new, exciting public health theme—sitting was being described as the new smoking! Evidence and critical thought on this topic was therefore much needed. The idea to have a conference and book on sedentary behavior and health was immediately supported by experts around the world and this book's publisher, Human Kinetics. Due to perhaps the tough economic times over the past several years, putting this conference and book together was rather challenging. Eventually, we made it through endless hours of hard work with the great support received. I would like to take this opportunity to express my sincere appreciation to the following people and organizations:

- The Society of Health and Physical Educators (SHAPE America) and the American College of Sports Medicine (ACSM) for their support of the conference, especially CEO E. Paul Roetert and executive vice-president James R. Whitehead
- All sponsors for their financial contributions and support
- Fujian Normal University, Nanjing Sport Institute, and Shanghai University of Sport in China for their conference participation from the other side of the globe
- Philip Lockwood of Voice of Movement for his support and enthusiasm
- Nate Hartmann and the staff of Yellow Box Advertising for their skillful support of the conference
- UIUC, especially Michael Miller, Tedra Tuttle, Barb Jewett, and Danny Powell at the National Center for Supercomputing Application, for their support and assistance
- Graduate students and visiting scholars in my kinesmetrics laboratory for their hard work and great support, especially Yan Yang, Hai Yan, and Zezhao (Jack) Chen
- All the contributing authors for their time, expertise, great presentations at the conference, and excellent chapters
- Human Kinetics' leadership and staff, especially Amy Tocco and Judy Park, for their support of both the conference and the book
- Professor Neville Owen, the coeditor of this book, for his leadership in the field of sedentary behavior research and his 110% support of the conference and this book project.

Finally, I want to extend special appreciation to Heidi A. Krahling, the visiting research specialist who coordinates everything in my kinesmetrics lab, for her extremely hard work, excellent support, and skillful proofreading and editing. Without her great efforts, the success of the conference and book would have been impossible.

Weimo Zhu

First and foremost, I must thank my coeditor, Weimo Zhu. His vision for what this book could be has resulted in a stimulating and original set of contributions to the emerging field of sedentary behavior and health. This book is also a tribute to the organizational skills and support of his team at the University of Illinois, especially Heidi A. Krahling. Thanks particularly to our contributors for their generosity in devoting their precious time, funds of knowledge, and intellectual resources and perspectives to each of their chapters.

I have had the good fortune to have many excellent research collaborators in my exploration of sedentary behavior and health: present and former PhD students, fellows, and other team members at Deakin University, the University of Queensland, and the Baker IDI Heart and Diabetes Institute. I have also had the joy of working with international collaborators, including in the United States (with many good people at Jim Sallis' program in San Diego and with Chuck Matthews at the National Cancer Institute), Belgium (Ilse DeBourdeaudhuij, Greet Cardon, Benedicte Deforche and their team), and Japan (through the programs of Koichiro Oka, Ai Shibata, and Shige Inoue at Waseda and Tokyo Medical universities).

My initial explorations of sedentary behavior and health started at Deakin University with my PhD student and now senior collaborator Jo Salmon, whose insights and acumen did so much to initiate our public health approach to sedentary behavior research. Jim Sallis and Adrian Bauman helped me muddle my way into this new approach to thinking about physical activity and public health. Len Epstein's elegant experimental work and seminal ideas on sedentary behavior were a shining light on our scientific horizon.

The Queensland Government's generous funding and Alan Lopez's leadership and practical support of the Cancer Prevention Research Centre at the University of Queensland provided me and Elizabeth Eakin with the opportunity to build a research team, including Genevieve Healy, whose findings have been fundamental to building the sedentary behavior and health research field. The many contributions of our program administrator, Cathy Swart, and of our research support staff, fellows, visiting scholars, and PhD students—including Elisabeth Winkler, Sheleigh Lawler, Marina Reeves, Katrien Wijndaele, Karin Proper, Ding Ding, Corneel Vandelanotte, Bronwyn Clark, Satyamurthy Anuradha, Paul Gardiner, Ruth Mabry, and Maike Neuhaus—can be seen in their excellent research publications.

The National Health and Medical Research Council (NHMRC) of Australia has been the major supporter of my research program through a Center of Research Excellence and Program and Project Grant support, as well as providing personal salary support through a Senior Principal Research Fellowship. The National Heart Foundation of Australia has also been a highly valued supporter. Two successive five-year NHMRC Program Grants have allowed my team to work with the teams of Adrian Bauman at Sydney University and Wendy Brown at the University of Queensland—both of whom deserve special mention and thanks.

The leadership of Garry Jennings and Tom Marwick at the Baker IDI Heart and Diabetes Institute has provided me with enviable freedom and an interdisciplinary scientific and intellectual environment to develop my sedentary behavior research program. Thanks especially to my good colleagues David Dunstan, Orly Lacham-Kaplan, Ruth Grigg, Bronwyn Kingwell, Brigid Lynch, Alicia Thorp, Takemi Sugiyama, Robyn Larsen, Megan Grace, Javad Koohsari, Karl Minges, Bethany Howard, Nyssa Hadgraft, Paddy Dempsey, and to the other excellent students and research staff who have contributed to our program. Billie Giles Corti and her team at the University of Melbourne and Ester Cerin and Takemi Sugiyama now at the Australian Catholic University also deserve special mention.

Thanks particularly to my close family: Sue, Alice, Derek, Beth, Angus, Cate, John, George, Eric, Chio, and Ruby.

Neville Owen

PART I

SEDENTARY BEHAVIOR CONCEPTS AND CONTEXT

Part I has six chapters dealing with the key concepts and scientific underpinnings of sedentary behavior. These chapters set the scene for what follows in the other four parts of the book. Here, the focus is on background issues, mechanisms, and the broad context of sedentary behavior and health. Chapter 1 deals with the more recent and immediate background of research on sedentary behavior and health. Over the past 15 years, there has been a rapid accumulation of research studies addressing the health consequences of sedentary behavior, particularly from the point of view of chronic disease prevention. In chapter 1, Neville Owen provides a perspective of research and practical and policy concerns about sedentary behavior and chronic disease risk. He reviews some key aspects of the epidemiological, behavioral, and experimental research that has emerged, puts forward concepts from behavioral epidemiology and ecological models of health behavior as organizing principles, and proposes directions for future research.

In chapter 2—Gravity, Sitting, and Health—Joan Vernikos provides important context and background. She does so in depth and focus, illustrating

the significant and highly informative precursors for the new sedentary behavior and health field that are apparent in research associated with the U.S. and international space programs. Chapter 3 then focuses on a stream of experimental research that has begun to identify the metabolic and other biological consequences of reducing and breaking up prolonged sitting time. David W. Dunstan and colleagues address key aspects of study design and other methods required for conducting human experimental research on sedentary behavior and health. They highlight several new research findings and provide some compelling hints about the mechanisms by which sedentary behavior exerts adverse influences on health outcomes.

Chapters 4, 5, and 6 provide a provocative and informative perspective on determinants of sitting, which can be both more and less difficult to change. In chapter 4, sociologist and designer Galen Cranz provides a novel and engaging perspective on the history of the chair, its many manifestations, and its role in making prolonged sitting such a ubiquitous contemporary attribute of human life. In chapter 5, Jorge A. Banda and Thomas N. Robinson

1

address the particular effects on children of another major environmental determinant of sedentary behavior—the screen. Chapter 6 takes a broader perspective as Kenneth A. Glover and Weimo Zhu address how sitting has become the default option in many contexts and why it is in many circumstances inextricably and unavoidably embedded in daily life.

Together, these six chapters provide the broad context for the rest of the book. The editors, however, must confess to a sin of omission—not address-ing the role of the automobile as a major source of sedentary behavior in modern life. Several recent studies have identified time spent sitting in cars as a significant source of sedentary behavior, with unique adverse health outcomes. We nevertheless are confident that the reader will come away from part I of the book with many new insights into sitting, its health consequences, and contexts and will gain a broader perspective on which to build a more detailed understanding of sedentary behavior and health.

CHAPTER 1

EMERGENCE OF RESEARCH ON SEDENTARY BEHAVIOR AND HEALTH

Neville Owen, PhD

The reader will gain an overview of the scientific background and context of sedentary behavior research and its potential to inform future chronic disease prevention initiatives. By the end of this chapter, the reader should be able to do the following:

▸ Understand how *too much sitting* may be defined as a behavioral attribute that is distinct from physical inactivity or too little exercise

▸ Describe some key characteristics of the rapidly evolving body of contemporary research evidence on sedentary behavior and health

▸ Provide a brief historical perspective and concepts to guide the development of research on sedentary behavior and health

▸ Outline research priorities for sedentary behavior and health within a behavioral epidemiology framework

---

What is sedentary behavior? Put simply, sedentary behavior may be characterized as too much sitting, as distinct from too little exercise. There is a rapidly emerging body of evidence on sedentary behavior and health that links back to a strong science base in space-flight and bed-rest studies (Vernikos 2004; Vernikos 2011; see also chapter 2). The term *sedentary behavior* requires some clarification, given that the term *sedentary* has been used previously to describe those who do little or no physical activity or who do not meet physical activity and health guidelines (see as an example Owen and Bauman 1992). Now, the recommendation is to use the term *sedentary* to characterize behaviors involving prolonged sitting and the term *inactive* in the context of doing little physical activity or not meeting activity guidelines (Owen, Healy, et al. 2010; Owen 2012; Pate et al. 2008).

To be more specific, sedentary behaviors typically involve sitting or reclining in the energy-expenditure range of 1.0 to 1.5 METs (metabolic equivalents; multiples of the basal metabolic rate). By contrast, physical activity (moderate- to vigorous-intensity physical activity [MVPA]; exercising) such as brisk walking or running typically requires an energy expenditure of 3 to 8 METs. Those with no participation at this level have in the past been described as sedentary (Pate et al. 2008). Now, especially since a focus on reducing sedentary behavior has been proposed as a potential new element of physical activity recommendations (Garber et al. 2011), the term *inactive* is preferable for describing those who do not engage in MVPA (Owen, Healy, et al. 2010).

A helpful definition comes from the Sedentary Behaviour Research Network:

Any behavior during waking hours that is characterized by energy expenditure less than or equal to 1.5 METs, while in a sitting or reclining posture; the term "inactive" should thus be used to describe those who are performing insufficient amounts of MVPA (i.e., not meeting specified physical activity guidelines) (2012, page 540).

An energy-expenditure perspective highlights how sitting time is important to consider in the context of physical activity and health. The objective measurement of all movement during every minute of waking hours is highly informative in this context. Studies using accelerometers with large population samples have shown that typical adults in the United States and Australia, for example, on average engage in only 20 to 30 minutes of MVPA, sit up to 10 hours of each day, and spend the balance of their waking hours in light-intensity activity (Healy, Clark, et al. 2011; Healy, Matthews, et al. 2011; Owen, Sparling, et al. 2010).

Reducing sitting time has emerged as a potential new strategy for physical activity and chronic disease prevention initiatives. Sitting time reflects the accumulated hours spent each day in the numerous sedentary behaviors during commuting and leisure time, and at school, in the workplace, and in the domestic environment. Even those who meet the public health recommendation (for adults, 30 min of MVPA on most days each week; for children and youth, 60 min daily) can be exposed each day to the deleterious metabolic consequences of *7 to 10 hours of sitting* (Healy, Matthews, et al. 2011; Salmon et al. 2011). Figure 1.1 shows objective-measurement findings from the 2003-2006 U.S. National Health and Nutrition Examination Survey (CDC 2011). It illustrates how adults, youth, and children in the United States allocate their time, based on accelerometer-derived time spent in sedentary activities, in light-intensity activity, and in MVPA.

The proportions shown in figure 1.1 are compelling. They illustrate that the majority of the day is spent in sedentary activity or in light-intensity physical activity. Although MVPA represents less than 3% (approximately) of waking hours, it has been the main focus of public health efforts to promote physical activity to date. Substantial opportunities exist for reducing sitting time throughout the day among children, youth, and adults.

Time spent sitting displaces time spent in higher-intensity activities, thereby contributing to a reduction in overall energy expenditure. So, substituting 2 hours of this high volume of sitting time with light-intensity activity (2 hr * (2.5 METs − 1.5 METs) = 2.0 MET-hr) would significantly increase energy expenditure. This would be greater than the additional energy expenditure associated with 30 minutes of walking, which we would assume to displace either sitting time (0.5 hr * (3.5 METs − 1.5 METs) = 1.0 MET-hr) or light-intensity time (0.5 hr * (3.5 METs − 2.5 METs) = 0.5 MET-hr). Thus, 2 additional hours of sitting each day, in simple energy-expenditure terms, would negate what is achieved by meeting the basic physical activity and health recommendation through walking.

Prolonged sitting is now understood to be a significant and distinct behavioral attribute that

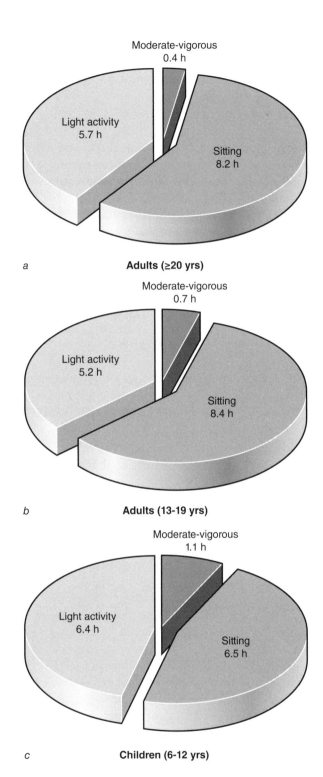

Moderate-vigorous
0.4 h

Light activity
5.7 h

Sitting
8.2 h

a   **Adults (≥20 yrs)**

Moderate-vigorous
0.7 h

Light activity
5.2 h

Sitting
8.4 h

b   **Adults (13-19 yrs)**

Moderate-vigorous
1.1 h

Light activity
6.4 h

Sitting
6.5 h

c   **Children (6-12 yrs)**

Figure 1.1 How U.S. adults (*a*), youth (*b*), and children (*c*) allocate their time, based on average population values for sedentary time, light-intensity physical activity, and moderate- to vigorous-intensity physical activity.

Data from Centers for Disease Control and Prevention 2011.

is manifested in multiple life contexts. Identifying sedentary behavior as a novel term within the physical activity and health equation does not, however, contradict or negate what is well understood about the health benefits of participation in moderate-intensity and vigorous-intensity physical activity. Rather, understanding sedentary behavior in this context broadens our perspective on the health benefits of physical activity and identifies novel targets for health promotion and disease prevention initiatives.

Contemporary Sedentary Behavior Research and Concepts

Sedentary behavior has its recent historical roots in the physical activity and health field. Research on physical activity and health gained much of its early impetus from epidemiological studies with members of active and inactive occupations in the UK (Morris et al. 1953) and the United States (Paffenbarger et al. 1997). Early studies were conducted with British civil servants—bus drivers and desk-bound workers—who primarily sat at work, compared to their occupational counterparts—bus conductors and mail delivery workers—who were on their feet for most of their working days. Morris and colleagues (1953) demonstrated significantly reduced cardiovascular disease risk in those who were more active, interpreting the findings as showing the beneficial effects of physical activity. However, an alternative perspective is that these early physical activity epidemiology studies showed deleterious health consequences of prolonged occupational sitting. Brown and colleagues (2009) argued that with burgeoning research attention on sedentary behavior, the physical activity and health field is now revisiting some of its fundamental epidemiological bases within the new sedentary behavior perspective.

Understanding the broader conceptual and scientific background to the current interest in sedentary behavior research is helpful. Research on sedentary behavior can be traced back to the history of behaviorist underpinnings, particularly in relation to the social and environmental determinants of behavioral choice shaped by thinking in the subdisciplines of behavioral economics and behavioral epidemiology. A focus on environmental determinants of sitting time emphasizes the limitations on individual initiative for many health-related behaviors (Owen et al. 2000; Sallis, Owen, and Fisher 2008). This is an important consideration in the context of physical activity and health research, where the concept of individual responsibility for exercising or otherwise choosing to be physically active has been the dominant paradigm (Sallis and Owen 1999).

Ecological Model

An ecological model of sedentary behavior (Owen et al. 2011; Sallis and Owen, 2015) proposes that environmental contexts are significant determinants of sedentary behaviors. It seems probable that sedentary behaviors will be determined more strongly by the situations people are in than by their individual characteristics. *Behavior settings* (Barker 1968) are the social and physical situations in which behaviors take place, and ecological models open the possibility of intervening on these environments. As Wicker (1979, page 4) notes, "The importance of behavior settings is they restrict the range of behavior by promoting and sometimes demanding certain actions and by discouraging or prohibiting others." Environmental contexts can shape or constrain individual-level initiative—for example, prolonged sitting may be unavoidable in most office, classroom, and transportation settings.

Factors at the intrapersonal level—particularly psychological factors, individual skills, and motivation—are one component within the multiple levels of influence on behavior. Figure 1.2 provides a simplified schematic for an ecological model of health behaviors. Strategies based on individual responsibility—persuading and encouraging people to pull themselves up by their personal-motivational bootstraps—are unlikely to be an effective public health approach to reducing sedentary behavior.

Behavioral Choice Theory

The behavioral epidemiology framework (Owen, Healy, et al. 2010; Owen et al. 2000; Owen et al. 2011) that we have proposed for understanding and influencing sedentary behaviors has been strongly flavored by the seminal work of Len Epstein

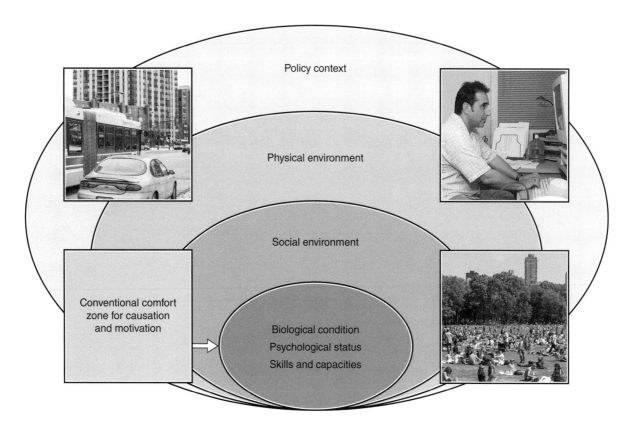

Figure 1.2 Simplified schematic for an ecological model of sedentary behavior emphasizing the breadth of relevant influences on behavior.

Based on Owen et al. 2011.

(1998), who drew from behavioral economics to analyze the determinants of choices made between participating in sedentary and physically active behaviors. Identifying factors associated with the choice to participate in either physical activity or in sedentary behaviors can inform the development of relevant intervention strategies. Behavioral choice theory (BCT) explicitly incorporates environmental influences (Rachlin et al. 1980). Epstein integrated BCT with the behavioral economics model in studies conducted in controlled laboratory settings (Epstein et al. 1991; Epstein 1998). Applications of BCT may have significant unrealized potential for informing public health strategy by providing a better understanding of the personal and environmental factors that can influence how adults in the general population choose to allocate time between physically active and sedentary behaviors (Epstein 1998).

Research on physical activity has predominantly been focused on individual-level and social influences (Sallis and Owen 1999; Trost et al. 2002). The constructs employed in BCT, however, have the potential to provide insights of greater public health relevance into the environmental determinants of sitting time in populations, particularly how behaviors may be determined by the simple availability of amenities such as chairs, but also on other environmental factors such as constraints on and ease of access (Lappalainen and Epstein 1990; Rachlin et al. 1980). Thus, individually focused interventions for reducing extremely common sedentary behavior in the natural environment may simply lead to substitution of these behaviors for other less preferred sedentary behaviors. These may be significant as determinants of the low rates of physical activity and the high rates of participation in sedentary behavior in the adult populations of industrialized countries (Salmon et al. 2003).

Sedentary Behavior and Health

The significance for health of too much sitting is now being acknowledged within the sports medicine and public health constituencies as a concern that is additional to the deleterious health consequences of insufficient physical activity.

In the United States, for example, the *Quantity and Quality of Exercise for Developing and Maintaining Cardiorespiratory, Musculoskeletal, and Neuromotor Fitness in Apparently Healthy Adults: Guidance for Prescribing Exercise* position stand of the American College of Sports Medicine acknowledged that "in addition to exercising regularly, there are health benefits in concurrently reducing total time spent in sedentary pursuits and also by interspersing frequent, short bouts of standing and physical activity between periods of sedentary activity, even in physically active adults" (Garber et al. 2011, page 1334).

In the United Kingdom, the *Start Active, Stay Active* document addressed the volume, duration, frequency, and type of physical activity across the life course needed for achieving broad-based health benefits. This national document makes the case for the importance of reducing sedentary behavior, albeit with a quite general message intended to be applied across the various age groups from children to older adults on the importance of minimizing extended periods of time spent being sedentary (sitting) (Davies et al. 2011).

Notably, such recommendations are at this point rather broad, endorsing the importance of reducing sitting time. These documents do not identify what might be an unsafe or detrimental amount of overall daily sitting time, nor do they specify how frequently sitting time should be broken up or the type and intensity of activity that would be desirable in doing so.

With the growing interest in sedentary behavior and health, it is clear that there are new research agendas to be addressed, particularly in identifying dose–response relationships and the mechanisms through which prolonged sitting can result in adverse health outcomes.

Sedentary Research Agenda

The behavioral epidemiology (Sallis and Owen 1999; Sallis et al. 2000) research agenda on too much sitting also includes conducting measurement studies, understanding the relevant determinants of sedentary behavior, developing effective interventions, and evaluating the outcomes of environmental and policy initiatives. The strategic and conceptual basis for this research agenda has been articulated for sedentary behavior (Owen, Healy, et al. 2010) and includes an ecological model of behavioral determinants (Owen et al. 2011).

- ▶ Associating sedentary behaviors with biomarkers and health outcomes; identifying dose–response relationships and mechanisms
- ▶ Developing measurements (device based and self-report) for sedentary behaviors

- ▸ Characterizing population prevalence, trends, and variations in sedentary behaviors
- ▸ Identifying the relevant determinants of sedentary behaviors in multiple contexts
- ▸ Conducting laboratory and field-based intervention trials on sedentary behavior change
- ▸ Informing and evaluating large-scale innovations and policy initiatives

Emerging evidence and implications of the behavioral epidemiology framework as it may be applied to understanding and influencing sedentary behavior are described in detail elsewhere (Owen 2012; Owen, Healy, et al. 2010).

Observational Studies and Experimental Findings

The AusDiab studies (which examine obesity, diabetes, and risk factors with a large national sample of adults) have shown an ubiquitous leisure-time sedentary behavior—TV viewing time—to be associated with the metabolic syndrome and its components (Dunstan et al. 2005; Thorp et al. 2010), disordered insulin and glucose metabolism (Dunstan et al. 2007; Dunstan et al. 2004), and adverse retinal vascular indices (Anuradha et al. 2011). Related Australian studies have also identified prospective relationships of TV viewing time with weight gain (Ding, Sugiyama, and Owen 2012), declines in MVPA (Lakerveld et al. 2011), risk biomarker changes (Wijndaele et al. 2010), and premature cardiovascular mortality (Dunstan et al. 2010). It was also estimated that for every hour of TV time watched after age 25 years, Australian adults can expect a 22-minute reduction in their life expectancy (Veerman et al. 2012). It is now reasonable to conclude that sedentary behavior is associated with adverse biomarker profiles and the risk of developing major chronic diseases (Hamilton et al. 2008; Hamilton and Owen 2012; Owen, Healy, et al. 2010; Thorp et al. 2011).

The relevant epidemiological evidence includes findings from a population-based sample of 222,497 middle-aged and older Australian adults (the *45 and Up Study*). High levels of overall daily sitting time were found to be related to all-cause mortality risk (Van Der Ploeg et al. 2012). From the United States, findings from a follow-up of more than 240,000 adults initially aged 50 to 71 years (from the National Institutes of Health-American Asso-

ciation of Retired Persons Diet and Health study) showed that adults who watched television for 7 or more hours per day and also reported high levels of MVPA (more than 7 hr/week) during leisure time had a 50% greater risk of death from all causes and twice the risk of death from cardiovascular disease compared to those who undertook the same amount of physical activity but watched television for less than 1 hour per day (Matthews et al. 2012).

Participation in physical activity may not therefore necessarily be protective for those who spend large amounts of time in sedentary behaviors. Studies have identified that dietary interactions with sedentary time in relation to biomarkers for cardiometabolic risk—poor diet quality (Reeves et al. 2013) and higher levels of snack-food consumption (Thorp et al. 2013)—together with higher television viewing time can be associated with more adverse biomarker profiles. Further research is needed on sedentary behavior–diet interactions, particularly to identify potential synergistic risk and protective exposures. The deleterious health effects of sitting may be strongly influenced by concurrent dietary practices.

Cross-sectional studies using accelerator-based measurement of sedentary time (Healy, Dunstan, et al. 2008; Healy, Matthews, et al. 2011; Healy, Wijndaele, et al. 2008) are also providing new insights. For example, in the U.S. National Health and Nutrition Examination Survey (NHANES), those in the lowest quartile of breaking up sedentary time had a more than 4 cm (1.6 in.) greater waist circumference than those in the highest quartile of breaks (Healy, Matthews, et al. 2011). Further analyses of the accelerometer data from NHANES have shown high levels of sedentary behavior in cancer survivors (Lynch et al. 2010; Lynch, Dunstan, et al. 2011; Lynch, Friedenreich, et al. 2011) and also relationships between sedentary time and measures of depression (Vallance et al. 2011).

This body of evidence from observational studies has generated hypotheses that have been tested in an experimental study with middle-aged and older overweight adults (Dunstan, Kingwell, et al. 2012). The effects of prolonged uninterrupted sitting on plasma glucose and serum insulin were compared with those of sitting interrupted by short 2-minute bouts of activity (treadmill walking) in overweight middle-aged adults. Compared to results from uninterrupted sitting, blood glucose was reduced after both activity-break conditions (light: 24%; moderate: 30%) and insulin was reduced by 23%.

No statistically significant differences were found between the two activity conditions, suggesting that brief interruptions to sitting can lead to significant reductions in glucose and insulin. This may be independent of activity intensity. Further analyses of the blood and tissue samples from participants showed effects of these activity-break conditions on hemostatic markers (Howard et al. 2013) and systematic relationships with gene expression in skeletal muscle (Latouche et al. 2013).

Measurement-Development Research

Measurement development is a key element of the sedentary behavior and health research agenda (Clark, Thorp, et al. 2011; Clark et al. 2009; Gardiner, Clark, et al. 2011; Winkler et al. 2011). For example, an initial study using multiple self-report measures suggested that TV time may be a marker of overall sedentary time (Sugiyama et al. 2008); however, accelerometer-assessed sedentary time was subsequently shown to be positively but only weakly related to television viewing time (Clark, Healy, et al. 2011). Although device-based measurement is leading to significant progress, self-report methods nevertheless remain essential elements of population-prevalence studies (Healy, Clark, et al. 2011; Troiano et al. 2012). Using the iPAQ instrument, wide international variations in the prevalence of prolonged sitting have been identified (Bauman et al. 2011). The employment of appropriate self-report methods in context-specific studies is crucial for documenting the prevalence and variations in sedentary behavior and developing and evaluating the outcomes of specific initiatives for behavioral change (Chau et al. 2011; Chau et al. 2012; Clark, Healy, et al. 2011; Marshall et al. 2010; Oliver et al. 2010).

Environmental Determinants of Sedentary Behavior

The ecological model of sedentary behavior described previously has set a strong environmental-determinants agenda that has the potential to inform environmental and policy initiatives. Evidence is emerging from cross-sectional studies in multiple countries on the environmental correlates of sedentary behavior, using self-report (Kozo et al. 2012; Van Dyck et al. 2011) and device-based measurement (Van Dyck et al. 2010). Much of this

evidence has come from cross-sectional studies, so our understanding to date tells us more about the correlates than about the determinants of sedentary behavior (Bauman et al. 2002). Intriguingly, relationships of neighborhood walkability attributes with device-measured sedentary time have emerged that are the inverse of what has been observed for self-reported sedentary behaviors. For Belgian adults, accelerometer-measured sedentary time was higher in highly walkable neighborhoods (Van Dyck et al. 2010). Among Australian adults living in lower-walkability neighborhoods, TV time was initially higher (Sugiyama et al. 2008) than in high-walkability neighborhoods and it increased more over 4 years (Ding et al. 2012).

A review of the relevant evidence published up to late 2014 identified 17 studies where 89 instances of such relationships were examined (Koohsari et al. 2015). Significant associations were found in 28% of instances and nonsignificant associations were found in 56%. Lower levels of sedentary behavior among residents of urban compared to regional areas were most consistently observed. It was concluded that a modest and mixed pattern of findings was available on associations of urban environmental attributes with adults' sedentary behaviors. That review describes a research agenda involving focusing efforts toward measurement and concept development, gathering international evidence to provide a wide range of environmental exposures, and strengthening the logical inferences that can be made through gathering data from prospective studies.

Controlled Intervention Studies of Behavioral Change

Studies gathering experimental evidence and findings from real-world intervention trials are crucial elements of the sedentary behavior research agenda. Further human experimental studies are needed (Dunstan, Kingwell, et al. 2012), particularly on dose–response relationships and underlying mechanisms, the feasibility of changing prolonged sitting in workplaces and other contexts (Alkhajah et al. 2012; Gardiner, Eakin, et al. 2011; Healy et al. 2013; Neuhaus et al. 2014), and how to best promote maintenance of the relevant sedentary behavior changes as well as the health benefits of doing so. These initial studies, with the exception of the trial by Gardiner and colleagues (2011) that used an informational-motivational intervention, have used height-adjustable workstations and demonstrated reductions of an hour or more in workplace sitting time. They have also provided evidence that additional reductions in sedentary time can be brought about through the use of behavioral coaching in combination with these simple workplace environmental changes (Healy et al. 2013; Neuhaus et al. 2014).

Sedentary Behavior Research Priorities

We have previously proposed 11 research questions (see sidebar) for a population-health science of sedentary behavior (Owen et al. 2010).

Evidence addressing several of these questions can now be found in the research literature. Nevertheless, further research findings are needed to better understand the relationships of sedentary behavior with health outcomes. Also needed are questions on measurement, the determinants of sedentary behavior, and the effectiveness and benefits of interventions for addressing changing

sedentary behaviors in multiple contexts. New evidence arising out of device-based measurement studies will provide further perspectives on the health consequences of different patterns of movement and posture (Healy, Clark, et al. 2011). This research is delivering novel insights into the ubiquitous nature of prolonged sitting time and its determinants. Research to develop evidence-based methods for changing sedentary behavior is at an early stage, but it is progressing rapidly.

However, much remains to be understood about sedentary behavior and health. Evidence from future mechanistic and dose–response studies might point to harmful or beneficial aspects of sedentary time that are not yet anticipated. If the relevant confirmatory evidence does continue to accumulate, there is a challenging research-translation agenda to be pursued (Dunstan, Howard, et al. 2012). Emerging evidence on the social and environmental determinants of prolonged sitting will inform future intervention trials, which will deliver invaluable evidence and insights. It seems likely that we will see many future public health

QUESTIONS FOR SEDENTARY BEHAVIOR RESEARCH

1. Can further prospective studies examining incident disease outcomes confirm the initial sedentary behavior and mortality findings?

2. Can sedentary behavior and disease relationships be identified through reanalysis of established prospective epidemiological data sets, by treating sitting time as a distinct exposure variable?

3. What are the most valid and reliable self-report and objective measures of sitting time for epidemiological, genetic, behavioral, and population-health studies?

4. Are the TV time–biomarker relationships for women pointing to important biological or behavioral gender differences?

5. What amounts and intensities of activity might be protective in the context of prolonged sitting time?

6. What genetic variations might underlie predispositions to sitting and greater susceptibility to the adverse metabolic correlates?

7. What is the feasibility of reducing or breaking up prolonged sitting time for different groups (older, younger) in different settings (workplace, domestic, transit)?

8. If intervention trials show significant changes in sitting time, are there improvements in the relevant biomarkers?

9. What are the environmental determinants of prolonged sitting time in different contexts (neighborhood, workplace, at home)?

10. What can be learned from the sitting time and sedentary time indices in built-environment and physical activity studies?

11. Can evidence on behavioral, adiposity, and other biomarker changes be gathered from natural experiments (for example, the introduction of height-adjustable workstations or new community transportation infrastructure)?

initiatives, environmental and policy changes, and clinical guidelines being informed by sedentary behavior and health research.

Summary

This chapter starts with a definition of sedentary behavior and clarification of the distinction between being sedentary and physically inactive. The basic idea is that too much sitting is distinct from too little exercise. Highlights of the rapidly growing interest in sedentary behavior research are presented, together with compelling population-based findings derived from large-scale use of objective measurement devices. These findings show the large proportions of waking hours that adults and children spend primarily sitting—contrasting the daily average of 10 hours of sitting time with around 20 minutes of MVPA—are striking. A perspective on sedentary behavior research in epidemiology and public health is provided, with some conceptual background showing how ecological models and behavioral choice theory can guide research on the social and environmental determinants of sitting time. Recent findings and research priorities are reviewed, emphasizing the need for further evidence on health consequences, the crucial role of measurement development (both device based and self-report), the importance of building a body of evidence on the determinants of sedentary behavior, and the contributions of experimental studies and real-world intervention trials in developing the evidence base on the feasibility and benefits of changing sitting time.

KEY CONCEPTS

▸ **Behavior settings:** Within an ecological model of sedentary behavior, the primary determinants of whether or not people sit or engage in physical activity are the attributes of the settings in which they spend time (for example, office-based work typically mandates sitting, as does driving in a car).

▸ **Behavioral epidemiology:** The systematic study of health-related behaviors addressing evidence on health benefits, measurement, determinants of behavior, intervention-derived evidence, and implications for public-health policy.

▸ **Correlates and determinants of sedentary behavior:** Identifying what needs to be changed in interventions in order to reduce or break up sedentary time in different contexts is the key aspect of the current research agenda. However, much of the observational-study research conducted to date has used cross-sectional designs, which allow inferences about correlates. Prospective study designs provide stronger grounds from which to infer that certain factors will determine sedentary behavior.

▸ **Experimental studies:** A small number of recent laboratory-based studies with humans have systematically manipulated sedentary time and breaks from sedentary time, providing some initial experimental confirmation of the hypotheses generated about sedentary behavior and health through the use of observational study methodologies.

▸ **Field-based intervention trials**: A small number of real-world intervention studies have demonstrated the feasibility of reducing time spent sitting, particularly in workplaces. Evidence from larger-scale trials is now needed to demonstrate the broader feasibility of initiatives for reducing sitting time, particularly through the more widespread use of height-adjustable workstations.

▸ **Observational study designs:** Strong clues to the importance of sedentary behavior for health outcomes have come from both cross-sectional and prospective observational studies. These studies typically involve large groups of people, either measured at one point in time or measured at multiple time points. Cross-sectional studies can identify associations and generate hypotheses. Examining prospective relationships of sedentary behavior with subsequent development of disease or cause-specific mortality allows stronger inferences to be made about the likely causal relationship between sedentary behaviors and poor health outcomes.

▸ **Sedentary behavior:** The Sedentary Behaviour Research Network (2012) defines this as any behavior during waking hours that is characterized by energy expenditure less than or equal to 1.5 METs while in a sitting or reclining posture. The term *inactive* should thus be used to describe those who are performing insufficient amounts of MVPA (i.e., not meeting specified physical activity guidelines).

▸ **Self-report and device-based measurement:** Epidemiological and behavior-change research on physical activity—and more recently on sedentary behavior—has largely relied on self-report measures of the key exposure and outcome variables. Self-report inevitably has been influenced by social desirability and other forms of recall bias, but nevertheless provides valuable contextually anchored information. Device-based measurement, typically using accelerometers or inclinometers, provides objective data but little information on contexts and other variables. The concurrent use of self-report and device-derived measures is desirable in most sedentary behavior research.

STUDY QUESTIONS

1. Why should people who spend long periods of time sitting not necessarily be described as physically inactive?
2. List (separately for children and adults) the settings in which sitting is either mandated or so strongly encouraged that alternative more active behaviors are unlikely.
3. Devise two questions that could be asked specifically of an office worker that would identify the average amount of time spent sitting each day.
4. Devise three questions that could be asked specifically of drivers of delivery trucks that would identify the number, volume of time, and physical activity level of breaks taken from driving.
5. Separately for children, working adults, and retired older adults, list the following factors in order of their likely strength as determinants of sedentary behavior: physical characteristics of the environment, the habitual behaviors of others, social norms, knowledge of health risks, and motivation to change.
6. For a laboratory-based experimental study to identify the possible benefits of breaking up prolonged sitting time, what would you prescribe that people do during their breaks from sitting?
7. List the reasons for and against using individual-motivational strategies to persuade people to reduce the time they spend sitting at home and at work. Do a similar for-and-against listing in relation to the use of environmental-change strategies.
8. In a real-world experiment in a workplace, what would be the three most effective elements to include in an intervention for reducing and breaking up prolonged sitting time?
9. In the future, if strong evidence on the adverse health outcomes of prolonged sitting continues to accumulate, what changes would you expect in the design of office-work and school environments?

The support of the National Health and Medical Research Council of Australia Program Grant (NHMRC # 569940) and Senior Principal Research Fellowship (NHMRC #1003960) and the Victorian Government's Operational Infrastructure Support Program are gratefully acknowledged. The author has no conflicts of interest to declare. Thanks to Bethany Howard for graphic and bibliographic support in the preparation of this chapter.

CHAPTER 2

GRAVITY, SITTING, AND HEALTH

Joan Vernikos, PhD

The reader will gain an appreciation of the role of gravity as a fundamental physiological stimulus in maintaining overall health, and in how exposure to lower gravity conditions, such as in space or sedentary behavior on Earth, lead to similar adverse consequences with common mechanisms that can lead to specific effective solutions. By the end of this chapter, the reader should be able to do the following:

▸ Discuss the history of the associations among space, reduced gravity, sitting, and health

▸ Understand gravity as a universal stimulus, as well as its relationship to physiology, form, and function

▸ Show how using ground analogs of space, such as bed rest, developed the context for understanding the responses to sitting

▸ Discuss the reasons for the limited effectiveness of current exercise or activity approaches in treating sitting

▸ Define and describe gravity deprivation syndrome (GDS)

▸ Explain the mechanisms by which GDS and the effects of sitting are regulated by gravity-perceiving central and peripheral systems

▸ Discuss the differences between activities that enrich gravity perceiving systems and exercise

▸ Outline paths for solutions through the development of research and technology

Because we live on planet Earth, development, growth, and span of life are influenced by our environment. Gravity (G) and light, two major forces of the universe, have emerged as crucial determinants of behavior and health. Less is known about the influence of magnetic fields and energy, the other two forces of the universe, because they have been harder to study. Gravity and light influence how we have evolved, as well as how we develop, grow, look, and function. As the Earth rotates around the sun, day–night cycles are roughly 24 hours. When it is dark, we lie down to sleep. As daylight awakes us, we get up, stand, sit, and move about the business of living until the cycle repeats itself. Integral to this day and night, light and dark, awake and asleep daily routine is the experience of various intensities and exposures to Earth's gravity vector.

When we stand up, gravity is experienced in the head-to-toe direction (Gz); less Gz is felt during sitting because the body's vertical column aligned with gravity is shorter and supported. When we lie down, we minimize Gz. Gravity now pulls across the chest (Gx), with minimal physiological influence that we know of.

As a function of light, we change our posture relative to the gravity vector (Gz), moving throughout the day until it is time again to lie down at night. The unidirectional downward gravity force does not change. However, we vary the influence of this gravity vector on our body throughout the day by virtue of what we do and how we move. In this way, we use Gz as an intermittent stimulus to keep our body systems primed and tuned so that they can be reflexively responsive to any demands.

Until the invention of the electric bulb, these 24-hour cycles of day and night, light and dark, activity and sleep, and +Gz versus Gx were maintained fairly universally. Industrialization, shift work, and more recently a flood of electric conveniences, appliances, transportation, and electronic devices have diverted the need to move during daylight hours. Today's sedentary working society, on the road as well as at home, no longer needs to move for essential activities, thus our bodies have become out of tune with nature. Health issues of metabolic syndromes followed, including type 2 diabetes, obesity, cardiovascular disease, cancer, and immune disorders, as well as sleep, emotional, and cognitive issues. Whether sitting causes some or all of these disorders is not unequivocally proven. Nevertheless, now ample evidence exists that a sedentary lifestyle exacerbates all disorders.

Though attempts to compensate for this daily movement deficit have focused on replacing it with structured exercise, usually once a day for 3 to 5 days per week, this approach alone appears to be inadequate. Frequent change in posture is a crucial factor. In space as in bed rest, exercise without the change in posture signal is inadequate.

By going into space, astronauts showed how sitting makes us sick and ages us faster. We learned that gravity is a universal stimulus, there to be used. Living in and using gravity on Earth helps us grow, develop, and stay healthy, mobile, and youthful throughout life.

This chapter discusses how taking it easy with continuous sitting works through benign neglect—reducing the input to the central nervous system that moving in gravity provides. When the G-perceiving system goes silent or is damaged, the rest of the body atrophies and prepares metabolically to shut down. It is a kind of total or partial vestibular and proprioceptive deafferentation. It is not that too much sitting, too little standing, or too little exercise are bad. Inadequate use of gravity by uninterrupted sitting is the cause of today's health problems.

Gravity and Spaceflight

Gravity is the force that keeps us rooted on Earth. It keeps the stars in their courses and the planets in their orbits. The gravitational pull of the moon, nearly 386,243 km (240,000 mi) away from Earth, causes the regular ebb and flow of the tides. Gravity is measured in units known as Gs, and the force that normally operates on Earth is designated as 1 G. For a rocket to break free from Earth's gravitational field, it has to reach a speed of more than 40,000 km per hour (25,000 mph). There is no such thing as zero gravity. We come near to it in space as the spacecraft free-falls around the Earth's orbit; gravity is then reduced to microgravity levels, approximately 10^{-5}. This gravity level is considered below the threshold of human perception, as evidenced by the familiar images of astronauts appearing to float in space—they still have mass but no weight. Equally, pictures of unstable Apollo astronauts hopping on the moon's 0.16th gravity surface are below G-threshold, whereas the 0.33 G on Mars may be getting closer to the gravity threshold.

Although extensive work with plants on Earth had established the significant influence of gravity on their growth and development, little was known about other biological systems. To understand gravity's role, we had to go into space as far away from Earth's 1 G as we could. The Space Race made it possible for the first time to explore what happens to the human body living in the microgravity of space. The answers led to an astonishing insight for those of us living down here on Earth, one that established the fascinating link between gravity and aging (Vernikos and Schneider 2010).

Movement in the presence of gravity imposes a physical stress that results in increased energy exchange, evidenced by a dramatic increase in oxygen uptake, respiration, heart rate, stroke volume, cardiac output, and sweating. Muscles required to perform various physical activities, such as moving one's body, lifting, or throwing objects, depend on the level of gravity opposing these actions. Gravity has therefore traditionally been considered the primary constant stress factor determining adaptation and maintaining health on Earth.

The very first clue to what and how human health would be affected to shifting to below G-threshold came from the immediate nausea with some vomiting (resulting from sensory conflict between visual and vestibular input) and diuresis, followed by drastically reduced blood volume. These initial responses focused attention on the brain's G-perceiving balance center and on fluid balance as key players in the physiological changes that followed.

Long before humans ever went into space, clinical observations of loss of calcium and bone in polio victims (Dietrick et al. 1948) led to the question of whether the bone loss was the result of the infectious disease or of the immobilization due to the paralysis. To answer this, studies in healthy students immobilized in lower body casts in bed confirmed that lying in bed for 30 days in the horizontal position caused severe calcium and bone loss. Since sending humans to space was being discussed, it was therefore hypothesized that astronauts would show similar calcium and bone loss in microgravity, where they would become virtually inactive. This theory was confirmed in 1964 in two astronauts on Gemini VII, the first 14-day mission in space, bringing attention to the bone-loss problem (Lutwak et al. 1969) that remains unresolved to this day.

It was not till the 1970s when three sequential Skylab missions of increasing duration of 28, 54, and 84 days, with three astronauts in each, validated hypotheses and generated new observations. Negative calcium balance; loss of bone density, muscle mass, and strength; fluid shifts; cardiovascular, hematological, metabolic, and endocrine changes; and disturbed sleep were some of these.

Other factors include shifts in hydrostatic pressure on the cardiovascular system, decreased weight load on muscles and bones (requiring lower energy needs or output), the removal of the sense of direction and acceleration, and the absence of the change in position and posture mediated on Earth by the vestibular system (Vernikos 1996).

Returning to Earth after adaptation to microgravity in space was in turn characterized by maladaptive responses to Earth's gravity—orthostatic hypotension (OH) on first standing up, reduced heart size and volume (which impaired cardiac output, stroke volume, and aerobic capacity), atrophy and weakness of supporting postural muscles and bones, back pain from vertebral compression, visual acuity problems during walking, immunodeficiency, viral reactivation, consequences of disturbed biological rhythms such as nocturnal diuresis, and balance and coordination issues (Vernikos 1996). Animal space research documented an alarming reduction in vascular endothelium within a few days in space (Delp 2007).

Medical observers commented that astronauts must be growing old faster in space since their symptoms were similar to those seen in the elderly. This unpopular conclusion was swiftly dismissed as soon as it was clear that astronauts recovered when they returned to Earth.

Head-Down Bed Rest Studies

Before the 19th century, sick people took to bed only when they were too weak to sit or stand. Primarily, this was because working people were afraid of losing income critical to survival as well as the superstition that if you went to bed, you would never get up again. How right they were! All this changed in 1863 when Hilton hypothesized that if immobilization could heal a broken leg, it should help in treating other problems as well. This was so heartily adopted by the physicians of the time that they often prescribed bed rest for almost anything to patients who often would have been much better off up and about. Not infrequently, bed rest was prescribed until patients died.

About 70 years ago, a few physicians began to question the accepted practices of 4 to 6 weeks in bed after surgery or treatment of myocardial infarction and pointed out the risks of prolonged bed rest (Asher 1947). World War II experience confirmed these findings when men who by necessity got out of bed and moved about had fewer problems than those who rested in bed for extended periods (Browse 1965). Yet because all observations were made in sick people whose basic illness was the cause of going to bed, the direct link between their sedentary status and the observed findings took time to be recognized.

The advent of the space program necessitated the study in healthy volunteers during ground simulation of the features of living in space, mainly inactivity and the reduction of the physiological influence of gravity. These methods to simulate reduced gravity on Earth included water immersion and bed or chair rest. Immersion in water soon proved impractical. A few earlier studies had used chair-sitting for up to 3 days to study the adverse cardiovascular effects of military jobs that required too much sitting. For practical reasons, healthy volunteers lying continuously in bed became the model of choice. In the late 1960s, cosmonauts returning from longer missions complained that on their return from space, they had a hard time sleeping because they felt as if they were sliding off the foot of the bed. They corrected this by raising the foot of the bed until it felt horizontal and they could get back to sleep. Every night they lowered the bed a little until lying horizontal felt normal again. Russian researchers took note of this observation, surmising that perhaps lying head down approximated what it felt like to sleep in space. The Soviets tested –15°, –10°, or –5° for comfort and acceptability. Head-down bed rest (HDBR) at –6° became the model of choice for studies of longer duration and evaluations of countermeasures.

Ground research in space analogs, mainly HDBR, provided the justification and the resources for studying the time course and the mechanisms of the reduced influence of the Gz vector in large numbers and controlled conditions of otherwise completely normal men and women confined to bed for prolonged periods. Results showed that all physiological systems of the body change with continuous lying in bed. The onset and the severity of the changes depend on how long the individual stays in bed rest. This body of data reinforced the clinical observations of the early 20th century: that the weeks of bed rest practiced postsurgery, post childbirth, and for the recovery from illness in general were counterproductive to health.

For a period of roughly 40 years, shorter bed-rest recovery and rehabilitation after surgery or illness

in the clinical setting resulted in increased health benefits. However, with the advent of modern technological inventions in the Space Age, the changing office and home environments have taken their toll. Entertainment and appliances designed to make life easier and communication technology have further encouraged sedentary habits among otherwise healthy young people. The result of this new, overwhelmingly sedentary lifestyle saw a reappearance of disability and an exacerbation of the diseases of the 19th and early 20th centuries. However, the prescribed clinical bed rest practice has been replaced by palliative short-term solutions, including medicinal, surgical, dietary, or a variety of intense once-a-day exercise approaches. These solutions have had limited or short-term success and led to an abundance of injuries.

Physiological changes in space and its analog HDBR are remarkably similar in the changes they induce (Pavy-LeTraon et al. 2007). They are very similar to sitting, though sitting is less severe. HDBR induces a headward shift of fluids, relieves the body from its usual head-to-toe Gz and weight-bearing position, and precludes changes in posture, leading to unloading and possibly inactivity as well (Vernikos 1996; Weinert and Timiras 2003). By inducing many of the changes observed in spaceflight, HDBR affords a means of mapping the time course of these changes, exploring the mechanisms under controlled conditions and evaluating means of preventing or reducing the adverse side effects of prolonged space flight. Equally, data from HDBR studies as well as space-related ground and flight animal research were considered relevant to the relatively new field of sedentary physiology.

Space, HDBR, and Aging

Initially dismissed as coincidental, the intriguing observation that space, HDBR, and aging share similar symptoms has been gaining ground. It was argued at first that although astronauts in space (or volunteers in HDBR) and the elderly showed similar changes, these were not the same because astronauts and bed-rest volunteers recover once they return back to Earth or reambulate. It was presumed that one does not recover from aging. Nevertheless, as spaceflight exposures increased to 6 months, recovery of astronauts seems slower and less complete.

After HDBR, just as after spaceflight, people must again adapt to an erect body posture and to moving in Earth's gravity. This is not as readily achieved as is the rate of change in response to going into space or when first lying in bed during HDBR. Why some people readapt more readily than others is not clear. So far all volunteers and astronauts have eventually recovered, yet the return of various physiological systems to normal is variable and may require days, weeks, or even years. For example, changes in the case of bone such as its density may appear restored within 2 years, though its architecture is not restored (Lang et al. 2004).

Similarly, aging and deconditioning in space or HDBR or in sedentary people cause a range of changes, such as hypovolemia, reduced aerobic capacity ($\dot{V}O_2$max), and baroreflex sensitivity (Convertino et al. 1990; 1991), as well as metabolic, cardiovascular, musculoskeletal, and balance and coordination problems. Ben Levine's group at Southwestern University College of Medicine (McGavock et al. 2009) showed that the decrease in cardiovascular functional capacity at the end of 3 weeks of HDBR as measured by $\dot{V}O_2$max and cardiac output was equivalent to that seen in the same subjects 30 years later. These findings suggested that 3 weeks of HDBR in 30-year-olds results in cardiovascular changes equal to 30 years of aging.

Spaceflight and to a less dramatic extent HDBR accelerate the onset and the rate of identical changes observed on Earth over decades of aging. Uncorrected, these changes not only hasten aging, but are often associated with chronic diseases. Whereas on Earth we expect to lose about 1% bone density a year from age 20 on, a 4-year study on the long-term effects of microgravity on ISS astronauts showed that on average they lost 11% (range 0-24%) of their total hip bone mass over the course of 4 to 6 months (Vernikos and Schneider 2010).

Newer techniques and longer durations in space are revealing that contrary to what was previously thought, living in microgravity accelerates 10- to 20-fold the normal rate of bone loss that happens with aging, enough to raise concern about the ability of astronauts to recover (Keyak et al. 2009). Furthermore, this rate of loss does not level off after 6 months. Such rapid and sustained changes could be explained by the acute and maintained near-total withdrawal of the Gz signal in space or in HDBR.

The less dramatic change in bone loss with age on Earth must reflect a gradual reduction of the use of gravity, by sitting more over decades. Older generations are now living longer, perhaps because they are not the ones who were exposed to the dramatic increase in sedentary behavior in their early and mid-life years. The active lifestyle habits of the longer-living generation have generally persisted in spite of modern lifestyle, since older people have been less consumed by the electronic age. However, the increasingly sedentary lifestyle of coming generations may in fact reduce life span or at the very least increase incapacitation in older years.

Relationship Between Exercise and Inactivity

It has generally been assumed that the primary common variable to space, bed rest, HDBR, and sitting was inactivity (Sandler and Vernikos 1986). And though activity in the form of exercise is doubtless a significant factor, in spite of 55 years of research using a variety of extensive and intense exercise approaches, the broad spectrum of physiological changes in space persist. Similarly, inadequate prevention of the effects of bed rest with similar exercise regimes has been tested. In addition, the postexercise sequence of changes in response to exercise usually observed on Earth is not experienced during recovery in space. Astronaut Steve Hawley described his amazement at this absolute lack of postexercise carryover after exercising in space as hard as he could. This observation, if pursued, could offer useful insights.

However, some forms of activity are effective in HDBR. After 16 days in bed, a single maximal, but not a submaximal, bout of exercise restored plasma volume and baroreflex sensitivity and prevented OH, but this benefit lasted only 24 hours (Engelke et al. 1995). Reasons for the failure of preventive or corrective approaches to yield effective solutions are likely due to targeting specific body systems and functions, overlooking integrated approaches, as well as ignoring the consequences of other variables on the experimental outcomes.

Approaches to transposing to a low-gravity environment have been found to be effective in Earth's gravity. Once-a-day exercise may be effective in maintaining good health in an otherwise active person, but appears to be inadequate both in space and HDBR (Vernikos et al. 1996), and even with people who exercise daily but are sedentary the rest of the time.

At least four factors are removed by hours of sitting: inactivity, a reduced gravity column and use of gravity, lack of postural change, and usually poor sitting posture or slouching, which has been found to influence cognitive function as well as strength

(Peper et al. 2014). By focusing on sitting as tantamount to inactivity and its metabolic consequences, researchers ignore the participation or significance of other variables to the health outcomes and assume that exercise is the sole solution.

A Swedish study of sitting time and physical activity reported that a generally active daily life was, regardless of exercising regularly, more beneficial on reducing waist circumference, HDL, cholesterol, and triglycerides in both sexes, with lower insulin, glucose, and fibrinogen (clotting factor) levels in men. Nonexercise activity was associated with a lower risk of a first cardiovascular event and lower all-cause mortality (Ekblom-Bak et al. 2014).

With respect to health in general, sedentary behavior may reflect an exchange of sedentary activity for moderate to vigorous activity. Sedentary behavior may also be a separate risk factor altogether. In a U.S. study of 2,286 adults aged over 60 who sat an average of 9 hours per day, Dunlap and colleagues (2015) found 46% greater disability in coping with normal daily activities of living for each daily hour spent sitting. This was independent of time spent in moderate or vigorous activity.

Two factors emerge worthy of note in resolving this issue. First, is once-a-day vigorous exercise less effective than an equal duration and intensity of activity distributed over the entire day or at least part of the day? Second, since sitting not only results in reduced activity but also eliminates postural change, does interrupting sitting with a change in posture at critical frequencies with or without activity prevent the deleterious effects of continuous sitting?

In a randomized crossover study, we (Vernikos et al. 1996) questioned whether exercise spread throughout the day might be more effective than the once-a-day exercise we had used to prevent the effects of being in HDBR the rest of the 24 hours. Since standing up provides the G-related stimulus with negligible energy expenditure and is inherent to normal upright exercising, we compared standing up with and without exercise every hour or every other hour throughout each day in the same nine subjects at monthly intervals in 4-day HDBR studies. Surprisingly, standing up 16 times per day was more effective than walking on a treadmill at 5 km (3 mi) per hour for an equivalent duration. It was more effective in preventing the post-bed-rest OH as well as the decrease in blood volume and $\dot{V}O_2$max. In other words, the gravitational stimulus of standing up was even more effective than stand-

ing up with walking exercise in these parameters. On the other hand, walking was more effective than standing in preventing calcium loss. Since the time course of the response in circulating hormones such as norepinephrine, angiotensin, cortisol, and vasopressin to standing lasts only 20 to 30 minutes, it was tempting to speculate that the posture stimulus would be most effective administered every 20 to 30 minutes instead of hourly. We recommended this self-directed activity of standing up every 30 minutes to six people with limited mobility (five men and one woman, aged 78-92 years of age). Five years later, all had regained considerable mobility (from wheelchair to standing upright to using a walker).

Dunstan and colleagues (2012) were the first to show that distributing activity at intervals during the day was more effective on plasma glucose, insulin, and lipids. This was followed by Peddie and others (2013), who showed that as little as 1 minute 40 seconds of activity with each posture change in both preprandial situations or in response to a meal or oral glucose tolerance test (OGTT) was more effective than once-a-day exercise. Duvivier and colleagues (2013) similarly confirmed in sitting studies that once-a-day short exercise activity was less effective than walking at intervals throughout the day. However, none of these studies included a posture change control without activity. In studying the relationship of exercise and gravity, Kolegard and colleagues (2013) investigated whether exercise training for 6 months would improve tolerance to G-acceleration. Neither endurance nor strength training had any effect on gravity tolerance, though the expected pressor responses to the exercise remained. Exercise appeared to have little effect on the sensitivity of the G-sensing system. The type of activity relevant to addressing the sitting dilemma may be different from the exercise we are accustomed to (Ekblom-Bak et al. 2014). The results of these few pertinent studies are encouraging but incomplete, and more targeted research along these lines is needed in this crucial area, taking into account all aspects of exercise, energy expenditure, as well as a change in posture signal.

Gravity Deprivation Syndrome

Although we are surrounded by gravity on Earth, we can nevertheless deprive ourselves of its benefits. These are evident in a growing child as she intuitively experiences gravity for the first time or in an astronaut returning from space who must relearn how to use gravity in order to recover from the microgravity experience. Gravity deprivation syndrome (GDS) conditions fall on a continuum of reduced gravity exposure as well as compromised physiological integrity that would prevent full gravity benefit. Such conditions could range from sitting to inactive lifestyles, such as lying in bed because of sickness, surgery, or injury and the limited mobility of aging. They could also be secondary to congenital birth defects, injury, or chronic disease. The extreme state would be characterized by sarcopenia and frailty.

Adverse consequences of GDS are the opposite of gravity's benefits. They affect all physiological systems and act through common pathways and mechanisms across conditions ranging from space to aging, cerebral or spinal injury to unloading, and sedentary lifestyles, as well as conditions that deprive sensory and postural stimulation signals involved in maintaining resilient health. This composite of consequences forms the GDS.

Excessive sitting where gravity is used inadequately also induces a cascade of changes similar to those of aging. Body composition, metabolism, wasting of the musculoskeletal system and connective tissue, and balance and coordination problems are only some of these. Both in space and in HDBR, bone and muscle not only atrophy, but they do so much faster than in ambulatory people on Earth.

When astronauts return from space, they have to relearn to live, move, and balance in gravity. Between these extremes, other conditions that use gravity less have become evident at an increasingly younger age as our modern lifestyle has become more sedentary. In today's modern life, we may inevitably spend part of the day lying in bed reading, watching TV, sitting at the office or at home in front of the computer or with a tablet in our lap, or driving or riding in a car. Yet in the process of adapting to modern conveniences designed to make life easier, hardly realizing it, we are aging faster and becoming unhealthier. In fact, from peak development on, our health declines. This decline is only accelerated by sitting and lying in bed. The common denominator among these conditions is the virtual absence of gravity in space, or from peak development on, or of using gravity increasingly less over decades as we age. Alexandre Kalache of the World Health Organization (WHO) presented a hypothetical chart to depict this concept that I later adapted (Vernikos 2011) (see figure 2.1).

Take any example, for instance, bone loss or poor balance. The downward slope in health or deconditioning usually begins at peak development around age 20, and will cross a risk zone characterized by falls or fractures. The acceleration of this decline in space or in poor-G users (sedentary people) on Earth suggests that this risk zone may

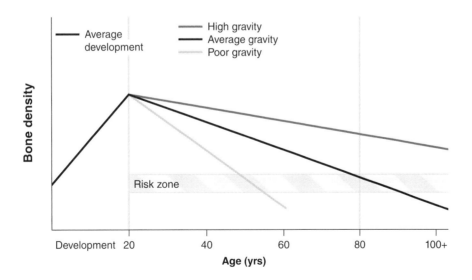

Figure 2.1 Conceptual model of effects (e.g., on bone growth) during development and from peak development on of using gravity increasingly less or more over decades as we age. The risk zone here would represent decreased bone density with greater risk of fracture.

be crossed at age 50, well ahead of today's normal aging. Equally, high-G users could put off reaching this risk zone to well beyond 100, and therefore extend their life.

Thus, sitting, lying down, aging, and spending time in space form a continuum of gravity deprivation that shares the same characteristic composite of disorders and disabilities. This downward slope is the reverse of what a child goes through as he plays, grows, and flourishes, intuitively using gravity to its fullest until development peaks. If children are G-deprived during childhood, then development and later health will be expected to be compromised. The image of today's children stooped over an electronic text-messaging device is cause for alarm.

Strong evidence exists that sedentary habits lead to reductions in the ability to develop and maintain dynamic muscle forces, bone strength, cardiovascular function, balance and coordination integrity, as well as the rest of the known consequences discussed previously from living with reduced availability or use of gravity. There may be others not yet identified.

GDS is potentially the 21st century's greatest health problem, its main contributing factor being too much sitting and poor postural use of gravity in general. The epidemiological data are there to support it. More directed research is needed. Yet by addressing the cause of the problem and identifying the basic mechanisms involved, solutions and technologies can be found. The challenge is to find ways of building G-use back into daily living habits.

Health Consequences of Prolonged Sitting and Gravity

Lack of gravity or reduction of the influence of gravity (unloading with ineffective activity, reduced cardiovascular need for work, and lack of postural change signals) more than likely affects all physiological systems, with broad consequences.

What was seen in space, HDBR, and as we age has also been seen (or should be expected to be seen) from sitting as well. These changes are generally characterized by the rapid onset of an overall metabolic disorder characterized by loss of blood volume and red cell mass, fluid and electrolyte shifts, and a reduction in endothelium lining affecting the integrity of blood vessels, bone, and other systems that depend on the nitric oxide (NO) generated by shear forces, which are seriously reduced in GDS.

Central among these metabolic changes are insulin resistance, hyperlipidemia, decreased fat oxidation, a shift in substrate use toward glucose, reduced protein synthesis, loss of collagen, muscle atrophy with a shift in muscle-fiber type from slow to fast, ectopic fat storage with fatty infiltration of the liver and bone marrow with a consequent form of anemia, and reduced anabolic neuroendocrine secretions such as growth hormone, testosterone, and leptin. Rapid bone loss with possible ectopic calcium deposits round off the metabolic picture. Reduced sensitivity of sensory systems and reflexes, with decreased sensitivity of central and peripheral balance and coordination systems, is a prime feature of reduced gravity consequences as well. In addition, viral reactivation, immune deficiency with resistance to antibiotics, inflammation, and a reduction in telomere length and telomerase activity have all been observed.

Metabolism

Muscle, the chemical factory of the body, produces energy for the body's needs. With loss of muscle tissue, there is a negative protein balance; in HDBR studies of 7 to 14 days, this begins with an acute decrease in protein synthesis followed by increased breakdown (Leblanc et al. 2000). Body composition shifts as fat stores increase and infiltrate muscle (Biolo et al. 2004; Krebs et al. 1990). Although humans obviously do not become obese in space or during bed rest, energy requirements are reduced to the basal metabolic rate plus a small percentage of calories needed for small residual movements and thermogenesis.

Prediabetic conditions with insulin resistance appear almost immediately with the onset of bed rest or sitting. Reduced glucose tolerance and hyperinsulinemia in response to a carbohydrate load and insulin resistance became evident within 3 days of bed rest (Smorawinski et al. 2000; Yanagibori et al. 1994). This hyperinsulinemia and insulin resistance probably occurs much sooner since it is seen within a few hours of sitting. Duvivier and colleagues' (2013) data show significant insulin resistance 30 minutes after a glucose meal in subjects after 14 hours of sitting.

Deprived of the daily challenge of gravity, metabolism is changed. The oxidation of fatty acids is reduced as are enzymes needed for fatty acid metabolism, indicating a decreased capacity to use fat for energy. Lipoprotein lipase (Bey and

Hamilton 2003) and high-density lipoproteins (HDL) decrease, whereas low-density lipoproteins (LDL) increase (Bergouignan et al. 2011). Increased C-reactive protein blood levels and decreased glucose transporter protein in gastrocnemius muscle biopsies have been measured in HDBR after as few as 6 days of bed rest (Mikines et al. 1991). One possibility for the rapid onset of insulin resistance with inactivity may result from liver disturbances or endothelial dysfunction. Alternatively, increased inflammation and oxidative stress arising during bed rest or inactivity could induce insulin resistance (Gratas-Delamarche et al. 2014).

Moving about in gravity has a major influence on the secretion of the anabolic growth hormone (GH) that is so important in keeping up muscle mass. GH is reduced in space, in HDBR, during prolonged inactivity, and with aging. GH that increases normally in response to exercise is not increased by exercise during spaceflight nor during HDBR of 14 days' duration. This response is still absent for at least 4 days after return to Earth or when reambulating after bed rest.

Cardiovascular System, Fluid Shifts, Electrolyte Balance, and Aerobic Capacity

Immediately on transitioning to microgravity in space or when lying down in HDBR, the shift in hydrostatic pressure gradients within the cardiovascular system causes a redistribution of body fluids, with increased perfusion in the upper regions and decreased perfusion in the lower body. Increased filling of the heart and central circulation trigger volume receptors and neuroendocrine, fluid, and electrolyte-regulating mechanisms (inhibition of vasopressin and renin-angiotensin-aldosterone systems) resulting in diuresis and natriuresis (Vernikos et al. 1993). Within 48 hours, plasma volume is reduced, hematocrit is increased, and erythropoietin is inhibited, inducing a gradual decrease in red cell mass and a resetting of blood volume by a 10% to 15% reduction (Dallman et al. 1984). This results in decreased cardiac filling and cardiac mass that progresses to significant change in heart shape and heart muscle atrophy (Levine et al. 1997).

Without the dynamic stimulation of the baroreceptors induced by changes in posture on Earth, their sensitivity is compromised (Convertino et al. 1990). With greater venous compliance of the lower extremities, which diverts blood away from the brain and heart, peripheral vascular constriction is compromised, often leading to OH, an inability to maintain blood pressure on standing or on return to Earth (Cooke and Convertino 2002).

Arteries no longer see the shear forces that stimulate arterial walls. Experiments in rats deconditioned by aging or hind-limb suspension, the rat analog of HDBR and microgravity, respond to reduced volume with diminished microvascular endothelial function. Rapid and dramatic thinning, weakening, and stiffening of arteriolar walls appear when shear forces and the resulting NO chemical signals that keep them responsive are reduced (Delp 2007; Muller-Delp et al. 2002).

In contrast, the same team found that chronic cephalic fluid shifts increased basal tone and vasoconstriction of the middle cerebral arteries through activation of the eNOS (endothelial nitric oxide synthase) signaling mechanism (Wilkerson et al. 2005). The potential functional consequence of these vascular alterations with head-down tilt in rats is regional elevation in cerebrovascular resistance and corresponding reductions in cerebral perfusion. This is consistent with measurements of decreased cerebral blood flow in the middle cerebral artery measured in humans with transcranial Doppler during HDBR (Sun et al. 2005).

Astronauts returning from space, or volunteers after as little as 4 days of HDBR, experience more than a 25% reduction in their maximal oxygen uptake ($\dot{V}O_2$max, aerobic capacity). This reduction can be explained entirely by a decrease in cardiac filling and stroke volume associated with lower circulating blood volume. The cardiovascular effect of the reduction of $\dot{V}O_2$max on returning to 1 Gz is highlighted depending on posture when tested with higher heart rates and lower stroke volumes measured when exercising upright rather than supine.

Anemia

Reduced red cell mass and erythropoietin were one of the earliest observations in spaceflight. Since then, an anemia sometimes called *anemia of immobility* has been described in spinal cord injury or other lower-limb unloading causes in elderly people with limited mobility, astronauts, and bed rest volunteers. It is characterized as low-grade, chronic, normocytic, normochromic anemia with no obvious etiology other than accumulation of fat in the bone marrow or a chronic inflammatory condition, both of which can limit erythrocyte generation (Payne et al. 2007).

Musculoskeletal System

The sedentary lifestyle that comes beyond age 20, in space, or lying in bed results in the deterioration of muscle quantity, quality, and metabolic function. Muscle strength, energy balance, and bone health affect the ability to perform the daily tasks of living. Sedentary lifestyle, even in healthy people, rapidly results in a setback in mobility and independence that normally would come only with advancing age (Vernikos 2004). The frailty that comes from steady bone loss that frequently leads to a greater incidence of fractures caused by falls from loss of balance, muscle weakness, or torqued motions may lead to a downhill health spiral compounded by additional immobilization.

Bone

Bone's major role is to support the mechanical needs of the body to move. During development, it grows by increasing in length. The size and shape of the mature skeleton is influenced by the forces applied to it by moving within the 1 G environment. After development peaks, the epiphyses close, youthful energy and activity begin to wane, and bone is steadily lost until the appearance later in life of fragility, structural reorganization, or osteoporosis (Schild and Heller 1982). Bone responds to loading in the Gz vector as well as to the tension that muscles, tendons, and ligaments apply with contracting muscles. Blood flow, neuromuscular messages, contracting muscle, and endocrine and nutritional factors all contribute to healthy and strong bones (Leblanc et al. 2000).

Bone formation is inhibited and bone resorption is increased in HDBR as well as in space, primarily in the legs and spine. The absorption of calcium from the gut is also reduced in HDBR as is the synthesis of vitamin D_3 that is crucial to this absorption. Intercellular signaling is an important physiological phenomenon involved in maintaining homeostasis. In bone as in other tissues responsive to reduced gravity signals, intercellular communication through chemical signals like NO plays a critical role in bone remodeling (Bacabac et al. 2004). Under normal conditions, gravity loads bones mechanically and fluid flows through minute channels in the bone matrix, resulting in shear stresses on the cell membrane that activate the osteocyte. Activated osteocytes modulate both bone-forming and bone-resorbing cell activity through NO-controlling bone mass and structure. Therefore, here, too, the removal of shear forces and reduced NO production result in impaired bone structure and remodeling (Klein-Nulend et al. 2014).

The observations of calcium and bone loss in astronauts in the early 1960s provided motivation and funding to the understanding of the importance of gravity for bone health. Even more significant was the impetus provided to the development of improved measurement technology tools. Computer tomography used to measure bone mineral density (BMD) in four cosmonauts who spent up to 7 months on the Russian space station *Mir* showed that all had lost BMD, mainly from the posterior vertebra; dual X-ray photon absorptiometry showed loss in the spine, femoral neck, trochanter, and pelvis of about 1% to 1.6% per month and 0.3% to 0.4% per month in the legs and whole body, but no loss at all in the forearm in 1- to 6-month missions (Sibonga et al. 2007).

A 4-year study on astronauts on the ISS (Keyak et al. 2009; Lang et al. 2004) showed that on average they lost 11% (0–24%) of their total hip bone mass over the course of 4 to 6 months. Thus, better techniques and longer stays in microgravity are showing that unlike what was previously thought, living in space accelerates 20-fold the normal rate of bone loss that happens on Earth, for instance, with aging. In trying to assess the severity of such BMD loss in these astronauts, what ultimately matters is how bone structure is affected. They lost both trabecular (spongy layer) and cortical (outer layer) bone in the hip. A gradient of mineral loss appears to begin at the lumbar spine and increase in the hip, underlining the role of gravity in this pattern.

Studies have found remarkably similar losses in bone during bed rest as in space (LeBlanc et al. 1990; Vico et al. 1987). Bone mineral content loss in the tibia of healthy males after 90 days of bed rest largely recovered within 1 year and was estimated to be fully recovered within 2 years with a structured, supervised exercise protocol. The initial reaccrual rate of bone was remarkably high, as compared to that during the development growth spurt, suggesting that the adult skeleton is capable of responding and readapting to gravity (Rittweger and Felsenberg 2009).

Muscle

In the microgravity of space, blood supply to the legs is reduced with reduced capillary-to-fiber ratio and reduced cross-sectional areas of both slow- and fast-twitch muscle fibers of the vastus lateralis. The overall decrease in limb circumference has been used as a gross index of atrophy.

Neuromuscular innervation to the legs is minimally activated because there is no requirement for the legs to contract, leading the muscles to atrophy. Disuse of muscles and unloading that comes from HDBR or increased sitting results in muscle atrophy and loss of strength of skeletal muscles—a 13% reduction in calf muscle volume, particularly those like the soleus (15% reduction over 6 months compared to 10% reduction in the gastrocnemius) involved in supporting the body's weight and erect posture, as well as muscles in the spinal cord and neck, which are both chronically bent forward during sitting and aging (Trappe et al. 2009; Vernikos 2004).

Across the velocity spectrum, force-velocity characteristics were reduced by 20% to 29% in space as well as in HDBR. A shift in the myosin-heavy chain (MHC) fiber type of 12% to 17% in both the soleus and the gastrocnemius, with a decrease in MHC I and redistribution among faster phenotypes, indicated that together with the decrease in muscle mass and performance, there was a shift from slow- to fast-twitch fiber type in both muscles. This is a characteristic adaptation associated with unloading of any kind in humans.

In a 90-day HDBR study, knee extensor and plantar flexor muscle volume decreased by 18% and 29%, respectively. Torque or force and power decreased by 31% to 60% (knee extension) and 37% to 56% (plantar flexion); EMG activity decreased 31% to 38% and 28% to 35%, respectively (Alkner and Tesch 2004a; 2004b). Equally similar but smaller changes in the back muscle groups were noted in a 17-week HDBR study (LeBlanc et al. 1992). These and similar studies collectively showed that antigravity extensors of the knee and the ankle are the most affected.

Although no significant changes occur in anaerobic, glycolytic enzyme activities in muscles after space flight, enzymes associated with aerobic metabolic pathways (succinate dehydrogenase, citrate synthase, b-hydroxyacyl-CoA dehydrogenase) and the use of oxygen are reduced in both slow- and fast-twitch muscle fibers.

The atrophy and fatigue of postural muscles can limit the ability to function during simple standing. This significant loss of muscle structure and function can predispose people to serious injury (Narici et al. 2003; Prisby et al. 2004) during physical activities. The changes might render people incapable of carrying out routine tasks required for normal living, such as standing, stair climbing, or simply getting out of bed.

Rhythms and Sleep

In space, one day and night are compressed into 14 90-minute cycles. The only time continuous monitoring of body temperature (BT) was done in space in humans was with astronaut Jerry Linenger aboard the Russian space station *Mir*. Even though in the spacecraft, the light–dark cycle is regulated at 24 hours daily, Linenger's BT and alertness rhythms, though normal for the first 90 days, thereafter (days 110 to 120) were considerably weaker, with consequent disruption in sleep (Monk et al. 2001). These changes suggested that gravity and light cycles work together to reinforce the signal needed to synchronize sleep. Rhythm desynchronization, particularly internal uncoupling of rhythms such as BT with heart rate (HR), has been seen in bed rest of 56 days (Winget et al. 1972) and usually becomes evident after 20 days.

Balance and Coordination

In the microgravity of space, there is no up or down. Coordination of movement and sensory organization of postural control are affected by this absence or reduction in information from the inner ear and the proprioceptors, the cells and nerve endings in the muscles, tendons, and joints that normally tell the body where it is relative to its surroundings. Initial exposure results in conflicting information until the astronaut learns in a couple of days how to move in space. Greater reliance on other senses, like vision and hearing, take over until it is time to return to Earth.

Once back in Earth's gravity, it is more difficult to maintain a steady gaze, measured by a visual acuity test taken while walking on a treadmill. Peripheral vision is reduced. After HDBR, stance and gait are also affected and resemble a 1-year-old's—feet placed wide apart to maintain balance, short, wide, often shuffling steps. Depth perception is affected, and people have problems judging how to negotiate a corner. Rats flown for 14 days first walk back on Earth by dragging the upper side of each foot before picking it up to place it down. Posturography, which involves standing on a sway platform with eyes open or shut, has proven a sensitive diagnostic test for the extent of balance issues (Paloski et al. 1993). Healthy volunteers who spent 30 days of HDBR also show decreased stability, stand with their feet wide apart, take small steps, walk with a careful wide gait, experience trouble with corners, and have tender foot soles, just like astronauts.

Perceiving Gravity

A fine-tuned nervous system determines the body's ability to respond. Achieving this requires frequent stimulation, that is, a series of challenges with time allowed between them for recovery. The frequency, intensity, and the pattern of the stimulus determine how effective it will be in keeping all systems sharp. Such tuning keeps blood pressure sensors sensitive and memory and reaction time sharp. Hormone and immune systems must be responsive and balance and coordination of movement primed, ready to prevent a fall. Body systems have evolved to use gravity as that stimulus. In space, this stimulus is absent or below threshold, in bed rest minimized, and during sitting muted, though it is optimized during development.

The human body perceives gravity in at least four ways. It is likely that all these mechanisms are involved and interact in keeping the body tuned, responsive, and resilient to changes in its relationship to the environment, direction, and acceleration

(Vernikos 2004). Though these mechanisms interact, they may be affected differently among people based on their history and characteristics of muscle strength, athletic ability, adaptability, intact senses, prior experience, and the demands placed on them.

Hydrostatic Pressure

Fluids in the body shift with changes in relation to the direction of gravity. Fluids are normally drawn to the feet in 1 Gz or shifted upward to the chest and head when gravity is withdrawn. The fluid shifts contained within the closed cardiovascular system and their consequences are discussed earlier. *Proprioception* is the most important sense for the control of equilibrium since it is impossible to balance against gravity without it. The subconscious awareness tells you where different parts of your body are located, both in relation to one another and to the surrounding environment. It is what enables you to walk without looking at your feet, to position yourself appropriately. A fast reaction is essential to any sports performance.

Within the body's complex neuromuscular system, there is two-way communication. Proprioceptor sensors in the muscles relay information to the brain, which in turn feeds back the awareness necessary for muscle and joint motion control. Their sensitivity is dulled in reduced gravity in HDBR and is unused or less used in a sedentary lifestyle or in the microgravity of space. Areas rich in proprioceptors include the palms of the hands, soles of the feet, and the glutes. Pilots refer to "flying by the seat of their pants" as that sensation of knowing where they

---

NEED FOR GRAVITY CHALLENGES IN BALANCE CONTROL

The extent of this postural disability and the role living in microgravity plays was evident even after 7 days in space on SLS-2 in 1993. Then-pilot Rick Searfoss was being tested post flight on the platform for balance. With eyes shut, he fell forward without putting his arms out and without, as he told us, experiencing any sensation of falling. Fortunately, his fall was stopped. This reaction has been observed consistently since then. It underlines the rapidity with which the lack of gravity reduces the sensitivity of G-sensing mechanisms in the inner ear, proprioceptor systems, and associated brain pathways, as well as their restoration. It also reinforces the need

in daily life of challenging gravity continuously as a basic requirement for maintaining the integrity of responses.

When Senator John Glenn took part in the 1998 flight on STS-95, he and the other much younger astronauts (aged 38-42) took the platform test three times before and four times after the flight (Paloski et al. 2004). Before the flight, the ability of the 78-year-old Glenn to control his posture in this test was well above average for his age group. After landing, his postural stability was seriously compromised, but no worse than any of the others. They all recovered by the fourth day after return.

are and how their plane is behaving as they take a turn "pulling Gs."

Increased sensitivity and tenderness of the soles of the feet is common after being in space, in bed rest for periods as short as a week, or even after sitting for mere hours as in care facilities. It is not uncommon in postsurgery rehabilitation. Some elderly people may refuse to get out of their chair or bed, not because they cannot but because the soles of their feet hurt.

Mechanotransduction

From birth, mechanical forces provided primarily by gravity are crucial to normal development and evolution of the extracellular matrices found in connective tissue or its loss (Silver et al. 2003). As body mass and its weight—a function of the gravity we live in—increases, musculoskeletal tissues and other extracellular matrixes adapt their size to meet increasing mechanical demands. Integrity theory and research (Ingber 2008) provide the framework for understanding how external (push and pull) and internal mechanical forces influence biological control at the molecular and cellular level. Molecules, cells, tissues, organs, and our entire body use tensegrity architecture to mechanically stabilize their shape and seamlessly integrate structure and function to all size scales. This explains how, at a mechanistic level, intermittent mechanical forces applied externally, such as vibration (Rubin et al. 2002; Rubin et al. 2007), movement or exercise, centrifugation (Vernikos 2004), and push-or-pull or intermittent tension can influence cell and tissue growth, biochemistry, and physiology (Pietramaggiori et al. 2007).

A key element in mechanotransduction relies on fluids within cells and organs, blood vessels (endothelium), channels (bone), and the inner ear of the vestibular system, to name a few, that use G-dependent shear forces generated by the swishing fluid to transmit signals for chemical production of signals such as NO required to maintain tissue integrity.

Vestibular System

The control center of the perception of gravity is the inner ear's vestibular system, an elegant series of fluid-filled canals strategically positioned at roughly right angles to each other. All share a common type of cell, a hair cell that receives and transmits information to the brain about the movement of the head, up or down, side to side toward the shoulders,

or left and right. With each head movement, fluid swishes over the hairs. Depending on the motion—up, down, left, right, or fast forward rotation—this makes them bend. This bending sends signals to the brain's vestibular nucleus and nerve fibers about the nature of the motion, resulting in an internal representation of the position of the head relative to gravity during the movement (see figure 2.2). The brain uses this information along with messages from the other senses (sight, hearing, and touch proprioceptors) to tell muscles what to do in order to maintain balance and stay upright. These representations, sometimes referred to as brain maps, were once thought to be developed during development to last for life. Astronauts showed us that these maps are G-dependent. They are erased in as little as 10 days in space and are rebuilt on return to normal locomotion on return to Earth. HDBR has the same effect. Too much sitting or illness or injury that results in reduced mobility would be expected to produce similar changes in the viability of these brain maps. It would therefore appear imperative for optimal mobility at any age to continually reinforce these maps throughout life.

It was once thought that the main role of the vestibular system was strictly for balance and coordination of gait, direction and acceleration of movement, as well as perception and coordination with vision and the other senses. It is now clear that its control is much broader.

The vestibular system is crucial to the regulation of blood pressure and blood supply to the brain in response to postural change and OH after space or HDBR. The sympathetic and parasympathetic nerves are stimulated, leading to constriction or relaxation of blood vessels for the purpose of maintaining blood pressure, speeding up or slowing down the heart, and maintaining adequate perfusion of the brain to prevent fainting. Yates (2000) has elegantly shown that in response to tilting, the vestibular system activates autonomic nervous system pathways through vagal stimulation, bradycardia, and OH as well as muscle sympathetic nerve stimulation to increase BP through noradrenergic mechanisms that maintain blood pressure. Hyper- or hypoactivity of one or the other pathway determines the outcome, such as OH after spaceflight or HDBR.

Studies have indicated that the vestibular system is also involved in other G-sensitive systems affected by space or HDBR, such as bone and muscle. Vestibular lesions in rats resulted in significant bone loss of weight-bearing bones with reduced bone

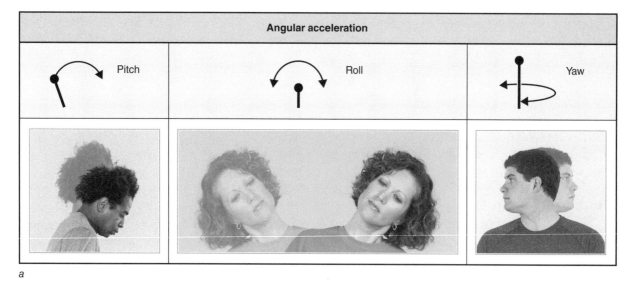

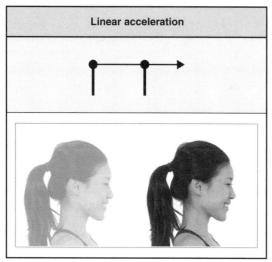

Figure 2.2 Fluid swishes over the hairs of the inner ear, which bend and send signals to the brain through nerve fibers, resulting in an internal representation of the position of the head relative to gravity during movement. This is illustrated for (*a*) angular acceleration and (*b*) linear acceleration.

formation (Vigneaux 2013). The bone loss did not result from reduced locomotor activity or metabolic changes, but was related to sympathetic outflow. Similarly, vestibulo-autonomic mechanisms were shown to be involved in antigravitational soleus muscle atrophy in response to neurovestibular deafferentation. These included high yields of hybrid fiber formation and reduced NFATc1 accumulation as signs of slow-type myofiber atrophy (Luxa et al. 2013). Prolonged but not short-term bed rest may also affect responses by attenuating the sensitivity of the vestibular-sympathetic reflex itself (Dyckman et al. 2012).

Gravity Intervention Design and Implementation

Counteracting the consequences of GDS is literally child's play. The simplest answer to how best to use gravity is to mimic a child at play. Like a child, you need to move all day long, whether you exercise once a day or not. Applying motor skills now advocated for young children (Robieson et al. 2012)—squatting, jumping, kicking, and throwing—makes for beneficial lifetime habits. Understanding how the system works further raises awareness of the most effective G-interventions.

The principles and hypotheses presented here provide a basis for developing a range of solutions to the health consequences of a sedentary lifestyle. Movement of any kind is good. Focusing on keeping the gravity-sensing and control systems sharp and responsive is optimal. G-tuning of this sort forms the foundation of resilience and mobility. It also leads to obvious practical solutions. Traditional exercise for endurance and strength could and should be added to this foundation.

Gravity stimulation, such as with gravity machines, may be directly provided by the following:

▸ *Centrifuge or human-powered centrifuge.* Centrifuges provide acceleration and gravity to those who cannot stand up on their own. They also provide hypergravity for added stimulation. You can lie down on a spinning wheel and get whole body weight training.

▸ *GyroGym*. This is a three-ring gimbaled device powered by the rider to control pace and movement with slight shifts in body weight. There is no motor involved. You drive it by your movement. Your motion moves the rotor, which spins about its axis. Movement can be head up, down, or at any angle. The other two axes also create a harmonic motion alternating motion and relaxation. Most space museums or space centers (Kansas, Houston, or Amsterdam) have one. They are also available commercially.

▸ *Vibration*. Not all vibrators are created equal. In fact, most do not provide sufficient frequency and strain to have any effect. The Galileo, designed to help European astronauts maintain bone strength, meets the requirements as does the HyperVibe from Australia.

Several studies suggest that the rate of the mechanical strain is more important to bone formation, for instance, than static Gz loading (as in standing) or the magnitude of the strain. Bone exposed to vibration, for instance, or exercise responds better to faster stimuli. Bone cells exposed to vibration stress over a wide range of frequencies from 5 to 100 Hz released more NO at the highest acceleration rate (Bacabac et al. 2006; Rubin et al. 2002). The increase in NO—the signaling molecule in osteocytes—correlated linearly to the rate of fluid shear stress in bone cells, *calyculi*. This resulted through the expression of several mechanosensitive genes such as ALP, runx2, osteomodulin, parathyroid hormone receptor 1, and osteoglycin. *In vivo* studies provided evidence that the rate of strain or movement is more important to building bone than the amplitude or power required. Low magnitude (<10 microstrains), high-frequency (10-100 Hz) loading has been found to stimulate bone growth and decrease disuse osteoporosis (Rubin et al. 2002). Detailed discussion on gravity machines can be found in *The G-Connection: Harness Gravity and Reverse Aging* (Vernikos 2004).

Since the G-vector is unidirectional, it is the movement and orientation we make in relationship to this vector that provide the physiological benefit. No movement equals no stimulation. Most benefit comes from movement in relationship to gravity and challenging Gz:

▸ Vertical jumping games make the most of the Gz vector. The greater the vertical trajectory, the greater the gravity load. Moving from a squat to a full jump can generate 6 G, jumping on a trampoline 4 to 4.5 G, and skipping rope, playing hopscotch, or doing jumping jacks could generate 2.5 to 3 G. Lower levels are attained during walking, bending over, reaching up, dancing, doing housework, and gardening.

▸ In addition to the level of gravity, the benefit of vertical shifts comes from the alternating change in posture signal that such movement around the gravity vector provides through major shifts in blood flow to the head and limbs. Work attitudes and environments should be changed to discourage sitting and encourage standing up often.

▸ Equally, moves that involve balance and coordination, acceleration, and stop-and-start motions of low intensity but high frequency, such as skating, dancing, squatting and standing, walking, hiking, and biking, can provide challenging and change-in-direction motion. Daily practices such as tai chi and yoga, qigong, or foundation training can help align with the Gz vector, improve posture, or increase vestibular system sensitivity.

▸ Adding an occasional G-dependent social sport, such as the rhythmic motion of riding, tennis, golf, dancing, sprinting, skiing, sailing, in-line skating, or snowboarding, is also beneficial.

Acceleration is G-dependent. It also is a fundamental source of fun, thus enhancing the G-stimulating value. Any playground provides fun and G-stimulation. Next time you are bored, try a swing for great vestibular stimulation. Germany and Finland have playgrounds for seniors. Merry-go-rounds and roller coasters are great gravity machines. In-line skating, ice skating, juggling, skiing, and snowboarding all depend on a good sense of gravity.

Today, numerous technologies are available that trigger self-awareness, including alerts of time spent sitting, accelerometers to measure gravity value, seating that encourages good Gz posture or core building like the Swopper chair, or variable height stand-up desks that move up and down with you in preprogrammed intervals.

Opportunities to move throughout the day are virtually unlimited, whether at home or at work. Studies in astronauts and healthy bed-confined volunteers collectively indicated that solutions to the sitting problem should encourage frequently interrupting sitting throughout the day every day, rather than interrupting rest once a day every few days or weeks. It appears that the Gz-stimulus of posture change may be crucial to the benefits of any activity that follows. It also suggests that the response to activity or inactivity (as in GDS) may be G-mediated. Identifying the mechanism of the consequences of uninterrupted sitting as G-related leads to creative technological options and combinations. Virtual environments perhaps could be enriched with vibration or motion.

Summary

Sitting for periods longer than 1 hour at a time is an independent risk for poor health and premature aging. Long hours of uninterrupted sitting are not the opposite of continuous standing, nor are they the same as lack of exercise once a day.

Research in reduced gravity environments or inadequate use of gravity has shown that the body declines rapidly when G-deprived, such as in sitting excessively, lying in bed, or living in the microgravity of space. Research shows that conditions of relative gravity deprivation from sitting and lying down, the reduced mobility of aging and other reduced mobility conditions, and the relative weightlessness of space are on a continuum on the gravity scale, and respond in a uniformly similar way to gravity deprivation. This response is characterized by a broad underlying metabolic dysfunction, as evidenced by insulin resistance, insulin-mediated inflammation, oxidative stress, ectopic fat storage, and organ infiltration. Disturbed substrate oxidation affects not only mobility but health in general.

A silent or reduced input to the vestibular system will not transmit normal G-mediated stimulus directives to bone, muscle, and metabolic pathways. Instead, the response may be an alert, triggering defenses through inflammation and shutting down peripheral systems.

Based on the pivotal role of G-sensing balance regulating systems and of the vestibular system in particular, it is proposed that the single common pathway for GDS is centered on or heavily involves vestibular-autonomic pathways. Effective treatment would entail low-intensity, high-frequency activities throughout the day every day, perpetual motion with enhanced gravity use, acceleration activities, and frequent change in posture, balance, and coordination. All of us suffer from some degree of GDS, and an assessment of GDS status should form part of patient history. The solution is not exercising once a day but rather moving frequently throughout the day, every day of the week. This can be achieved only by turning G-using movement into habits. Interrupting sitting by simply standing frequently every 10, 20, or 30 minutes throughout the day is a powerful antidote, as well as the most efficient way of using gravity.

KEY CONCEPTS

▸ **Bed rest:** Used to study the effects of reducing the influence of gravity on the body from 1 Gz (perpendicular force pulling head to toe) to Gx (pulling across the chest) in healthy human volunteers lying in bed continuously in a horizontal position.

▸ **Gravity deprivation syndrome:** The set of physiological changes resulting from reduced influence of gravity, either by living in reduced gravity or microgravity (as in space) or in conditions where the effect of gravity is reduced, by changing the orientation of the body to gravity (Gx), sitting in the buoyancy of water as in immersion, or not using gravity by not moving against the force of gravity.

▸ **Force of gravity:** On Earth, this is attributed a 1 G value.

▸ **Head-down bed rest:** Used to study changes that are even more similar to spaceflight than horizontal bed rest in healthy volunteers, who lie continuously in bed at a –6° head-down position.

▸ **Microgravity:** The reduced gravity experienced in Earth orbit that is approximately 10^{-5}G.

STUDY QUESTIONS

1. What are the clinical consequences of sitting and what is the evidence?

2. How does gravity relate to sitting?

3. How can we be deprived of gravity on Earth and what can we do about it?

4. What is gravity deprivation syndrome (GDS) and what conditions can you think of that might produce it?

5. What are the primary physiological consequences of GDS that lead to clinical conditions?

6. What is the relationship of gravity to health and fitness?

7. If you were to prescribe a program to counter the effects of sitting, what would you recommend based on the concepts presented here?

8. What do you understand by body tuning? What activities would best represent what you were trying to achieve?

CHAPTER 3

PHYSIOLOGICAL EFFECTS OF REDUCING AND BREAKING UP SITTING TIME

David W. Dunstan, PhD; Bethany J. Howard, B Ex Sport Sci, Hons;
Audrey Bergouignan, PhD; Bronwyn A. Kingwell, PhD; and Neville Owen, PhD

The reader will gain an overview of the physiological implications of sedentary behavior with a specific focus on the emergence of recent human experimental studies examining potential causal relationships and effective solutions for mitigating the adverse health consequences of prolonged sitting. By the end of this chapter, the reader should be able to do the following:

▶ Better understand the scientific, public health, and clinical benefits of reducing sitting time

▶ Identify key aspects of study design, control conditions, and methodologies required for human experimental studies on the physiological implications of reducing sitting time

▶ Describe recent human experimental studies on the physiological implications of reducing and breaking up sitting time

▶ Identify directions for future research on the potential biological mechanisms that underlie sedentary behavior and health

The rapid accumulation of epidemiological evidence over the past decade indicating that time spent in sedentary behavior (sitting) is a distinct risk factor for several adverse health outcomes has stimulated broad scientific interest on sedentary behavior and health. As highlighted in several reviews in the last 10 years (Dunstan, Howard, et al. 2012; Owen et al. 2009; Owen et al. 2010; Thorp et al. 2011), a high priority for the sedentary behavior and health research agenda is to generate new evidence from human experimental studies on the benefits of reducing and breaking up sitting time and to better understand potential biological mechanisms underlying the associations of sedentary behavior or sitting time with adverse health outcomes. As demonstrated by the significant contributions of exercise physiology studies to informing public health and clinical exercise guidelines, human experimental evidence is essential for informing and targeting prevention efforts to reduce the deleterious health effects of this highly prevalent risk behavior.

Reviews by Hamilton and colleagues (2004; 2007) have highlighted the need for studies to examine the potentially unique molecular, physiological, and clinical effects of engaging in too much sitting and, alternatively, the potential effect of increases in nonexercise movements (described as inactivity physiology), separate from the responses elicited through structured exercise (exercise physiology). The authors proposed the concept that some of the specific cellular and molecular processes explaining the responses during inactivity versus adding vigorous exercise training on top of the normal level of nonexercise activity are qualitatively different from each other and that maintaining daily low-intensity postural and ambulatory activity may significantly mitigate the detrimental effects induced by inactivity. To support this concept, the authors presented the emerging evidence from a series of animal experimental models indicating that the activity of some health-related proteins in skeletal muscle, such as lipoprotein lipase (LPL), is rapidly suppressed during inactivity (reduced standing or low-intensity ambulation). In contrast, protein activity is profoundly influenced by lower-intensity muscle contractile effort more than by intense exercise training.

Additionally, significant scientific efforts have been directed at understanding the physiological, clinical, and molecular effects of imposed or enforced physically inactive states (e.g., bed rest, reductions in habitual stepping, space flight). Collectively, these studies have provided unique insights into the potential causal relationship and possible underlying mechanisms through which physical inactivity may contribute to chronic disease development. Reviews have provided an extensive account of the evidence generated so far on the many physiological responses related to imposed physical inactivity (see Bergouignan et al. 2011 and Thyfault and Krogh-Madsen 2011), including a reduced capacity to use fat as a substrate or produce ATP, muscle atrophy, a shift in muscle fibers toward fast-twitch glycolytic type, muscle insulin resistance, ectopic fat storage, and increased central and peripheral adiposity.

Our key purpose in this chapter is to examine the effect of reducing and breaking up sitting time and the likely influence on health of doing so. This focus is in keeping with recently revised public health guidelines for physical activity that have highlighted the importance of not only engaging in regular moderate- to vigorous-intensity physical activity, but also reducing sedentary time. Specifically, the UK (Davies et al. 2011) and Australian (Australian Government 2014) physical activity guidelines advocate minimizing sitting for prolonged or extended periods, with the Australian guidelines further recommending breaking up sitting time as often as possible. Within this operational framework, we have identified three fundamental considerations for human experimental models targeting the reduction and breaking up of sitting time, all of which will affect the relevance of the knowledge for population health initiatives aimed at chronic disease prevention:

1. Evidence from population studies that have employed accelerometer (and more recently, inclinometer) assessment of active versus sedentary and sitting patterns indicates that time spent in sedentary behavior dominates the typical daily life of the average adult (Healy et al. 2008) (figure 3.1). As such, there is strong rationale for experimental studies to focus on addressing (i.e., reducing) the current behaviors of a large proportion of the population—that is, sitting for very high volumes of time.

2. We acknowledge the nuance between experimental models comparing normal activity to imposed or enforced physical inactivity versus those experimental models directed at reducing and breaking up sitting time. As we illustrate in figure 3.2, a key distinction is that the imposed or enforced physical inactivity approach is a model of transitioning from an active state (typically young, healthy, active people) to an inactive or less active state (e.g., bed rest, reductions in habitual stepping); this approach is essential for understanding the physiological consequences of inactivity. In contrast, we argue that experimental models of reducing and breaking up prolonged sitting are more solutions focused; that is, they investigate the effects of transitioning from an inactive (sitting) to an active (reduced or nonsitting) state. This latter model is considered to be less extreme than previous bed rest models, and it is likely to have high relevance to the large proportion of the population in which sitting time, not active time, predominates.

3. For most people, a large proportion of their waking hours—following breakfast, lunch, and the evening meal, plus between-meal snacking—coincides with the postprandial state (i.e., after the meal) rather than the fasted state. Given that up to three-quarters of each day can be spent in a postprandial state, examination of the effects of prolonged sitting and reduced sitting in the postprandial state has high relevance to the daily-life scenario for the majority of the adult population. This third consideration is central to understanding the health risks of sedentary behavior. It is well documented that daily ingestion of high-calorie meals—rich in processed carbohydrate and saturated fat—can lead to transient spikes in glucose and lipids, which promote metabolic and oxidative stress that triggers a biochemical inflammatory cascade, endothelial dysfunction, and sympathetic hyperactivity. Since such postprandial excursions, when repeated multiple times each day, can create a milieu conducive to the development of cardiometabolic diseases, in a solutions-focused research approach, it is important to investigate lifestyle modifications that may be effective for reducing exaggerated postprandial dysmetabolism.

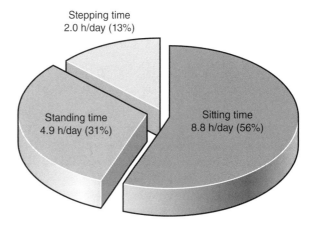

Figure 3.1 Objectively measured (inclinometer) distributions of sitting time, standing time, and stepping time during waking hours in the 698 Australian adult (36-80 years) participants from the 2011/2012 Australian Diabetes, Obesity and Lifestyle Study (AusDiab3) who wore the posture-based ActivPal3 activity monitor for at least 1 day.

Data from G. Healy, University of Queensland.

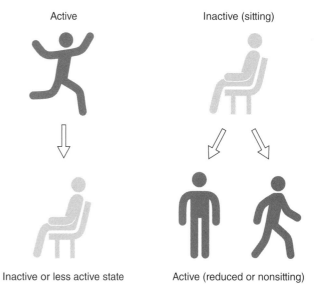

Figure 3.2 Simplified schematic depicting the distinction between an experimental model comparing normal physical activity to imposed or enforced physical inactivity versus an experimental model focusing on reducing and breaking up sitting time through replacing sitting with standing or ambulation.

Methodological Considerations for Studies of Sedentary Behavior

As for all human physiological investigations, it is important to conduct protocols under controlled environmental conditions in order to well observe the effects induced by the intervention free of any confounding effects. In the case of metabolic studies, control of ambient temperature, pressure, sleeping pattern, energy input in terms of both quality and quantity, and energy outputs are factors that need to be taken into consideration. Although temperature, pressure, and daylight are unlikely to be altered in a laboratory facility, diet and physical activity can vary considerably and have a huge effect on the obtained results. In the sidebar Key Methodological Considerations, we have identified some of the methodological considerations in relation to conducting experimental studies on reducing and breaking up sitting time. Understanding these pertinent methodological considerations from the studies conducted so far is essential for identifying where current gaps exist and shaping future experimental studies in this field.

In this chapter, we provide a summary synthesis of the key studies that have sought to understand the influence of reduced states of sitting on indicators of cardiometabolic health. Accordingly, we considered only those studies in which exposure to prolonged sitting within the experimental condition was explicitly detailed or those studies that compared reduced sitting to prolonged sitting. For this summary, we have concentrated only on those studies that have examined the effects on cardiometabolic risk factors.

The studies described in this chapter have employed experimental conditions involving short-term exposures to prolonged sitting or reduced sitting conditions (range: 2 to 24 hr), with the exception of two studies that have investigated the effects of the experimental conditions over repeated days (up to 5 days) (Duvivier et al. 2013; Thorp et al. 2014). Most of the studies identified have examined participants with younger mean ages (< 30 years); only one study was undertaken in older adults (>65 years) (Van Dijk et al. 2013). In general, normal weight adults have been examined, although seven studies focused on overweight or obese adults (Blankenship et al. 2014; Dunstan, Holmstrup et al. 2014; Howard et al. 2013; Kingwell et al. 2012; Larsen et al. 2014; Lunde et al. 2012; Thorp et al. 2014) and one investigated overweight or obese men with type 2 diabetes (Van Dijk et al. 2013). Eleven studied both male and female participants (Bailey and Locke 2015; Blankenship et al. 2014; Buckley et al. 2013; Dunstan, Kingwell et al. 2012; Duvivier et al. 2013; Holmstrup et al. 2014; Howard et al. 2013; Larsen et al. 2014; Peddie et al. 2013; Thorp et al. 2014; Stephens et al. 2011), two studied male participants only (Miyashita et al. 2013; Van Dijk et al. 2013), and two studied female participants only (Nygaard et al. 2009; Lunde et al. 2012). None however studied gender differences. Most conducted the experimental conditions in a laboratory-based setting; three studies utilized the workplace setting (Blankenship et al. 2014; Buckley et al. 2013; Nygaard et al. 2009), while another undertook the experimental condition in the free-living condition (Duvivier et al. 2013). With one exception (Buckley et al. 2013), all utilized a randomized crossover study design in which the experimental conditions have been applied in a counterbalanced approach.

Methodological considerations for these key studies include the following:

▸ *Inclusion criteria.* Volunteers characterized as being insufficiently active (i.e., not meeting minimum recommended physical activity levels) were included across all but two (Holmstrup et al. 2014; Stephens et al. 2011) of the studies, although a

---

KEY METHODOLOGICAL CONSIDERATIONS

- Inclusion criteria consistent with active and sedentary patterns observed in population-based surveys
- Familiarization with testing procedures prior to experimental conditions

- Standardization and control of physical activity and exercise
- Standardization and control of dietary intake
- Standardization and control of energy balance

number did not describe the pre-experiment activity levels of participants. In concordance with the high frequency of sitting time observed in population studies, five studies specifically targeted volunteers employed in sedentary occupations (Blankenship et al. 2014; Dunstan, Kingwell, et al. 2012; Nygaard et al. 2009; Peddie et al. 2013; Thorp et al. 2014).

▶ *Familiarization with testing procedures prior to experimental conditions.* Several studies (Bailey and Locke 2014; Blankenship et al. 2014; Dunstan, Kingwell, et al. 2012; Holmstrup et al. 2014; Miyashita et al. 2013; Peddie et al. 2013; Stephens et al. 2011; Van Dijk et al. 2013; Thorp et al. 2014) used a familiarization session as an additional control measure in the lead-in to the experimental conditions. Typically, this involved familiarization with the testing equipment and experimental protocols (e.g., treadmill walking) or preliminary testing to ascertain individualized workloads at the appropriate intensity to be applied within experimental conditions.

▶ *Standardization and control of physical activity and exercise.* All studies restricted nonexperimental exercise within the preceding 24 to 72 hours of each trial condition. Intensity of activity during the experimental conditions in some trials was prescribed based on aerobic fitness testing (Blankenship et al. 2014; Miyashita et al. 2013; Peddie et al. 2013; Van Dijk et al. 2013), leading to a relative intensity depending on the exercise capacity of each subject (Dunstan, Kingwell, et al. 2012; Duvivier et al. 2013; Lunde et al. 2012; Nygaard et al. 2009; Stephens et al. 2011) and resulting in a same absolute workload for all study participants regardless of their individual fitness. To ensure compliance and to monitor and potentially control for any activity-induced variability, six studies incorporated objective monitoring of sedentary and physical activity patterns during and between conditions (Blankenship et al. 2014; Dunstan, Kingwell, et al. 2012; Duvivier et al. 2013; Miyashita et al. 2013; Stephens et al. 2011; Thorp et al. 2014).

▶ *Standardization and control of dietary intake.* Diet, including alcohol and caffeine consumption, can induce varied metabolic responses. Any differences in the diet of participants can mask the effect of physical activity on metabolism or induce high interindividual variability. Diet-induced variability was minimized in four studies through the provision of one or several standardized test meals prior to each experimental condition (Dunstan, Kingwell, et

al. 2012; Stephens et al. 2011; Thorp et al. 2014; Van Dijk et al. 2013). In other studies, participants were instructed to replicate their diet based on 24-hour dietary records prior to condition one (Buckley et al. 2013; Holmstrup et al. 2014; Miyashita et al. 2013; Peddie et al. 2013) or to keep their diet as similar as possible (Duvivier et al. 2013; Lunde et al. 2012; Nygaard et al. 2009). All but three studies (Blankenship et al. 2014; Lunde et al. 2012; Nygaard et al. 2009) restricted alcohol intake for at least 24 hours, while several studies also restricted caffeine intake (Bailey and Locke 2014; Dunstan, Kingwell, et al. 2012; Holmstrup et al. 2014; Stephens et al. 2011; Thorp et al. 2014).

During the experimental conditions, standardized test meals (Blankenship et al. 2014; Buckley et al. 2013; Lunde et al. 2012; Miyashita et al. 2013; Nygaard et al. 2009; Stephens et al. 2011; Van Dijk et al. 2013) or liquid meals (Bailey and Locke 2014; Dunstan, Kingwell, et al. 2012; Holmstrup et al. 2014; Peddie et al. 2013; Thorp et al. 2014) were provided to examine postprandial responses. Most of these respected the macronutrient composition recommended by the World Health Organization (i.e., 55% carbohydrate, 30% fat, and 15% protein of total energy intake). Marked variations in the macronutrient composition can, however, challenge metabolism and enhance variations in metabolic postprandial response. With this in mind, two studies opted for a high-carbohydrate, high-fat liquid meal used as a combined oral glucose and fat tolerance test (Bailey and Locke 2014; Dunstan, Kingwell, et al. 2012; Thorp et al. 2014).

▶ *Standardization and control of energy balance.* In addition to food quality, the quantity of food provided can affect metabolism and physiology. Energy balance is defined as the relationship between energy intake and energy output. When energy intake is greater than energy expenditure, individuals are overfed and will gain weight over the long term. On the contrary, when energy intake is lower than the amount of energy expended, the system is in energy deficit, which results in weight loss over time. In studies that manipulate physical activity (i.e., one of the two sides of the energy balance equation), it is evident that tightly controlling food intake is of great importance in data interpretation. So far very few studies, however, have considered energy balance within their designs. Stephens and colleagues (2011) factored in energy balance by comparing the relative effects of 1 day of sitting with or without a concomitant reduction in energy intake (leading to energy balance or surplus) to the day of minimal sitting. Blankenship and others (2014) factored in energy balance by matching total daily energy expenditure across two of the conditions (continuous walking bout and frequent long breaks ~ 300 kcal), with the third (frequent short breaks) having a lower energy expenditure. By doing so, these studies avoided the effect of overfeeding as a confounding factor.

The early insights obtained from the human experimental studies described are promising, showing that the various strategies that have specifically compared prolonged sitting to reduced states of sitting and the breaking up of prolonged sitting time can elicit favorable changes in cardiometabolic biomarkers, at least in the short term. In particular, several studies have demonstrated a positive influence on postprandial glucose and insulin responses, while some have demonstrated improved responses in blood pressure, lipids, and hemostatic markers.

Metabolic Effects of Reduced Sitting and the Postprandial State

Several studies have investigated the effects on cardiometabolic biomarkers of short episodes (2- to 9-hr, single-day experiment) of prolonged uninterrupted sitting versus various manipulations of reduced sitting during the postprandial period. Although the findings from the experimental studies that have specifically addressed the cardiometabolic consequences of prolonged sitting and reduced sitting are promising, there is still a clear need for the development of further high-quality research evidence. In addition to examining the effect of longer-term exposures (i.e., weeks or months), the various perturbations in the frequency (high versus low), length (short versus long), and type (ambulation versus standing) of activity interruptions to prolonged sitting and interactions with moderate- to vigorous-intensity physical activity, dietary intake, and meal patterns need to be examined.

Furthermore, there are likely to be effects of reducing and breaking up sitting time on multiple body tissues, organs, and systems (e.g., vascular and hemodynamic mechanisms, cognitive function, musculoskeletal adaptations). Establishing the dose–response relationships among interrupting sitting, risk markers, and physiological adaptations also has the potential to inform further work in specific disease groups—for example, among patients with hypertension, peripheral artery disease, osteoarthritis, overweight and obesity, metabolic syndrome and diabetes, and cognitive impairment, and among those with elevated thrombotic risk.

Prolonged Slow Walking Post Meal

Within the work-office setting, a randomized crossover trial by Nygaard and colleagues (2009) investigated the capillary (finger-prick) blood glucose response to a carbohydrate-rich meal over a 2-hour period (see table 3.1). The study compared, in healthy women aged >50 years, uninterrupted sitting to reduced sitting achieved through initial 15- and 40-minute bouts of slow, very light walking followed by sitting. The 40-minute walking condition, but not the 15-minute walking condition, induced a significant decrease in the 2-hour incremental glucose area under the curve (AUC), leading the authors to suggest that a dose response between the duration of slow walking (and the resultant increase in energy expenditure) and reductions in postprandial glycemia may exist. However, a subsequent study by Lunde and others (2012) using a similar study design and methodologies in female Pakistani immigrants (most of whom had abnormal glucose tolerance) demonstrated reductions in the 2-hour incremental area under the curve for both the 20-minute (by 30.6%) and 40-minute (by 39.0%) walking conditions relative to the control day. A significant reduction in systolic blood pressure was also observed after the 40-minute walking condition. The discrepancies between the results in these two studies suggest that a greater workload in terms of duration of the bout of activity or in terms of energy expenditure is required in metabolically unhealthy people. An interaction between extrinsic factors (i.e., physical activity) and genetic background (Caucasians versus Asians) may also influence the dose–response relationship between physical activity and metabolic health.

High-Frequency Brief Activity Bouts

Building on the observational-study findings showing beneficial health associations with breaking up sedentary time, Dunstan, Kingwell, and colleagues (2012) conducted an experimental study with overweight middle-aged adults (see table 3.2). In a randomized crossover trial, they examined the effects of uninterrupted sitting compared with sitting

Table 3.1 Reduced Sitting Through Prolonged Slow Walking Post Meal

Nygaard 2009	
Experimental conditions	Findings
1. Seated office work: 120 min	
2. Slow walking: 15 min walk, 105 min sit	VS condition 1 ↑ time to peak glucose
3. Slow walking: 40 min walk, 80 min sit	VS condition 1 ↓ 2 hr glucose iAUC by 31.2% ↑ time to peak glucose

Lunde 2012	
Experimental conditions	Findings
1. Sit: 120 min	
2. Slow walking: 20 min, 100 min sit	VS condition 1 ↑ time to peak glucose ↓ 2 hr glucose iAUC by 31%
3. Slow walking: 40 min, 80 min sit	VS condition 1 ↓ 2 hr glucose iAUC by 39% ↑ time to peak glucose ↓ postprandial glucose peak ↓ 2 hr systolic BP VS condition 2 ↓ postprandial glucose peak

iAUC = incremental area under the curve, BP = blood pressure, VS = versus (i.e., control condition 2 versus control condition 1)

Table 3.2 Reduced Sitting Through High-Frequency Brief Activity Bouts

Dunstan, Kingwell, et al. 2012; Howard 2013; Larsen 2014	
Experimental conditions	Findings
1. Uninterrupted sit: 300 min	
2. Sit + light-intensity activity breaks: 14 × 2 min light walk, 272 min sit	VS condition 1 ↓ 5 hr glucose iAUC by 24% ↓ 5 hr insulin iAUC by 23% ↓ plasma fibrinogen ↓ hematocrit, hemoglobin, and red blood cell count ↑ plasma volume ↓ systolic BP by 3 mmHg ↓ diastolic BP by 3 mmHg
3. Sit + moderate-intensity activity breaks: 14 × 2 min moderate walk, 272 min sit	VS condition 1 ↓ 5 hr glucose iAUC by 30% ↓ 5 hr insulin iAUC by 23% ↓ 2 hr insulin by 37 pmol/L ↓ hematocrit, hemoglobin, and red blood cell count ↑ plasma volume, mean platelet volume, and white cell count ↓ systolic BP by 2 mmHg ↓ diastolic BP by 2 mmHg VS condition 2 No significant effects

iAUC = incremental area under the curve, BP = blood pressure, VS = versus (i.e., control condition 2 versus control condition 1)

interrupted by short 2-minute bouts of activity (either light- or moderate-intensity treadmill walking) on postprandial glucose and insulin levels (Dunstan, Kingwell, et al. 2012), hemostatic markers (Howard et al. 2013), and blood pressure (Larsen et al. 2014). Relative to the uninterrupted sitting condition, significant reductions of a similar magnitude were observed in the 5-hour incremental glucose and insulin area under the curve and systolic and diastolic blood pressure in both of the activity break conditions. The significant increase in plasma fibrinogen with prolonged sitting was attenuated only in the light-activity break condition. Notably, no statistically significant differences between the two activity conditions were observed, supporting the hypothesis that brief interruptions to sitting time with a minimum of light-intensity physical activity can attenuate acute postprandial glucose and insulin and blood pressure responses during prolonged sitting. This suggests that many of the benefits of breaking up sitting time occur at a relatively low threshold in terms of activity intensity. These insights into the possible benefits of activity behaviors considered to be at the lower end of the physical activity spectrum

(i.e., breaking up of sitting time via light-intensity physical activity) provided the initial foundation for future physiological research endeavors that are distinct from the traditional approaches employed within exercise physiology–type studies.

Continuous Postmeal Exercise Bout or Brief Activity Bouts

In the largest experimental study on prolonged sitting undertaken to date, Peddie and colleagues (2013) investigated the effects of regularly breaking up prolonged sitting with activity over a 9-hour period in 70 healthy younger adults of normal weight (see table 3.3). A meal-replacement beverage was provided at 1 hour, 4 hours, and 7 hours. In a novel approach, the effects of interrupting prolonged sitting with frequent short bouts of brisk treadmill walking every 30 minutes over the 9-hour period were also compared to a condition whereby participants walked briskly for 30 minutes and then sat continuously for the remainder of the condition. Of note, these two conditions were isocaloric (i.e., a similar amount of energy was expended), since participants worked out for a total duration of 30 minutes at an exact same intensity. Consistent with the findings from Dunstan, Kingwell, and colleagues (2012) in overweight adults, the regular brief interruptions to prolonged sitting lowered 9-hour postprandial plasma glucose and insulin concentration relative to prolonged sitting. Notably, the regular activity breaks condition was shown to be more effective than sitting preceded by a continuous bout of physical activity at lowering both postprandial glucose and insulin; in contrast, the 9-hour triglyceride postprandial concentration was higher with the activity breaks condition relative to the continuous physical activity bout condition. Further studies are required to elucidate the differential effects of breaking up sitting time and continuous moderate- to vigorous-intensity physical activity on the relative consumption of glucose and fat throughout the day.

In another randomized crossover trial, Van Dijk and others (2013) compared the effects of prolonged sitting to reduced sitting states achieved through the introduction of less frequent (three in total over the 10.5 hr) but longer duration (15 min) bouts of slow-paced strolling in older adults with type 2 diabetes. Additionally, another condition examined the effects of an initial 45-minute continuous bout of moderate-intensity exercise followed by prolonged sitting. Significant reductions were observed in the 10.5-hour postprandial glucose and insulin responses following both activity conditions, with the magnitude of change for glucose (36% vs. 19%) and insulin (32% vs. 14%) greater with the continuous exercise bout condition, likely because of the greater effect on intensity of the exercise and on the amount of energy expended. No significant effects were seen for total cholesterol and blood pressure.

Increased Standing

Two studies have examined the single-day effects of reducing sitting time through increased standing. In a repeated measures study undertaken in a real office environment using height-adjustable workstations in 10 desk-based office workers, Buckley and colleagues (2013) reported significantly attenuated blood glucose excursions (assessed by using a continuous monitoring device) following one afternoon of standing work compared to an afternoon of seated work (see table 3.4). A randomized crossover trial undertaken by Bailey and Locke (2015) in 10 healthy young participants compared the effects of reducing sitting time through frequent 2-minute bouts

Table 3.3 Reduced Sitting Through Continuous Post-Meal Exercise Bout or Brief Activity Bouts

Dunstan, Kingwell, et al. 2012; Howard 2013; Larsen 2014	
Experimental conditions	Findings
1. Uninterrupted sit: 300 min	
2. Sit + light-intensity activity breaks: 14 × 2 min light walk, 272 min sit	VS condition 1 ↓ 5 hr glucose iAUC by 24% ↓ 5 hr insulin iAUC by 23% ↓ plasma fibrinogen ↓ hematocrit, hemoglobin, and red blood cell count ↑ plasma volume ↓ systolic BP by 3 mmHg ↓ diastolic BP by 3 mmHg
3. Sit + moderate-intensity activity breaks: 14 × 2 min moderate walk, 272 min sit	VS condition 1 ↓ 5 hr glucose iAUC by 30% ↓ 5 hr insulin iAUC by 23% ↓ 2 hr insulin by 37 pmol/L ↓ hematocrit, hemoglobin, and red blood cell count ↑ plasma volume, mean platelet volume, and white cell count ↓ systolic BP by 2 mmHg ↓ diastolic BP by 2 mmHg VS condition 2 No significant effects
Peddie 2013	
Experimental conditions	Findings
1. Uninterrupted sit: 540 min	
2. Sit + one continuous physical activity bout: 510 min sit, 30 min walk	VS condition 1 No significant effects
3. Sit + regular activity breaks: 18 × 15 min sitting initially followed by 100 sec moderate walk (510 min sit, 30 min walk)	VS condition 1 ↓ 9 hr glucose iAUC by 39% ↓ 9 hr insulin iAUC by 26% VS condition 2 ↓ 9 hr glucose iAUC by 37% ↓ 9 hr insulin iAUC by 18% ↓ 9 hr triglyceride iAUC by 31%
Van Dijk 2013	
Experimental conditions	Findings
1. Uninterrupted sit: 650 min	
2. Sit + ADL bouts: 3 × 15 min slow-paced strolling (605 min sit, 45 min walk)	VS condition 1 ↓ 10.5 hr glucose iAUC by 19% ↓ 10.5 hr insulin positive iAUC by 14%
3. Sit + exercise bout: 1 × 45 min moderate-intensity cycling (605 min sit, 45 min cycle)	VS condition 1 ↓ 24 hr prevalence of hyperglycemia by 30% ↓ 10.5 hr glucose iAUC by 36% ↓ 10.5 hr insulin positive iAUC by 32% VS condition 2 ↓ insulin positive iAUC

iAUC = incremental area under the curve, BP = blood pressure, VS = versus (i.e., control condition 2 versus control condition 1) of light-intensity walking over 20-minute intervals and, separately, the effects of a similar frequency of short stationary standing breaks for 2 minutes every 20 minutes over the 5-hour observation period. Although no significant effects were observed for total cholesterol, HDL-C, or blood pressure, a reduction in sitting time induced through the incorporation of frequent light-intensity walking breaks led to significantly lower postprandial glucose response relative to the uninterrupted sitting and the standing breaks conditions. The findings suggest that the magnitude of skeletal muscle activation that occurs during the break condition may influence the subsequent metabolic response, since interrupting sitting time with frequent light-intensity activity imparted beneficial postprandial glucose responses, but interrupting sitting with frequent standing (characterized by its diminished relative skeletal muscle activity) did not.

Cardiometabolic Effects Following Exposure to Reduced Sitting

To investigate the acute (1 day) effects of prolonged sitting on glucose and insulin metabolism on the day following exposure to experimental conditions, Stephens and others (2011) compared the effects of

Table 3.4 Reduced Sitting Through Increased Standing

Buckley 2014	
Experimental conditions	Findings
1. Seated desk work: 185 min	
2. Standing desk work: 185 min	VS condition 1 ↓ 185 min in glucose AUC by 43%
Bailey and Locke 2015	
Experimental conditions	Findings
1. Uninterrupted sit: 300 min	
2. Sit + light-intensity activity breaks: 300 min (14 × 2 min bouts of light walking at 20 min intervals)	VS condition 1 ↓ 5 hr blood glucose iAUC by 15.9%
3. Sit + standing breaks: 300 min (14 × 2 min bouts of standing still at 20 min intervals)	VS condition 1 No significant effects VS condition 2 ↓ 5 hr blood glucose iAUC by 16.7%

iAUC = incremental area under the curve, VS = versus (i.e., control condition 2 versus control condition 1)

1 day of predominately sitting (16.9 hr sitting) to 1 day of minimal sitting (5.8 hr sitting) in 14 active, normal-weight young adults (see table 3.5). In one condition, they replaced the energy expended during the extra physically active time to place subjects in stable energy balance conditions. In a second condition, they did not match energy intake for energy expenditure, inducing an energy deficit in participants. When increased physical activity was not compensated for by food intake, minimal sitting improved insulin action compared to prolonged sitting. When calories expended during the physical activity were replaced, the decline in insulin action observed following prolonged sitting (approximately 17 hr, measured objectively) was significantly attenuated by breaks but was not completely prevented. These results indicate that the magnitude of the benefits of breaking up sitting time are dependent on energy balance, with greater benefit achieved when food intake is less.

In 18 young participants, Miyashita and colleagues (2013) used a 2-day experimental design to compare the effects of prior (total: 7.5 hr) exposure to uninterrupted sitting versus reduced sitting through intermittent 45-minute bouts of standing or the inclusion of a 30-minute brisk walk immediately before the bout of sitting. Participants returned the following day to undertake postprandial blood measurements (in response to a standardized test meal). Significant effects were observed only following the walking condition, with a reduction in the 6-hour postprandial glucose response compared to uninterrupted sitting and reductions in the 6-hour triglyceride area under the curve relative to the uninterrupted sitting and the standing breaks conditions, respectively. Either the energy expended during the multiple bouts of standing was not sufficient or the beneficial effects of standing last for a shorter amount of time than those of a more intense physical activity. Determining the period of action of bouts of activity according to their nature, volume, intensity, and duration will be of great importance in developing future recommendations and establishing the minimum amount of time allowed between two sets of activity.

To compare the effects of adding exercise as opposed to reducing sitting, but maintaining a constant energy expenditure, Blankenship and others (2014) examined 10 sedentary overweight or obese office workers who were exposed to three experimental conditions within the office setting. The examination was administered in a randomized order across an 8-hour workday followed by a mixed

Table 3.5 Cardiometabolic Effects Following Exposure to Reduced Sitting

Stephens 2011	
Experimental conditions	Findings
1. Prolonged sit: 16.9 hr sit, 0.2 hr stand, 0.1 hr step	
2. Active condition with reduced sit: 5.8 hr sit, 9.8 hr stand, 2.2 hr step	VS condition 1 ↓ insulin action by 39%
3. Prolonged sit + reduced energy intake: 16.8 hr sit, 0.3 hr stand, 0.1 hr step	VS condition 2 ↓ insulin action by 18%
Miyashita 2013	
Experimental conditions	Findings
1. Uninterrupted sit: 7.5 hr	
2. Sit + standing: 6 × 45 min stand, 3 hr sit (3.5 hr stand, 3 hr sit)	VS condition 1 No significant effects
3. Sit + 1 continuous walking bout: 7 hr sit, 30 min walk	VS condition 1 ↓ 6 hr serum triacylglycerol total AUC by 18% ↓ 6 hr total glucose AUC by 7% VS condition 2 ↓ 6 hr serum triacylglycerol total AUC by 18%
Blankenship 2014	
Experimental conditions	Findings
1. One continuous walking bout (30 min) + sit: 8 hr	
2. Sit + frequent long breaks: 8 hr (uninterrupted sit limited to <20 min, interruptions of standing or walking ~300 kcal)	VS condition 1 ↓ glycemic variability (all measures) ↓ nocturnal elevated glycemia
3. Sit + frequent short breaks: 8 hr (uninterrupted sit limited to <20 min, interruptions of standing or walking, equal number but shorter breaks condition 2)	VS condition 1 ↓ glycemic variability (CONGA) ↓ glucose AUC for evening meal (CGM) VS condition 2 ↓ glycemic variability (SD) ↓ elevated glucose (CGM)

CGM = continuous glucose monitoring, CONGA = continuous overlapping net glycemic action, SD = standard deviation

meal tolerance test performed in the laboratory at the end of the workday. Glycemic variability (using continuous glucose monitoring) and postprandial glucose and insulin responses were examined after a day spent taking either frequent long breaks (FLB) from sitting (incorporating standing or stepping) versus taking fewer breaks (walking as per activity guidelines; AWG), with total energy expenditure matched between conditions. The third condition containing the same number of breaks as FLB but lower energy expenditure (frequent short breaks [FSB] involving standing and stepping) was included to examine whether energy expenditure or simply altering body position frequently mediated the responses. Although no differences were observed between all conditions for the evening postmeal glucose and insulin responses, glycemic variability was more effectively lessened in the breaks conditions compared to the AWG condition; nocturnal duration of elevated glucose was also shorter after the FLB (2.5 min) than the AGW (32.7 min) or FSB (45.6 min) conditions. In the presence of equivalent effects from breaks in sitting and the moderate-intensity exercise bout on postmeal glucose and insulin responses, yet more effectively constrained glycemic variability from the breaks despite their matched energy expenditure, it was interpreted that frequent breaks in sitting of sufficient duration may be more effective in reducing glycemic variability than one bout of exercise in sedentary people. Additionally, since glycemic variability was highest in the AGW condition, it was suggested that, at least in the short term, structured exercise may not completely negate the effects of sedentary behavior on cardiometabolic health.

Cardiometabolic Effects of Repeated-Day Exposure to Reduced Sitting

A randomized crossover study undertaken by Duvivier and colleagues (2013) compared the effects of 4 consecutive days of sitting with two separate reduced sitting conditions under free-living conditions in 20 healthy university students (see table 3.6). In the sitting condition, across all 4 days, subjects were instructed to sit for 14 hours, walk for 1 hour, stand for 1 hour, and to spend 8 hours per day sleeping or supine. In the exercise condition, on each day, 1 hour of sitting was replaced by

1 hour of vigorous supervised cycling, with the rest of the day spent in a similar manner to the sitting condition. In the minimal-intensity physical activity condition, subjects were instructed to replace 6 hours of sitting with 4 hours of walking at a leisurely pace and with 2 hours of standing on each of the 4 days. During the 4 days of each condition, participants wore an inclinometer continuously for 24 hours to quantify daily physical activity and postural allocation. Laboratory measurements were undertaken on day 5 after each condition. Relative to the sitting condition, significant reductions were observed following the minimal-intensity physical activity condition for the 2-hour insulin area under the curve, fasting plasma triglycerides, non-HDL-cholesterol and Apo B (cardiometabolic biomarkers). Although a significant reduction in the postmeal insulin concentration was observed following the exercise condition relative to the sitting condition, it was reported that greater reductions in the insulin area under the curve, fasting plasma triglycerides, and fasting plasma non-HDL cholesterol, as well as an increase in the insulin sensitivity index, were evident for the minimal-intensity physical activity versus the exercise condition.

In a simulated office environment within the laboratory setting, Thorp and colleagues (2014) compared the effects of repeated days (5 days) of prolonged seated work (8 hr/day) to a similar period of alternating between standing and seated work, using a height-adjustable workstation every 30 minutes (4 hr standing, 4 hr sitting) in 23 office workers. Using a randomized crossover design, laboratory measurements were performed on day 1 and day 5 of each condition. The introduction of 30-minute bouts of standing work each hour resulted in a significant attenuation in the postprandial blood glucose response (incremental area under the curve) relative to the seated condition. No such attenuations were observed for insulin or triglycerides.

Public Health and Clinical Guidelines

The emerging evidence from experimental studies is supportive of recent calls for practitioners and public health experts to expand their thinking beyond just purposeful health-enhancing exercise and give serious consideration to advocating reductions in sitting time. Already, some leading health agencies have taken a proactive stance on this issue

Table 3.6 Cardiometabolic Effects of Repeated-Day Exposure to Reduced Sitting

Duvivier 2013	
Experimental conditions	Findings
1. Sit: sit 14 hr/day, walk 1 hr/day, 8 hr/day sleeping or supine	
2. Exercise: replaced 1 hr sit with 1 hr vigorous supervised cycling	VS condition 1 ↓ 2 hr insulin total AUC by 7%
3. Minimal intensity PA: replaced 6 hr of sit with 4 hr of light walking and 2 hr stand	VS condition 1 ↓ 2 hr insulin total AUC by 13.2% ↓ fasting plasma triglyceride by 22% ↓ fasting plasma non-HDL cholesterol by 10% ↓ fasting plasma Apo B by 8% VS condition 2 ↓ 2 hr insulin total AUC by 19% ↑ insulin sensitivity index (ISI) by 15% ↓ fasting plasma triglyceride by 17.6% ↓ fasting plasma non-HDL cholesterol by 6.7%
Thorp 2014	
Experimental conditions	Findings
1. Seated only work: 560 min	
2. Seated and standing work: height-adjustable workstation, interchanging every 30 min (240 min sit, 240 min standing)	VS condition 1 ↓ 4 hr glucose total AUC by 11.1%

AUC = area under the curve, ISI = insulin sensitivity index, HDL = high-density lipoprotein

through the release of new advice within physical activity recommendations on the likely importance of reducing sedentary behavior.

The 2011 United Kingdom *Start Active, Stay Active* document (Davies et al. 2011) and the 2014 Australian Physical Activity and Sedentary Behavior guidelines (Australian Government 2014) present recommendations on the volume, duration, frequency, and type of physical activity required across the life span to achieve general health benefits. In addition, attention is also directed at reducing sedentary behavior across all age groups, with the nonspecific and sufficiently broad message to minimize the amount of time spent being sedentary (sitting) for extended periods and break up long periods of sitting as often as possible applied across the various age groups from the early to later years.

From the United States, the *2011 Quantity and Quality of Exercise for Developing and Maintaining Cardiorespiratory, Musculoskeletal, and Neuromotor Fitness in Apparently Healthy Adults: Guidance for Prescribing Exercise* position stand of the American College of Sports Medicine acknowledges that

> *In addition to exercising regularly, there are health benefits in concurrently reducing total time spent in sedentary pursuits and also by interspersing frequent, short bouts of standing and physical activity between periods of sedentary activity, even in physically active adults.* (Garber et al. 2011, page 1334)

The UK *Start Active, Stay Active* document, the 2014 Australian Physical Activity and Sedentary Behavior guidelines, and the American College of Sports Medicine position stand do, however, indicate that in the absence of an extensive body of experimental evidence allowing stronger causal inferences about the health effects of too much sitting, such recommendations relating to sitting will continue to remain general and tentative. Furthermore, the 2010 *Global Recommendations on Physical Activity for Health* document from the World Health Organization is explicit about the potential importance for health outcomes of too much sitting, yet stops short of making specific recommendations around sitting.

Reducing and breaking up sitting time is a new approach to enhancing daily physical movement, and relatively little is known regarding the mechanisms of benefit. In the absence of such evidence, public health guidelines for reducing sitting time and acceptable upper limits of accumulated or sustained sitting time will continue to remain nonspecific. Rigorously designed human experimental research is therefore crucial for developing specific recommendations on sitting that are needed in future clinical and public health guidelines and informing a range of related initiatives.

Summary

Within this chapter, we have highlighted several study design features and methodological elements that will be relevant for future research endeavors directed at understanding the physiological implications of sedentary behavior. Notwithstanding the importance of employing strict and population-relevant study entry criteria, strategic decisions relating to the nature of the physical activity substitute for achieving a reduced state of sitting (likely to be contingent on the physiological and metabolic outcomes to be assessed), and the methods for obtaining strict control of dietary and physical activity patterns and energy balance will be paramount for all researchers in this field.

The emerging evidence arising from the human experimental studies targeting reducing and breaking up sitting time is supportive of the observational study evidence linking sitting time and breaks in sitting time with significant compromises in cardiometabolic health. Yet, despite the promising findings, it is still too early to generate definitive recommendations on how long people should sit or how often people should break up their sitting time and how this should be achieved. Additional evidence, particularly from longer-term intervention studies (i.e., chronic trials), is needed to reliably inform specific guidelines and advice that can be given to patients and the general population. Nevertheless, at this stage—on the basis of observational study findings and the early-stage human experimental evidence—broad advice can be given with reasonable confidence. There are likely to be beneficial effects and no harm done if adults create opportunities to limit their sitting time while at home, at work, and during transportation in addition to breaking up prolonged periods of sitting through frequent transitions from sitting to standing or ambulating throughout the day. A simple message that could be put forward is, Stand up, sit less, move more, move more often. However, the specifics of such messages remain to be delineated by future experimental studies.

KEY CONCEPTS

- **Area under the curve (AUC):** The integrated expression of the cumulative area under the plasma or serum concentration curve of a selected biomarker (e.g., glucose, insulin). Frequently used to assess the responsiveness to a stimulus (e.g., glucose load, meal), expressed as incremental area under the curve, which takes into account area below baseline (fasting or premeal) levels.

- **Blood glucose:** Also known as blood sugar, glucose is a fuel source that is absorbed into the blood stream following consumption of carbohydrate.

- **Crossover trial:** Study design in which the participants are their own control. Each participant completes all conditions, usually in a random order separated by a washout period. This design therefore allows for the comparison of both within- and between-group effects (Mills et al. 2009).

- **Insulin:** A hormone made by the pancreatic beta cells that is secreted into the bloodstream after eating. Insulin aids in glucose uptake into liver, adipose, and muscle cells for energy (ATP) production or storage as glycogen.

- **Postprandial state:** The American Diabetes Association (2001) defines this as the time after a meal. The postprandial state is often related to the plasma glucose profile after eating. Typically, plasma glucose rises 10 minutes after a meal and peaks around 60 minutes after, returning to premeal levels within 3 hours.

STUDY QUESTIONS

1. Why are experimental models of reducing and breaking up sitting time considered to be more solutions focused than other experimental models?

2. For a laboratory-based experimental study to identify the possible benefits of breaking up prolonged sitting time, what could you prescribe that people do during their breaks from sitting?

3. What are the key methodological or design considerations of human experimental studies on the physiological implications of sedentary behavior?

4. Why is it important to control for food intake and food quality within experimental studies on the physiological implications of sedentary behavior?

5. What findings from human experimental studies would be most informative in helping to provide more specific public health recommendations and clinical guidelines on too much sitting?

The following support is gratefully acknowledged: National Health and Medical Research Council of Australia Senior Research Fellowship (Dunstan), National Health and Medical Research Council (NHMRC) of Australia Senior Principal Research Fellowships and Program Grants (Owen, Kingwell), an Australian Government Endeavour Research Fellowship Award (Bergouignan), NHMRC/National Heart Foundation Postgraduate Research Scholarship (Howard), and the Victorian government's Operational Infrastructure Support Program (all authors). The authors have no conflicts of interest to declare.

CHAPTER 4

RETHINKING THE CHAIR AND SITTING

Galen Cranz, PhD

The reader will gain an overview of why right-angle chair sitting is intrinsically problematic and why designing for movement and diverse postures is preferable. By the end of this chapter, the reader should be able to do the following:

▸ Summarize the history of the chair

▸ Outline the biomechanical and ergonomic problems of chair sitting

▸ Appreciate how chair designers have tried to solve the ergonomic problems

▸ Understand how right-angle chair designs move problems around the body but never eliminate them

▸ Use alternatives to the classic right-angle chair (the lounge, the perch, sit-to-stand solutions, adjustability, continuous movement, job redesign, and postural education)

Westerners are now worrying that we are too sedentary, so let us consider the material artifact that allows us to sit so much: the chair. Before considering the anatomical and physiological problems associated with chair sitting, let's glance backward to see where the chair came from and why we have come to rely on it.

History of the Chair

We may never know the exact origin of the chair, although we do know that chairs are older than most furniture histories indicate. Most scholars start with Egyptian pharaohs or possibly kings from the Mesopotamian Fertile Crescent, which would make chairs about 5,000 years old. An archeological find from the former Yugoslavia offers evidence of a much longer history (Cranz 1998). Kiln-fired models of women seated on chairs from the Neolithic era (7,500 BCE) have been found in graves. This means that chairs are at least 10,000 years old and possibly even older. The primary material record from the Paleolithic era (about 40,000 years ago) is cave art, which shows mostly animals, only occasionally a human, less often a tool, and never a chair (Cranz 1998), so exact dating of the first chair seems unlikely.

This earliest evidence of chair sitting from the Neolithic era suggests that chairs were associated with role differentiation and social status; they remain so today. In classical Greece, the *klismos* chair was developed for domestic life, but in the Roman Empire, social life was conducted on flat platforms, beds, and *triclinia*. The *triclinium* was a specialized three-sided, U-shaped platform for upper-class banquet dining while semirecumbent. The Last Supper would have taken place on a *triclinium*, not at tables and chairs. During the so-called Dark Ages, furniture was uncommon, but reinvented during the Renaissance, first with simple three-legged stools, then chairs with backs, and finally in the 18th century with the refined works of Chippendale, Sheraton, and others. Furniture historians (Giedion 1948; Lucie-Smith 1990) consider the 18th century the apex of chair design for its aesthetic integration of physical comfort and cultural symbolism. Up until this point, chairs were relatively expensive handmade objects and therefore relatively rare compared to today, when industrial manufacturing has made them cheap and plentiful. With industrialization came the first spring coil upholstery, despised by Modernists who want to

see structure, not have it hidden by deep cushioning and fabric. Industrialization also made possible bent wood chairs, which Modernists like because the structure becomes the decoration. Giedion (1948) blamed the World Exposition of 1893 for the split between chairs as high art and the chairs for work settings that dominated most of the 20th century. Modernist chairs do not use ergonomic criteria, and no one would put an office chair in their living room or even in the lobby of their corporate headquarters. The 20th century was a time of artistic experimentation with new processes of assembly and new materials, like steel and plastic; however, aesthetically speaking, the body was left out of the picture. Yet dimensions for chair designs were standardized midcentury, and ergonomics with applications for seating emerged as a special field after World War II.

The economic shift to office work has meant that a larger and larger portion of the population sits in chairs. Before the days of repetitive strain injuries, the average work chair was not particularly ergonomic. That is, adjustable chairs were considered expensive, so most workers made do with the chair they were given. These chairs were possibly on wheels, but not likely to be scaled to a worker's physique. Computers and lawsuits have changed all that. Now companies do not think twice about investing in $1,000 (USD) chairs for their employees. Suddenly $1,000 seems cheap compared to the medical costs of rehabilitation caused by the anatomical and physiological problems associated with chair sitting.

Problems With Sitting in Chairs

To start, sitting is hard work; it puts 30% more pressure on the intervertebral discs than standing (Andersson 1980; 1981; 1985; Andersson, Ortengren, and Nachemson 1982; Andersson et al. 1974; "Sitting down on the job" 1981; Zacharkow 1988). It strains the spinal column, back muscles, lower back nerves, and diaphragm. Those who squat report less compression of the spine than Europeans who sit (Hettinger 1985) and lower rates of disc degeneration (Gross 1990).

A team of Swiss researchers were the first to show that sitting at video display terminals and full-time typing were associated with physical impairment of hands, arms, shoulders, and neck (Hunting, Laubli, and Grandjean 1981). Chairs are designed for a stable upright posture with legs at right angles to the torso. Holding still is a strain in itself; in particular the right-angle posture between the thighs and torso strains the pelvis and lumbar spine. Distortion of the diaphragm and intestines creates a variety of breathing and digestion problems. Sometimes people experience sciatic nerve pain down the legs, which is best relieved by standing, walking, or lying down, but not by sitting. Varicose veins occur in chair-sitting cultures, not commonly in cultures where people sit on the ground. Chair seats that are too high for a person press the muscles under the thighs, reducing circulation of blood and lymph (possibly a contributing cause to cellulite). Overly padded chairs also press on muscles, and give them a load-bearing function they cannot sustain; weight is best transferred down through bones. Sitting still means that one usually does not pump the ankles; as a result blood pools, impeding venous return. Eventually, pressure builds up to force the blood back up the veins with such a strong force as to damage the valves that keep blood from falling back down to the feet. This has been linked to deep vein thrombosis (Levine 2007).

If these biomechanical problems were not enough, research on the adverse metabolic consequences and premature mortality associated with too much sitting means the chair is virtually a coffin. Saunders (2011) commented in *Scientific American* on research studies with large samples around the world about correlations with the absolute number of hours seated and mortality from stroke, heart attack, and cancer. Others have argued that sitting can be more dangerous than smoking (Ravn 2013). The plethora of adverse health consequences from too much sitting is addressed in several other chapters in this book.

Chair Designers' Responses

Chair designers have chased physical problems through the body but have never been able to eliminate them completely. Solving one problem has created problems elsewhere.

Height

When we sit on chairs that are too tall, the musculature on the back of the thighs is pressed, and even gouges the popliteal region (sometimes referred to colloquially as the *knee pit*). If a tall person sits on a chair that is too short, (usually) the knees are positioned higher than the hip joints; the pelvis

tips backward, rounding the spine and losing the lumbar curve that allows all of us to sit upright. The global average height for women is 160 cm (5'3") and 175 cm (5'9") for men, so the average person could be said to be 168 cm (5'6". Most chair seats in the United States are 46 cm (18 in.) from the floor, which is too tall for most people who are 168 cm tall (in other words, for more than half of all adults). One of the earliest chair researchers, Akerblom, argued in 1948 that chair height should be lowered to 41 cm (16 in.), but his advice has been ignored, possibly because designers have been responding to the taller male rather than the shorter female part of the population.

Height was one of the basic adjustments in the evolution of chair design, because a good height for some is problematic for others. Making early office chairs adjustable was an advance, but eventually the furniture industry learned that few users bother to make adjustments, especially if they have to get out of the chair to make them. Consequently, levers that adjust height while the user is seated in the chair became the norm. Still, the industry observed that users do not often make adjustments, so height remained problematic. In response, some designers engineered chairs that adjust the relationship between seat and back automatically with the sitter's movements. Some have added footrests, including treadle-like ones that involve movement, to help shorten the distance to the floor for many in the office workforce. Despite these adaptations, each sitter personally has to attend to the issue of seat height. If the seat is too low, one's knees are higher than the hips, which tips the pelvis back and reverses the lumbar curve. More commonly, if the seat is too high, the musculature and blood vessels on the back of the thighs are compressed, which creates circulation problems.

At first, ergonomic chairs were not considered beautiful, but eventually designers tried to give the mechanisms of adjustability aesthetic properties. Ambasz and Piretti used accordion-like tubing that visually expressed the idea of adjustability in their Vertebra chair of 1976. The Aeron chair's mesh fabric largely accounts for its enormous market success; it fit in with the zeitgeist of the 1990s—spare, taut, sheer, black.

Seat Tilt

In order to stop the forward slide intrinsic to leaning back in a chair, some designers have canted the seat pan up in front. However, this runs the danger of increasing pressure on the underside of the thighs. Further, it reduces the angle between thigh and trunk to less than 90°, which rounds the lumbar spine even more than the right angle chair already does. In response some designers tilted the back backward to open the angle to greater than 90°, but this creates problems for the shape of the spine, neck, and head. Some designers favor a flat seat. Yet others, who have become aware of how the top of the pelvis rolls backward in the classic right-angle seated posture, choose to create a slight forward tilt to the seat pan. This runs the risk of making the sitter slide off the seat, so the angle cannot be very great (less than 10.5° for a slight person, possibly steeper for a heavier person) and the surface needs to provide enough friction to deter sliding forward. Using the legs to stop sliding forward can be a strain, or activating leg muscles could be a benefit if doing so stimulates the pancreas to produce the key enzyme lipase needed by the liver for fat metabolism. Activating leg muscles without straining them requires attention to the variation in human size and proportions, possibly different seat heights, and different degrees of seat tilt. Solving the problem of the retroverted pelvis and rounded lumbar spine by tilting the seat can create other problems.

Back

Designers pursue markedly different strategies regarding the height and shape of the chair back, and the amount of lumbar support it provides. Earlier ergonomics researchers (Grandjean 1980) observed that the right-angle seated posture tends to round the lower back, so they recommended lumbar support: a curve in the seat back that would mimic the shape of the spine's lumbar curve. They lamented that people do not often sit far enough back into a chair to make contact with the lumbar curve in the seat back. At first they recommended instructions but eventually came to recommend mechanisms that synchronize the movement of the seat and back. The right-angle seated posture is what rounds the lumbar spine, so opening the angle between the thigh and trunk is more efficient than trying to get people to push their lumbar curve back into shape mechanically with the chair's so-called lumbar support. In 1999, designers at Steelcase told me that what I was saying about the folly of lumbar support was correct, but that the market wasn't ready to give it up.

They said that people still expect lumbar support in a chair considered ergonomic.

Another problem with chair back design is that if the sitter brings his or her back all the way to the seat back, this posture pushes the large gluteus maximus muscles (buttocks) forward, further flattening the pelvis and lumbar spine. Hence, in the better designs the back does not meet the seat back; rather, they create space for the buttocks. Back support actually weakens the torso, which means that in the long run, most sitters would be better off on stools. However, if we do want back support, it would be best to maintain the balance between the lumbar and thoracic curves. Accordingly, some chair designers use only a bar or circle at the transition midback between the spine's concave and convex curves.

Arms

Little weight (4%) is transferred to the ground through arm support and few office tasks require arm support, so arm features have been optional in chair design. Sometimes chair arms get in the way of movement, especially in task chairs, but sometimes they contribute to the symbolism of comfort and ease, and can even serve as side tables for a drink. In office settings, the increase in carpal tunnel problems has directed attention to the support of hands and wrists more than arms and elbows. To move wrists into their most neutral position, some ergonomic specialists advocate reshaping the keyboard into two parts and lowering and slightly rotating both halves, which may require rethinking the issue of arm and elbow support.

Perch

Sitting on seats tall enough to create an obtuse angle between the thighs and trunk automatically preserves the lumbar curve, but few designers have been willing to think outside the right-angle paradigm until quite recently. Cranz (1998) termed this position the perch position; F.M. Alexander (1918) called it the position of mechanical advantage, and National Aeronautics and Space Administration (NASA) called it neutral body posture. This position requires raising the height of our work surfaces from 70 cm (27 in.) to closer to 90 cm (36 in.), which has met cultural resistance. Few customers have been willing to invest in new tables and desks, as well as new chairs. Manufacturers and retailers have not yet figured out how to get customers to change everything, demonstrating how conservative culture can be.

For this reason, Norwegian architect and furniture designer Peter Opsvik designed the Balans chair (known in the United States as the kneeling chair; see figure 4.1) to take advantage of the obtuse angle between the torso and thighs while lowering the body in space enough to slide under existing table and desktops. This meant folding the legs at the knees so that one kneels on pads. Kneeling can be stressful to knees, and losing proprioceptive feedback from the soles of the feet is not ideal. Opsvik went on to design chairs to support the perch posture, namely the Capisco, manufactured by HAG. The Danish surgeon A.C. Mandal designed school furniture for the perch position with an elevated forward-slanted work surface to bring the head and neck into a neutral rather than drooped position.

Footwear designer Martin Keen went on to design a moveable seat for the perch position with an appropriately raised forward-sloping work surface, called the Focal Upright, which was marketed in 2012 (see figure 4.2). This combination fulfills the criteria from my research and writing about chairs. Specifically, it allows people to keep their feet on the floor and their knees significantly lower than the hips; sit without their pelvis rolling backward; hold their spines upright while retaining both its lumbar and thoracic curves; keep their chests open; balance their heads actively on the top of their spines without moving the head back and down;

and see the work surface without having to bend the neck forward.

Lounge

The perch position, when rotated in space, turns into a lounge position (see figure 4.3). This changes the way gravity works on the spine and allows one to rest while still keeping the head and eyes upright enough to read, use a keyboard in front of a computer monitor, and maintain social contact with others . Cheap lounge chairs raise the torso, but support the legs extended out straight, rather than flexed, which is unfortunate because straight legs pull the pelvis backward and flatten the lumbar curve. The Corbusier and Perriand *chaise longue* (Corb lounge) of 1925 and contemporary folding deck chairs by Lafuma and Caravan Canopy both offer the support for flexed knees that make this position so comfortable. Even in a comparatively hard material like wood the lounge configuration is surprisingly comfortable, which I demonstrated in a chair of my own design. Opsvik designed the

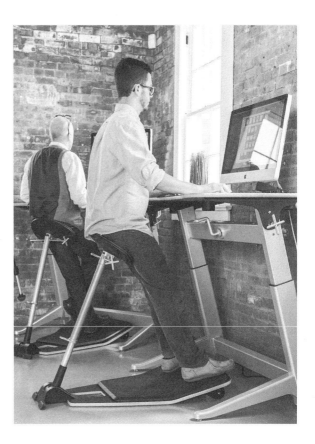

Figure 4.2 Focal Upright workstation.
Courtesy of Focal Upright.

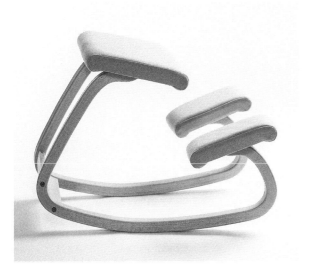

Figure 4.1 Balans chair by Peter Opsvik.
Courtesy of Peter Opsvik, designer; Tollefsen, photographer.

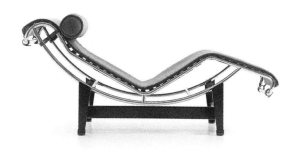

Figure 4.3 Optimal lounge chair design.
Courtesy of Haworth.

Gravity lounge chair manufactured by Stokke that has four positions: conventional right angle, kneeling, and lounging in two angles of recline. The only problem with the lounge position is that it distributes gravitational force so evenly through the entire skeleton that it may not stimulate bone formation, thereby leading to osteoporosis, but this negative possibility has not been measured.

Standing Workstations

Designers have created high stools and adjustable work surfaces for sit-to-stand workstations. Ten years ago, this was still a fringe option associated with the brilliant eccentricities of Churchill and Hemingway. Today the research on the adverse health outcomes of prolonged sitting has galvanized the thinking of designers and customers to consider stand-up workstations. When we stand, gravity loads the bones and activates the muscles that stimulate the pancreas to produce the key enzyme lipase, needed for the liver to process fat. Without lipase, undigested fats enter the bloodstream, thereby leading to premature mortality from causes including heart attack, stroke, and cancer. Standing solves the back problems of chair sitting, but it is tiring to the legs. There is no perfect posture. Humans are designed for movement, so changing postures is ideal.

Adjustability

Adjustability appears to be a transition between the search for the *right* posture, on the one hand, and the recognition that humans are designed for *ongoing* movement, on the other. Adjustability allows users to change the height of their chair or desk, the

relationship between depth of the seat and the chair back, and the position of the arms. In some cases, adjustability has also meant being able to change the location and shape of the lumbar curve in the seat back. Peter Opsvik (1997) has quipped, "The best posture is the next posture." Accordingly, his office chair, the Capisco by HAG, accommodates different postures and movements. The chair swivels and its seat goes up and down; the sitter's thighs are free to assume several different positions because the cutaways at the corners of the seat pan allow the thighs to fall away from the torso and bring the pelvis forward, creating a lumbar curve without requiring the sitter to lean back into a molded curve in the chair back. For conventional right-angle seating, Opsvik argued that conventional sitting could be improved through movement. Thus, his Flysit chair has springs at the bottom of the legs that invite rocking backward and forward, and the Actulum has a faceted rocker. He designed a table with cross bars on the legs so that sitters can reach out with their feet and push against the bars to activate the movement potential built into these two dining room and conference table chairs. The Focal Upright by Keen is also adjustable in the height of the seat, work surface, and degree of slant. The Finnish designer Vessi Jalkanen also has created active seating, the Salli chair-stool, with two separate seat pans—one for each pelvic half—that allow the pelvis to constantly make micro-movements. These solutions are the best to date because they challenge the ideal of sitting still.

Although production is limited, readers are directed to the designers' websites to view these designs:

▸ www.opsvik.no/works/industrial-design
▸ www.focaluprightfurniture.com
▸ www.salli.com

Continuous Motion

Because no single posture is perfect for any length of time, designing for movement is even more advanced than designing adjustable chairs. Several options have emerged recently. Activity balls (or physioballs) have been appropriated as seating by those who appreciate the advantages of needing to use the legs and fine spinal muscles to keep balance while working. June Ekman, a teacher of the Alexander Technique—a mind–body system focusing on posture and movement—and others have designed chairs around balls to stabilize them in order to reduce the amount of active balancing needed for the legs while still taking advantage of fine movement in the spine. The designer of the ErgoErgo thought activity balls were ugly and so created a more articulated and stylized form that still took advantage of the movement of a ball (see figure 4.4). The German Swopper has a rounded top in suede that promotes forward tilt of the pelvis but provides enough friction to stop slipping off the seat; the pedestal stem of the chair flexes side to side and front to back, and the height can be adjusted (see www. swopper.com). These options include movement, but the chair may be too demanding to those not used to using their legs or might seem too unusual for those who want a conventional look. The Pony by Haworth is a backless seat that one straddles; it rocks back and forth to allow continuous motion. Many people like this chair-stool because it makes sitting up straight easy, but some are not used to spreading their legs and using them actively. Over a decade ago, only an eccentric few might work at a computer while walking on a treadmill, but now that many have learned about the mortal dangers of sitting, the biggest U.S. office furniture provider, Steelcase, markets a treadmill workstation. Similarly, inexpensive bike racks can be used to convert commuting bicycles into desk chairs at raised desks. Thus, a bike formerly used to get to work serves as a machine for moving while working at a desk, thus fusing the ecology movement regarding transit at a city scale with the fitness movement at an individual scale.

Designing a slow-motion continuous-movement chair and table combination would be ideal, but this design has yet to be produced. Although Keen's Focal Upright may be the best product on the market to date, we are waiting to see a continuously moving, slow-motion desk and screen combination that *engages the feet* in a lounge position. In such a device, joints, muscles, and organs would have the simultaneous benefit of movement and rest, while legs and skeleton would have the benefit of gravitational loading to promote bone building.

Postural Education

Rather than redesign the chair, a different solution to the backaches and other problems associated with chair sitting is to educate the sitter. A century ago, the movement educator F.M. Alexander (1918, page 2) disparaged chair design in favor of education about how to use one's body:

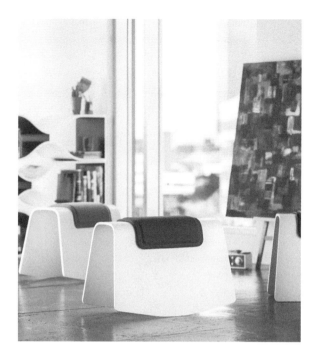

Figure 4.4 ErgoErgo chair design.
Courtesy of Haworth.

JOB REDESIGN

Equipment and furniture can be improved, but underlying the need for comfort and movement is the need to design the rhythm of the workday so that no one is expected to perform the same activity repeatedly for many hours. This becomes a question of managerial style and policy, not physical design. This in turn suggests that management should recognize that people's needs vary and that employees are the ultimate source of authority regarding their needs. Locating authority in the employee rather than a supervisor or boss may require a change in organizational culture.

"Let us waste no valuable time, thought or invention in designing furniture, when by a smaller expenditure of those three gifts we may train the child to win its own conscious control, and rise superior to any probable limitations imposed by ordinary school fittings."

His dismissal of the importance of design did not anticipate the increasing number of hours spent in chairs over the last century. In fact, people are hurt by sitting in chairs for as long as we do today. Nor could he appreciate the ensuing scholarship about the power of the silent language of design and the built world; because a designer's consciousness is communicated nonverbally, below the level of conscious awareness, it can be especially persuasive (Cranz 1998).

Alexander was correct that education is important. Today most movement and fitness systems pay attention to how to sit. Now instructors of the Alexander Technique (along with those who teach yoga, Gyrotonics and Gyrokinesis, and the Feldenkrais Method) teach people to sit directly on and over the sit bones (ischial tuberosities) instead of on either the tailbone (slumping the spine) or the pubic arch (arching the spine). Typically, movement education systems deliberately develop the student's awareness of the subtle differences between sitting on the back edge, middle, or front edge of the ischial tuberosities. Some difference of opinion about the use of the sit bones does exist. Many assume that one sits centered on the sit bones, but others differ. For example, some teachers of Eutony, a century-old system from Danish-German teacher Gerda Alexander, recommend sitting far forward all the way to the pubic ramus so that the top of the pelvis tilts forward and the lumbar curve is correspondingly arched. Similarly, today in Palo Alto, California, Jean Couch teaches modern sitters to model themselves after native people who sit with the top of their pelvis tipped forward and the sit bones pointing backward into the chair seat. In the same vein, Esther Gokhale teaches people to sit with a J-shaped spine, with the tail of the J going back into the chair seat and the spine stacking on top of that. The Swiss movement educator Benita Cantieni also advocates sending the sit bones back in order to keep the front of the torso upright. In these cases, the sit bones point backward as much as transfer weight downward, which may or may not be problematic. What is certain is that whether balanced on the centers of the sit bones or rocked further forward, all of these systems share the idea that being educated to use the body on any surface encountered is more efficient and important than the design of that surface.

Educating the body presumes that humans do not automatically know what feels best physically. We cannot always rely on our felt experience to show us what is best for us. Our nervous systems get used to inefficient movements and postures so that efficient ones do not always feel right at first. Alexander teachers call this distortion in perception "faulty sensory awareness" and Alexander himself called it "debauched kinesthesia" (Alexander 1923). There is a paradox here if we simultaneously affirm that people should have personal control over their work environment and also that people do not always sense what is physically most healthful.

Thus, the body is not an infallible touchstone from which to evaluate alternative environments. Instead of relying on unconscious habit or the illusion of pure sensation, we need a normative ideal rooted in anatomy and physiology. This ideal emerges from interplay among cognition, perception, and sensation. Hence, education is still needed. Design alone does not guarantee healthy sitting behavior.

Summary

We cannot design our way out of the problems associated with chair sitting by making better chairs. Admittedly, it is possible to improve chairs, and some chairs are emphatically better than others. Nevertheless, structural and consequently health strains are intrinsic to the right-angle seated posture. The cultural idealization and naturalization of this posture is a problem.

Further, being still is a deadly problem, no matter what posture we hold. A new seating paradigm that includes sitting, standing, perching, and lounging is preferable to the conventional right-angle seated posture. Even more desirable is rethinking workplace and job design to include movement. Such a change is likely to shift authority from external to internal, that is, from institution to individual. Reconceiving work routines will require education in sensory awareness. Physical redesign, public education, and new policies are all needed to address the problems associated with sedentary behavior.

KEY CONCEPTS

▸ **Adjustability:** The ability to change the ratios of elements of seats or work surfaces, either mechanically with cranks or pegs, or with motorized controls.

▸ **Continuous motion:** Changing angles between seat, back, and work surfaces so that the body has to follow and thereby gets exercise without thinking about exercise as a separate activity.

▸ **Ergonomic:** The study of how the human body interacts with the machines in the near environment, especially in work settings (hence, the literal meaning of *ergo* as work).

▸ **Job redesign:** Analyzing the postures needed to accomplish the work of an enterprise and distributing tasks throughout the workday so that no one holds the same posture all day.

▸ **Lounge:** A seat design that accommodates the human body in a semireclined position with an obtuse angle between the torso and thighs, with bent knees, and with head up high enough to read and have eye contact with others. The entire back reclines.

▸ **Perch:** Any seat design that accommodates the human body in a vertical position halfway between sitting and standing, with an obtuse angle between the torso and thighs. The spine is upright without back support, and weight is more evenly distributed between sit bones and feet than in right-angle sitting.

▸ **Postural education:** Learning about physiologically and anatomically beneficial postures and movements; for example, the Alexander Technique, Cantienica, Feldenkrais, GyroKinesis Pilates, tai chi, and yoga.

▸ **Right-angle chair:** The classical chair design with the body arranged so that the lower leg and thigh are at a right angle to one another and the torso is at a right angle to the thigh. About 60% of weight is transferred to the seat through the sit bones and another 40% is transferred to the feet.

▸ **Sit-to-stand workstations:** A work surface and seat support that adjust so a person can choose to sit in the right-angle position, or stand, or perch anywhere between the two extremes.

STUDY QUESTIONS

1. List the biomechanical and ergonomic problems of chair sitting.

2. What was the purpose of chairs in ancient history?

3. How have chair designers tried to solve the ergonomic problems?

4. How has each design solution produced another ergonomic problem?

5. How does each of the following solve the ergonomic problems of the right-angle chair: the lounge, the perch, sit-to-stand, adjustability, continuous movement, job redesign, and postural education.

CHAPTER 5

CHILDREN AND SCREEN TIME

Jorge A. Banda, PhD; and Thomas N. Robinson, MD, MPH

The reader will gain an overview of the effects of screen time exposure, including television, video game, and computer use, on child health. By the end of this chapter, the reader should be able to do the following:

- ▶ Describe U.S. children's screen media use
- ▶ Identify the effects of recent technological advances in personal media on children's screen media use
- ▶ Understand epidemiological research on screen time, obesity, and cardiometabolic health
- ▶ Discuss hypothesized mechanisms linking screen time to obesity and other cardiometabolic risk factors
- ▶ Better understand randomized controlled trials examining the effects of reducing screen time on obesity and health

The relationship between children's use of screen media, such as televisions, computers, and video games, and their health is complex. Screen media can have a positive influence on children's health by increasing knowledge and awareness of health information, fostering social connectedness, and teaching prosocial attitudes, such as empathy, tolerance, and respect toward others (Strasburger, Jordan, and Donnerstein 2010). However, screen media can also negatively affect children's health in terms of aggression, sexual behavior, substance use, consumerism, academic performance, obesity, and other health outcomes (Strasburger, Jordan, and Donnerstein 2010). The full potential of screen media to positively affect child and adolescent health has not been substantially realized; therefore, public health strategies have been primarily focused on limiting children's screen media use (Strasburger, Jordan, and Donnerstein 2010).

Screen Time Exposure

The American Academy of Pediatrics advises parents to limit children's total entertainment screen time to less than 2 hours per day, to discourage screen media exposure for children less than 2 years of age, and to avoid placing televisions and Internet-connected devices in children's bedrooms (Council on Communications and Media 2013). Healthy People 2020 highlights the importance of reducing screen time in children by setting objectives to increase the proportion of children and adolescents aged 2 to 18 years who

1. view television and videos or play video games for no more than 2 hours per day and

2. use a computer or play computer games outside of school (for non-school work) for no more than 2 hours per day (U.S. Department of Health and Human Services n.d.).

Despite these recommendations, average children in the United States spend more than a quarter of their waking lives, from age 2 to 18 years, watching screen media (Rideout 2015; Rideout, Foehr, and Roberts 2010; Robinson 2001).

In the 2013 Common Sense Media (CSM) Study, involving a nationally representative sample of parents of children aged 8 years and younger in the United States, young children spent an average of 1.85 hours per day viewing television content, using computers, and playing video games, accounting for 70% of total media exposure (Rideout 2013). In the 2015 Common Sense Census (CSC) Study, involving a nationally representative sample of 8- to 18-year-olds in the United States, 8- to 12-year-olds reported an average of 4.6 hours per day viewing screen media (accounting for 78% of total media exposure), while 13- to 18-year-olds reported an average of 6.67 hours per day viewing screen media (accounting for 75% of total media exposure) (Rideout 2015). In the 2015 CSC Study, media exposure included watching television, movies, and videos; playing video, computer, and mobile games; listening to music; using social media; reading; and using digital devices for entertainment purposes (e.g., browsing websites, video chatting, or creating digital art or music), while screen media exposure included time spent in visual media activities on screen devices, including watching television or videos, playing games, video chatting, searching the Internet, and reading or writing on a computer, tablet, or smartphone for entertainment purposes (does not include time spent listening to music through screen devices) (Rideout 2015).

Prevalence data demonstrate that racial/ethnic minority and low socioeconomic status children have more screen time than their white and high socioeconomic status counterparts. Data from the 2015 CSC Study sample found that white, black, and Hispanic 8- to 12-year-olds reported an average of 4.00, 6.37, and 5.30 hours per day viewing screen media, and that white, black, and Hispanic 13- to 18-year-olds reported an average of 6.30, 8.43, and 6.48 hours per day viewing screen media (Rideout 2015). Consistent with these results, data from the 2009 Kaiser Family Foundation (KFF) Study, involving a nationally representative sample of 8- to 18-year-olds in the United States, found that white, black, and Hispanic 8- to 18-year-olds spent an average of 5.82, 8.72, and 8.75 hours per day viewing television content, using computers, and playing video games (Rideout, Foehr, a nd Roberts 2010).

Data from the 2015 CSC Study sample found that 8- to 12-year-olds from families with lower, middle, and higher family incomes reported an average of 5.53, 4.53, and 3.77 hours per day viewing screen media, while 13- to 18-year-olds from families with lower, middle, and higher family incomes reported an average of 8.12, 6.52, and 5.70 hours per day viewing screen media (Rideout 2015). Data from the 2004 Youth Media Campaign Longitudinal (YMCL) Survey, involving a nationally representative sample of 9- to 15-year-olds in the United States, found the odds of exceeding 2 or more hours per day in screen time were significantly higher for children in households with annual incomes ≤ $25,000 than for children in households with annual incomes > $75,000 (Carlson et al. 2010). In addition, the odds of exceeding 2 or more hours per day in screen time were significantly higher for children with a household income of $25,001 to $50,000 and $50,001 to $75,000 than for children with a household income > $75,000 (Carlson et al. 2010). Similar results were found among 2- to 15-year-olds in the 2001-2006 NHANES, which showed that 51% of children from low- and middle-income households engaged in 2 or more hours per day of screen time compared to 43% of children from high-income households (Sisson et al. 2009).

Television

Television content is the largest source of media exposure among children aged 8 years and younger in the United States (followed by reading or being read to, listening to music, playing video games, and using computers), accounting for 55% of total media exposure and 78% of total screen media exposure among children (Rideout 2013). In the 2013 CSM Study sample, parents of children 8 years and younger reported their child spent an average of 1.45 hours per day viewing television content, which included programming viewed on a television set, On Demand programming, programming recorded and viewed at a later date, DVDs, television or videos viewed on a computer, television or videos viewed on mobile devices, and television or videos streamed (Rideout 2013).

Television content is also the largest source of media exposure among 8- to 12-year-old children (followed by playing video games, listening to music, and reading) and among 13- to 18-year-old children (followed by listening to music, playing video games, and using social media) in the United States (Rideout 2015). In the 2015 CSC Study, television content included programming viewed as broadcasted on a television set, programming recorded and later viewed on a television set (e.g., recorded on a DVR, viewed On Demand, streamed through a program such as Netflix), programming viewed online (e.g., downloaded or streamed to a computer, tablet, or smartphone), DVDs, and online videos (e.g., from websites such as YouTube) (Rideout 2015).

In the 2015 CSC Study sample (Rideout 2015), 8- to 12-year-olds reported an average of 2.43 hours per day viewing television content, accounting for 41% of total media exposure and 53% of total screen media exposure, while 13- to 18-year-olds reported an average of 2.63 hours per day viewing television content, accounting for 30% of total media exposure and 39% of total screen media exposure. It's important to note that these data represent the average hours per day of television content viewing among all children, including those who report viewing no television content. When examining television content use only among users (85% of 8- to 12-year-olds and 81% of 13- to 18-year-olds), 8- to 12-year-olds reported 2.85 hours per day viewing television content, and 13- to 18-year-olds reported 3.25 hours per day viewing television content.

These recent data also demonstrate that racial/ethnic minority and low socioeconomic status children view more television content than their white and high socioeconomic status counterparts. In 2015, black and Hispanic 8- to 12-year-olds viewed more television content (3.37 and 2.82 hr/day) than white 8- to 12 year-olds (2.08 hr/day), and black and Hispanic 13- to 18-year-olds viewed more television content (3.68 and 2.78 hr/day) than white 13- to 18-year-olds (2.37 hr/day). In addition, 8- to 12-year-olds from lower- and middle-income families viewed more television content (2.85 and 2.55 hr/day) than 8- to 12-year-olds from higher-income families (1.82 hr/day), and 13- to 18-year-olds from lower- and middle-income families viewed more television content (3.40 and 2.53 hr/day) than 13- to 18-year-olds from higher-income families (2.20 hr/day) (Rideout 2015).

A large level of background television among children in the United States (i.e., when children are in a room with a television that is turned on, but no one is watching) is indicative of the central role televisions play in families' lives. Data from a 2009 nationally representative sample of children aged 8 months through 8 years in the United States found that younger children were exposed to an average of 3.87 hours per day of background television (Lapierre, Piotrowski, and Linebarger 2012). In a case study that videotaped 10 subjects (8- to 10-year-olds watching television in their own homes) over 10 days, providing an objective measure of actual viewing and background viewing, children were not looking at the screen for a median of only 18% of the time they were in a room with the television on (Borzekowski and Robinson 1999).

In the 2015 CSC Study sample, 34% of 8- to 12-year-olds and 37% of 13- to 18-year-olds indicated the television was on all or most of the time in their home (Rideout 2015). Similar results were found in the 2009 KFF Study sample, with 45% of 8- to 18-year-olds indicating the television was on most of the time even if no one was watching, and another 34% indicated the television was on some of the time even if no one was watching. As expected, reported exposure to background television is associated with increased reported television viewing. In that same 2009 study, 8- to 18-year-olds reporting high amounts of background television also reported more time watching live television than children exposed to low amounts of background television (3.28 versus 1.70 hr/day) (Rideout, Foehr, and Roberts 2010).

Although television content accounts for the largest proportion of total screen media and total media, it is not listed as children's favorite media activity. Among 8- to 12-year-olds, 13% identified watching television as their favorite media activity, with playing video games (22%) and reading (16%) being more popular choices. Among 13- to 18-year-olds, 9% identified watching television as their favorite media activity, with listening to music (30%), playing video games (15%), reading (10%), and using social media (10%) being more popular choices. In addition, 61% and 45% of 8- to 12-year-olds and 13- to 18-year-olds, respectively, indicated they enjoyed watching television a lot, and 46% and 45% of 8- to 12-year-olds and 13- to 18-year-olds indicated they enjoyed watching online videos a lot (Rideout 2015).

Video Games

Video games are the second largest source of screen media among children aged 8 years and younger, accounting for 16% of total screen media exposure. In the 2013 CSM Study sample, children 8 years and younger spent an average of 0.30 hours per day playing video games, which included the amount of time spent playing on a console player connected to a television set, on a handheld gaming device, and on mobile devices, but not the amount of time spent playing computer games (Rideout 2013).

Although television viewing is a larger source of screen media among children in the United States, video game use accounts for 29% of total reported screen media exposure among 8- to 12-year-olds and 20% of total reported screen media exposure among 13- to 18-year-olds. In the 2015 CSC Study, video game use included the amount of time spent playing on a console video game player (e.g., Wii, Xbox, PlayStation), on a handheld device (e.g., Nintendo DS, Game Boy, LeapPad), on mobile devices, and on a computer (Rideout 2015).

In the 2015 CSC Study, 8- to 12-year-olds reported an average of 1.32 hours per day playing video games, while 13- to 18-year-olds reported an average of 1.35 hours per day playing video games. Again, it's important to note that these data represent the average hours per day playing video games across all children, including children who do not play video games. In 2015, 66% of 8- to 12-year-olds and 56% of 13- to 18-year-olds reported playing video games, and when examining video game use only among users, 8- to 12-year-old video game players reported an average of 2.00 hours per day playing video games and 13- to 18-year-old video game players reported 2.42 hours per day playing video games (Rideout 2015).

In 2015, boys reported more time playing video games than girls (1.67 versus 0.95 hr/day for 8- to 12-year-olds and 2.02 versus 0.65 hr/day for 13- to 18-year-olds). The association between time spent playing video games and race/ethnicity is less consistent, with results differing by age group. That same year, black and Hispanic 8- to 12-year-olds spent more time playing video games (1.43 and 1.38 hr/day) than white 8- to 12-year-olds (1.33 hr/day). In contrast, white 13- to 18-year-olds spent more time playing video games (1.45 hr/day) than black and Hispanic 13- to 18-year-olds (1.32 and 1.18 hr/day) (Rideout 2015).

Similar to television viewing, low socioeconomic status children reported spending more time playing video games than their higher socioeconomic status counterparts. In 2015, 8- to 12-year-olds from lower- and middle-income families spent more time playing video games (1.37 and 1.32 hr/day) than 8- to 12-year-olds from higher income families (1.28 hr/day). In addition, 13- to 18-year-olds from lower-income families spent more time playing video games (1.45 hr/day) than 13- to 18-year-olds from middle- and higher-income families (1.32 and 1.32 hr/day) (Rideout 2015).

Computers

Computer use is a smaller source of screen media than television viewing and video games among children aged 8 years and younger, accounting for

5% of total screen media exposure. In the 2013 CSM Study sample, parents of children 8 years and younger reported their child spent 0.10 hours per day using a computer, which included time spent using a computer for entertainment purposes, such as viewing photos or graphics, playing games, visiting social networking sites, and visiting other websites, but did not include time spent using a computer for educational purposes or to watch television or videos, listen to music, or to read (Rideout 2013).

In contrast to younger children, computer use is a large source of screen media among 8- to 18-year-olds. In the 2015 CSC Study, computer use accounted for 11% of total screen media exposure among 8- to 12-year-olds, with television sets (32%), tablets (20%), and smartphones (17%) accounting for more screen media exposure. However, computers accounted for 24% of total screen media exposure among 13- to 18-year-olds, behind only smartphones (40%) as a percentage of screen media exposure (Rideout 2015).

In the 2015 CSC Study, computer use included all time spent using a computer for non-homework purposes, including time playing computer games, watching online videos, watching television online, browsing websites, listening to music, using social media, making digital art or music, video chatting, writing, and reading. In these recent data, 8- to 12-year-olds reported an average of 0.52 hours per day using a computer, while 13- to 18-year-olds reported an average of 1.62 hours per day using a computer. However, when limited to the 22% of 8- to 12-year-olds and 38% of 13- to 18-year-olds who reported using computers at all, 8- to 12-year-old computer users reported an average 2.43 hours per day and 13- to 18-year-old computer users reported an average of 3.13 hours per day (Rideout 2015).

Playing computer games accounted for the largest proportion of computer use among 8- to 12-year-olds (35%) and 13- to 18-year-olds (20%), with social media accounting for 4% and 14% of computer use among 8- to 12-year-olds and 13- to 18-year-olds (Rideout 2015). These reports differ from prior studies of U.S. children, demonstrating changes in the way children interact with media. In the 2009 KFF Study, visiting social networking websites accounted for the largest proportion of computer use among 8- to 18-year-olds (25%), followed by playing games (19%), visiting video websites (16%), and instant messaging (11%) (Rideout, Foehr, and Roberts 2010). Additional changes in children's use of media devices are discussed later in this chapter.

In contrast to television viewing, prevalence data demonstrate that in 2015, white 8- to 12-year-olds reported more time using a computer (0.57 hr/day) than black and Hispanic 8- to 12-year-olds (0.40 and 0.45 hr/day). White 13- to 18-year-olds also reported more time using a computer (1.77 hr/day) than black and Hispanic 13- to 18-year-olds (1.20 and 1.30 hr/day). The relationship between socioeconomic status and computer use is more complex, however. In 2015, 8- to 12-year-olds from lower-income families reported about the same or more time using a computer (0.58 hr/day) as 8- to 12-year-olds from middle- and higher-income families (0.55 and 0.42 hr/day). However, 13- to 18-year-olds from higher-income families reported more time using a computer (1.73 hr/day) than 13- to 18-year-olds from middle- and lower-income families (1.58 and 1.57 hr/day) (Rideout 2015).

Social Media

Social media accounts for a large proportion of child screen media exposure, accounting for 6% among 8- to 12-year-olds and 18% among 13- to 18-year-olds (Rideout 2015). In the 2015 CSC Study, 8- to 12-year-olds reported an average of 0.27 hours per day of social media use, while 13- to 18-year-olds reported an average of 1.18 hours per day of social media use, which included time spent on social networking sites and mobile apps such as Facebook, Twitter, or Instagram (Rideout 2015). However, when limited to the 15% of 8- to 12-year-olds and 58% of 13- to 18-year-olds who report using social media, 8- to 12-year-old social media users report an average time of 1.72 hours per day and 13- to 18-year-old social media users report an average of 2.07 hours per day.

Similar to video game playing, large differences in social media use occur by gender. In 2015, 8- to 12-year-old girls spent more time using social media (0.43 hr/day) than 8- to 12-year-old boys (0.10 hr/day). Similarly, 13- to 18-year-old girls spent more time using social media (1.53 hr/day) than 13- to 18-year-old boys (0.87 hr/day). Racial/ethnic minority children also report using more social media than their white counterparts. In 2015, black 8- to 12-year-olds reported more time using social media (0.58 hr/day) than Hispanic and white 8- to 12-year-olds (0.40 and 0.13 hr/day), and black 13- to 18-year-olds reported more time using social media (1.72 hr/day) than Hispanic and white 13- to 18-year-olds (1.10 and 1.10 hr/day) (Rideout 2015).

Mobile Devices and Screen Time Changes

Large changes are occurring in the way children view television content and play video games. From 2011 to 2013, the percentage of children 8 years and younger using mobile devices increased substantially for viewing videos (20% versus 47%), watching television and movies (11% versus 38%), and playing video games (33% versus 63%) (Rideout 2013). Similar changes have occurred among older children.

Although television sets are still widely used to view screen media among children, interactive devices such as smartphones and tablets are also commonly used among children. Data from the 2015 CSC Study indicate that television sets account for the largest proportion of screen time among 8- to 12-year-olds (32%), followed by tablets (20%), smartphones (17%), and computers (11%). In contrast, smartphones account for the largest proportion of screen time among 13- to 18-year-olds (40%), followed by computers (24%), television sets (23%), and tablets (11%) (Rideout 2015).

In the KFF Study, live television programming (i.e., watching regularly scheduled programming on a television set) accounted for 80%, 81%, and 59% of 8- to 18-year-olds' television content in 1999, 2004, and 2009 (Rideout, Foehr, and Roberts 2010). However, live television programming still accounted for 50% of 13- to 18-year-olds' television content in the 2015 CSC Study (Rideout 2015). Although these data come from different nationally representative samples of U.S. children, they provide evidence that large shifts are occurring in the way children view television content.

Data from the KFF Study show that console players that connect to television sets accounted for 65% and 49% of video game use in 2004 and 2009 among 8- to 18-year-old children (Rideout, Foehr, and Roberts 2010). Data from the 2015 CSC Study indicate that these declines in console player use are continuing, since console players accounted for 36% of video game use among 8- to 12-year-olds and 39% of video game use among 13- to 18-year-olds (Rideout 2015). In line with these data, a greater proportion of video games are being played on mobile devices. Data from the 2010 KFF Study showed that cell phones accounted for 23% of video game use among 8- to 18-year-old children in 2009. Data from the 2015 CSC Study indicate that mobile devices accounted for 42% of video game use among 8- to 12-year-olds and 31% of video game use among 13- to 18-year-olds.

As more children gain access to computers and mobile devices, more content is made available for them, screen media become more interactive, and new technologies emerge; these trends are anticipated to continue. Therefore, it will be necessary to examine the effects these trends and new uses of screen media have on children's health. For example, some families have reported replacing Lego and similar building block toys with electronic building block games; one of these products has been downloaded more than 20 million times (Nunneley 2013). As more children move away from television sets, desktop computers, and video game console players toward mobile devices, there also may be changes in the contexts of screen viewing (i.e., what, when, where, how, and with whom they are viewing) that influence child health and development. These changes will need to be examined.

Parental Rules and the Home Environment

Survey data demonstrate that many parents take an active role in their children's media use by having conversations with them on the subject. In 2015, 84% of 8- to 12-year-olds and 66% of 13- to 18-year-olds reported that their parents had talked with them about the types of media they can use, and 72% of 8- to 12-year-olds and 53% of 13- to 18-year-olds reported their parents had talked with them about how long they can spend using media. Among children who said they often or sometimes view television, 78% of 8- to 12-year-olds and 58% of 13- to 18-year-olds reported their parents knew a lot about the television shows they watch (Rideout 2015).

Screen-Time Use Rules

Survey data demonstrate that only about half of children in the United States report that their families have screen viewing rules and that children are more likely to have rules limiting screen media content than screen time. In the 2009 KFF Study sample, 46% of 8- to 18-year-olds reported having rules about what they were allowed to watch on television, 52% about what they were allowed to do on a computer, and 30% about which video games they were allowed to play. In comparison, only 28%

had rules about how much time they could spend watching television, 36% about how much time they could spend using a computer, and 30% about how much time they could spend playing video games (Rideout, Foehr, and Roberts 2010).

Similar to screen time viewing, there is an association between race/ethnicity and socioeconomic status with screen viewing rules. White and high socioeconomic status children are more likely to report screen viewing rules than their racial/ethnic minority and low socioeconomic status counterparts. In the 2009 KFF Study sample, the proportion of white, black, and Hispanic 8- to 18-year-olds with screen viewing rules was 29%, 26%, and 26% for television; 37%, 34%, and 33% for computers; and 31%, 27%, and 28% for video games, respectively. In the 2004 KFF Study sample, the proportion of children with screen viewing rules from low, middle, and high parental education households was 9%, 15%, and 16% for television; 23%, 27%, and 32% for computers; and 22%, 19%, and 26% for video games, respectively (Roberts, Foehr, and Rideout 2005). A similar pattern but much higher rates of rules was found in the Neighborhood Impact on Kids (NIK) Study, a longitudinal, observational cohort of 6- to 11-year-olds in Washington and California, where 70% of children from low and middle parental education households had rules limiting television and video game use to less than 2 hours per day, compared to 76% of children from high parental education households (Tandon et al. 2012). One possible explanation for the difference in prevalence of rules between these two samples is that the KFF Study data are from child reports while the NIK data are from parent reports.

Evidence suggests that screen time rules are inversely associated with the amount of screen time reported by children. In the 2009 KFF Study sample, 8- to 18-year-olds who reported having some media use rules reported less total media exposure (2.87 hr/day less) than those with no media rules (Rideout, Foehr, and Roberts 2010). Similar results were found in the 2004 YMCL Survey (Carlson et al. 2010), where the odds of having more than 2 hours per day of screen time were significantly lower for children who "really agreed" their parents had rules limiting their television time than for children who "really disagreed." In addition, the odds of having more than 2 hours per day of screen time were significantly lower for children who "really agreed" their parents had rules limiting their video game time than for children who "really disagreed." These findings suggest that screen time rules may play an important role in limiting screen time viewing among children.

Media Environment

The media environment can also influence children's screen media exposure. Most children in the United States report being surrounded by a large number of media devices in their home. In addition, media devices have become more interactive in recent years, leading to large changes in children's media environment. Data from a nationally representative sample of parents of children 8 years and younger showed large increases from 2011 to 2013 in home ownership of smartphones (41% versus 63%), tablets (8% versus 40%), and iPods or similar devices (21% versus 27%) (Rideout 2013).

Data from a nationally representative sample of 8- to 12-year-olds in 2015 showed home ownership was high for television sets (94%), video game consoles (81%), tablets (80%), smartphones (79%), laptop computers (73%), desktop computers (56%), and portable game players (53%). Similar results were found for 13- to 18-year-olds, where home ownership was also high for television sets (95%), smartphones (84%), video game consoles (83%), laptop computers (77%), tablets (73%), desktop computers (63%), and portable game players (45%) (Rideout 2015).

Data from separate sets of nationally representative samples indicate that personal ownership of smartphones and tablets have increased in recent years. Survey data from 12- to 17-year-olds in 2012 showed that 37% owned a smartphone and 23% owned a tablet computer (Madden et al. 2013). However, survey data from 8- to 12-year-olds in 2015 showed that 24% owned a smartphone and 53% owned a tablet, and that 67% of 13- to 18-year-olds owned a smartphone and 37% owned a tablet (Rideout 2015). These ownership data are in line with prevalence data demonstrating children's increased use of mobile devices to view screen media (Rideout 2015; Rideout, Foehr, and Roberts 2010).

The 2013 CSM Study found that 36% of children age 8 years and younger had a television in their bedroom (Rideout 2013). In addition, the 2015 CSC Study found that 47% of 8- to 12-year-olds and 57% of 13- to 18-year-olds had a television in their bedroom (Rideout 2015). These rates are dramatically counter to the American Academy of Pediatrics recommendation to avoid placing televisions and

Internet-connected devices in children's bedrooms (Council on Communications and Media 2011).

Similar to screen time viewing and screen viewing rules, the presence of a television in the bedroom is associated with race/ethnicity and socioeconomic status. Data from the 2013 CSM Study sample found that among children 8 years and younger, the proportion of white, black, and Hispanic children with a television in their bedroom was 28%, 61%, and 50%, and the proportion from high, middle, and low parental education households with a television in their bedrooms was 16%, 46%, and 56% (Rideout 2013). Data from the 2015 CSC Study found that among 8- to 12-year-olds, the proportion of white, black, and Hispanic children with a television in their bedroom was 37%, 77%, and 59%, and the proportion of white, black, and Hispanic 13- to 18-year-olds with a television in their bedroom was 54%, 76%, and 58%. In addition, the proportion of 8- to 12-year-olds from higher-, middle-, and lower-income families with a television in their bedroom was 29%, 47%, and 66%, and the proportion of 13- to 18-year-olds from higher-, middle-, and lower-income families with a television in their bedroom was 46%, 57%, and 69% (Rideout 2015).

As expected, having a television in the bedroom is associated with increased screen time among children. In the 2009 KFF Study sample, 8- to 18-year-olds with a television in their bedroom spent more time watching live television than children without a television in their bedroom (2.97 versus 1.90 hr/day) (Rideout, Foehr, and Roberts 2010). Similar results were found in the 2007 National Survey of Children's Health (Sisson and Broyles 2012) and in a large epidemiological study of 4- to 8-year-olds in the Netherlands (de Jong et al. 2013). These findings are consistent with the suggestion that children with greater environmental access to media devices will spend more time using them.

Screen Time and Body Weight

The relationship between screen media exposure and obesity is one of the most studied areas of media and health research. Epidemiological studies have generally observed positive associations between screen time and obesity (Chaput, Klingenberg, et al. 2011; Council on Communications and Media 2011). For example, a 4-year longitudinal cohort study of a nationally representative sample of 10- to 15-year-olds in the United States observed a strong dose–response relationship between the number of hours per day children viewed television and the prevalence of overweight; the odds of being overweight were significantly higher for children who viewed television for more than 5 hours per day than for children who viewed television for 2 or less hours per day. In addition, estimates of attributable risk demonstrated that 60% or more of the overweight incidence observed in this study sample was potentially linked to excess television viewing (Gortmaker et al. 1996). Similar results were found in a study using pooled data from four population-based German studies of 3- to 18-year-olds, where less than 1 hour per day of television and computer screen time was associated with an 11% lower prevalence of overweight in the study sample (Plachta-Danielzik et al. 2012).

Long-term cohort studies have also demonstrated that increased television viewing during childhood is a significant predictor of overweight and obesity in adulthood. Data from the 1970 British Birth Cohort Study found that greater total hours per day of weekend television viewing at 5 years of age predicted higher body mass index (BMI) at 30 years of age. In addition, each additional hour of television viewed on weekends at 5 years of age was associated with a 7% increased risk of obesity at 30 years of age (Viner and Cole 2005). Similar results were found in a longitudinal birth cohort study of New Zealand children, where greater hours per day of weekday television viewing between 5 and 15 years of age predicted higher BMI at 26 years of age. Estimates of attributable risk in this study indicated that up to 17% of the overweight prevalence observed at 26 years of age was potentially linked to viewing television for more than 2 hours per day on weekdays during childhood and adolescence (Hancox, Milne, and Poulton 2004).

In contrast to the television viewing research literature, the research examining associations between computer use and video game playing with overweight and obesity is more limited, and has produced inconsistent results. However, observational studies indicate there may be a direct association between computer use (Russ et al. 2009) or video game playing (Chaput, Klingenberg, et al. 2011) with overweight and obesity. It is likely this research has been hampered by limitations in accurately measuring computer and video game use. As a result, improving the measurement of screen media use in children will be important for understanding

MECHANISMS LINKING SCREEN TIME AND OBESITY AND OTHER CARDIOMETABOLIC RISKS

Five mechanisms have been hypothesized to explain screen media viewing's contribution to obesity and other cardiometabolic risk factors (Council on Communications and Media 2011; Robinson 2001):

1. Screen media viewing decreases metabolic rate.

2. Screen media viewing displaces sleep or disturbs sleep patterns.

3. Screen media viewing displaces physical activity, resulting in reduced energy expenditure.

4. Dietary energy intake increases and dietary quality decreases during screen media viewing.

5. Dietary energy intake increases and dietary practices worsen in response to advertising.

Although all of these mechanisms may be playing at least some role in the development of obesity and other cardiometabolic risk factors, limited evidence exists for the first three mechanisms. To date, the bulk of epidemiological and experimental studies are providing the greatest support for the fourth and fifth mechanisms.

whether computer and video game use influence overweight and obesity and child health.

Screen Time and Cardiometabolic Risk Factors

In addition to the relationships with overweight and obesity, there is mounting evidence that screen time is associated with other cardiometabolic risk factors such as hypertension, high cholesterol levels, insulin resistance and type 2 diabetes mellitus, and metabolic syndrome (Council on Communications and Media 2011). A study of 6- to 19-year-olds in the 2003-2004 and 2005-2006 NHANES found that the odds of having a higher cardiometabolic risk score (calculated from waist circumference, resting systolic blood pressure, non-high-density lipoprotein cholesterol, and C-reactive protein) were significantly higher for children who viewed 4 or more hours per day of television than for children who viewed less than 1 hour per day, adjusting for demographic characteristics, smoking, total calories from fat, total calories from saturated fat, dietary cholesterol intake, sodium intake, and physical activity (Carson and Janssen 2011). Similar results were found in a population-based sample of Portuguese 2- to 12-year-olds in the 2009 and 2010 Portuguese Prevalence Study of Obesity in Childhood, which found that higher television viewing time was significantly associated with an unfavorable cardiometabolic risk score (calculated from resting heart rate, resting diastolic blood pressure, resting systolic blood pressure, BMI, and skinfold thickness), adjusting

for age, gender, parental education, parental BMI, perceptions of crime in the area, sleep duration, birth weight, duration of breastfeeding, a "bad diet" score, number of fruit portions eaten per week, and physical activity. This study also found significant positive associations between television viewing and resting systolic blood pressure and resting diastolic blood pressure (Stamatakis et al. 2013). In addition, a cross-sectional study of overweight and obese 14- to 18-year-olds found a significant positive association between television viewing and fasting insulin and HOMA-IR (indicators of insulin resistance), adjusting for demographic characteristics, waist-to-hip ratio, total caloric intake, percent of caloric intake from carbohydrate, and physical activity (Goldfield et al. 2013).

Although more limited than the television viewing research literature, studies provide some evidence for associations between computer use and video game playing with cardiometabolic risk factors. A cross-sectional study of overweight and obese 12- to 18-year-olds found a significant positive association between computer use and total cholesterol and low-density-lipoprotein cholesterol, adjusting for age, gender, pubertal stage, race/ethnicity, and physical activity (Altenburg et al. 2012). Another cross-sectional study of overweight and obese 14- to 18-year-olds found a significant positive association between video game playing and systolic blood pressure and ratio of total cholesterol to high-density lipoprotein, adjusting for demographic characteristics, BMI, sexual maturity, total caloric intake, percent of caloric intake from dietary fat, and physical activity (Goldfield et al. 2011).

Screen Time, Physical Activity, and Cardiorespiratory Fitness

The research literature examining the effects of screen media viewing on physical activity has been inconsistent, with many observational studies showing that greater screen time is associated with less physical activity, and many others finding no relationship between screen time and physical activity (Council on Communications and Media 2011). Because the research literature consists primarily of observational studies, and only experimental studies can establish a causal relationship between screen time viewing and physical activity, more experimental studies are needed to better understand the effects of screen time viewing on physical activity.

Results from experimental studies provide limited evidence that decreasing screen time results in increased physical activity. For example, Epstein and colleagues (2005b) examined how experimental changes in screen media viewing (i.e., watching television or videos, playing video games, and using a computer recreationally) might influence physical activity. In a crossover design with three 3-week phases (baseline, increasing screen media viewing by 25%-50%, and decreasing screen media viewing by 25%-50%) among 8- to 16-year-olds, there was a significant decrease in accelerometer-measured physical activity when screen media viewing was increased, but no significant change in accelerometer-measured physical activity when screen media viewing was decreased. Further, children with a greater BMI were more likely to decrease physical activity when screen media viewing increased.

Results from screen-time-reduction interventions also provide limited evidence that decreasing screen time results in increased physical activity. For example, a school-based randomized controlled trial among third and fourth grade children found that although treatment participants significantly reduced their self-reported television viewing and computer use compared to control participants, there was no significant difference between treatment and control participants for changes in self-reported moderate- to vigorous-intensity physical activity (Robinson 1999). Similar results were found in a separate randomized controlled trial of 4- to 7-year-olds and their families; although treatment participants significantly reduced their self-reported television viewing and computer use compared to control participants, there was no significant difference between treatment and control participants for changes in accelerometer-measured physical activity (assessed as mean counts per min) (Epstein et al. 2008).

In contrast to these findings, some studies have indicated that screen time viewing is negatively associated with cardiorespiratory fitness independent of physical activity. The United Kingdom's East of England Healthy Hearts Study, a cross-sectional school-based study of 10- to 16-year-olds, found that the odds of being physically fit (based on age- and gender-specific cut points for the 20 m shuttle run) were significantly lower for children who had more than 4 hours per day of screen time than for children who had less than 2 hours per day, adjusting for age, gender, socioeconomic status, race/ethnicity, BMI, and physical activity (Sandercock and Ogunleye 2013). Further, a longitudinal study using a subsample of children from the East of England Healthy Hearts Study (mean baseline age = 11.5 years) found that the odds of becoming physically unfit at a 2-year follow-up were significantly higher for children who had 2 or more hours per day of screen time than for children who had less than 2 hours per day (Aggio et al. 2012). Similar results were found in a longitudinal sample from the HEALTHY Study, a cluster randomized controlled trial of middle schools in the United States, where there was a significant negative association between screen time and cardiorespiratory fitness (measured with the 20 m shuttle run test) from ages 11 to 13 years, adjusting for household education, child BMI, and physical activity (Mitchell, Pate, and Blair 2012). These results are important because they suggest that the relationship between screen media viewing and cardiorespiratory fitness may be independent of any changes in physical activity. However, experimental studies are needed to determine whether causal relationships exist.

Screen Time and Dietary Habits

Epidemiological studies have found that increased screen media viewing in children is associated with worse dietary habits, including less fruit and vegetable consumption and greater consumption of energy-dense snacks, energy-dense drinks, fast food, and total energy intake (Pearson and Biddle 2011). A cross-sectional study using 2003-2006 NHANES data found that compared to viewing television for 4 or more hours per day, viewing television for less than 1 hour per day was significantly associated with a healthier diet (i.e., higher Healthy Eating Index 2005) among 2- to 5-year-old, 6- to 11-year-old, and 12- to 18-year-old children, adjusting for demographic characteristics, BMI, physical activity, and total energy intake (Sisson et al. 2012). Similarly, a study using data from the 2009 Health Behavior in School-Aged Children Study (Lipsky and Iannotti 2012), a nationally representative sample of children in the 5th through 10th grades in the United States, found that television viewing was significantly negatively associated with daily fruit consumption and significantly positively associated with daily consumption of candy and chocolate, soft drinks with sugar, and fast food, adjusting for demographic characteristics, computer use, physical activity, and family affluence. In addition, computer use was significantly positively associated with daily consumption of candy and chocolate, soft drinks with sugar, and fast food, adjusting for demographic characteristics, television use, physical activity, and family affluence.

A prospective observational study of children (mean age = 11.7 years) living in Massachusetts found that a 1-hour increase in television viewing was significantly associated with an average 106 kcal per day increase in total energy intake, adjusting for demographic characteristics, BMI, and change variables for other behaviors (i.e., reading or doing homework, playing video and computer games, and doing physical activity) (Sonneville and Gortmaker 2008). Further, a 1-hour increase in video and computer game playing was significantly associated with an average 92 kcal per day increase in total energy intake, adjusting for demographic characteristics, BMI, and change variables for other behaviors (i.e., reading or doing homework, watching television, and doing physical activity). A longitudinal study of Norwegian 11- to 13-year-olds in the Health in Adolescents intervention study also found that changes in television and DVD use over 20 months was significantly negatively associated with changes in vegetable consumption and significantly positively associated with changes in consumption of soft drinks with sugar and unhealthy snacks. In addition, changes in computer and game use over 20 months were significantly negatively associated with changes in fruit and vegetable consumption and significantly positively associated with changes in consumption of soft drinks with sugar and unhealthy snacks (Gebremariam et al. 2013).

Experimental research has demonstrated increased energy intake in response to screen media use. For example, in a randomized crossover design study of healthy normal-weight adolescents (mean age = 16.7 years), ad libitum energy intake after 1 hour of video game playing was an average of 80 kcals greater than ad libitum energy intake after 1 hour of rest (Chaput, Visby, et al. 2011). Importantly, the increased food intake with video game playing was observed without increased sensations of hunger and was not compensated for during the rest of the day (Chaput, Visby, et al. 2011). In a crossover design with three 3-week phases (baseline, increasing screen media viewing by 25–50%, and decreasing screen media viewing by 25–50%) among 8- to 12-year-olds, there was a significant 281 kcal per day decrease in caloric intake when screen media viewing was decreased, but no significant change in energy intake when screen media viewing was increased (Epstein et al. 2002). Similar results were found in a separate crossover design with three 3-week phases (baseline, increasing screen media viewing by 25–50%, and decreasing screen media viewing by 25–50%) among 12- to 16-year-olds, where there was a significant 463 kcal per day decrease in energy intake when screen media viewing was decreased, but no significant change in energy intake when targeted screen media viewing was increased (Epstein et al. 2005a).

Screen-time-reduction interventions have also shown reductions in energy intake in response to reductions in screen time. A randomized controlled trial of screen time reduction among 4- to 7-year-olds and their families found that treatment participants significantly reduced their self-reported television viewing and computer use and their self-reported energy intake compared to control participants (Epstein et al. 2008). Results from these epidemiological and experimental studies demonstrate that decreasing screen viewing time can reduce dietary energy intake and can be an important component of obesity prevention interventions (Epstein et al. 2005a).

Eating While Viewing

One of the ways that screen media use may lead to increased energy consumption and poor nutrition is from eating while viewing. Research demonstrates that children consume a large proportion of their daily calories and meals while watching screen media. For example, an ethnically diverse sample of third grade children and a predominately Latino sample of fifth grade children in California consumed 18% and 26% of their total daily calories while watching television on weekday and weekend days, respectively, and consumed 18% to 23% and 37% to 51% of breakfast meals, 36% to 45% and 31% to 34% of dinner meals, and 59% to 67% and 39% to 45% of snacks while watching television on weekdays and weekends (Matheson, Killen, et al. 2004). Similarly, 8- to 10-year-old African American girls in the Girls Health Enrichment Multisite Studies in four cities across the United States consumed 27% to 35% of their total daily calories while watching television and consumed 19% to 46% of breakfast meals, 40% to 50% of dinner meals, and 22% to 44% of snacks while watching television (Matheson, Wang, et al. 2004).

Some excessive eating during viewing may simply be due to the large amount of time spent in screen media viewing and the types of foods and beverages that are easier to consume while viewing. In addition, there is a building body of evidence that screen media viewing may have specific effects in increasing energy consumption, with several different mechanisms having been proposed. Screen media viewing may trigger eating independent of hunger (e.g., prompting eating by the association of television viewing with eating), extend the duration of eating (e.g., eating until the television show is done or the game is over), or obscure self-monitoring of eating and awareness of satiety cues (Wansink 2004). Watching screen media may also impair the development of satiety by interfering with the habituation of gustatory and olfactory cues and may shift attention away from processing food and satiety cues, slow the rate of habituation of food cues, and lead to additional eating after habituation has occurred (Epstein et al. 1997; Temple et al. 2007). Evidence also exists that eating may be more susceptible to distraction among obese than normal-weight people (Rodin 1974), leading to greater overconsumption of calories while watching television or other screen media.

Food Advertising to Children

Food advertising is the other factor thought to explain increased energy consumption and poor dietary practices due to screen media viewing. The Federal Trade Commission reported that in 2009, $9.65 billion was spent marketing food in the United States. Of this spending, $1.79 billion was spent

marketing to 2- to 17-year-olds, with quick service restaurant food and carbonated beverage marketing accounting for $1.10 billion of spending in children. Television marketing accounted for the largest proportion of spending on advertising to children in 2009 (35%) (Leibowitz et al. 2012). Nielsen data demonstrated that in 2011, 2- to 11-year-olds and 12- to 17-year-olds viewed an average of 13.1 and 16.5 food, beverage, and restaurant advertisements per day on television, respectively (Dembek, Harris, and Schwartz 2014).

The Federal Trade Commission reported that food marketing to children on new media (e.g., mobile, online, viral marketing) accounted for 7% of total food marketing spending to children in 2009, an increase of 50% from 2006 (Leibowitz et al. 2012). As noted previously, children are moving away from traditional screen devices (e.g., television sets and video game consoles) toward mobile devices and online viewing. Unfortunately, little is known about the effects of Internet (Blades, Oates, and Li 2013) and mobile advertising on children. As a result, examining the effects of advertising on these media on child health will be important as more children increase their use of mobile devices and consumption of online content.

Data from the 2002 Panel Survey of Income Dynamics, a longitudinal study of 7- to 13-year-olds in the United States, found that viewing television with in-program advertisements was significantly positively associated with BMI z-scores, adjusting for demographic characteristics, mother BMI, and average sleep duration (Zimmerman and Bell 2010). In contrast, viewing television without in-program commercials was not associated with BMI z-scores (Zimmerman and Bell 2010).

The most convincing evidence that advertising has a large effect on children's eating behaviors and food preferences comes from experimental studies. For example, a randomized controlled trial among 7- to 11-year-olds demonstrates the power of food advertising to prime automatic eating behaviors (Harris, Bargh, and Brownell 2009). Children were randomly assigned to view either a 14-minute cartoon embedded with four 30-second food commercials or a 14-minute cartoon embedded with four 30-second non-food commercials. Children in both conditions were presented with a large bowl of cheddar cheese goldfish crackers and a glass of water, which were not advertised to either group, and were told they could have a snack while watching. The results showed that children randomly assigned to the food commercial group consumed 45% more crackers than children who saw the same cartoon without food commercials.

Another randomized controlled trial among 2- to 6-year-olds demonstrates that even a single exposure to food commercials can influence children's food preferences (Borzekowski and Robinson 2001). Children were randomly assigned to view either two 13-minute animated programs embedded with a 2.5-minute education segment on sea creatures between the programs or two 13-minute animated programs embedded with 10- to 30-second food commercials between the programs and at the end of the programs. After viewing the animated programs, children were asked to pick from nine pairs of photos of similar looking brands, matched for packaging color, shape, and content, and state which product they would like (i.e., prefer). The results show that children exposed to food commercials were significantly more likely to choose the advertised food items than children who saw the same program without commercials.

Finally, an experimental trial among 3- to 5-year-olds demonstrated that branding alone can strongly influence young children's actual taste perceptions, even beyond their preferences. Children were asked to taste five randomly ordered, side-by-side pairs of identical foods and beverages with McDonald's packaging and matched but unbranded packaging. Children were then asked to indicate whether the foods tasted the same or whether one tasted better. The children significantly preferred the taste of foods and drinks if they thought they were from McDonald's, and effects of branding were significantly greater among children with more television sets in their homes (Robinson et al. 2007).

Experimental Studies of Reducing Screen Time

Only experimental studies can establish causal relationships between screen media viewing and health. With the average child's screen media exposure currently at such high levels, the question of greatest practical and public health policy significance is not whether increased screen media use will harm health, but whether reducing screen media exposure will lead to health and developmental benefits (Robinson 1999). There have now been a number of experimental trials of reducing children's screen time that start to answer this question.

The first to address screen time exclusively was a 7-month, school-based, randomized controlled trial among third and fourth grade children from two schools in San Jose, California (Robinson 1999). Schools were randomized to either an assessment-only control group or to a treatment condition consisting of an 18-lesson screen time reduction curriculum delivered by the regular classroom teachers. The lessons included a television turnoff that challenged children to not watch television or videotapes or play video games for 10 days. Classroom activities focused on topics such as self-monitoring television, videotape, and video game use to motivate children to reduce time spent in these activities; teaching children to become "intelligent viewers" by using their viewing and video game time selectively; and enlisting children as advocates for reducing media use. In addition, families received an electronic television time manager to assist with screen-time budgeting and instructional newsletters to assist them in helping their children stay within their viewing time budgets and promote strategies for limiting television, videotape, and video game use for the entire family. Over the 7 months of the trial, participants randomized into the treatment condition significantly reduced their self-reported television viewing, video game use, and number of meals eaten in front of the television and significantly slowed their gain in BMI, triceps skinfold thickness, waist circumference, and waist-to-hip ratio compared to controls. Additional analysis found that, compared to control participants, participants randomized into the treatment condition also significantly decreased their aggressive behaviors (Robinson, Wilde, et al. 2001) and their consumeristic behaviors (Robinson, Saphir, et al. 2001).

The longest screen-time-reduction study to date was a 2-year randomized controlled trial among 70 4- to 7-year-olds and their families (Epstein et al. 2008). Participants were randomized to either a control group, where they received parenting newsletters but were allowed free access to television and computers, or to a treatment condition that involved installing an electronic television time manager to each television and computer monitor in the participant's home. The treatment consisted of study staff setting weekly time budgets for television viewing, computer use, and associated sedentary behaviors. The budget was reduced by 10% of its baseline viewing level once a month until it was reduced to 50% of the baseline level. In addition, parents were instructed to praise their child for reducing television viewing and engaging in alternative behaviors. Decreases in screen time were reinforced with the use of a star chart, in which participants were praised by study staff during home visits on the number of stars they had earned. Once participants reached a 50% decrease in screen time, the star chart was discontinued and changes in screen time were supported through tailored monthly newsletters and parental praise. Compared to control participants, participants randomized to the treatment group had significant decreases in television viewing and computer use, BMI z-score, and caloric intake that persisted for 2 years. Mediational analysis suggested that the effects on BMI were associated with reductions in dietary intake rather than increased physical activity.

Together, these and other experimental studies of reducing screen time as part of multiple-component interventions (Epstein et al. 2005b; Gortmaker et al. 1999) demonstrate the causal relationship between screen media viewing and weight gain and show that reducing screen time results in significant reductions in BMI gain in children. There is great promise in applying this experimental model to test the effects of reduced screen time on other risk factors and outcomes, overcoming the many limitations of observational studies.

Summary

National survey data demonstrate that children in the United States spend a large portion of their lives using screen media—an average of more than 7 hours per day viewing television content, using computers, and playing video games among 8- to 18-year-old children. These data also indicate that racial/ethnic minority and lower socioeconomic status children spend disproportionately more time viewing screen media. Screen time has been identified as one of the most modifiable causes of obesity and other cardiometabolic risk factors in children. The American Academy of Pediatrics advises parents to limit total entertainment screen time to less than 2 hours per day, discourage screen media exposure for children less than 2 years of age, and avoid placing televisions and Internet-connected devices in children's bedrooms. Despite these recommendations, only about half of children in the United States report having time use rules for screen time, and the vast majority have televisions in their bedrooms.

Evidence from epidemiological studies and experimental trials indicates that screen media viewing contributes to obesity and other cardiometabolic risks. The mechanisms appear to be primarily through increased dietary energy intake and poor dietary practices during screen time viewing and in response to food advertising. Novel randomized controlled trials have been successful in reducing screen time and BMI gain in children. Additional experimental trials are needed to test the effects of reducing screen media viewing on other child health characteristics.

An important area of uncertainty is the effects of newer and often more interactive forms of screen media use, including online viewing, mobile phones, tablet computers, and handheld video games. National survey data demonstrate that large changes are occurring in the way children use media, shifting from more traditional passive viewing (e.g., television sets, video game console players) toward interactive and mobile devices. The effects of these new types of screen media use on child health are still unknown, and should be prioritized in future research. In addition, the potential of using screen media, new and old, to promote positive benefits to children's health and behaviors has been mostly unrealized to date and may represent an important opportunity.

KEY CONCEPTS

▸ **American Academy of Pediatrics Recommendations:** The American Academy of Pediatrics advises parents to limit children's total entertainment screen time to less than 2 hours per day, discourage screen media exposure for children less than 2 years of age, and avoid placing televisions and Internet-connected devices in children's bedrooms.

▸ **Healthy People 2020 Screen Time Objectives:** To increase the proportion of children and adolescents aged 2 to 18 years who view television and videos or play video games for no more than 2 hours per day and use a computer or play computer games outside of school (for nonschool work) for no more than 2 hours per day.

▸ **Media exposure:** Commonly described as time spent watching television, movies, and videos; playing video, computer, or mobile games; listening to music; using social media; reading; and using digital devices for entertainment purposes (e.g., browsing websites, video chatting, or creating digital art or music).

▸ **Screen media exposure:** Commonly described as time spent in visual media activities on screen devices, including watching television or videos, playing games, video chatting, searching the Internet, and reading or writing on a computer, tablet, or smartphone for entertainment purposes (does not include time spent listening to music through screen devices).

STUDY QUESTIONS

1. Describe positive and negative effects of screen media on child health.

2. State the American Academy of Pediatrics' three screen time exposure recommendations.

3. State the largest source of media exposure among children.

4. Explain why age 13 appears to be a pivotal age for greater reported screen media use.

5. Discuss changes taking place in the way children view and interact with screen media.

6. Explain how parental screen media rules may play an important role in limiting screen time viewing among children.

7. Discuss limitations affecting the understanding of the relationship between computer use and video games with child health, and how these limitations can be addressed in future research.

8. State five mechanisms hypothesized to explain screen media viewing's contribution to obesity and other cardiometabolic risk factors.

9. State a hypothesized mechanism explaining how screen media viewing may have specific effects on children's increased energy consumption.

10. Explain how food advertisements prime automatic eating behaviors and influence children's food preferences and how branding influences children's taste perceptions.

This work was supported in part by U.S. Public Health Service grant number T32 HL007034 (Banda) and grant numbers RO1 HL096015 and UO1 HL103629 (Robinson) from the National Heart, Lung, and Blood Institute, National Institutes of Health, and the Child Health Research Institute at Stanford University (Robinson).

CHAPTER 6

REGULATED SEDENTARY BEHAVIOR IN OCCUPATIONS

Kenneth A. Glover, MS, MBA; and Weimo Zhu, PhD

The reader will gain an overview of the influence of economic forces and governmental regulation on sedentary behavior. By the end of this chapter, the reader should be able to do the following:

- ▶ Identify the three economic sectors
- ▶ Describe how the U.S. economy has changed over time
- ▶ Define deindustrialization
- ▶ Discuss how economic change has influenced occupational physical activity
- ▶ Describe how energy expenditure affects health risks
- ▶ Identify strategies employers use to combat the health effects of physical inactivity
- ▶ Discuss the U.S. government's regulatory process
- ▶ Explain how regulation promotes innovation
- ▶ Discuss why regulation is imperfect
- ▶ Illustrate how regulation can produce unintended social consequences
- ▶ Identify methods for enhancing the regulatory decision-making process
- ▶ Discuss how nudges can be used to improve physical activity
- ▶ Summarize the effects of government regulation on occupational physical activity

This chapter defines *regulated sedentary behavior* as that caused by a regulation, a policy, or an involuntary environment.

Over the past century, the United States has experienced remarkable social and economic transformations that have been attributed to technological advancements, consumer affluence, and global competition (Kollmeyer 2009). To remain competitive, businesses invest in technology to improve work efficiencies, reduce production costs, and increase production outputs (Bell 1973). Unfortunately, these same technologies that make our lives easier and promote economic growth can have important societal costs in the forms of reduced occupational energy expenditure and increased obesity rates (Philipson and Posner 2003).

To remain competitive in a global economy, businesses depend on the expansion of human knowledge to innovate and create new technologies (Drucker 2001; Kuznets 1973). The U.S. government encourages innovative growth through regulatory processes to ensure economic competitiveness and protect social welfare (Executive Order 13563 2011). Regrettably, the current regulatory process is imperfect and creates unintended social consequences (Joskow 2010; Orbach 2013; Sunstein 2002). One of the unintended social consequences of innovation—through regulation—is the increase in sedentary occupations that have emerged from economic restructuring.

Today, developed societies are spending more time engaged in sedentary behaviors due to reductions in physical work, increases in labor-saving technologies, greater reliance on motor transportation, increases in modern conveniences, and decreases in walking and cycling (Brownson, Boehmer, and Luke 2005; Fox and Hillsdon 2007). Objective and subjective studies have shown that today's work environment contributes to high volumes of time performing sedentary work, requiring prolonged periods of time spent sitting (Clemes, O'Connell, and Edwardson 2014; Thorp et al. 2011; Tudor-Locke et al. 2011). Sedentary work leads to negative health consequences because it elevates the risk for all-cause cardiovascular mortality (Katzmarzyk et al. 2009; Morris et al. 1953).

Economic Sectors

The agricultural, manufacturing, and service industries are the three main economic drivers in the U.S. economy (Kuznets 1973). These three productive economic sectors are referred to as primary, secondary, and tertiary. The primary sector includes industries such as agriculture, fisheries, mining, and timber. The secondary sector includes manufacturing industries such as automobile, construction, utilities, pharmaceuticals, electronics, and petroleum. The tertiary sector includes service industries such as transportation, marketing, and retailing (Kenessey 1987; Wolfe 1955).

Profound changes to both economic and social structures occur as a country progresses through the three economic structures and new technologies are introduced. A country's economic development starts with the majority of its gross domestic product (GDP) and employment in the agricultural sector. In the next stage of economic development, the manufacturing sector begins to rise while agricultural employment rates decrease and production volumes increase. As technology increases, manufacturing efficiencies emerge and employment begins to shift to the service sector (Pilat et al. 2006).

Structural Change

The transition from one sector to another creates structural change that leads to the transformation of industries and displacement of workers (Bell 1973). Industrial transformation often leads to the permanent removal of manufacturing jobs. As jobs are eliminated and workers are displaced, workers are compelled to seek other employment opportunities (Groshen, Potter, and Sela 2004).

Today, farmers use more efficient production methods to plant, grow, and harvest crops through mechanization and automation and take advantage of economies of scale (Dimitri, Effland, and Conklin 2005). These efficiencies have contributed to decreases in agricultural U.S. employment rates from 12.2% in 1950 to 2.0% in 2000 (Brownson, Boehmer, and Luke 2005). The manufacturing industry has also experienced declines in employment as a result of economic restructuring and technological advancements (Blakely and Shapira 1984). Between 1960 and 2008, for example, manufacturing jobs decreased from 30% to 12% of the United States' workforce (Church et al. 2011).

With economic structural change, some sectors will grow faster than other sectors over time. These economic structural changes are influenced by unbalanced productivity growth, growing affluence of consumers, and economic globalization (Kollmeyer 2009). To remain competitive, businesses seek to adapt to these changes and optimize performance by adjusting labor needs and production levels (Clark 1957). This often results in the offshoring of low-skilled, labor-intensive jobs to developing countries (Kollmeyer 2009).

Deindustrialization

During the 1980s, American manufacturing jobs were displaced by new technologies resulting in industrial restructuring (Blakely and Shapira 1984). Bluestone and Harrison (1982) define this process as *deindustrialization*, "a widespread, systematic shift away from a nation's industrial productive base" (page 4). Shrinking employment opportunities in the manufacturing sector make it difficult for workers with industry-specific skills to find comparable employment in other industries (Masur and Posner 2012). Blakely and Shapira also argue that displaced workers are forced to pursue other (lower paying) careers or relocate to other communities. These types of economic events create serious socioeconomic problems such as rising income inequality and severe community decline.

Social costs are particularly high in deindustrialized areas. Recognized industrial cities like Detroit, Michigan, have experienced high unemployment rates and other failures due to deindustrialization. In 1950, Detroit reported a population high of just over 1.8 million people. In 2010, after declaring bankruptcy, the city's population had declined to about 700,000 people (Bluestone 2013). Huntington, West Virginia, and a host of other industrial cities have experienced similar social and economic effects as a result of deindustrialization (Ermolaeva and Ross 2010; Gordus, Jarley, and Feman 1981).

The United States is not the only country experiencing significant declines in manufacturing as a result of economic structural change and deindustrialization (Brady and Denniston 2006). England has also been affected. Manual labor has decreased significantly in the agricultural, manufacturing, and mining sectors as a result of growing industrial innovations. Occupational physical activity levels have decreased, socioeconomic inequalities have increased, and environments that promote physical activity have been threatened in the wake of deindustrialization (Rind, Jones, and Southall 2014).

Reduced Occupational Physical Activity and Fitness

Structural change through deindustrialization influences not only the health of the economy, but also societal behavior norms. Researchers have demonstrated that goods-producing industries like agriculture and manufacturing require greater amounts of physical labor (Lakdawalla and Philipson 2009; Philipson and Posner 2003). Economic restructuring has created shifts away from goods producing and manual labor occupations to service sector occupations (Cerina and Mureddu 2013). These shifts have been attributed to advancements in labor-saving technologies by way of automation, mechanization, and computerization, each of which have improved manufacturing output (Kollmeyer 2009).

Adding to the complexity of structural change, technological advancements (i.e., computers, dishwashers) have increased the amount of time people spend engaged in sedentary behaviors at work and home (Brownson, Boehmer, and Luke 2005; French, Story, and Jeffery 2001). Changes in land-use patterns, urban design factors, and the transportation system influence energy expenditure levels (Brownson et al. 2009). These changes in the physical environment present challenges in the fight to increase energy expenditure.

Studies exploring long-term changes in occupational physical activity levels shed light on how much physical behavior can change in the workforce. In just 50 years, high-activity occupations in the United States decreased from 30% to 22.6%. In the same period, low-activity occupations increased from 23.3% to approximately 41.0% (Brownson, Boehmer, and Luke 2005). In a separate study, following changes in the United States from 1960 to 2008, occupations requiring moderate physical demands decreased from 48% to 20%, whereas sedentary and low-activity jobs slowly increased during this same time frame (Church et al. 2011). These occupational shifts have contributed to 79% of employees working in sedentary or light-intensity jobs (Tudor-Locke et al. 2011).

Based on the number of hours spent in the workplace, occupational physical activity can have a significant effect on total daily caloric expenditure (Church et al. 2011). Full-time U.S. employees spend an average of 8.09 hours working each workday (U.S. Department of Labor 2013). Workers are spending up to 71% of working hours performing sedentary tasks (Clemes, O'Connell, and Edwardson 2014).

Increasing the amount of time performing sedentary work leads to decreased metabolic energy expenditure, resulting in a caloric surplus.

Prolonged seated sedentary behavior (i.e., computer use) results in an energy expenditure of ≤1.5 times resting energy expenditure. To put this into perspective, light-intensity activities (i.e., standing) require no more than 2.9 times resting energy expenditure, while moderate- to vigorous-intensity activities require 3 to 8 times resting energy expenditure (Owen et al. 2000). Increased time spent performing sedentary work can lead to unintended health consequences.

Workers in predominantly sedentary occupations are at greater risk for all-cause cardiovascular mortality when compared with workers in more active job functions (Morris et al. 1953; Palmer et al. 2007). The health implications associated with sedentary occupations is of paramount concern because today's society is spending increasing amounts of time in environments that limit physical activity through prolonged sitting (Hill et al. 2003). These trends in occupational and domestic activities are likely to continue to decline and trends in sedentary behaviors are likely to continue to increase over the coming years (Pronk 2015; Ng and Popkin 2012) unless new systematic regulatory processes are developed.

Economics of Inactivity

Efficiencies gained from technological enhancements have led to reductions in food prices and physical energy expenditure in the workplace (Hill et al. 2003; Philipson and Posner 2003). As such, the cost of consuming calories has decreased and the cost of burning calories has increased (Philipson and Posner 2003). Reductions in energy expenditure are evident even in occupations that have been traditionally recognized as requiring high energy expenditure (Hill et al. 2003). This is an important issue because energy balance through caloric intake or caloric expenditure is needed to prevent weight gain and obesity (Hill, Wyatt, and Peters 2012).

Obesity has been referred to as an outcome of economic factors that lead to both food consumption and physical activity decisions (Finkelstein, Ruhm, and Kosa 2005). As trends and sedentary behaviors increase, obesity rates follow. Since 1960, obesity rates have increased from 13.4% to 35.1% of the U.S. population (Flegal et al. 2010). Obesity is a major health concern that has been linked to a greater

prevalence of multiple comorbid conditions (Guh et al. 2009). The incidences of type 2 diabetes, cardiovascular disease, various cancers, musculoskeletal disorders, sleep apnea, and gallbladder disease have increased as the disease prevalence of obesity has increased (Must et al. 1999).

As a result of these comorbidities, obese patients contribute to a large amount of the annual health care costs, pharmacy costs, and primary care costs in the United States (Thompson et al. 2001). This places an economic strain on health care by increasing overall costs on a system that spends more per capita on health care than any other country (Bodenheimer 2005). Obesity-related conditions account for roughly 20.6% of U.S. health care expenditures (Cawley and Meyerhoefer 2012). Annual health care costs for obese people are estimated to be between $1,429 (Finkelstein et al. 2009) and $2,741 per person per year (Cawley and Meyerhoefer 2012).

Worksite Health Promotion

To control rising health care costs, employers are exploring comprehensive approaches to better manage the direct (medical) as well as indirect (productivity) costs that hamper global competitiveness (Loeppke et al. 2007). Direct health care costs for employers continue to rise. From 2004 to 2014, U.S. health care costs increased from $11,192 to $23,215 for a family of four (Girod et al. 2014).

Indirect costs associated with employee health can also have a profound effect on business performance. Work quality and performance are influenced by employee physical activity levels (Pronk et al. 2004). Physically inactive workers have been shown to have higher absenteeism rates than physically active workers (van Amelsvoort et al. 2006). Lack of physical activity, be it through work or leisure, has also been associated with a higher prevalence of lower back pain symptoms and sick leave (Hildebrandt et al. 2000). Overall health risks are also strongly associated with lost productivity through increased absenteeism and presenteeism (Boles, Pelletier, and Lynch 2004).

In response to these direct and indirect health care costs, many businesses are investing in health promotion solutions to prevent and manage chronic medical conditions (Claxton et al. 2013). Goetzel and Ozminkowski (2008) define these worksite health promotion programs as "employer initiatives directed at improving the health and well-being of workers" (page 304). These investments are based on the assumption that reducing health risks will result in reductions in the organization's overall health care cost (Nyce et al. 2012).

Refocusing on disease prevention rather than treatment is supported by the economic burden associated with unhealthy behaviors. Employers have a larger financial incentive to keep employees healthy through disease prevention as opposed to disease reduction programs. For example, preventing a disease leads to $145 return on investment whereas reducing a disease leads to a $105 return on investment (Nyce et al. 2012). The average return on investment for worksite health promotion is estimated to be $3.27 saved for every $1.00 spent (Baicker, Cutler, and Song 2010).

Regulation and Innovation

Historically, industry, economic, and policy leaders have espoused the notion that the enactments of environmental regulations impose excessive costs to businesses, thus hindering global competitiveness

GOVERNMENTAL REGULATION

Government agencies and regulations continue to expand to protect consumers, workers, the environment, and other natural resources. The following are examples of three prominent U.S. agencies and their respective social actions taken from the Federal Regulatory Directory (2009).

- The Clean Air Act (CAA) of 1970 is enforced by the Environmental Protection Agency (EPA). The CAA protects society from harmful air pollutants such as those emitted from manufacturing plants and automobiles.

- The Food, Drug, and Cosmetic Act (FDCA) of 1938 is enforced by the Food and Drug Administration (FDA). The FDCA protects society from hazardous and misrepresented products.

- The Occupational Health and Safety Act of 1970 is enforced by the Occupational Health and Safety Administration (OSHA). OSHA protects worker health and safety through the enforcement of occupational health and safety standards.

Title VII of the 1964 Civil Rights Act, the 1967 Age Discrimination in Employment Act (ADEA), and the 1990 Americans with Disabilities Act (ADA) are other regulation examples directly related to physical aspects of the workforce. The federal guidelines, standards, and rules derived from the 1964 Civil Rights Act and 1990 ADA regulations, for example, prohibit employment discrimination on the basis of race, color, religion, sex, or national origin, including the designing and applying of pre-employment physical testing.

The disparate impact theory was used to establish discrimination under these regulations, usually having a three-part burden of proof, according to Jackson (2006, 317):

1. The plaintiff (employee) must establish a disparate impact on a protected group, e.g., the passing rate for a protected group is less than four-fifths, or 80%, of the group with the highest passing rate;

2. The defendant (employer) must justify the business necessity, as well as selection method and standards are job related;

3. If #2 is established, the plaintiff has to demonstrate that the employer failed to use a selection method that is equally effective, but with less disparate impact.

In 2011, President Obama issued Executive Order 13563 to enhance the regulatory process established by his predecessors (Carey 2013). The directive requires executive agencies "to use the best available techniques to quantify anticipated present and future benefits and costs as accurately as possible" and to "maximize net benefits (including potential economic, environmental, public health and safety and other advantages; distributive impacts; and equity)" (Executive Order 13563 2011, page 3821).

In its simplest form, Executive Order 13563 highlights the processes and systems that should be applied by regulators to protect public health, welfare, safety, and the environment while promoting economic growth, innovation, competitiveness, and job creation. Executive Order 13563 provides a declaration that regulatory agencies will ensure open exchange of information to the public, simplify rules to promote innovation, reduce burdens, promote freedom of choice, ensure regulations are supported by science, and conduct retrospective analyses of existing regulations.

(Ambec et al. 2013). The classical view contends that if a revenue-generating opportunity existed, companies would have already found a way to profit from it (Palmer, Oates, and Portney 1995). The contemporary view contends that introducing strict social regulations is required for influencing technological innovation and enhancing economic competitiveness (Porter 1991). Porter's hypothesis suggests that the government's role is to create optimal conditions for citizens to achieve higher standards of living by creating opportunities for industry to succeed in the global markets.

In his State of the Union address on January 25, 2011, President Obama highlighted the importance of innovation to ensure America remains competitive both domestically and globally:

> The first step in winning the future is encouraging American innovation. None of us can predict with certainty what the next big industry will be or where the new jobs will come from. Thirty years ago, we couldn't know that something called the Internet would lead to an economic revolution. What we can do—what America does better than anyone else—is spark the creativity and imagination of our people. We're the nation that put cars in driveways and computers in offices; the nation of Edison and the Wright brothers; of Google and Facebook. In America, innovation doesn't just change our lives. It is how we make our living. (2011, para. 23)

Government regulation can be viewed as an imperfect system resulting from failures of decision-makers to appropriately act in response to economic or social issues (Joskow 2010; Orbach 2013). It is unlikely that these failures can be prevented; however, adequate processes can help mitigate the costs of these failures (Orbach 2013).

It is likely that government officials and industrialists become fixated on immediate issues while paying little attention to the unforeseen consequences that arise from new systems (Bell 1973). Foreseeing all consequences of regulation is impossible; therefore, retrospective analysis can be used to help mitigate the risk of unintended consequences (Council of Economic Advisers 2012).

Poorly designed regulations can have devastating unintended social consequences (Thornton 2011; Hazlitt 1979). Intrusion of unintended consequences frequently accompanies well-meaning regulatory policies (Orbach 2013). The following examples demonstrate how some policymakers have failed to examine direct and indirect effects of regulations. Although policymakers did not intend for these events to occur, a more systematic, circumspect analysis may have alerted them to these risks.

- ▶ *Example A.* A manufacturing firm chooses to offset regulatory costs by passing the additional costs off to consumers. The price increases lead to a reduction in consumer demand, slowing plant production. As a result, the firm chooses to lay off workers to remain profitable (Masur and Posner 2012).

- ▶ *Example B.* To protect the environment, the FDA banned the use of chlorofluorocarbons as propellants in medical inhalers in 2005. As a result, the price of asthma inhalers tripled. The increase will likely deter many lower-income patients from treating their asthma condition (McLaughlin and Greene 2014).

- ▶ *Example C.* Globalization, technological advancements, and environmental regulations drive deindustrialization in blue-collar communities like Huntington, West Virginia. Deindustrialization contributes to reductions in manual occupations, increases in worker displacement, and increases in obesity rates (Ermolaeva and Ross 2010).

Even regulations developed intentionally for the purpose of protecting employees' health could have a negative effect if work tasks are modified to require lower levels of physical fitness and the increase of sedentary behavior in occupational settings. For example, there are usually three ways to reduce job-related injuries and workers' compensation costs, including ergonomics (i.e., redesign the work), wellness and training (i.e., change the worker's required fitness level or work habits), and pre-employment testing (i.e., hire those with the physical ability to perform the work). Although the pre-employment test approach has been the most effective of the three (Driessen et al. 2010), employers often decide to use the less effective and more expensive approaches of ergonomics along with wellness and training (Daltroy et al. 1997) to avoid possible legal challenges of the disparate effect associated with pre-employment testing (Jackson 1994). As a result, physically demanding jobs are disappearing quickly from occupational settings.

Cost–benefit analysis (CBA) is one technique used by government agencies to assess the potential social and economic effects of policy (Robinson 1993; Sunstein 2002). According to Robinson, a CBA attempts to monetize the effects of regulation on inputs (costs) and outputs (benefits) for society. Conducting a CBA provides a rational approach to the political decision-making process. The U.S. government has established requirements for federal agencies to follow when conducting a CBA prior to and following social regulatory interventions (Executive Order 13563 2011).

The influence of social and economic trade-offs resulting from regulations should be assessed proactively and retroactively. This is because regulations passed today may or may not interact well with evolving social and economic changes of the future. Retrospective CBAs are needed for evaluating and preserving the beneficial aspects of regulations by providing the opportunity to address any negative unintended costs before they outweigh the benefits (McLaughlin and Williams 2014). However, when a CBA focuses only on productivity or similar outcomes, its finding and recommendation may bring unintended negative social consequences (Sunstein 2002), such as increases in sedentary behavior resulting from innovation and technology and discouraging physical activity breaks for employees. Thus, CBA should take the economic benefits of enhanced fitness into consideration (Shephard 1986).

Proper design considerations must be made when developing new technologies and systems to prevent negative social and environmental externalities (Schinzinger 1998). *Externalities* are defined as spill-over costs created by the production or consumption of a good; however, these costs are not considered in the price of the good (Sturm 2005). Porter and van der Linde (1995) argue that the government is best equipped to manage external costs through social regulation.

Classical economists, however, do not support government intervention through regulatory action as a means of correcting sedentary behaviors or the pursuant health-related outcomes (Bleich and Sturm 2009). As such, a nonregulatory approach from government agencies and businesses would be to use social nudges to modify unhealthy behaviors. Nudges are a result of designing choices (choice architecture) to alter behaviors in a predictable way without introducing paternalistic policies (Thaler and Sunstein 2008).

Choice Environment and Architecture

Environments that promote physical activity can be used to nudge people toward healthy choices (French, Story, and Jeffery 2001; Kremers, Eves, and Andersen 2012; Pronk and Kottke 2009). For example, making stairs more prominent while reducing the number of motorized lifts, providing cycling opportunities instead of motorized transport (Marteau et al. 2011), and replacing conventional desks with walking workstations (Torbeyns, Bailey, and Bos 2014) are forms of choice architecture. Nudges such as these create a sustainable worksite environment that encourages physical activity and counteracts the unintended consequences of sedentary work (Pronk and Kottke 2009).

Recently, efforts have been made to understand the effects of indoor built environments on physical activity and sedentary behavior. For example, a special issue of *Building Research & Information* (May 2015) examined possible factors correlated to indoor sedentary behaviors that promote the indoor built environment as a tool for change:

▶ Duncan and colleagues (2015) demonstrated that individual, workplace, and spatial configuration factors are associated with the frequency of breaks in sitting, but that breaks were affected by office type (e.g., participants working in shared offices reported a high level of physical activity and higher frequency of breaks).

▶ Ucci and others (2015) reported that a radical change in elementary school classrooms may increase physical activity. They found that stand-biased desks may be promising and that height-appropriate standing workstations can be successfully integrated into classrooms to increase overall standing and decrease sitting time.

These findings were well supported by the works by Rashid and others (Rashid, Craig, et al. 2006; Rashid, Kampschroer, et al. 2006; Rashid, Wineman, and Zimring 2009), who found that office movement is positively affected by integration and connectivity, sedentary activities increase when workspace's degree and closeness are high, and the amount of time employees spend in team spaces is positively affected by how they are connected to their neighbors and to all others in the workplace social network. (Note: The degree of a workspace is the number of other workspaces visible from that space, which may be a source of stress due to lack of privacy. The closeness of a workspace describes how close the workspace is to all other workspaces in the visibility network; high closeness therefore means more exposure to all workspaces in a setting.)

Summary

Technological advancements spurred by regulation and innovation have created economic shifts from the primary to secondary to tertiary sectors (Bell 1973). This economic restructuring creates a division of labor that changes the occupational structure by decreasing blue-collar manual occupations and increasing white-collar knowledge occupations (Janowitz 2010). As a result of the transition from physical work to knowledge work, employees are spending more time engaged in sitting and sedentary activities (Church et al. 2011; Clemes, O'Connell, and Edwardson 2014; Harrington et al. 2014; Kirk and Rhodes 2011; Matthews et al. 2008; Tudor-Locke et al. 2011). This is a national health concern because sedentary occupations lead to increased risk of all-cause and cardiovascular mortality (Morris et al. 1953).

Technological advancements have led to a transition from a high-energy expenditure economy to a low-energy expenditure economy, thus increasing obesity rates (Lakdawalla and Philipson 2009; Philipson and Posner 2003). The rise in obesity is accompanied by a rise in obesity-related comorbidities (Guh et al. 2009; Must et al. 1999). These comorbidities contribute to a large amount of the annual health care costs, pharmacy costs, and primary care costs (Bodenheimer 2005; Cawley and Meyerhoefer 2012; Finkelstein et al. 2009; Thompson et al. 2001). In response to increasing direct and indirect health care costs, many businesses are investing in health promotion solutions (Claxton et al. 2013).

To promote economic competitiveness and protect social welfare, the U.S. government uses regulation to encourage innovation (Executive Order 13563 2011; Porter 1991; Porter and van der Linde 1995). Industrial innovation not only improves efficiencies and performance (Porter 1991), but also alters the way in which work is performed (Bell 1973). The influence of social regulations has created a fundamental change in workplace activity, thus contributing to the reduction of total daily energy expenditure levels and the rise of obesity (Brownson, Boehmer, and Luke 2005; Church et al. 2011; Lakdawalla and Philipson 2009; Philipson and Posner 2003).

Cost–benefit analysis is a rational tool that government agencies use to help improve the regulatory decision-making process (Robinson 1993; Sunstein 2002). However, CBA is imperfect and still evolving (Joskow 2010; Orbach 2013; Sunstein 2002). In lieu of a fail-safe system, other strategies focus on nudging society to become more active (Marteau et al. 2011; Pronk and Kottke 2009; Thaler and Sunstein 2008). To offset costs associated with an imperfect regulatory system and its effects on occupational physical activity, government agencies should investigate and implement new strategies to better predict both foreseeable and unforeseeable risks.

KEY CONCEPTS

▸ **Choice architecture:** An approach that influences the decisions people make through the careful design of environments in which people make choices (Thaler and Sunstein 2008). Choice architecture is a nonpaternalistic way to nudge society toward healthier habits.

▸ **Cost–benefit analysis (CBA):** A decision-making process used by government agencies to proactively or retroactively assess the social and economic consequences of government policy. CBA, however, often fails to measure the negative externalities resulting from government regulation (however well intentioned).

▸ **Deindustrialization:** "A widespread, systematic shift away from a nation's industrial productive base" (Bluestone and Harrison 1982, page 4) that results in decreased employment opportunities for blue-collar workers.

▸ **Knowledge worker:** "The man or woman who applies to productive work ideas, concepts, and information rather than manual skill or brawn" (Drucker 1968, page 264).

▸ **Labor saving technologies:** Advancements made in automation, mechanization, and computerization for the purpose of improving manufacturing output (Kollmeyer 2009) and reducing labor requirements, thus increasing the amount of time people spend engaged in sedentary behaviors.

▸ **Regulated sedentary behavior:** The sedentary behavior caused by a regulation, policy, or an involuntary environment.

▸ **Social regulations:** Government regulations that attempt to correct externalities that have the potential to negatively affect public interests such as health, safety, and the environment. The economic effects of social regulation can often be unforeseen and produce unintended consequences.

▸ **Structural change:** The change in the relative size of a nation's economic sectors (primary, secondary, tertiary) as a result of advancements in technology, wealth, and globalization.

STUDY QUESTIONS

1. What are the three main factors driving economic structural shifts?
2. How might technological advancements contribute to decreased caloric expenditure in the workplace and in the home?
3. How might economic restructuring and deindustrialization lead to reductions in physical activity?
4. How might innovation through regulation lead to reductions in physical activity?
5. How can government regulations contribute to work-related physical inactivity?
6. Why is government regulation considered imperfect?
7. How can businesses use choice architecture to promote physical activity in and outside of the workplace?

PART II

SEDENTARY BEHAVIOR AND HEALTH

Part II has six chapters dealing with the main content focus of the book: sedentary behavior and health. The most immediate and obvious concern about *too much sitting* is lack of muscular work and prolonged periods of very low energy expenditure. Thus, in chapter 7, Michael L. Power deals with sedentary behavior and obesity from a broad-based ecological and comparative-biology perspective.

Concerns about sedentary behavior and health have arisen primarily as a result of compelling epidemiological evidence—initially from long-term prospective cohort studies demonstrating premature mortality and disease incidence related to TV viewing time. In chapter 8, Carl J. Caspersen and G. Darlene Thomas address sedentary behavior and incident diabetes. This is an important chapter, not only because it illustrates a key body of evidence but also because of the way in which the authors consider the logic of epidemiological studies and related methodological issues. They applied these insights to the capacity to infer a causal association. Sedentary behavior is also related to another major cause of premature mortality and morbidity: cardiovascular disease. In chapter 9, Edward Archer and colleagues provide a detailed exposition focused on epidemiological findings, identifying

the relevant evidence linking sedentary behaviors to adverse cardiovascular health outcomes. The role of sedentary behavior in promoting poor metabolic health—as the initial chapters in part I illustrate so compellingly—is of significant relevance for cancer causation. In chapter 10, Brigid M. Lynch and Christine M. Friedenreich provide a comprehensive review of the research on the relationship between sedentary behavior and cancer, the evidence for which is variable but consistent in demonstrating relevance for several types of cancers. They also highlight (as do the preceding two chapters) important nuances of epidemiological method in the context of understanding the relationship between sedentary behavior and health outcomes. For type 2 diabetes, cardiovascular disease, and cancer, it is important to note that the majority of well-conducted epidemiological studies have controlled for (albeit to varying degrees) the role of physical activity when identifying how sedentary behavior influences these health outcomes.

In chapter 11, Marco S. Boscolo and Weimo Zhu review evidence on sedentary behavior and lower back pain, a common complaint among those with occupations involving prolonged sitting. Chapter 12 addresses sedentary behavior and psychological well-being. Stuart J.H. Biddle and Stephan Bandelow address an element within the multiple health consequences of sedentary behavior that is less well understood but likely to have broad implications. Cognitive functioning and psychological health encompass important determinants, and likely outcomes, of sedentary behavior.

Taken as a whole, the chapters in part II illustrate the broad importance of sedentary behavior for major chronic diseases and other health problems. These chapters are particularly helpful in illustrating research strategies and methodological issues, including many of the challenges for future research on sedentary behavior and major health outcomes.

CHAPTER 7

SEDENTARY BEHAVIOR AND OBESITY

Michael L. Power, PhD

The reader will gain an overview of the biology of fat, metabolic consequences of obesity, and potential links between sedentary behavior and obesity. By the end of this chapter, the reader should be able to do the following:

▶ Understand some of the diverse functions that fat and adipose tissue perform

▶ Identify how fat in moderation is adaptive

▶ Explain the concept of allostatic load

▶ Identify the main health risks of obesity

▶ Better understand sex differences in fat metabolism and health risks

▶ Understand obesity and sedentary activity in an evolutionary perspective

▶ Discuss relationships among obesity, vitamin D, and sedentary behavior

▶ Articulate the major sources of the human obesity epidemic

Human obesity is old. There are historical references to obese people for essentially our entire written history. Carved artifacts that appear to represent obese people date back to approximately 25,000 years ago. What is new about human obesity is its prevalence. This implies that novel risk factors for obesity exist in the modern environment.

In the distant past, obesity in humans was rare and likely caused by metabolic dysregulation due to genetic or disease-related pathology. External factors precluded the ability of most people to overeat or underexert. Sociocultural obesity came about due to the rareness of obesity and how difficult it was to achieve. What is rare becomes valuable and what is difficult to achieve becomes a badge of prestige. Obesity was a status symbol in some cultures, something to be obtained as a sign of wealth and power. Today, obesity has become common. In many cultures, obesity is approaching the norm. As many as 1 in 3 adult women in the United States is thought to be obese (Flegal et al. 2010). Now that obesity has become so prevalent, perhaps we need a third category, environmental obesity, to account for the large number of otherwise physiologically normal people who become obese in modern society even though obesity has acquired a social stigma.

Obesity has a deceptively simple cause: consuming more calories in food than are expended in daily life, which results in positive energy balance over a sustained period of time. It is deceptively simple because the biology that underlies the regulation of all aspects of energy balance is extremely complex and not well understood (Power and Schulkin 2009). The advice to eat less and exercise more is easy to give, but difficult to follow.

Particular challenges also exist for the new public health and clinical agendas for addressing sedentary behavior—put simply, how to articulate the risks associated with too much sitting as distinct from those of too little exercise. As other chapters in this volume make clear, obese people sit more, and prolonged sitting results in less physical activity—especially light-intensity activity that can account for an important component of overall daily energy expenditure. In this context, it is helpful to have an informed understanding of obesity, especially from the point of view of the import and biologically adaptive roles of adipose tissue and how adipose tissue can influence the ways in which energy balance is regulated.

Role of Fat

Fat is an essential part of our bodies. Fats, or lipids, perform many functions: nutritional, hormonal, and even structural. Certain long-chain polyunsaturated fatty acids are essential for proper eye and brain development. Cell membranes are composed of phospholipids, glycolipids, and steroids. And of course the cholesterol-based steroid hormones such as estrogens, testosterone, and glucocorticoids perform vital functions necessary for life and reproduction. Fat is essential and adaptive.

Fat has significant advantages as an energy storage medium. It contains approximately twice the amount of metabolizable energy per gram of dry weight than does either carbohydrate or protein. Furthermore, it is stored on the body in association with very little water. In contrast, 1 g of glycogen is stored with anywhere from 3 to 5 g of water (Schmidt-Nielsen 1994). A single kilocalorie of glycogen will have a mass of about 1 g; 1 kcal of fat has a mass of 0.11 g (Schmidt-Nielsen 1994). The ability to store substantial amounts of energy in adipose tissue has many adaptive advantages. It buffers the organism from the effects of unpredictable and variable food supply. It allows available excess energy to be consumed and then used at a later time. It allows an animal to go longer between feeding. The ability to store fat increases the behavioral flexibility and the potential feeding strategies an organism can employ.

Several advantages exist to having both a greater capacity to store fat and a greater reliance on fat as a metabolic fuel during periods of sustained increased need, for example, during pregnancy and lactation. Upregulating fat metabolism spares glucose; during pregnancy, the glucose demands of the fetus and placenta must be balanced with the glucose need of the maternal brain. Increasing fat oxidation to provide fuel for maternal muscle and peripheral organs relieves some of this conflict (Peters et al. 2004).

After birth, the infant receives nutrition from milk. Maternal transfer of nutrients is delivered through the infant's digestive tract rather than through the placenta. Although energy requirements during the last trimester of gestation are certainly significant, women even in poor countries generally are able to gain maternal mass during early gestation. Appetite is usually increased during pregnancy, and energy expenditure is often reduced. Excess energy intake during early pregnancy can be stored as fat and then used during lactation.

Although fat has many beneficial functions in the body, fat is toxic to cells in high levels (Schrauwen and Hesselink 2004; Slawik and Vidal-Puig 2006). Lipid droplets that accumulate in cells and organs cause pathology (e.g., fatty liver). To prevent the adverse effects of lipotoxicity, fatty acids must be either oxidized or sequestered. There are limits to metabolism and the rate of energy that animals can process in any given time. If fat cannot be oxidized, it must be safely stored. Adipocytes are cells specially adapted for fat storage; fat is preferentially stored in adipose tissue, and thus less fat accumulates in muscle and organs, where it would cause morbidity. Adipocytes store fat for the positive benefit associated with its energy value, storing energy that can be later used far away in space and time from the act of ingestion. Adipocytes also sequester excess fat to prevent lipotoxicity (Slawik and Vidal-Puig 2006).

Adipose tissue is not just a passive organ, however. It actively regulates metabolism through multiple pathways. Indeed, adipose tissue contains more than just adipocytes. A large number of nonfat cells are also found in adipose tissue, including fibroblasts, mast cells, macrophages, and leukocytes (Fain 2006). Both adipocytes and these nonfat cells produce, regulate, and secrete active peptides and steroids (Kershaw and Flier 2004), as well as immune function molecules (Fain 2006). Adipose tissue is an active component of regulatory physiology.

It is the metabolically active functions of adipose tissue that are related to much of the pathology associated with obesity. The conception of adipose tissue as an endocrine and immune function organ gives insight into why excess adipose tissue can have important effects on physiology and metabolism. Just consider for a moment the expectations you would have if an animal's liver or adrenal gland doubled in size. Obesity is an increase in adipose tissue well beyond the functional range that was typically experienced during our past, and thus the secretions from adipose will likely be out of balance with those from other organ systems.

Adipose Tissue and Endocrine Function

The original notion of adipose tissue as a relatively metabolically inert store of energy has been replaced by a concept of adipose tissue as a metabolically active player in many physiological and endocrine processes (Kershaw and Flier 2004). Adipose tissue functions as an endocrine gland in three different ways. It stores and releases preformed steroid hormones. In addition, many of these steroid hormones are metabolically converted from precursors in adipose tissue, or the active hormones are converted to inactive metabolites. For example, estrone is converted to estradiol in adipose tissue. Most if not all circulating estradiol in postmenopausal women comes from their adipose tissue (Kershaw and Flier 2004). Adipose tissue expresses aromatase, 3α-hydroxysteroid dehydrogenase type 3 (3α-HSD3) and 17β-hydroxysteroid dehydrogenase (17β-HSD5), which are involved in androgen metabolism. These enzymes are increased in obesity (Wake et al. 2007). Adipose tissue also expresses 11β-hydroxysteroid dehydrogenase type 1 (11β-HSD1), which converts cortisone to cortisol (Seckl and Walker 2001), and 5α-reductase enzymes (Wake et al. 2007; Tomlinson et al. 2008), which convert cortisol to 5α-tetrahydrocortisol (5α-THF). Thus, adipose tissue regulates the local concentrations of glucocorticoids (Tomlinson et al. 2008; Stimson et al. 2009) and contributes to metabolic clearance of glucocorticoids (Rask et al. 2002). Obesity is associated with both increased adrenal glucocorticoid production and higher glucocorticoid metabolic clearance, which appear to result in normal plasma concentrations. In obese people, 11β-HSD1 activity is reduced in liver and the inactivation of cortisol by 5α-reductase is enhanced in both liver (Stewart et al. 1999; Rask et al. 2002) and adipose (Tomlinson et al. 2008). However, 11β-HSD1 activity is enhanced in adipose tissue of both obese men and women (Rask et al. 2001; 2002). Obese people have increased hepatic inactivation of cortisol, which is generally balanced by increased regeneration of cortisol in adipose tissue. The effect appears stronger in women compared to men (Rask et al. 2002), possibly due to the higher fat mass in women for a given BMI. Finally, adipose tissue produces and secretes numerous cytokines and peptide hormones, such as leptin, adiponectin, and many of the interleukins (e.g., IL-6, IL-8, and IL-10). A partial list of these bioactive molecules in adipose tissue is found in table 7.1. The hormones secreted by adipose tissue can act locally and on other end-organ systems (e.g., in autocrine, paracrine, or endocrine fashion).

Table 7.1 Fat-Derived Peptides and Steroid-Hormone-Converting Enzymes

Hormone	Function	Changes in obesity
Leptin	Effects on food intake, onset of puberty, bone development, immune function	Circulating leptin increased
Tumor necrosis factor α (TNF-α)	Represses genes involved in uptake and storage of nonesterified fatty acids and glucose	Adipose tissue expression of TNF-α increased
Adiponectin	Enhances insulin action	Circulating adiponectin lowered
Interleukin 6 (IL-6)	Involved in regulation of insulin signaling; central effects on energy metabolism	Circulating IL-6 increased; expression of IL-6 greater in visceral fat
Resistin	Effects on insulin action; linked with insulin resistance	Serum resistin is elevated in rodent obesity models
Aromatase	Converts androgens to estrogens	No change, but increased fat mass results in greater total conversion
17β-hydroxysteroid dehydrogenase (17β-HSD5)	Converts estrone to estradiol and androstenedione to testosterone	Same as aromatase
3α hydroxysteroid dehydrogenase type 3 (3α-HSD3)	Inactivates dihydrotestosterone	Increased
5α-reductase	Inactivates cortisol	Increased
11β-hydroxysteroid dehydrogenase type 1 (11β-HSD1)	Converts cortisone to cortisol	Increased activity in adipose tissue

Homeostasis

Homeostasis is a simple but powerful concept. The internal milieu must remain constant, despite external challenges:

> The organs and tissues are set in a fluid matrix. . . . So long as this personal, individual sack of salty water, in which each one of us lives and moves and has his being, is protected from change, we are freed from serious peril (Cannon 1935, page 1).

The concept of stability, of resistance to change, is fundamental to homeostasis. However, homeostasis is not synonymous with regulatory physiology, and stability is perhaps a misleading word when considering evolved physiological adaptations. Some of the changes are programmed, such as circadian or seasonal rhythms or the physiological changes associated with pregnancy and lactation. Others are acute responses to challenges. Many are anticipatory rather than reactive, occurring before the need has arrived. This is not an inherent contradiction of homeostasis, as Cannon quoting Richet noted: "We are only stable because we constantly change" (1935, page 2).

Stability is not the currency of evolutionary success. Viability, defined as the capability of success or ongoing effectiveness, is a better concept. Physiological regulation to maintain viability requires regulation of set points under some conditions and abandonment of set points under others. There must be physiological processes that are not homeostatic, and that oppose, at least temporarily, stability.

Allostasis

The concept of allostasis was proposed to account for regulatory systems that appeared to fall outside of the classic concept of homeostatic processes (Schulkin 2003). For example, regulatory systems in which there are varying set points or no obvious set points at all (e.g., fear), or where the behavioral and physiological responses are anticipatory and do not simply reflect feedback from a monitored parameter. Homeostasis and allostasis can be considered as complementary components of physiological regulation. Homeostatic processes maintain and regulate physiology around a set point, and allostatic processes change the state of the person, including changing or abandoning physiological set points. Homeostatic processes are associated with negative restraint and resistance to perturbations. Allostatic processes are associated with facilitating positive induction, perturbing the system, and changing the animal's state. Both types of processes evolved to enhance the viability of the organism.

The term *allostatic state* refers to chronic activation of regulatory systems due either to dysregulation or dysfunction of physiology or to conflicting, competing, or opposing demands (McEwen 1998). The term *allostatic load* refers to the strain on physiology and regulatory capacity due to sustained activation of regulatory systems. Many regulatory systems evolved to respond to acute or at least short-lived challenges to viability. Their activation generally results in a change of state that alleviates the challenge and thus allows the regulatory response to cease, at least temporarily. Sustained activation of these regulatory circuits is outside of the evolutionary experience. If these regulatory systems are chronically activated, either due to competing imperatives, conflicting signals, or the failure of the regulatory physiology to resolve the challenge, the associated costs can accumulate. The concept of allostatic load arises from the fact that many physiological adaptations are short-term solutions. They have a cost that can be borne over a limited time period, but will begin to lessen health if they remain continuously activated.

One mild criticism of the term *allostatic load* is that there is no particular reason why the regulatory circuits being chronically activated have to be allostatic in nature (Power 2004). Homeostatic systems that become chronically activated due to sustained external pressures, or simply because the regulatory system is failing to achieve the desired homeostatic state, will potentially have the same general long-term consequences, slowly degrading physiology and lessening health. Allostatic load might be more properly termed *regulatory load* or *metabolic load*. The basic concept rests on the fact that any regulatory system that remains continuously activated or activated to a level outside of its norm will eventually break down.

Mismatch Paradigm

The modern human environment differs substantially from the environment our early ancestors evolved under. Technological, economic, and cultural factors have created conditions that allow an increased incidence of overweight and obese people in the world. A complete understanding of our biology relevant to obesity requires a careful consideration of the evolutionary events and pressures that have shaped our adaptive responses to hunger, food, exertion, and energy stores that, in today's world, may not be as appropriate as in the past. Obesity, in many cases, is probably due to normal adaptive responses that encourage eating high-energy-density foods while limiting energy expenditure. Food is rewarding, and there was adaptive advantage in the past to restricting energy expenditure when possible. In many ways, our modern society is constructed to allow us to eat well while expending little; economic and business decisions reflect our evolved preferences. We have diligently worked to conquer the external constraints that forced our ancestors to expend considerable energy to obtain barely sufficient food; we are now seeing that, for many of us, the motivations and biological drives to obtain calories appear to exceed those to expend.

The mismatch paradigm (Gluckman and Hanson 2006) is a simple but powerful concept. Our biology evolved under particular sets of circumstances and to respond effectively to specific challenges. The modern environment differs substantially from the past environment. Our evolved biology is adapted to meet challenges that in today's world are markedly changed or even largely absent, and we are faced with novel challenges that were never faced in our evolutionary past. Thus, our evolved biological responses may be out of sync with our modern-day challenges.

Evolution has resulted in our bodies having some capability to respond metabolically and physiologically to circumstances and challenges. Thus, we don't have to have a perfect match between the expected environment (based on our past) and the actual one. The congruence between the mismatch paradigm and allostatic load is fairly straightforward; the more an organism's biology and physiology is a mismatch for its environment, the greater the effort or cost it will incur in its attempts to adapt physiologically, and the more likely that the physiological adaptations will be insufficient and even possibly inappropriate. The greater the mismatch, the greater the allostatic load. Normal adaptive (in the evolutionary sense) responses become maladaptive.

Obesity and Inflammation

Obesity is associated with chronic low-grade inflammation (Clement and Langin 2007). Obesity enhances adipose tissue secretion of proinflammatory cytokines, and is associated with lower secretion by adipose tissue of the anti-inflammatory hormone adiponectin (Denison et al. 2010). Adipose tissue in obese people is characterized by increased recruitment of adipose tissue macrophages (ATMs) with a shift toward a more proinflammatory ATM phenotype (Denison et al. 2010; Weisberg et al. 2003; Lumeng et al. 2008; Morris et al. 2011). Infiltration of adipose tissue by proinflammatory T-cells precedes the recruitment of and phenotypic changes in ATMs (Kintscher et al. 2008; Nishimura et al. 2009). The production of cytokines and other proinflammatory molecules from macrophages contributes to the pathologies associated with excess adipose tissue. Insulin resistance is particularly linked with the inflammation due to obesity (Roth et al. 2004).

Hypoxia might play a role in the inflammation due to excess adipose tissue. When adipose tissue mass increases to a great extent, some adipocytes and macrophages may not be well connected to the circulatory system and will suffer from hypoxia. These cells will begin to secrete the appropriate inflammatory cytokines in response. This response may be locally beneficial but systemically harmful, and will produce an allostatic load.

Central Versus Peripheral Obesity

Central obesity, excess adipose tissue in the abdominal region, is associated with higher risks of type 2 diabetes, hypertension, dyslipidemia, and cardiovascular disease in both men and women (Goodpaster et al. 2005; Karelis et al. 2004; Racette et al. 2006; Van Pelt et al. 2002; 2005). Abdominal obesity was found to be the strongest predictor of insulin resistance among men and women over 50 (Racette et al. 2006). Overweight and obese women and obese men with a higher proportion of fat in subcutaneous thigh adipose tissue were significantly less likely to display symptoms of metabolic syndrome (Goodpaster et al. 2005). Obese people with mostly peripheral fat, distributed in subcutaneous depots in the gluteal-femoral region are at lower risk of the common comorbidities of obesity than are obese people with a large proportion of their fat in intraabdominal depots (Van Pelt et al. 2005). In adult subjects with existing coronary heart disease, central obesity was associated with mortality regardless of body mass index (BMI) (Couthino et al. 2011). In children ages 4 to 18, waist-to-height ratio was a better indicator of adverse metabolic status (high LDL cholesterol, triglycerides, and insulin) than was BMI (Mokha et al. 2010).

Abdominal fat mainly consists of visceral and subcutaneous adipose tissue; the proportions of fat between these depots differ between men and women and also among racial/ethnic groups. The metabolic and health consequences appear to differ as well. Visceral fat is associated with a greater likelihood of adverse health conditions (Karelis et al. 2004; Racette et al. 2006), although excess subcutaneous abdominal fat has been implicated in poor glucose regulation (Garg 2004; Jensen 2006).

Visceral fat is found within the peritoneal cavity. Excess visceral fat is a significant risk factor for the metabolic and health complications of obesity (Fujioka et al. 1987; Karelis et al. 2004; Racette et al. 2006). About 20% of obese men and women have metabolically healthy profiles. These people generally have a significantly smaller proportion of adipose tissue as visceral fat (Karelis et al. 2004). Men and women with a higher proportion of adipose tissue as visceral fat can exhibit an unhealthy phenotype even if they are not technically obese (Karelis et al. 2004). A higher proportion of fat as visceral adipose tissue significantly increases the risk for metabolic syndrome (insulin resistance, dyslipidemia, and hypertension) in older men and women, even among those of normal weight (Goodpaster et al. 2005). Visceral fat also is associated with dysregulation of cortisol production and metabolism. Urinary excretion of cortisol and its metabolites is increased in women with excessive visceral adipose tissue (Pasquali et al. 1993). Arterial stiffness, a risk factor for cardiovascular disease, is associated with increased truncal fat, while increased peripheral fat confers a small degree of protection (Ferreira et al. 2004).

Although the accumulation of subcutaneous fat in the lower body might represent a healthier regulation of fat stores compared with abdominal fat, excess adipose tissue is still associated with poor health outcomes. Metabolically healthy obese people may be less at risk than other obese people, but they still appear to be more at risk than the general population (Karelis et al. 2004).

There appear to be racial differences in the susceptibility to acquiring visceral fat. Asians have a higher percent of body fat for any given BMI than do Caucasians or people of sub-Saharan African descent (Deurenberg et al. 2002), carrying a greater proportion of fat in visceral adipose tissue (Park et al. 2001; Yajnik 2004). Obese postmenopausal African-American women have less visceral fat for any given BMI than do postmenopausal Caucasian women, but a higher proportion of subcutaneous abdominal fat (Conway et al. 1995; Tittelbach et al. 2004). Young African-American men and women have less visceral adipose tissue on average than do their Caucasian counterparts, despite African-American women generally having higher total fat (Cossrow and Falkner 2004). Interestingly, African-Americans and Caucasians differ in their susceptibility to different aspects of metabolic syndrome: Caucasians are more likely to express dyslipidemia (e.g., unfavorable cholesterol pattern and high triglycerides), and African-Americans appear more susceptible to dysregulation of glucose metabolism (Cossrow and Falkner 2004).

Sex Differences in Fat Storage and Mobilization

Men and women differ in their patterns of fat deposition, fat mobilization, use of fat as a metabolic fuel, and the consequences of both excess and insufficient fat stores. Many of these differences may reflect evolved adaptive differences that stem from the differences in male and female reproductive costs. The costs of gestation and lactation dwarf the energy costs of male reproductive effort. This asymmetry in reproductive cost is reflected in the asymmetry in fat storage and in the use of fat as fuel.

Women have greater adipose stores than men, even after correcting for BMI. This is true for all races and all cultures. Indeed, the mean percent of body fat for normal-weight women (BMI between 18 kg/m^2 and 25 kg/m^2) is similar to the percent body fat of men who are classified as obese (BMI > 30 kg/m^2) (Nielsen et al. 2004). This is partly explained by higher muscle mass in men, but women often have more total fat than men, even given male–female size differences. This sex difference in adiposity is present at birth. Female babies have more subcutaneous fat than male babies for all gestational ages (Rodriguez et al. 2005). Prepubertal girls have more fat in their legs and pelvis than do prepubertal boys (He et al. 2004).

Body fat also is distributed differently between men and women (see figure 7.1). Men are more susceptible to abdominal adiposity (Nielsen et al. 2004), while women have greater adipose stores in the thighs and buttocks (Williams 2004). Women have larger stores of subcutaneous fat; men are more likely to have visceral fat (Lemieux et al. 1993). Men have also consistently been shown to have greater

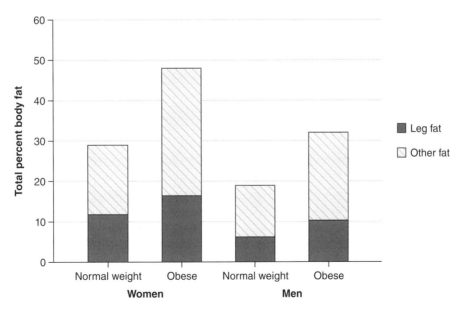

Figure 7.1 Women have higher total percent body fat and a greater proportion of fat in the legs than do men.

Data from Nielsen et al. 2004.

rates of both fatty acid release (lipolysis) and fatty acid uptake (lipogenesis) in visceral fat compared with women (Williams 2004). Thus, in addition to men being more susceptible to excess visceral fat, the effects of visceral fat on health may differ between the sexes.

Waist circumference is a significant risk factor for the comorbidities of obesity. Waist circumference in men and women is significantly associated with abdominal subcutaneous and visceral fat; however, the relationship between circumference and fat differs significantly between the sexes. The regression lines of waist circumference against subcutaneous abdominal fat for men and women are parallel; however, women have on average 1.8 kg (4 lbs) more subcutaneous abdominal fat than men for any given waist circumference (Kuk et al. 2005). In contrast, the slope of the regression line of waist circumference against visceral fat is significantly greater for men than for women (Kuk et al. 2005). Age and menopausal status also have significant effects on the relationship between waist circumference and visceral fat. Older men and women have significantly higher regression slopes than do their younger counterparts. The slopes of the regression lines for men are greater than for women standardized to any age; however, the standardized slope for 40-year-old women is the same as the standardized slope for 25-year-old men. The slope for menopausal women is greater than the slope for premenopausal women, and approaches the male pattern (Kuk et al. 2005).

Sex Hormones

Not surprisingly, sex hormones affect adipose tissue metabolism and appear to play significant roles in the resulting distribution and consequences of stored fat. Testosterone acts to increase lipolysis, inhibit lipoprotein lipase activity, and decrease triglyceride accumulation in adipose tissue. Lowering circulating testosterone levels in healthy young men increases total adipose tissue; raising circulating testosterone decreases total adipose tissue (Woodhouse et al. 2004). Estrogens play multiple roles in the regulation of adipose tissue in both men and women. Androgens appear to block proliferation and differentiation of preadipocytes (Singh et al. 2006). Estradiol enhances proliferation of preadipocytes from both men and women in vitro (Anderson et al. 2001). The effect was greater in preadipocytes from women compared to those from men.

Estradiol favors the deposition of subcutaneous fat; lack of estrogen in women leads to both weight gain and a larger proportion of fat gain stored as visceral fat. Menopausal women have higher visceral fat mass than do premenopausal women for the equivalent percent body fat (Tchernof et al. 2004). Estradiol-treated postmenopausal women have lower lipoprotein lipase (LPL) activity (Pedersen et al. 2004). Adipose tissues express both androgen and estrogen receptors. Both the alpha and beta estrogen receptors are found in adipose tissue (Pedersen et al. 2004). Visceral fat has higher levels of androgen and estrogen receptors than subcutaneous fat, and this is true for both men and women (Rodriguez-Cuenca et al. 2005).

Fat Metabolism

Fat metabolism in women and men differs in a number of ways consistent with the differences in body fat percentage and adipose tissue distribution between men and women. Women appear to be more metabolically inclined to store fat than are men. At rest, women shunt more circulating free fatty acids into re-esterification pathways than do men (Nielsen et al. 2003). Women have higher VLDL-triglyceride production rates than do men, but similar circulating concentrations (Mittendorfer 2005). This is further evidence that women have higher rates of re-esterification and thus re-uptake of free fatty acids into adipose tissue than do men. In the basal condition, women are more physiologically adapted to store fat than are men.

The rates of fatty acid uptake and release depend on the type of adipose tissue as well as sex, and this is reflected in the differing patterns of fat deposition between men and women. Women have higher rates of fat uptake into leg fat depots than do men (Votruba and Jensen 2006). Rates of fatty acid release from abdominal adipose tissue are higher in women than men, but they are lower from gluteal or femoral adipose tissue (Williams 2004). After feeding, fatty acid uptake is higher in abdominal adipose tissue relative to gluteal or femoral adipose tissue in both men and women. However, in women, the majority of fatty acid uptake in abdominal adipose tissue is into subcutaneous fat, while in men a larger proportion goes into visceral fat (Williams 2004). These findings are consistent with women being more likely to store fat subcutaneously and preferentially in the gluteal and femoral regions compared with men.

Interestingly, women also appear to use fat as an energy substrate during periods of sustained exertion more than men do. Women have higher rates of fat oxidation than men during sustained bouts of increased energy expenditure such as endurance training. Men are more likely to upregulate glucose and amino acid metabolism during sustained exercise bouts (Lamont et al. 2001; Lamont 2005). The difference is associated with estrogen. Giving exogenous estrogen to men decreases carbohydrate and amino acid metabolism during exercise and increases fat oxidation (Hamadeh et al. 2005). It would appear that women are more physiologically geared to use fat as a metabolic fuel under conditions of sustained increased demand, while men rely more on glucose and protein metabolism. This difference is mediated by sex hormones.

Despite the greater increase in fat oxidation with sustained exercise by women, men are more likely to lose fat through a program of increased exercise (Ross 1997; Donnelly et al. 2003). This puzzling result is not well understood. The studies to date have not shown that men are more motivated or dedicated when exercising to lose weight. A possibility is that although women may burn more fat through exercise than do men, afterward they may be more likely to replenish their adipose stores during recovery.

Differences in fat metabolism between men and women during sustained exertion probably relate to differences in past evolutionary pressures between men and women. Male metabolism may reflect selective pressures primarily based on muscular activity, both intense and sustained. Our female ancestors also expended large amounts of energy in physical tasks; we are not suggesting that women did not physically work as hard as men, though there are and always have been differences between the sexes in physical capability. More importantly, however, women differed from men in that they expended large amounts of energy during pregnancy and lactation. Pregnancy and lactation were perhaps the most energetically costly events in the lives of our female ancestors. The demands of reproduction

IS BEING LAZY ADAPTIVE?

Animals in the wild act according to evolved behavioral strategies that have, on balance, produced the highest fitness. Anyone who has observed wild animals for any length of time knows that doing nothing appears to be a remarkably common strategy. Many animals spend a good part of their day simply resting; for example, colobus monkeys spend more than half of their waking time resting (Wong and Sicotte 2007). Performing calisthenics, expending energy for the sole purpose of exercising one's muscles, is largely a human endeavor. Of course, many animals expend energy in physical play, both social and solitary.

Sedentary behavior can have adaptive value. It reduces energy expenditure as well as the risks of acute injury. In our evolutionary past, the opportunities to engage in sedentary behavior were usually limited, both in total amount and, perhaps most importantly, in the duration of any sedentary behavior episode. For our human ancestors, important survival tasks such as eating were intrinsically linked with exertion. Short periods of sedentary behavior may have been important as rest and recovery times for the necessary efforts to sustain life, but the number and duration of sedentary bouts were constrained. In the modern environment, we have seen increases in both the opportunity to engage in sedentary behavior and the requirement for sitting time in order to function in society.

Human beings vary in how energetically they choose to live their lives. Some people are always doing something; others are quite content to kick back whenever the opportunity arises. It is interesting to consider that both strategies would have had adaptive advantages in our past. One of the asymmetries that likely contributes to overweight and obesity is that motivation to indulge in food can be greater than motivation to indulge in physical activity.

NHANES performed one study measuring not only the amount of steps taken, but the intensity of those actions, and found that less than 5% of people meet the recommended 30 minutes of moderate- to vigorous-intensity physical activity 5 days per week. Self-report of physical activity was significantly less accurate than direct measures, with individual reports indicating that 30% of people believed they met current exercise guidelines. Perhaps this discrepancy reflects a bias within our cognitive system in which effort is assessed as a higher cost than food is a benefit.

were more likely to be the important selective pressures in women, and thus had a larger influence on female metabolism.

Vitamin D, Adipose Tissue, and Sedentary Behavior

Vitamin D was not a required nutrient for most of our evolutionary past. Our ancestors produced sufficient vitamin D through a photosynthetic reaction in skin in which 7-dehydrocholesterol is converted to previtamin D by absorbing ultraviolet B radiation (UVB). Previtamin D spontaneously converts to vitamin D at mammalian skin temperatures. Rather than being a nutrient, vitamin D is an endogenously produced precursor to a steroid hormone. It is converted in the liver by an unregulated hydroxylation to 25-hydroxyvitamin D, the main circulating form and the best measure of vitamin D status, and then again in the kidney, through a tightly regulated reaction to 1,25-dihydroxtvitamin D, which is the form with the highest bioactivity. Vitamin D deficiency is a disease of modern humanity related to reduced sunlight exposure that first emerged during the industrial revolution and is still present today. Although frank deficiency is rare, large segments of the human population have low levels of circulating 25-hydroxyvitamin D (van Schoor and Lips 2011) and might suffer lessening of health because of it (Holick and Chen 2008).

Both obesity and sedentary behavior are associated with low vitamin D status and increased risk of vitamin D deficiency (Wortsman et al. 2000; Brock et al. 2010). The proposed underlying causes for low vitamin D status in sedentary people include low exposure to sunlight, low intakes of foods rich in vitamin D, and the interaction of excess adipose tissue with vitamin D storage and metabolism. It appears that a large mass of adipose tissue leads to excess vitamin D metabolites becoming sequestered in adipose tissue, and thus circulating levels are decreased. There also appears to be a direct effect of high physical activity on vitamin D status. Higher physical activity is associated with better vitamin D status even after accounting for sun exposure and diet (Bell et al. 1988; Brock et al. 2007), though the mechanism is unknown.

Adipose tissue acts as a storage depot for vitamin D metabolites and other fat-soluble molecules. This is one reason why vitamin D deficiency takes a long time to develop and why humans far from the equator can remain vitamin D sufficient through the winter even with low dietary vitamin D. High sun exposure during the summer months would result in several months' supply of vitamin D and its metabolites being stored in body fat. This mechanism is potentially important for infant health as well. Infants are born with several months' supply of vitamin D transferred in utero across the placenta and stored in adipose tissue. Even though breast milk is deficient in vitamin D (Hillman 1990), a solely breast-fed infant has enough stored vitamin D to avoid frank deficiency for many months. And of course if the infant is exposed to intense enough sunlight (or another source of UVB radiation), endogenous photosynthetic production will be sufficient. However, it appears that above some thresholds, adipose tissue acts to reduce vitamin D availability by effectively trapping it (Worstman et al. 2000).

Low vitamin D status is associated with increased risk for a number of diseases besides the bone diseases of rickets and osteoporosis. Low vitamin D status is strongly associated with colorectal cancer (Garland and Garland 1980; Grant and Garland 2004; Jenab et al. 2010). Indeed, low vitamin D status appears to be a risk factor for many cancers; this is not surprising considering that 1,25-dihydroxyvitamin D is a potent hormone in the regulation of cell growth (Zhang and Naughton 2010). Low circulating 25-hydroxyvitamin D is associated with an increased risk of cardiovascular disease (Anderson et al. 2010). Vitamin D supplementation reduces inflammation, possibly by its effect on cytokine profiles, increasing anti-inflammatory cytokines such as IL-10 (Schleithoff et al. 2006). Although the mechanisms are uncertain, low vitamin D status is associated with poor glucose metabolism, impaired insulin secretion, and insulin resistance (Roth et al. 2011). Increasing circulating 25-hydroxyvitamin D levels improved insulin sensitivity in obese women (Tzotzas et al. 2010). Thus, vitamin D insufficiency appears to be linked with the development of diabetes, both type 1 and type 2 (Osei 2010). Vitamin D appears to have potent effects on immune function, and low vitamin D status increases the risks of contracting infectious disease, including higher risk for contracting tuberculosis (Zhang and Naughton 2010). Overall mortality risk declines with increasing circulating 25-hydroxyvitamin D up to a threshold of 87.5 nmol/L (Zittermann et al. 2012). Finally, low vitamin D status is associated with significant cognitive decline in the elderly (Llewellyn et al. 2010). The extent to which a sedentary lifestyle contributes to vitamin D insufficiency and thus to the associated disease risks is uncertain, but the evidence suggests that a sedentary lifestyle can contribute to a lessening of health through its negative effect on vitamin D status, both directly and through the increased risk of obesity from a sedentary lifestyle.

Obesity Prevalence

Is obesity really at epidemic levels? Throughout history and likely extending into prehistory, there have been obese human beings. In the past, obesity was rare, and represented highly unusual metabolic or cultural circumstances. External factors generally restricted the obesity phenotype from being expressed. Today obesity has become common. In 1994, more than half of the American states had a prevalence of obesity among adults of less than 15%. By 2000, only 1 state was below 15%. By 2005, all 50 states had higher than 15% obesity prevalence and 3 states were over 30%. In 2009, the number of states with an obesity prevalence of 30% or higher had increased to 9. Five years later, in 2014, no state had an obesity prevalence less than 20% and 22 states had an obesity prevalence greater than 30%. The lowest state obesity rate in 2014 was Colorado at 21.3%; the highest was Arkansas at 35.9% (see table 7.2). Globally, between 1980 and 2008, the obesity prevalence among adult men doubled and the prevalence among adult women increased by 75%. In 1980, no major region of the world had an adult female obesity prevalence above 25%. The obesity prevalence among adult women now exceeds 30% in North America, Central America, the Middle East, and North and Southern Africa (Malik et al. 2012). This is extraordinarily rapid phenotypic change in a population. It cannot be caused by genetic change; rather, the modern environment is interacting with our evolved biology in ways that create large groups of people who are vulnerable to sustained weight gain. Human cultural and technological abilities have allowed obesity to become common. The modern human environment has become obesogenic.

The word *epidemic* conjures up visions of substantial numbers of healthy people suddenly being stricken with some affliction. Human obesity does not fit that definition. However, Flegal (2006) care-fully reviewed definitions of the word *epidemic* and concluded that the recent changes in human obesity prevalence do indeed have characteristics of an epidemic. She relied mainly on the epidemiological definition of epidemic, in which the salient point is that an epidemic is an occurrence of "health related events clearly in excess of normal expectancy" (page 72). She concluded that the extent of the increase in the prevalence of obesity was not predictable from the obesity prevalence data prior to 1980. Changes in the prevalence of obesity occur on the timescale of human generations. On that timescale, the increase in number of obese people over the last 20 to 30 years is indeed dramatic, and would not have been predicted from an examination of data from the previous hundreds of years.

Others have criticized the use of the word *epidemic* in regard to human obesity, arguing that it inappropriately raises the level of concern around this health issue. They argue that the rise in overweight and obesity is not rapid and dramatic enough and the health consequences not so dire as to justify the notion of an obesity epidemic. Campos and colleagues (2006) caution that many economic interests (e.g., the diet industry, health food industry, and even biomedical researchers) have a vested interest in an exaggerated concern over humanity's increase in body weight. Of course others (e.g., Kim and Popkin 2006) have pointed out that there are equally economically powerful groups that would benefit from a lack of concern (e.g., fast food and soft drink companies).

Still, the word *epidemic* does suggest a crisis, and scientists especially should be careful of contributing to the crisis mentality that seems to permeate our culture these days. The norms of body form and adiposity have changed many times over history. Some of the changes, especially as they have related to women, are not biologically sound or health based, and health-based guidelines for human adiposity are what is needed. Still, as Flegal (2006, page 74) noted, the increase in human obesity "does have some characteristics of an epidemic." This conclusion does not negate or override the cautions brought up by researchers who disagree. Health is a multidimensional parameter; BMI and even percent body fat will explain only part of the variation in people's health. What is true is that humanity has changed quite dramatically in BMI over the last few decades, and this change appears likely to continue worldwide for the near future.

Table 7.2 U.S. 2014 Obesity Prevalence by State and the District of Columbia

State	Obesity prevalence (%)	State	Obesity prevalence (%)
Colorado	18.6	Illinois	26.5
Washington, D.C.	19.7	Delaware	27.0
Connecticut	20.6	Georgia	27.2
Massachusetts	21.4	Nebraska	27.2
Hawaii	22.3	Pennsylvania	27.4
Vermont	22.8	Iowa	27.9
Oregon	23.0	North Dakota	27.9
Montana	23.2	Kansas	28.1
New Jersey	23.3	Texas	28.7
Utah	23.5	Wisconsin	28.7
New York	24.2	Ohio	28.8
Idaho	24.5	North Carolina	29.3
Minnesota	24.6	South Carolina	29.4
Rhode Island	24.6	Indiana	29.5
Wyoming	24.6	Michigan	29.6
Alaska	24.8	South Dakota	29.6
California	24.8	Missouri	30.0
Virginia	25.0	Arkansas	30.5
New Mexico	25.1	Alabama	31.0
Florida	25.2	West Virginia	31.1
Arizona	25.5	Oklahoma	31.4
New Hampshire	25.7	Kentucky	31.5
Maine	25.8	Tennessee	32.3
Nevada	25.8	Louisiana	33.0
Maryland	26.2	Mississippi	34.4
Washington	26.4		

Data from CDC 2015.

Summary

Human obesity has ancient origins but was at low prevalence for most of our evolutionary history. The rapidly increasing prevalence of obesity indicates that novel risk factors have been created in the modern world. Adipose tissue sequesters lipid (fat) to prevent lipotoxicity and provide a store of metabolic energy for periods of deprivation. Adipose is endocrinologically active, and can affect metabolism and physiology directly and indirectly by the release of hormones and cytokines. These are all adaptive functions necessary for health. Obesity is an unhealthy excess of adipose tissue. It is associated with an increased inflammatory state, in part due to inflammatory cytokines released by adipose. The metabolic dysregulation from obesity creates an allostatic load on the individual's physiology, leading to eventual pathology. Men and women differ in their proportion of adipose tissue, its distribution on the body, and the propensity to store, mobilize, and metabolize fat. On average, women have larger stores of subcutaneous fat, are more likely to have large adipose stores in thighs and buttocks, and are less likely to have abdominal fat than are men. Central obesity, excess adipose tissue in the abdominal region, is associated with higher risks of metabolic disease. Sedentary behavior may have had adaptive value in the past, when it was constrained by circumstances to be infrequent and of short duration. The modern environment allows and even requires more sedentary behavior of longer duration. Obesity and sedentary behavior are risk factors for each other. Both obesity and sedentary behavior also are associated with an increased risk of vitamin D deficiency. The epidemic of obesity and the substantial increase in the amount of time people spend sitting are both important factors in the unfortunate increase in the prevalence of metabolic disease in modern humans.

KEY CONCEPTS

▶ **Adipose tissue:** The main depot for fat storage on the body. It consists of adipocytes that store lipid, connective tissue, and macrophages and other cells that produce immunological and endocrine factors. Adipose tissue is thus an endocrine organ as well as a fat storage organ.

▶ **Allostatic load:** The breakdown of physiology and even tissue due to the continuous upregulation of regulatory mechanisms attempting to maintain physiology and metabolism within viable parameters. Allostatic load is often referred to as the wear and tear on the body due to adaptive physiological responses that become dysregulated or upregulated beyond their normal levels or timescales. Circumstances under which the maladaptive upregulation of these adaptive responses can arise include repeated or chronic challenges to the organism's viability, a failure of the adaptive regulatory response to solve the challenge that results in continual activation of a normally short-term physiological response, and uncertainty in the environment that causes habitual anticipatory responses to challenges that might not then occur.

▶ **Body mass index (BMI):** The body mass of a person in kg divided by their height in m^2. Normal BMI is generally defined as between 18 and 25 kg/m^2, overweight between 25 and 30 kg/m^2, and obesity as 30 kg/m^2 or greater; below 18 kg/m^2, a person can be considered unhealthily lean.

▶ **Central obesity:** Excess adipose tissue in the abdominal region, often with substantial visceral fat in addition to subcutaneous fat. Associated with higher risks of type 2 diabetes, hypertension, dyslipidemia, and cardiovascular disease in both men and women.

▶ **Epidemic:** A rapid spread or increase in the occurrence of something, affecting or tending to affect a disproportionately large number of people within a population, community, or region at the same time.

▶ **Mismatch paradigm:** Because the modern environment differs substantially in many ways from that of our ancestors, our evolved biological responses may be out of sync with our modern-day challenges. Our physiological responses to modern circumstances may not always be appropriate. We are evolved to respond to challenges that rarely occur in the modern world (e.g., extreme hunger, the need for constant exertion) and have not evolved responses to some of the challenges to health we now face (e.g., moderating intake of highly palatable foods, sitting for long periods of time). The congruence between the mismatch paradigm and allostatic load is fairly straightforward; the more an organism's biology and physiology is a mismatch for its environment, the greater the allostatic load.

▶ **Obesity:** An unhealthy excess of adipose tissue on the body. In epidemiology, it is often measured by use of BMI, with a BMI equal to or greater than 30 kg/m^2 defined as obese.

STUDY QUESTIONS

1. What are the differences among metabolic obesity, sociocultural obesity, and environmental obesity?

2. What is the difference between homeostasis and allostasis?

3. Describe the concept of the mismatch paradigm within the context of obesity.

4. List three adaptive functions of adipose tissue.

5. How do men and women generally differ in the patterns of fat deposition on their bodies?

6. Are some patterns of fat deposition considered healthier than others?

7. Describe at least two ways adipose tissue influences circulating steroid hormones.

8. How might sedentary behavior contribute to vitamin D deficiency?

9. Is the rate of increase in worldwide obesity sufficient to be labeled an epidemic?

CHAPTER 8

SEDENTARY BEHAVIOR AND INCIDENT DIABETES

Carl J. Caspersen, PhD, MPH; and G. Darlene Thomas, BA

The reader will gain an overview of epidemiological evidence from prospective observational cohort studies of sedentary behavior and incident diabetes and its potential relevance to public health. By the end of this chapter, the reader should be able to do the following:

▸ Understand the public health burden of diabetes in the United States

▸ Identify risk factors that influence the development of diabetes

▸ Understand what epidemiologic evidence reveals about the association between sedentary behavior and incident diabetes, especially regarding dose response

▸ Understand what other variables and biases may explain the association between sedentary behavior and incident diabetes

▸ Understand the use of criteria for inferring a potential causal association between sedentary behavior and incident diabetes

In 1996, the United States Surgeon General's Report on Physical Activity and Health (U.S. Department of Health and Human Services 1996) concluded that physical activity reduces the risk of incident diabetes. This association compared population levels of the least active with the most active people on a physical activity continuum assessed mainly during leisure time. From this evidence, it became clear that being the least active person in one's society increases one's future diabetes risk. More recently, it has been noted that there is a very weak correlation between time spent being physically active in leisure time versus time spent in sedentary pursuits like television (TV) viewing (Hu et al. 2003). This suggests that there might be a unique association between sedentary behavior and diabetes incidence. Such an association is important because Americans spend large amounts of time in sedentary pursuits. For example, Americans spent almost 34 hours per week watching TV in 2012 (Nielsen Company 2012). Also, from 1960 to 2008, the prevalence of sedentary (<2.0 METs) jobs increased from about 15% to 23% (Church et al. 2011) (a MET represents the metabolic cost of resting quietly). As Ainsworth et al. note, "For a reference adult, 1 MET is approximately 3.5 ml oxygen·kg^{-1} body weight·min^{-1} or 1 kcal·kg^{-1}·h^{-1} body weight" (2011, page 1577). Also, McKenzie and Rapino (2011) indicated that American workers reported a mean one-way travel time to work of slightly under 22 minutes in 1980, which increased to roughly 25 minutes by 2005 and remained at that level until 2009. For that final year, slightly more than 2% of workers spent 90 minutes or more traveling to work.

Understanding the unique influence of sedentary behavior on diabetes may help in identifying and implementing public health efforts that could reduce the future burden of diabetes in the United States or any other modern society. This chapter examines epidemiological evidence from four prospective observational cohort studies detailing multiple levels of sedentary behavior and incident type 2 diabetes with a goal of identifying dose–response relationships while highlighting limitations that might explain noted associations. This chapter concludes by applying criteria to assess whether a causal inference exists for the association between sedentary behavior and diabetes that might warrant public health action.

Diabetes and Its Public Health Burden

The Centers for Disease Control and Prevention (CDC) defines diabetes mellitus as a condition characterized by high amounts of blood glucose arising from defects in insulin production, insulin action, or both that occurs when there is limited production of, or reduced capacity to use, insulin (a hormone that facilitates the transfer of glucose into cells to be converted to energy) (2014). The American Diabetes Association (ADA) has established that diabetes is determined by a blood glucose test result of ≥126 mg/dl following an overnight fast or ≥200 mg/dl after a 2-hour oral glucose tolerance test or a hemoglobin A1c level of ≥6.5% (2013a). The latter test does not require fasting. Along with diabetes symptoms (e.g., frequent urination, excessive thirst, unexplained weight loss), a casual plasma glucose value of ≥200 mg/dl may also reveal the presence of diabetes. Two principle types of diabetes exist. Type 1 usually presents during childhood or adolescence and occurs through autoimmune destruction of pancreatic beta cells, making insulin unavailable. Type 2 is associated with obesity and physical inactivity and usually appears in adults 40 years and older. Type 2 arises when cells become resistant to the effects of insulin and when there is a relative insulin deficiency. Type 2 accounts for 90% to 95% of all cases. Thus, this chapter is limited to type 2 diabetes.

In 2012, 29.1 million Americans (or 9.3% of the U.S. population) had diabetes (CDC 2014). In 2012, about 1.7 million diabetes cases were newly diagnosed among American adults aged 20 years and older (CDC 2014). National survey data from 1997 to 2003 suggest that the incidence of diagnosed diabetes among American adults aged 18 to 79 years increased by 41% (from 4.9 to 6.9 per 1,000 population) (Geiss et al. 2006). Projections that allow for increased aging of Americans and expected changes in race/ethnic composition suggest that diabetes prevalence of adults ages 18 to 79 years will rise to as much as 33% by 2050 (Boyle et al. 2010). Normal aging processes are hastened among people with diabetes (Aronson 2003; Ulrich and Cerami 2001), resulting in shorter life expectancy of as much as 8 years for adults aged 55 to 64 years and 4 years for those aged 65 to 74 (Gu et al. 1998; Narayan et al. 2006).

Unfortunately, diabetes and its complications (e.g., cardiovascular, physical function, problems with feet, eyes, and kidneys) produce large economic costs (Engelgau et al. 2004). In 2012, total diabetes costs in the United States amounted to almost $245 billion, with $176 billion attributed to direct medical costs and $68.6 billion to indirect costs (ADA 2013b). The latter costs include disability, work loss, and premature death. For the same year, Americans with diagnosed diabetes had medical expenditures estimated to be 2.3 times higher than for expenditures among people without diabetes, with annual diabetes-related expenditures higher still for older diabetic patients due to more use of medications, medical services, and home care.

Key Risk Factors

Current risk tests from the National Diabetes Education Program include questions on these factors and on sex, blood pressure, and inactivity (2012). Risk factors for type 2 diabetes include race/ethnicity, family history of diabetes, history of gestational diabetes, impaired glucose metabolism, older age, physical inactivity, and obesity (CDC 2014). However, a recent systematic review examined 145 risk prediction models and scores and determined that "there is no universal ideal risk score, as the utility of any score depends not merely on its statistical properties but also on its context of use" (Noble et al. 2011, page 6). Regardless of presumed relative importance of diabetes risk factors, only impaired glucose metabolism, BMI, and inactivity are modifiable; therefore, these factors are likely candidates for targeted public health interventions that improve diet and increase leisure-time activity. Independent of the use of physical inactivity in general, other things like sedentary behavior are not yet considered as risk factors.

Sedentary Behavior as Distinct From Physical Activity

For sedentary behavior to be seen as a unique risk factor, some definitions are helpful. Physical activity has been defined as "any bodily movement produced by skeletal muscles that results in energy expenditure" (Caspersen et al. 1985, page 126). Physical activity in daily life can be categorized into occupational, sports, conditioning, transportation,

household, or other activities. Recently, a group of 52 researchers published a letter to the editor stating the following:

> We suggest that journals formally define sedentary behaviour as any waking behaviour characterized by an energy expenditure ≤ 1.5 METs while in a sitting or reclining posture. In contrast, we suggest that authors use the term "inactive" to describe those who are performing insufficient amounts of MVPA [moderate to vigorous physical activity] (i.e., not meeting specified physical activity guidelines). (Sedentary Behavior Research Network 2012, page 544)

Because of the recency of this definition, it may not correspond to the definition of physical inactivity in the U.S. Surgeon General's Report on Physical Activity and Health (U.S. Department of Health and Human Services 1996). Likewise, earlier researchers could not use this definition; hence, we relied on their operational definitions and measures of sedentary behavior in our chapter.

Epidemiological Diabetes Research

We examined prospective epidemiologic evidence of sedentary behavior and incident diabetes. We found four cohort studies that measured multiple levels of baseline sedentary behavior among participants without previously diagnosed diabetes and with incident diabetes cases ascertained prospectively. Table 8.1 provides an overview of the measures of sedentary behavior for each study. When choosing from multiple models that have differing amounts of confounding variables, we selected those that included age, smoking, alcohol use, physical activity, dietary factors, and BMI.

Health Professionals Follow-Up Study

In 1986, the U.S. Health Professionals Follow-Up Study began following 37,918 men ages 40 to 75 years who were initially free of diabetes, cardiovascular disease, and cancer (Hu et al. 2001). In 1988, these men self-reported average weekly hours spent viewing TV or videos. Men reporting a diagnosis of diabetes received a supplemental mail

Table 8.1 Four Prospective Observational Cohort Studies Examining the Association Between Sedentary Behavior and Incident Diabetes

Study	Measures of sedentary behavior and physical activity

Health Professionals Follow-Up Study, United States (Hu et al. 2001)	▸ TV viewing (average hr/week) using the 1988 baseline questionnaire (and every 2 years thereafter) in categories of 0-1, 2-10, 11-20, 21-40, and >40
	▸ Weekly physical activity energy expenditure (MET-hr) calculated from 1986 baseline questionnaire responses (and every 2 years thereafter)
	  - Average weekly time spent walking, jogging, running, bicycling, doing calisthenics or using a rowing machine, lap swimming, or playing squash, racquetball, or tennis
	  - Walking pace (in mph) was assessed as easy or casual (<2), normal (2-2.9), brisk (3-3.9), or striding (≥4).

Nurses' Health Study, United States (Hu et al. 2003)	Time (average hr/week) from 1992 baseline questionnaire (and every 2 years thereafter) in categories of 0-1, 2-5, 6-20, 21-40, >40 for:
	  - TV or VCR viewing
	  - Other sitting at home (e.g., during reading, meal times, at desk)
	  - Sitting at work or away from home or while driving
	▸ Weekly physical activity energy expenditure (MET-hr) calculated from questionnaire responses at 1992 baseline (and every 2 years thereafter)
	  - Average weekly time spent walking, jogging, running, bicycling, doing calisthenics, aerobics, or aerobic dance, using rowing machine, lap swimming, or playing squash, racquetball, or tennis
	  - Walking pace (in mph) was assessed as easy or casual (<2), normal (2-2.9), brisk (3-3.9), or very brisk or striding (≥4).

Black Women's Health Study, United States (Krishnan, Rosenberg, and Palmer 2009)	▸ TV viewing (hr/day) using biennial questionnaire in categories of 0-1, 1-2, 3-4, ≥5 ▸ Vigorous activity (hr/week) in categories of 0-<1, 1-2, 3-4, 5-6, ≥7 ▸ Walking (hr/week) in categories of 0-<1, 1-2, 3-4, ≥5, with pace (mph) assessed as no walking, casual/strolling (<2), average/normal (2-<3), and fairly brisk (3-<4)

European Prospective Investigation into Cancer and Nutrition (EPIC)–Potsdam study, Germany (Ford et al. 2010)	TV viewing (average hr/day) during the last 12 months using baseline questionnaire in categories of <1, 1-<2, 3-<4, ≥4
	Physical strain at work specific to the following categories:
	  - Manual work, including handling of heavy objects and use of tools (e.g., plumber, electrician, carpenter)
	  - Heavy manual work. including very vigorous activity such as handling of very heavy objects (e.g., docker, miner, bricklayer, construction worker)
	▸ Physical activity (hr/week) walking, gardening, bicycling, and performing sports using self-administered questionnaire at baseline followed by a personal interview

questionnaire to confirm a case through one or more of the following:

1. Classic diabetes symptoms plus a fasting glucose ≥ 7.8 mmol/L (≥140 mg/dl) or random glucose ≥ 11.1 mmol/L (≥200 mg/dl)
2. Without symptoms, having elevated glucose concentrations on two or more different occasions
3. Treatment with hypoglycemic medications

Over 8 years of follow-up, there were 767 cases of diagnosed type 2 diabetes for 249,617 person-years of TV or video exposure. Adjustment for confounders included age, study time periods, cigarette smoking, parental history of diabetes, alcohol consumption, and physical activity (see table 8.2). With these adjustments, the relative risk (RR) of diabetes increased with average weekly hours of TV viewing. Comparing extreme contrasts for this adjusted model but also including body mass index (BMI) reduced the RR by almost 20% to 2.31 (p for trend = 0.01), while added adjustments for dietary saturated fat, monounsaturated fat, polyunsaturated fat, trans-fatty acids, and cereal fiber reduced the RR by 22% to 2.23 (p for trend = 0.02). Evaluating adjustment for confounding variables is critical in any prospective observational cohort study to consider more correctly the veracity of the identified association. For example, when finding that adjustment for other variables substantially reduces or renders nonsignificant the effect (e.g., RR), then one must assume that these factors have importantly influenced the association between baseline exposure to sedentary behavior and incident diabetes.

Table 8.2 Health Professionals Follow-Up Study Analysis

TV viewing (hr/week) [%]	Relative risk of incident diabetes (95% CI) [change in risk (%)]	p-value for linear trend	Model adjustments for confounding variables
0-1 [6.7] 2-10 [57.1] 11-20 [25.1] 21-40 [10.5] >40 [0.7]	1.00 1.63 (1.13-2.35) [63] 1.61 (1.10-2.36) [61] 2.16 (1.45-3.22) [116] 3.02 (1.53-5.93) [202]	<0.001	Multivariate with age, study time, cigarette smoking, parental history of diabetes, and alcohol consumption
0-1 [6.7] 2-10 [57.1] 11-20 [25.1] 21-40 [10.5] >40 [0.7]	1.00 1.66 (1.15-2.39) [66] 1.64 (1.12-2.41) [64] 2.16 (1.45-3.22) [116] 2.87 (1.46-5.65) [187]	<0.001	Above multivariate model with PA quintiles
0-1 [6.7] 2-10 [57.1] 11-20 [25.1] 21-40 [10.5] >40 [0.7]	1.00 1.51 (1.05-2.19) [51] 1.44 (0.98-2.11) [44]nsd 1.83 (1.23-2.74) [83] 2.31 (1.17-4.56) [131]	0.01	Above multivariate model with PA quintiles and BMI
0-1 [6.7] 2-10 [57.1] 11-20 [25.1] 21-40 [10.5] >40 [0.7]	1.00 1.49 (1.03-2.15) [49] 1.39 (0.95-2.05) [39]nsd 1.77 (1.18-2.64) [77] 2.23 (1.13-4.39) [123]	0.02	Above multivariate model with PA quintiles, BMI, and dietary restrictions

BMI = body mass index, CI = confidence interval, nsd = nonsignificant difference, PA = physical activity

Data from Hu et al. 2001.

In the latter case, it may very well prove to be the primary variable explaining the association.

Hu and colleagues (2001) also examined RRs of incident diabetes for increasing quartiles of weekly TV viewing (hr/week) when stratified by quartiles of increasing physical activity (MET-hr/week categories) (see table 8.3). The referent category was the most active group (e.g., ≥46 MET-hr/week) having the lowest TV viewing rate (e.g., <3.5 hr/week).

Although neither error bars nor test statistics were offered to compare individual estimates, the tendency across rows was to see increasing RRs for increasing quartiles of TV viewing, with smaller estimates row to row as quartiles of physical activity increased. Interestingly, the lowest physical activity quartile (e.g., <10 MET-hr/week) included the minimal amount of physical activity currently recommended for health (e.g., 8.75 MET-hr/week for 2.5 hr/week of moderate-intensity activity of 3.5 METS) (U.S. Department of Health and Human Services, Physical Activity Guidelines, 2008), while the highest quartile (e.g., ≥46 MET-hr/week) was 5.4 times the recommended level. Hence, Hu's 2001 questionnaire results suggest an extremely active sample, which should be kept in mind when evaluating the generalizability of these data.

Nurses' Health Study

From 1992 to 1998, the Nurses' Health Study followed 68,497 women aged 30 to 55 years from 11 American states who were initially free of diabetes, cardiovascular disease, or cancer (Hu et al. 2003). These women self-reported their average hourly weekly sitting time while at home viewing TV or videos; at work, away from home, or driving; and at home while reading, eating, or sitting at a desk (see table 8.4). During follow-up, 1,515 women who reported having diabetes completed a supplemental questionnaire confirming diabetes using symptoms and reported blood tests or hypoglycemic medications, as Hu and colleagues (2001) also did. Average weekly TV viewing significantly increased type 2 diabetes risk following adjustment for physical activity. Additional adjustments for the dietary variables of glycemic load, polyunsaturated fatty acid, trans fat, and cereal fiber slightly reduced the RR by less than 4% to 1.70. Further adjustment for BMI substantially attenuated the RRs to nonsignificance. For extreme categories of sitting at work and also of other sitting at home exclusive of TV viewing, when adjusting for physical activity, there was a significantly increased diabetes risk of 1.51 for both sedentary behavioral definitions.

Table 8.3 Relative Risks for Incident Diabetes for Quartiles of TV Viewing and Physical Activity

Quartiles (Q) of physical activity [MET-hr/week]	Quartiles (Q) of TV viewing [hr/week]			
	Q1 [<3.5]	Q2 [3.6-8.0]	Q3 [8.1-15]	Q4 [>15]
Q1 [<10]	1.92	2.23	2.36	2.92
Q2 [10.0-23.5]	1.65	1.71	1.83	2.12
Q3 [23.6-45.9]	1.11	1.36	1.29	1.67
Q4 [≥46]	1.00	1.26	1.09	1.37

Data from Hu et al. 2001.

Additional adjustments for dietary variables produced no important changes in the RRs for the extreme contrast: 1.48 and 1.54, respectively. Adjustments for BMI were not discussed. Diabetes risk increased for each 2-hour increase in sitting during TV viewing of 14% (95% confidence interval [CI]: 5%-23%) increasing by 7% (95% CI, 0%-16%) for sitting while at work (that latter has a confidence interval whose lower bound represents no change, however).

Black Women's Health Study

From 1995 to 2005, the Black Women's Health Study followed 45,668 participants aged 21 to 69 years, during which 2,928 incident cases of type 2 diabetes emerged for 182,994 person-years of follow-up (Krishnan, Rosenberg, and Palmer 2009) (see table 8.5). The women of the sample "were enrolled through postal questionnaires mailed to subscribers of *Essence* magazine, members of several professional organizations, and friends and relatives of early respondents" (page 428). Using Cox proportional hazards models, women who reported ≥5 hours compared to <1 hour of daily TV viewing had an incidence rate ratio of 1.86 independent of physical activity levels (both vigorous physical activity and walking), energy intake, and other covariate adjustments (see table 8.5), but not adjusting for specific dietary variables or BMI. For the same extremes of TV viewing, the incident rate ratio was highest for those in the lowest BMI category (<25 kg/m²) (e.g., 2.49) compared with that for the highest BMI category (>35 kg/m²) (e.g., 1.59). Data for incidence rates were not offered, but this seemingly counterintuitive finding might have arisen, for example, when otherwise identical absolute changes between extreme BMI categories resulted in a higher rate ratio when lower rates of diabetes development occurred for the leaner context compared to higher rates for the heavier context. This, nonetheless, suggests that future research should try to replicate this finding with other data.

EPIC Potsdam Study

The European Prospective Investigation into Cancer and Nutrition (EPIC)–Potsdam Study (see table 8.6) followed 9,167 men aged 40 to 65 and 14,688 women aged 35 to 65 for an average of 7.8 years, during which 927 self-reported cases of incident diabetes were verified by contacting the patient's attending physician (Ford et al. 2010). There were 186,355 person-years of follow-up for this cohort. The adjusted hazard ratio (HR) for diabetes among those whose daily hours of TV viewing were ≥4 versus <1 was 1.84 when adjusting for age, sex, educational status, smoking status, alcohol use, and occupational and other physical activity (based on hr/week spent in walking, gardening, bicycling, and doing sport). When the model was additionally adjusted for total energy intake and a variety of dietary variables, including whole-grain bread, fruits and vegetables, and total fat, the HR was virtually unchanged (1.83). While maintaining these prior adjustments and adding BMI, the HR declined by 37% to 1.15, becoming a nonsignificant association.

Taken as a whole, the four prospective studies of sedentary behavior and incident diabetes were relatively recent findings—published between 2001 (Hu et al. 2001) and 2010 (Ford et al. 2010). Only one study gathered data beginning as far back as 1986 (Hu et al. 2001). The average years of follow-up from baseline sedentary behavior assessment to incident diabetes cases ranged from 6 (Hu et al. 2003) to 10 (Krishnan, Rosenberg, and Palmer 2009), for a total of 853,486 person-years of exposure for the TV viewing results alone. The four studies contained data from 176,938 men and women, with the latter contributing almost 73% to

Table 8.4 Nurses' Health Study Analysis

Time spent (hr/week) [%]	Relative risk of incident diabetes (95% CI) / [change in risk (%)]	p-value for linear trend	Model adjustments for confounding variables
TV viewing			
0-1 [7] 2-5 [24.6] 6-20 [52.4] 21-40 [13.9] >40 [2.1]	1.00 1.10 (0.86-1.41) [10][nsd] 1.33 (1.06-1.68) [33] 1.49 (1.16-1.92) [49] 1.77 (1.24-2.52) [77]	<0.001	Multivariate with age, hormone use, cigarette smoking, family history of diabetes, alcohol consumption, and physical activity (METs in quintiles)
0-1 [7] 2-5 [24.6] 6-20 [52.4] 21-40 [13.9] >40 [2.1]	1.00 1.09 (0.85-1.39) [9][nsd] 1.30 (1.03-1.63) [30] 1.44 (1.12-1.85) [44] 1.70 (1.20-2.43) [70]	<0.001	Above multivariate model plus dietary variables
Other sitting at home			
0-1 [3.7] 2-5 [25.9] 6-20 [56.3] 21-40 [11.6] >40 [2.5]	1.00 0.87 (0.67-1.13) [−13][nsd] 1.12 (0.77-1.28) [12][nsd] 1.13 (0.71-1.25) [13][nsd] 1.51 (1.10-2.19) [51]	0.003	Multivariate with age, hormone use, cigarette smoking, family history of diabetes, alcohol consumption, and physical activity (METs in quintiles)
0-1 [3.7] 2-5 [25.9] 6-20 [56.3] 21-40 [11.6] >40 [2.5]	1.00 0.87 (0.67-1.13) [−13][nsd] 0.98 (0.76-1.26) [−2][nsd] 0.94 (0.70-1.24) [−6][nsd] 1.54 (1.10-2.18) [54]	0.004	Above multivariate model plus dietary variables
Other sitting at work, away from home, and while driving			
0-1 [7.9] 2-5 [30.8] 6-20 [45.3] 21-40 [12.9] >40 [3.2]	1.00 1.00 (0.82-1.21) [0][nsd] 1.12 (0.92-1.35) [12][nsd] 1.13 (0.90-1.42) [13][nsd] 1.51 (1.11-2.04) [51]	0.004	Multivariate with age, hormone use, cigarette smoking, family history of diabetes, alcohol consumption, and physical activity (METs in quintiles)
0-1 [7.9] 2-5 [30.8] 6-20 [45.3] 21-40 [12.9] >40 [3.2]	1.00 0.99 (0.81-1.20) [−1][nsd] 1.10 (0.91-1.33) [10][nsd] 1.12 (0.89-1.41) [12][nsd] 1.48 (1.10-2.01) [48]	0.005	Above multivariate model plus dietary variables

CI = confidence interval, METs = metabolic equivalent hours, nsd = nonsignificant difference

Data from Hu et al. 2003.

the results and two studies based solely on women (Hu et al. 2003; Krishnan, Rosenberg, and Palmer 2009). This is important because the Potsdam study (Ford et al. 2010) noted that the proportion of women increased significantly for increasing TV viewing categories; hence, exposure may be higher for women than for men. Although not addressed in these four prospective studies, several cross-sectional studies suggest that the effects of TV viewing on glycemic status and insulin resistance may be greater for women than for men (Dunstan et al. 2004; Dunstan et al. 2005; Dunstan et al. 2007; Healy et al. 2008). As such, summary conclusions from the four studies might have been different had

they represented equal numbers of men and women. The age in years of study participants ranged from 21 (Krishnan, Rosenberg, and Palmer 2009) to 75 (Hu et al. 2003), with mean ages across TV viewing categories 53.1 to 60.8 years for male health professionals (Hu et al. 2001), 56.1 to 61 years for female nurses (Hu et al. 2003), 38.4 to 37.9 years for black women (Krishnan, Rosenberg, and Palmer 2009), and 46.8 to 54.1 years for German men and women (Ford et al. 2010). The size of RRs or HRs for TV viewing alone ranged from 1.77 (Hu et al. 2003) to 2.87 (Hu et al. 2001).

We also tabled estimates from models that included BMI or that used BMI as a stratifying variable.

Table 8.5 Black Women's Health Study Analysis

BMI (kg/m2) category	TV viewing (hr/day) [%]	Hazard ratio of incident diabetes (95% CI) [change in risk (%)]	p–value for linear trend	Model adjustments for confounding variables
All BMI groups	0-<1 [9] 1-2 [37.3] 3-4 [37.1] ≥5 [16.6]	1.0 1.43 (1.19-1.71) [43] 1.53 (1.28-1.83) [53] 1.86 (1.54-2.24) [86]	<0.0001	Multivariate with age, study time, cigarette smoking, family history of diabetes, alcohol consumption, years of education, family income, marital status, energy intake, coffee consumption, vigorous activity, and walking
<25	0-<1 1-2 3-4 ≥5	1.0 1.64 (0.84-3.19) [64]nsd 1.71 (0.87-3.34) [71]nsd 2.49 (1.24-5.02) [149]	0.01	Same as for all BMI groups
25-29	0-<1 1-2 3-4 ≥5	1.0 1.42 (1.01-2.00) [42] 1.41 (1.00-1.98) [41]nsd 1.57 (1.09-2.25) [57]	ns	Same as for all BMI groups
30-34	0-<1 1-2 3-4 ≥5	1.0 1.08 (0.78-1.49) [08]nsd 1.10 (0.80-1.52) [10]nsd 1.29 (0.92-1.81) [29]nsd	ns	Same as for all BMI groups
>35	0-<1 1-2 3-4 ≥5	1.0 1.37 (1.00-1.89) [37]nsd 1.35 (0.99-1.86) [35]nsd 1.59 (1.15-2.19) [59]	0.01	Same as for all BMI groups

BMI = body mass index, CI = confidence interval, ns = a nonsignificant dose response, nsd = nonsignificant difference

Data from Krishnan, Rosenberg, and Palmer, 2009.

In the specific case of the Black Women's Health Study (Krishnan, Rosenberg, and Palmer 2009), we selected adjusted results for the BMI category of 25 to 29 kg/m^2 (e.g., 1.57), because this category most reflected the mean BMI for all black women in the categories of <1 hour per day of TV viewing (26.5 kg/m^2) and ≥5 hours per day (29.1 kg/m^2). Across all four studies of TV viewing, the percent reductions in effect size after adjusting for BMI was –19.5% (2.87 versus 2.31) for Hu and colleagues (2001), –33.9% (1.77 versus 1.17) for Hu and colleagues (2003), –15.6% (1.86 versus 1.57) for Krishnan, Rosenberg, and Palmer (2009), and –37.2% (1.83 versus 1.15 for Ford et al. 2010)—roughly a 27% reduction across all four studies. Regardless, effect sizes following BMI adjustment remained significant only for Hu and colleagues (2001) and Krishnan, Rosenberg, and Palmer (2009). Hence, BMI may be explaining much of the noted association between TV viewing and incident diabetes.

Dose Response

Figure 8.1 presents the dose–response data for six sets of study estimates—one for TV viewing from each of the four studies and two for non-TV sedentary behavior from Hu and colleagues (2003). We graphed estimates from models using multivariate adjustment for age, physical activity, and other available confounders, but included diet-adjusted data only from Hu and colleagues (2003) and Ford and colleagues (2010). We could not include diet-adjusted data from Hu and colleagues (2001) because they simultaneously adjusted for BMI, which they presumed might be in the causal pathway. The lines generally show increases in incident diabetes risk for increases in sedentary behavior using Xs as markers to reflect point estimates that were significantly (p < 0.05) greater than the referent category (see black horizontal line). The referent group was set at 0.14 hours per day (e.g., 1 hr/week ÷ 7 days/week) for

Table 8.6 EPIC Potsdam Study Analysis

TV viewing (hr/day) [%]	Hazard ratio of incident diabetes (95% CI) [change in risk (%)]	p-value for linear trend	Model adjustments for confounding variables
<1 [11.5] 1-<2 [30.3] 2-<3 [34] 3-<4 [16.5] ≥4 [7.8]	1.00 1.23 (0.91-1.65) [23][nsd] 1.35 (1.01-1.80) [35] 1.86 (1.38-2.52) [86] 1.84 (1.32-2.57) [84]	<0.001	Multivariate with age, cigarette smoking, alcohol consumption, educational status, occupational activity, and physical activity
<1 [11.5] 1-<2 [30.3] 2-<3 [34] 3-<4 [16.5] ≥4 [7.8]	1.00 1.22 (0.91-1.65) [22][nsd] 1.34 (1.00-1.79) [34][nsd] 1.84 (1.36-2.48) [84] 1.83 (1.31-2.55) [83]	<0.001	Above multivariate model plus dietary variables
<1 [11.5] 1-<2 [30.3] 2-<3 [34] 3-<4 [16.5] ≥4 [7.8]	1.00 1.11 (0.82-1.50) [11][nsd] 1.12 (0.84-1.51) [12][nsd] 1.38 (1.01-1.88) [38] 1.15 (0.81-1.64) [15][nsd]	ns	Above multivariate model plus dietary variables, SBP, and BMI

BMI = body mass index, CI = confidence interval, ns = a nonsignificant dose response, nsd = nonsignificant difference, SBP = systolic blood pressure. Two models shown in the table adjusting for dietary variables consider different variables.

Data from Ford et al. 2010.

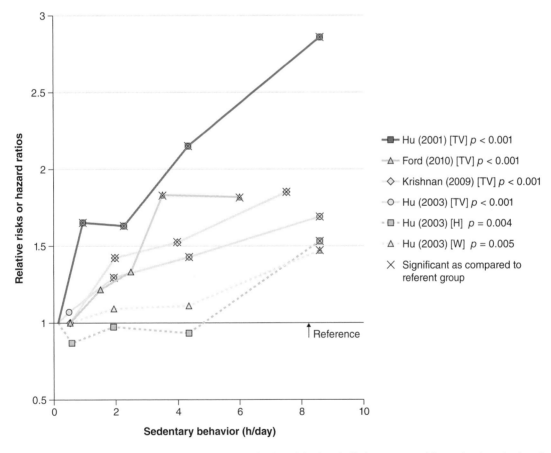

Figure 8.1 Partially-adjusted* dose–response relationship for daily hours spent in sedentary behavior with incident diabetes risk for six prospective study estimates of persons initially free of diabetes, 2001-2010.** TV = Television viewing, H = Sedentary at home, not TV, W = Sedentary at work or driving.

*Graphed results included adjustment only for age, family history of diabetes, smoking, alcohol, diet, physical activity, and other available confounders, except the results for Hu and colleagues (2001), which did not include diet, and for those of Ford and colleagues (2010), which did not include family history of diabetes. These lines do not include more complete adjustment for BMI.

**The p-values from tests for linear trends across time categories are < 0.0001 (Krishnan, 2009), < 0.001 (Hu, 2001; Ford, 2010; Hu 2003, *TV*), = 0.004 (Hu, 2003, *H*), and = 0.005 (Hu, 2003, *W*).

Hu and colleagues (2001) and Hu and colleagues (2003) and roughly 0.5 hours per day for Krishnan, Rosenberg, and Palmer (2009) and Ford and colleagues (2010). To create a single graphing point for all studies with unbounded upper categories, we used 1.5 times the value of the cut-off point demarcating the highest applicable TV viewing category. For example, for Ford and colleagues (2010), the largest category was ≥4 hours per day, so we used 6 hours per day. For non-TV sedentary behavior, only about 9 hours per day was a significant threshold for increased incident diabetes risk. Otherwise, for all four studies of TV viewing except one (Hu et al. 2001), there was a significantly increased risk for incident diabetes that most often was found at about 2 or more hours per day. Please note that this graph is a generous view of all of the associations because the graphed data were not adjusted for BMI, an important confounding variable that explains much or in some cases all of the effect (Ford et al. 2010; Hu et al. 2003).

Research Limitations

One potential limitation might arise for two studies that used extreme contrasts of TV viewing categories of ≥40 versus <1 hours per week (Hu et al. 2003; Hu et al. 2001). The highest category was composed of just 0.7% (Hu et al. 2001) and 2.1% (Hu et al. 2003) of their samples and the lowest category was composed of only 6.7% and 7.0%, respectively. Using these explicit categories of weekly TV viewing might seem more meaningful than using cut-off points to form quartiles from sample distributions that will vary from study to study and sample to sample. However, one must wonder if using such small proportions of sample participants for the highest viewing category (equivalent to weekly hours spent in a full-time job) might have spuriously inflated effect sizes to unrealistic levels. Another issue is that these two studies use different time groupings than Krishnan, Rosenberg, and Palmer (2009) and Ford and colleagues (2010), making it difficult to compare results across studies. This signals the need for less extreme time groupings and standardization for future studies.

Another limitation might be how one views evidence of a dose response. One study (Hu et al. 2003) presented a statistically significant linear dose response driven solely on the significant increased risk of developing diabetes when comparing hours per week of other non-TV activities—sitting at home, sitting at work, and driving (≥40 versus <1 hr/week)—because RRs for the two intermediate categories were at or below the risk for the referent category. As such, the significant extreme category is really an outlier (see lines for non-TV data in figure 8.1). For the linear trend to be useful, one should also report the interpolated relative risk for the extreme category, which would be closer to 1.1.

Confounding may have influenced the association between baseline exposure to sedentary behavior and incident diabetes. As noted earlier, we selected model estimates of incident diabetes risk that made adjustment at least for age, physical activity, BMI, and diet. Adjusting for age is critical in understanding the association between sedentary behavior and incident diabetes because average age tends to be higher with increases in TV viewing (Ford et al. 2010; Hu et al. 2001; Hu et al. 2003; Krishnan, Rosenberg, and Palmer 2009) and the risk of developing diabetes also increases with age (Noble et al. 2011).

Adjusting statistically for physical activity is important because there is competition for finite amounts of leisure time, particularly between total sedentary time and physical activity time. Most of the prospective studies usually adjusted for substantive amounts of moderate- to vigorous-intensity physical activity using questionnaires. Ford and colleagues (2010) additionally adjusted for occupational activity. Because questionnaire space is limited, light activities tend not to be measured, yet its adjustment is critical because light activities are the most likely behaviors by which one would break up time spent in sedentary behavior. When adjustment for light-intensity activity is not performed, it is not possible to argue sedentary behavior as a unique risk factor. Unfortunately, such adjustment will not be easy because Healy and colleagues (2011) found, when using accelerometers, near-perfect inverse collinearity of –0.96 between light-activity participation and sedentary behavior. The resulting problem is manifested by a quote from Maher and colleagues: "There is virtually no association between sedentary behaviour and cardiometabolic biomarkers once analyses are adjusted for total physical activity. This suggests that sedentary behaviour may not have health effects independent of physical activity" (2014, page 1).

The detailed TV viewing results across the four prospective studies revealed that confounder adjustment for BMI reduced risk estimates by more than 25% on average and washed it out completely in two instances (Ford et al. 2010; Hu et al. 2003). This implies that BMI has a very pronounced effect on the association and raises the question of whether sedentary behavior produces diabetes through its effect on BMI. If so, adjustment should not be performed because BMI is part of the causal path. However, increased BMI, which often leads to subsequent diabetes, may result in sedentary behavior. For example, Mortensen and colleagues stated, "Our findings suggest that a high BMI is a determinant of a sedentary lifestyle but do not unambiguously support that sedentary lifestyle has an effect on later BMI changes" (2006, page 1470), while Pulsford and colleagues concluded that "Sitting time was not associated with obesity cross-sectionally or prospectively. Prior obesity was prospectively associated with time spent watching TV per week but not other types of sitting" (2013, page 132). When BMI acts as an antecedent, sedentary behavior is in the middle of an association between BMI and diabetes, and a researcher studying the association between sedentary behavior and diabetes who chooses not to adjust for BMI is ignoring a legitimate and important confounder. In all, researchers should continue adjusting for BMI as a confounder in the association between sedentary behavior and diabetes to achieve a less biased estimate of effect.

As previously noted, dietary factors are important in the association between sedentary behavior and diabetes, with all but Krishnan, Rosenberg, and Palmer (2009) making some form of dietary adjustment. This is important because Bowman (2006) showed that the amount of total calories derived from snacks, a distinct contributor to dietary behavior, increases with increasing amounts of daily TV viewing. Unfortunately, this is not the same as studying the snacking that occurs during the act of TV viewing, which has been studied in children (Robinson 1999). This more precise behavioral interrelationship is critical because Ford and Caspersen noted that "disentangling the possible effects of sedentary behaviour from those of unhealthy dietary and snacking behaviour remains a critical challenge before reaching firm conclusions or stipulating guidelines for costly interventions" (2012, page 1347).

A few other limitations are worth noting. One is that there are many different measures of sedentary behavior whose reliability and validity are often uncertain (Clark et al. 2009), which may lead to misclassification (Ford and Caspersen 2012). Another is generalizability. Results of the four prospective studies of incident diabetes relied on women, who constituted almost 75% of the data, and may not apply well to men. Importantly, Krishnan, Rosenberg, and Palmer (2009) derived their sample from subscribers to a popular magazine for black women, members of

several professional organizations, and friends and relatives of early questionnaire respondents. Finally, Hu and colleagues (2001) and Hu and colleagues (2003) have samples that do not reflect adults who are not college educated, while Ford and colleagues (2010) examined German residents. In all, because these four studies did not sample many men or older or younger adults, their results do not reflect most U.S. adults in general.

Also, each prospective study excluded self-reported diabetes at baseline before ascertaining future incident diabetes. Hence, participants with undiagnosed diabetes were not fully and accurately identified, and they may have been more likely to become a detected incident case during follow-up when disease severity or symptoms evolved. To reduce such bias, only Hu and colleagues (2001) excluded participants during the first 2 years of monitoring, but only for their physical activity analyses. At present, none of the four detailed studies of sedentary behavior performed this maneuver. To avert this critical bias, Rockette-Wagner and colleagues (2015) recently excluded preexisting diabetes among adults at high risk of developing diabetes by using blood tests at baseline. They did not use multiple TV viewing categories like the other four prospective studies, but did find a significant 3.4% increased incident diabetes risk per each hour of daily TV viewing. Even using the very extreme category of 5.7 hours per day to equate to 40 hours per week of TV viewing of Hu and colleagues (2001) and Hu and colleagues (2003), incident diabetes risk would increase by only 19% (corresponding to a hazard ratio of about 1.19) without adjustment for weight (whose adjustment rendered the association nonsignificant). Importantly, this less biased estimate is closer to meta-analytic results of HRs for five measures for all-cause mortality, cardiovascular disease, and cancer, which ranged between 1.1 and 1.2 when comparing extreme contrasts of highest to lowest sedentary time (Biswas et al. 2015). Hence, all sedentary behavior effects are very small.

Six Criteria for Assessing if a Causal Inference Exists for Sedentary Behavior and Diabetes

In viewing the existing epidemiologic evidence from prospective studies of the association between sedentary behavior and incident diabetes, it might be informative to place it within the context of criteria devised to help reach a causal inference in the absence of a randomized controlled clinical trial. Such criteria were used in the 1960s to assess a broad set of evidence to establish a causal relationship between cigarette smoking and lung cancer (Hill 1965; U.S. Public Health Service 1964). Caspersen (1989) compared the use of six criteria (in italics in the following paragraphs) for an assessment of 43 observational studies examining the association between physical activity and incident coronary heart disease (CHD) end points (Powell et al. 1987) and contrasted the results for cigarette smoking and lung cancer studies. Here we compare the former evaluation with that for sedentary behavior and incident diabetes.

For CHD prospective studies, the results were (1) *consistent* in that more than two-thirds of the 43 studies reported statistically significant associations between physical activity and CHD (Powell et al. 1987). Each of the four prospective studies of incident diabetes showed a significant association with sedentary behavior, being 100% consistent, albeit from a very small body of evidence having limited generalizability (see previous).

For CHD studies, the (2) *strength* of the association was reasonably strong, having a median RR of 1.9 for the reviewed studies. For the four diabetes studies, the size of RRs or HRs for TV viewing alone ranged from 1.77 (Hu et al. 2003) to 2.87 (Hu et al. 2001). However, after ruling out the critical bias of undetected preexisting diabetes before follow-up, Rockette-Wagner and colleagues (2015) found an increased incident diabetes risk HR equivalent to about 1.19 even though they did not use multiple TV viewing categories. Also, two of the studies of incident diabetes had RRs arising from TV viewing that may actually be overstated because of extreme TV viewing categories having contributions of only 0.7% and 2% of their entire study samples (Hu et al. 2001; Hu et al. 2003). As such, it is difficult to argue public health effects from the tails of a distribution. In light of the unbiased results of Rockette-Wagner and colleagues (2015), all other studies reflect spuriously inflated relative risks and hazard ratios that are both inaccurate and unrealistic.

More than three-quarters of the 43 CHD studies demonstrated (3) an *appropriate temporal sequence* (e.g., the assessment of exposure predated the outcome), while all four detailed diabetes studies met this criterion.

Regarding (4) *dose–response effects*, more than two-thirds of CHD studies with relevant data met this criterion, and all four diabetes studies detailing TV viewing met this criterion, but not as much so for other types of sedentary behavior that nurses reported doing (Hu et al. 2003). However, without BMI adjustment, the dose–response attributions are moot.

Numerous scientific studies supported a (5) *plausible and coherent* set of physiologic mechanisms whereby increased physical activity might have a favorable effect on CHD (Powell et al. 1987), while a few physiological mechanisms existed to support potential unfavorable diabetes outcomes associated with sedentary behavior. For example, although extreme, 5 days of prolonged bed rest in humans results in insulin resistance, as evidenced by an almost two-thirds increase in insulin response to a glucose load (Hamburg et al. 2007), and skeletal muscle, the primary insulin-sensitive tissue, accounts for almost 80% of glucose uptake under euglycemic hyperinsulinemic conditions (de Fronzo et al. 2009). Otherwise, the simple act of standing rather than maintaining a sedentary posture may generate sufficient caloric expenditure to resist fat gain in humans (Levine et al. 1999), which places a sedentary person at greater risk of developing diabetes due to increased BMI. Also, a recent experiment found that breaking up 5 hours of prolonged sitting with 2-minute breaks of light- or moderate-intensity activity every 20 minutes can reduce postprandial glucose and increase insulin response following ingestion of a 200 ml test drink containing 75 g of glucose (Dunstan et al. 2012). Although compelling, this latter finding more aptly reflects a unique physical activity mechanism and not a physiological mechanism for sedentary behavior, per se.

Regarding (6) *experimental evidence*, no randomized controlled trials existed that assigned people to physical activity and control groups and then examined CHD events. Conducting such a trial was deemed infeasible by Taylor, Buskirk, and Remington (1973). A similar absence exists for incident diabetes end points. Also, the CHD studies that used better quality measures and study designs more often reported a statistically significant inverse association (Powell et al. 1987). A quality assessment is nonexistent for the limited studies of incident diabetes. This may be important because Caspersen (1989) noted that, in making

RESEARCH RECOMMENDATIONS

Research must better define dose–response relationships between sedentary behavior and physiologic mechanisms, especially for varying frequency, length, and total time spent in breaks intended to disrupt prolonged periods of sedentary behavior. It will be particularly important to examine varying combinations of sedentary behavior from multiple domains of time use (e.g., leisure, occupational, domestic, and occupation) and to establish their relative contribution to total sedentary behavior as an overall exposure measure. Such research is critical given the limited, extremely biased, and relatively recent data that exist today.

Also, although the use of physical activity bouts may be useful in offsetting the negative effects of prolonged sitting (Dunstan et al. 2012), one must temper enthusiasm for these encouraging findings because the bouts are still physical activity—a behavior that arises from "any bodily movement produced by skeletal muscles that results in energy expenditure" (Caspersen et al. 1985, page 126). Hence, one might view the bouts as simply making use of available energy substrate, which is especially plentiful in the postprandial state, as examined by the researchers (Dunstan et al. 2012).

Future epidemiologic research must clarify the dose response of sedentary behavior and incident diabetes along with disease outcomes among people with diabetes, explore all potential confounding and mediating variables that influence the association, and expand the research to more groups that vary by race/ethnicity, age, and socioeconomic characteristics that may have different types and patterns of sedentary behavior. For example, although one study sampled relatively young black women (Krishnan, Rosenberg, and Palmer 2009), the generalizability of that study sample is suspect. Also, at present, no prospective study has adjusted for specific confounding from physical activity of any intensity occurring in the same day during which large amounts of sedentary behavior also occur. Because recommendations allow for less regular patterns of behavior to reach 2.5 hours of weekly activity participation (U.S. Department of Health and Human Services, 2008), this distinction is an important research consideration that could address concerns of collinearity and independence (Maher et al. 2015).

Because it is likely that declines in physical activity are associated with increased incident diabetes risk and because this also may lead to the transition of increasing amounts of sedentary behavior (which is also associated with increased risk), future research should seek to separate the two events and establish the relative importance of each phenomenon.

In an experiment interrupting 5 hours of prolonged sitting with 2-minute activity breaks every 20 minutes to reduce postprandial glucose, Dunstan and colleagues (2012) used a sample of 19 men and women aged 45 to 65 (mean age 53.8 years) with an average BMI of 31.2 kg/m^2. Future studies should consider contrasting sex-specific groups of younger and older adults belonging to different BMI groups (e.g., normal weight, overweight, and obese) because it is likely that activity breaks intended to be performed at absolute intensities above resting metabolic rate (RMR) will produce greater benefits among those for whom RMR levels are lowest (e.g., those of higher age, higher BMI, and of female gender) (McMurray et al. 2014).

causal inferences, it may be best to focus most on study results deemed to be of highest quality.

In comparing the ability to reach a causal inference for physical activity and CHD versus sedentary behavior and incident diabetes, the evidence for the latter is not as compelling. This is due in part to a more limited number of studies, generalizability issues, uncertainty regarding complete adjustment for legitimate confounders (especially BMI), not having ruled out undetected diabetes as an extremely critical bias, and not having unique physiological mechanisms for sedentary behavior fully independent from mechanisms that also pertain to physical activity.

Summary

Being in the group that has the least amount of physical activity and the most sedentary behavior may increase risk for incident diabetes. In the absence of randomized controlled trials, the best evidence exists in the form of prospective epidemiological studies of incident diabetes. Unfortunately, these relatively recent data and other evidence are not plentiful enough to reach a causal inference, especially when the critical bias remains from not ruling out preexisting diabetes.

One might logically conclude that breaks in periods of sedentary behavior of moderate- and even light-intensity physical activity may be a potent intervention (Dunstan et al. 2012). However, establishing the association of such an intervention on reduced incident diabetes outcomes should also be a clear goal. Some might regard this as an unnecessary effort to prove a principle, yet such evidence is important in providing policymakers with more complete information that is relevant for the allocation of limited resources. Some intervention efforts are underway to combat sedentary behavior in places like worksites, yet they may not be able to reduce incident diabetes outcomes alone. Hence, efficacy data are needed, as well as studies for establishing the relative cost-effectiveness of intervention efforts for reducing incident diabetes. This and many other gaps in knowledge should be filled with future research findings to more fully understand the association between sedentary behavior and incident diabetes.

KEY CONCEPTS

▸ **Bias**: A factor that may influence the observation under investigation. For example, if undiagnosed diabetes is more common among those who have the most sedentary behavior, then a spuriously greater association will be found between sedentary behavior and incident diabetes. To help control for this specific bias, one might exclude cases found in the first several years of observation by assuming that those with undetected diabetes will manifest the disease early.

▸ **Confounding variable**: A factor that may influence the association between exposure to sedentary behavior and incident diabetes. For example, diabetes increases with age, while the average age tends to be higher among adults engaged in greater amounts of sedentary behavior, such as TV viewing. One must therefore control for the confounding effect of age when studying the association between sedentary behavior and incident diabetes.

▸ **Criteria for drawing a causal inference**: In the absence of definitive proof, six criteria are helpful in trying to infer a causal association: (1) consistent associations, (2) strength of the association, (3) appropriate temporal sequence with assessment of exposure predating the outcome, (4) dose–response effects, (5) plausible and coherent set of physiologic mechanisms, and (6) experimental evidence.

▸ **Diabetes mellitus**: A condition characterized by high amounts of blood glucose arising from defects in insulin production, insulin action, or both that occurs when there is limited production of or reduced capacity to use insulin (a hormone that facilitates the transfer of glucose into cells to be converted to energy).

▸ **Generalizability of population sample**: A sample should represent (or generalize to) the population from which it is drawn. Associations found in samples having limited generalizability tend to pertain only to people having similar characteristics of that group, and not to the population at large.

▸ **Hazard ratio**: A measure of how often an event occurs in one group compared to how often it occurs in another contrasting group over time. Within the context of a prospective cohort study conducted for a set period of time, survival analysis compares the hazard ratios of the instantaneous risk of the occurrence of an event (e.g., the hazard), for this example, incident diabetes. The hazard rates are compared for contrasting groups, creating a hazard ratio. A hazard ratio of 1 means that there is no difference in the likelihood of surviving the occurrence of incident diabetes between the two contrasting groups. A hazard ratio of greater than 1 would mean that there is less likelihood of surviving until the occurrence of incident diabetes, say, in the group with TV viewing of 6 or more hours per day made relative to the likelihood of surviving the occurrence of incident diabetes in the group having TV viewing, for example, less than 1 hour per day.

- ▸ **Prospective observational cohort study**: This type of epidemiologic study assesses exposure to a sedentary lifestyle among participants without preexisting diabetes and then follows them over time to ascertain incident cases of diabetes. This type of study is better than a cross-sectional study for drawing inferences of a causal association between sedentary behavior and diabetes and is especially important when experiments are not available to assess causality.

- ▸ **Relative risk**: A measure of the risk of an event occurring in one group compared to the risk of the same event occurring in a contrasting group. Within the context of a prospective cohort study conducted for a set period of time, the event may be the development of incident diabetes. The cumulative risk of incident diabetes in that period can be contrasted between, for example, a group with TV viewing of 6 or more hours per day made relative to TV viewing for, say, less than 1 hour per day. When the relative risk is 1, the risk of developing incident diabetes is the same irrespective of the amount of exposure to TV viewing. A relative risk greater than 1 means that the risk of developing incident diabetes is higher in the group, in this example, with the greater amount of TV viewing.

- ▸ **Sedentary behavior**: The Sedentary Behaviour Research Network (2012) defines this as any behavior during waking hours that is characterized by energy expenditure greater than or equal to 1.5 METs while in a sitting or reclining posture; the term *inactive* should thus be used to describe those who are performing insufficient amounts of MVPA (moderate- to vigorous-intensity physical activity) (i.e., not meeting specified physical activity guidelines). TV viewing is considered to be a component of this broader definition of sedentary behavior.

STUDY QUESTIONS

1. What was the percent of the U.S. population estimated to have diabetes in 2014?
2. In 2014, how many estimated cases of newly diagnosed diabetes occurred among American adults aged 20 years and older?
3. Name three risk factors for the development of diabetes.
4. How many of the four prospective studies of incident diabetes used measures of sedentary behavior congruent with the definition recommended by the Sedentary Behaviour Research Network in 2012?
5. Name one confounding variable and one biasing factor that influences the independent association between sedentary behavior and incident diabetes.
6. What study suggests that increases in BMI might lead to increases in sedentary behavior, and how would that affect the interpretation of BMI as part of a causal pathway between sedentary behavior and incident diabetes?
7. How many of the four detailed prospective studies of sedentary behavior and incident diabetes adjusted for light-intensity as well as moderate- to vigorous-intensity physical activity? Why is it important to adjust for light-intensity physical activity to understand the independent association between sedentary behavior and incident diabetes?
8. How does the percentage of women, and the overall composition of the study samples, affect the generalizability of results of the four prospective studies?
9. At how many hours per day of TV viewing did most of the four prospective studies show a significantly increased risk for the development of incident diabetes? About how many hours do you spend watching TV each day?
10. When applying the criteria for drawing a causal inference to existing scientific evidence, can one make a causal inference between sedentary behavior and incident diabetes?

We gratefully acknowledge the very kind help and support of William I. Thomas, MLIS, in conducting literature searches and retrieving important documents. *Disclaimer*: The findings and conclusions in this chapter are those of the authors and do not necessarily represent the official position of the Centers for Disease Control and Prevention.

CHAPTER 9

SEDENTARY BEHAVIOR AND CARDIOVASCULAR DISEASE

Edward Archer, PhD; Enrique G. Artero, PhD; and Steven N. Blair, PED

The reader will gain an understanding of the relationships between sedentary behavior and cardiovascular diseases. By the end of this chapter, the reader should be able to do the following:

▸ Define the various cardiovascular diseases (CVD)

▸ Describe the role that CVD plays in global disability and mortality

▸ Understand and identify the underlying pathologies of CVD

▸ List the risk factors for atherosclerosis

▸ Explain why the prevention of CVD must begin in childhood

▸ List the sequence of events that are antecedent to myocardial and cerebral infarctions

▸ Discuss the history of the associations of sedentary behavior and inactivity with health

▸ Articulate the mechanisms by which sedentary behavior contributes to CVD

▸ Differentiate the effects of excessive sedentary behavior and low physical activity (PA)

▸ Explain the mechanisms by which PA, exercise, and cardiorespiratory fitness (CRF) may partially ameliorate the effects of excessive sedentary behavior

▸ Describe the major correlates of sedentary behavior

▸ Discuss in detail the epidemiologic research examining sedentary behavior

Cardiovascular diseases (CVD) remain the leading cause of death in the United States and throughout the world. Recent data suggest that more than 2,100 Americans die of CVD each day, an average of more than one death per minute (Go et al. 2013; Roger et al. 2012). Globally, CVD accounts for more than 10% of the total disease burden and approximately 30% of all deaths. Of the more than 17 million CVD deaths that occurred in 2008, over 3 million were early mortality, (i.e., people < 60 years of age). Although the total number of deaths attributable to CVD are expected to pass 24 million by 2030 (Mendis, Puska, and Norrving 2011), a large portion of overall CVD mortality and the majority of early CVD deaths are preventable because many of the primary risk factors are modifiable through lifestyle choices such as increases in physical activity (PA) and decreases in sedentary behavior. As such, efficacious and cost-effective public health initiatives that result in more optimal lifestyles that include adequate levels of PA and decreases in sedentary behavior may lead to major reductions in CVD mortality.

Cardiovascular Diseases

The term *CVD* subsumes a number of pathological conditions of the heart and blood vessels (see table 9.1). The categorization of the specific diseases is complex because many of the underlying disease processes (e.g., arteriosclerosis, thrombosis) are multidimensional and interdependent. Nevertheless, >75% of all CVD mortality is attributable to coronary artery disease (CAD) and cerebrovascular disease culminating in myocardial or cerebral infarctions (i.e., heart attack or stroke, respectively) (Mendis, Puska, and Norrving 2011).

Major nonmodifiable risk factors for CVD:

- Age: There is an increased risk with advancing age.
- Sex: Men have an increased risk for early CVD death compared to women.
- Familial history: People with family members who suffer from CVD have a significantly increased risk.

Modifiable risk factors for CVD:

- Smoking
- Physical inactivity or low CRF
- Hypertension (i.e., high blood pressure)

- Dyslipidemia (e.g., high LDL cholesterol, low HDL cholesterol, high triglycerides)
- Excessive alcohol consumption
- Obesity
- Diabetes (elevated blood sugar)

With the exception of smoking and alcohol consumption, PA significantly affects each of the other modifiable risk factors (Archer and Blair 2011), and there is strong evidence that increased levels of PA that lead to improvements in physical fitness significantly ameliorate the effects of smoking and excessive alcohol consumption (Blair et al. 1995).

The prevalence of CVD varies by sex, ethnicity/race, and age. In the United States, the highest prevalence of CVD is among non-Hispanic blacks (45% of men and 47% of women) followed by non-Hispanic whites (37% of men and 34% of women) and Mexican-Americans (33% of men and 31% of women) (Roger et al. 2012). In 2009, the overall rate of death attributable to CVD in the United States was 236 per 100,000 people. Mortality rates also varied by sex and ethnicity/race and were 281 and 387 per 100,000 for white and black men, respectively, and a significantly lower 190 and 268 per 100,000 for white and black women, respectively. Although the relative rate of death attributable to CVD declined by ~33% from 1999 to 2009, it still accounted for ~32% of all deaths (787,931 of 2,437,163 deaths), or 1 out of every 3 deaths in the United States. More than 153,000 Americans suffered early CVD mortality (i.e., under the age of 65) and ~34% of all deaths attributable to CVD occurred before 75 years of age; these occurrences are well below the average life expectancy of 78.5 years (Roger et al. 2012).

Although each of the risk factors plays a role in the development of CVD, the primary underlying pathophysiological factor that results in the greatest mortality (i.e., heart attacks and strokes) is atherosclerosis. In the next section, we describe the conditions under which the major risk factors predispose people to atherosclerotic processes, the development of CVD, and early morbidity and mortality.

Atherosclerosis

Atherosclerosis is a progressive disease and the underlying pathology of more than 80% of all CVD deaths in developed societies (Mendis, Puska, and Norrving 2011; Lusis 2000). It is characterized by the inflammation-driven accumulation of lipids, cholesterol, and cellular detritus within the tunica

Table 9.1 Cardiovascular Diseases and Mortality

CVD	Percent of all CVD mortality	
	Men	Women
Ischemic heart disease or coronary artery disease (CAD)	46%	38%
Cerebrovascular disease	34%	37%
Hypertensive heart diseases	6%	7%
Inflammatory heart diseases (endocarditis, myocarditis, pericarditis)	2%	2%
Congenital heart disease	2%	2%
Rheumatic heart disease	1%	1%
Other cardiomyopathies & arrhythmias	<1%	<1%
Other cardiovascular diseases	11%	14%

Data from Mendis, Puska, and Norrving 2011.

intima (i.e., lining) of the major arteries. This buildup leads to both acute and chronic luminal obstruction, reducing blood flow to major organs such as the heart and brain. These pathological processes are progressive and symptomless, and begin in early childhood (Kones 2011; Ayer and Steinbeck 2010; Truong, Maahs, and Daniels 2012; Strong et al. 1999). Research suggests that intimal lesions may occur in more than 50% of people aged 15 to 19 years, and the prevalence and extent of these lesions increase with age. These results suggest that the pathophysiological processes that clinically manifest as CVD in later life are driven by lifestyle and behavioral choices of childhood (Strong et al. 1999).

Atherosclerotic processes are a pathological response to an injury of the endothelial cells of the vasculature (Lusis 2000). A layer of endothelial cells forms the intima of the major arteries and acts as a semiselective barrier between the vessel lumen and other vascular tissue such as the lamina, media, and adventitia. The endothelium, in concert with other vascular tissues (e.g., smooth muscle), control vasodilation and vasoconstriction as well as the movement of fluids and immune system components into and out of the bloodstream (Deanfield et al. 2005). The health and function of the endothelium have numerous determinants, but the predominant factor is the fluid shear stress produced by the flow of blood in the arteries. Increases in the volume and velocity of the flow of blood during activity (e.g., exercise) increase the shear stress on the intima and improve endothelial function in much the same way that stress of resistance training improves skeletal

muscular function (Nikolaidis et al. 2012). Improvements in endothelial function decrease the risk of pathologies such as diminished vasodilation or the development of intimal lesions (i.e., injuries) that are the antecedent of atherosclerosis. Endothelial dysfunction (i.e., the loss of healthy endothelial function) is predictive of future CVD (Martin and Anderson 2009).

Atherosclerotic processes begin with an injury to the intima and are most often the result of oxidative stress from smoking (Burke and FitzGerald 2003) or the glycoxidation and glycation of nutritive molecules (e.g., fatty acids, amino acids, glucose) (Halliwell 2000; Piarulli, Sartore, and Lapolla 2012; Coccheri 2007). Once an injury (lesion) to the intima occurs, numerous molecules (e.g., fatty acids, LDL-C molecules) and immune system components such as macrophages and T-lymphocytes migrate to the site. The immune system response and consequent inflammation associated with the injury, combined with the deposition of lipids and cellular debris, lead to increasing oxidative stress through reactive oxygen species. These progressive pathological processes stimulate gene expression, cellular proliferation, and programmed cell death. The incorporation of connective tissue into the lesion results in the development of an atheroma (i.e., vascular plaque). Plaques cause the intima to become irregular (thereby disturbing the flow of blood), decrease associated shear stresses, and predispose the artery to the loss of endothelial function. As plaques increase in size, they reduce the size of the lumen, making it more difficult for blood to travel through the artery. This leads to ischemia (i.e., reduced blood flow); if this occurs in the heart, it may result in angina (i.e., ischemia-induced chest pain).

Over time, atheromas become calcified and the associated vascular smooth muscle proliferates, leading to the hardening of the affected arteries. As the plaque increases in size, it undergoes remodeling and qualitative changes (e.g., increased rigidity) that culminate in the formation of a necrotic core that is characteristic of an advanced, unstable atheroma (Rosenfeld 1998). These alterations decrease the stability (i.e., structural integrity) of the plaque, predisposing a rupture. When the plaque is deformed or overstressed from the increased cardiac output necessitated by physical exertion, it will rupture and expose the systemic vasculature and blood to lipid-rich thrombogenic (clot-producing) material. The rupture and resulting emboli may precipitate thromboses (i.e., clots) anywhere in the systemic vasculature as the cellular debris from the rupture travels throughout the body. Occlusions from thromboemboli may significantly decrease or completely obstruct blood flow to the related tissues; if they occur in the heart or brain, they will result in a myocardial infarction (MI) or stroke, respectively (Strong et al. 1999). Although most ruptures occur only in advanced, unstable atheromas, an individual may develop a rupture in an atheromatous plaque at any stage of the continuum from lesion formation to advanced, unstable atheromas (Libby 2000). The reason why age is one of the greatest predictors of CVD is because the lifestyle-related development of advanced atheromas takes many years.

Epidemiological studies over the past five decades have demonstrated that numerous interdependent factors determine a person's propensity for the progression of atherosclerotic processes and the development of CVD once an injury has occurred (see table 9.2). The effects of any combination of these risk factors are multiplicative and not simply accumulative. For example, the effects of inactivity or hypertension on the progression of atherosclerotic processes and CVD are significantly amplified when dyslipidemia (e.g., high LDL cholesterol) is also present (Lusis, Weinreb, and Drake 1998).

Coronary Artery Disease

Coronary artery disease (CAD), also known as coronary artery atherosclerosis and ischemic heart disease, is the leading cause of death as well as sudden death for men and women worldwide. Approximately 14 million Americans have CAD, and it has been the number one cause of death since the 1920s, causing >20% of all deaths each year. In 2009, 386,324 Americans died of CAD. The incidence, prevalence, and manifestations of CAD vary significantly with age, sex, and race. Age is the strongest risk factor for the development of CAD, and ~82% of people who die of CAD are 65 years or older. Approximately 8.5% of all white men, 7.9% of black men, and 6.3% of Mexican-American men have CAD, while 5.8%, 7.6%, and 5.3% of white, black, and Mexican-American women, respectively, have CAD (Roger et al. 2012). Under the age of 60, men are twice as likely to have CAD as women. People of African and Asian Indian descent have higher CAD morbidity and mortality, even after corrections for education and socioeconomic status. The risk factors experienced by those of African descent differ from that of people of European descent, with the prevalence of hypertension, obesity, metabolic diseases, and physical inactivity being much higher in those of African descent (Roger et al. 2012).

CAD is caused by atherosclerotic processes and thromboemboli that reduce and occlude the blood vessels supplying the myocardium (i.e., heart muscle). The resulting ischemia (a lack of oxygen from reduced or inhibited blood flow) may initially lead to chest pain (angina), but is often symptomless. In situations in which myocardial oxygen consumption is dramatically increased, such as intense physical exertion (e.g., shoveling heavy snow, intense sexual activity, or emotional distress), the obstruction may lead to a myocardial infarction (heart attack), a condition in which a portion of the myocardium dies. If the victim survives, the affected myocardium is replaced with collagen, an inelastic scar tissue that may significantly reduce cardiac output. If the MI was severe, the resulting injury will limit the heart's ability to efficiently pump blood and support physical functioning, such as the ability to carry out the activities of daily living.

Myocardial Infarction

A myocardial infarction (MI), commonly known as a heart attack, is the result of an occlusion in the coronary arteries that limits the flow of blood to the heart. If deprived of oxygen for an extended period, the myocardial tissue dies. This process is irreversible, and cardiac output is permanently

Table 9.2. Factors Associated With Atherosclerosis and Cardiovascular Diseases

Risk factors	Evidence
Family history of CVD	A very significant risk factor, independent of other known risk factors (Goldbourt and Neufeld 1986)
Hypertension (elevated blood pressure)	Strong epidemiological evidence exists. Clinical trials have demonstrated benefits of reductions in hypertension, with consistently strong effects on stroke (Assmann et al. 1999).
Dyslipidemia (elevated levels of triglycerides or LDL/VLDL cholesterol with reduced levels of HDL cholesterol)	Strong epidemiological evidence and supported by studies of genetic diseases and animal models (Di Angelantonio et al. 2012; Assmann and Gotto 2004)
Elevated levels of lipoprotein	Mixed epidemiological and animal model research evidence (Nordestgaard et al. 2010)
Elevated levels of homocysteine	Some epidemiological evidence exists. Animal models suggest that homocystinuria results in occlusive vascular disease (Lewington, Bragg, and Clarke 2012).
Sex	Below 60 years of age, men develop CVD at approximately twice the rate of women (Vassalle et al. 2012).
Systemic inflammation and hemostatic factors	Elevated levels of inflammatory molecules (e.g., C-reactive protein) are associated with CVD (Tabas and Glass 2013).
Environmental factors	Evidence
Smoking or tobacco use	Very strong epidemiological evidence exists. Clinical trials have demonstrated the benefit of smoking cessation (Gupta and Deedwania 2011).
Low cardiorespiratory fitness, inactivity, or high sedentary behavior	Very strong epidemiological and clinical evidence exist (Lavie et al. 2013; Wei et al. 1999). Significant independent associations with CVD present after correcting for other risk factors (Archer and Blair 2011; Beaglehole et al. 2011; Blair, Cheng, and Holder 2001). Primary prevention necessitates increased activity (Gupta and Deedwania 2011).
High-fat diet	Some epidemiological evidence exists (Siri-Tarino et al. 2010). Activity moderates the relationship between diet and CVD (Blair et al. 1996a; Vuori 2001). The absence of exercise wheels is necessary for development of advanced atherosclerosis in wild-type experimental animal models.
Diabetes, metabolic syndrome, and obesity	Strong epidemiological and clinical evidence exist and in studies with animal models (Nikolopoulou and Kadoglou 2012). Activity moderates the relationship between metabolic diseases and CVD (Blair, Cheng, and Holder 2001; Earnest et al. 2013; LaMonte et al. 2005; Wei et al. 1999). This cluster of metabolic disturbances, with insulin resistance as a prominent feature, is strongly associated with CAD (Nikolopoulou and Kadoglou 2012).
Low antioxidant levels	Evidence is suggestive but not conclusive (Xu et al. 2014).

affected. Annually, >1.5 million Americans have an MI; approximately 500,000 will die as a result. In 2009, 785,000 Americans were estimated to have suffered a first MI and about 470,000 Americans were estimated to have had a recurrent event (Roger et al. 2012; Heron et al. 2009). Additionally, it is estimated that more than 150,000 silent heart attacks occur each year, and an American will have an MI roughly every 30 to 40 seconds. Globally, MI results in more than 7.3 million deaths annually (Mendis, Puska, and Norrving 2011).

Stroke

Cerebrovascular disease and stroke occur when the major arteries that supply the brain are affected by plaques that reduce blood flow. If an arterial plaque ruptures anywhere in the systemic vasculature, the resulting emboli may travel to the cerebral arterial system and cause an occlusion. The loss of oxygenated blood to the brain causes the death of neurons and supporting microglia; the result is a stroke and an associated loss of brain function. Of the 17.3 million CVD deaths in 2008 worldwide,

6.2 million were from strokes (Mendis, Puska, and Norrving 2011). From 1999 to 2009, the relative rate of stroke mortality fell by 37% and the actual stroke mortality declined by 23%. Yet annually ~800,000 people experience an initial or recurrent stroke. In 2009, stroke was the cause of 1 of every 19 deaths in the United States, and a stroke-related death occurs every 4 minutes. As with other forms of CVD, the occurrence of stroke varies by age, sex, and ethnicity/race. Non-Hispanic blacks suffer the highest rates of stroke mortality (62 and 53 per 100,000 for men and women, respectively), followed by whites (39 per 100,000 for both men and women), and Hispanics (33 and 29 per 100,000 for men and women). Each year, ~55,000 more women have a stroke than men. This is primarily due to the fact that a greater percentage of women reach the oldest age groups, which have the highest rates of stroke. The 2009 overall death rate for stroke was 39 per 100,000, and 37, 50, 30, and 28 per 100,000 for white, black, Asian, and Hispanic women respectively. In addition to the burden of stroke mortality, the global financial burden from stroke-induced disability is substantial and increasing as health care costs increase (Norrving and Kissela 2013).

Hypertension

Hypertension, also known as high blood pressure, is a highly prevalent and significant risk factor for most forms of CVD. Globally, hypertension is responsible for more than 9 million deaths (~17% of all deaths). It is defined by a systolic pressure of ≥140 millimeters of mercury (mmHg), a diastolic pressure ≥ 90 mmHg, the use of antihypertensive pharmaceuticals, and physician diagnosis. Based on recent data, well over 70 million Americans (33% of all U.S. adults ≥ 20 years of age) have hypertension, and the prevalence is nearly equal between men and women. Recent public health surveillance efforts suggest that the prevalence of hypertension is increasing and that rates of control of blood pressure among those diagnosed remain low. Among women age 20 and older, 31% of non-Hispanic whites, 47% of non-Hispanic blacks, and 29% of Mexican Americans are hypertensive. In 2009, more than 34,000 women died from hypertension, which represented 55% of all hypertension-related deaths. The overall 2009 death rate from hypertension was >18/100,000, with >14/100,000 for white women and >38/100,000 for black women (Roger et al. 2012).

The risk for fatal and non-fatal CVD, especially CAD and cerebrovascular disease (i.e., stroke), increases progressively with higher levels of systolic or diastolic blood pressure. At any level of elevated blood pressure, the relative risks of CVD when other risk factors are present are increased substantially. In addition to CVD, hypertension also affects renal disease and all-cause mortality in a progressive manner.

Occupational Physical Activity and CVD

From the beginning of the Age of Enlightenment (early 18th century) to the 19th century, there were frequent commentaries on the relationship between sedentary occupations and chronic disease. The deleterious effects of sedentary behavior on cardiovascular health have been in print for over a century. In 1843, Dr. W.A. Guy of King's College in London compared the rate of mortality of both male and female sedentary workers with those of more physically active workers. Guy posited that sedentary lifestyles affected women as much if not more than men and demonstrated that sedentary single women had much higher mortality rates than their married counterparts. This suggested that the chores associated with hearth and home provided more activity and allowed for less sedentary time. Modern research examining the effects of housework on health parallel Guy's keen observations (Archer, Shook, et al. 2013; Archer, Lavie, et al. 2013). Dr. Edward Smith of London, a contemporary of Guy, noted in 1864 that the mortality rate among sedentary tailors was much greater than that of the more physically active agricultural workers (Smith 1864).

In 1939, O.F. Hedley examined the CVD mortality of sedentary businessmen and found that it was significantly higher than those in occupations that demanded manual labor. Nevertheless, the celebrated cardiologist Dr. William Osler suggested that the disparity in mortality was not directly attributed to activity but rather emotional stress and societal factors (Nieto 1999). Given the prestige and position of Osler, Hedley's work was routinely ignored until the seminal work of the father of physical activity epidemiology, Jeremiah Morris (Blair et al. 2010). Morris and his collaborators (1953) examined a large cohort of London transport workers during 1949 and 1950. They discovered that the conductors who climbed

HISTORICAL PERSPECTIVE ON SEDENTARY BEHAVIOR AND CVD

Many of the earliest forms of deliberate exercise were specifically developed to offset the sedentary behavior of people who were able to avoid the physical toils of the common man (i.e., wealthy elite, monks, and holy men). As human societies evolved, the emergence of a leisure class supported by slave and peasant economies gave rise to the earliest instances of inactivity, excessive sedentary behavior, and hypokinetically induced diseases such as CVD. Many of the earliest physicians were not concerned with the conditions and diseases of the poor, but rather the preservation of health and longevity in wealthy clients. Sushruta, the famous Indian surgeon and father of Ayurvedic medicine, practiced around 600 BCE. His keen sense of observation led to the discovery that his most sedentary clients suffered from a number of classic hypokinetic diseases (Guthrie 1956). Sushruta chronicled his observations in the ancient text *The Sushruta Samhita*, cataloguing numerous diseases that are familiar to physicians today, such as stable angina (i.e., *hritshoola* or heart pain), *madhumeha* or "honey-like urine" (i.e., diabetes), *vataraka* (i.e., hypertension), and *medoroga* (i.e., obesity) (Dwivedi and Dwivedi 2007). For these conditions, he prescribed daily exercise. His experience taught that decreasing sedentary behavior forestalled disease and protected the body against physical and mental impairment (Guthrie 1956).

Centuries after Sushruta, the practice of Hatha Yoga was developed to overcome the sedentary spiritual pursuits of Indian Sadhus (i.e., holy men). The health decrements of long hours of sitting meditation (i.e., dhyana) were found to be offset by a simple series of asanas (i.e., Yoga postures) that stressed the musculoskeletal and cardiovascular systems. Buddhist monks became increasingly more sedentary as Chinese society prospered. The development of early forms of medical qigong was intended to counter the effects of spending many hours per day in zazen (i.e., Buddhist meditation).

Wushu (i.e., Chinese martial arts) was inspired by Chinese philosophies on health. The practitioners of ancient Chinese medicine such as Hua Tuo (2500 BCE) used patterns in nature as examples from which to draw inferences about health and well-being (Wai 2004). As a result, the animal mimicry of Kung Fu (developed during the late 16th century for the defense of the Shaolin monastery) was one of the first institutionalized forms of exercise that specifically emphasized the development of chi or qi (i.e., an inner energy or life force) to counter the effects of the monks' excessive sedentary behavior. Later forms of qigong (e.g., Tai Chi) are now practiced throughout China and the world (Wile 2007).

In the ancient Greco-Roman world, PA and exercise played a central role in culture and medicine (Green 1951). Like Sushruta, early Greco-Roman physicians were more concerned with the preservation of health than the treatment of disease. Hippocrates of Kos (460 BCE to 370 BCE) noted that "exercise should be many and of all kinds" and "eating alone will not keep a man well; he must also exercise...for food and exercise . . . work together to produce health" (Hippocrates 1868, pages 228-299). His perspective was based on simple observation and presaged the modern view that most chronic diseases are caused by lifestyle factors such as nutrition and habitual patterns of PA.

After Hippocrates, the most prominent figure in ancient medicine was the Roman physician Claudius Galen (210 CE). In his text *On Hygiene*, he extolled the virtues of activity (Green 1951). The observations and prescriptions for exercise by ancient physicians provide an interesting prelude to modern epidemiological evidence that supports the contention that the primary prevention of chronic disease requires the adoption of a physically active lifestyle.

and descended many hundreds of steps each day while collecting fares on London's double-decker buses had much lower rates of CVD mortality than sedentary bus drivers (annual incidence 1.9/1,000 versus 2.7/1,000, respectively). Morris and colleagues suggested that physically active work had cardioprotective effects that were exhib-ited principally through a decrement in sudden cardiac death.

They continued by examining other government employees in a variety of occupations. They discovered that the occupational sedentariness of office workers (e.g., clerks) led to much higher rates of CVD when compared to people with jobs that required more PA (e.g., postal workers who walked or cycled while delivering mail). Interestingly, Morris and his collaborators were the first to document a dose response for activity and sedentary behavior. Postal workers who performed at least some PA (e.g., counter workers, supervisors) had lower CVD rates than employees who were completely sedentary.

A great deal of criticism surrounded Morris' early work. When he and colleagues posited that "men doing physically active work have a lower mortality from coronary heart disease in middle age than men in less active work" (1953, page 1112), it was met with extreme cynicism and disbelief. Once again, the teachings of William Osler led many people to believe that CVD was a result of the psychological stressors of the employment environment rather than a lack of occupational physical exertion. The criticism abated when it was noted that the respective work environments of the postman and conductors were quite different, yet each had lower CVD mortality. Morris and colleagues' work ushered in the age of PA epidemiology and clearly established the relationship among sedentary behavior, PA, and CVD. Morris' seminal work was paralleled and extended by the investigations of Dr. Ralph Paffenbarger Jr.

In 1951, Paffenbarger and colleagues began an observational study of >3,000 San Francisco longshoremen who were 35 to 64 years of age. They examined nearly 45,000 man-years over the next 16 years. During that period, there were 888 deaths, of which 291 were coronary fatalities. The CVD death rate was significantly lower in the most active when compared with the more sedentary workers: 59 versus 80/10,000 man-years of work (Paffenbarger and Hale 1975).

Many investigations over the past 50 years have documented an inverse relationship between occupational sedentariness and overall CVD risk. The association has been replicated in U.S. railroad workers (Slattery, Jacobs, and Nichaman 1989), postal workers (Kahn 1963), Kibbutz workers (Brunner et al. 1974), and farm workers (McDonogh et al. 1965). With each empirical undertaking, death from CVD was two to four times more likely in sedentary workers. As the 20th century came to a close, research on the benefits of PA and cardiorespiratory fitness (Blair and Brodney 1999; Blair et al. 1996b; Blair et al. 1989) led the American Heart Association to report, "inactivity is a risk factor for coronary artery disease" (Fletcher et al. 1992, page 340; Fletcher et al. 1996).

Physical Activity and CVD

With the advent of objective protocols for measuring activity (e.g., accelerometry-based PA monitors), it is now clear that physical inactivity is one of the greatest public health problems facing developed and developing nations (Lee et al. 2012). Nevertheless, until recently, people who failed to meet PA guidelines were considered sedentary despite the lack of reliable measures of sedentariness (Pate, O'Neill, and Lobelo 2008). As such, sedentary behavior was imprecisely conflated with insufficient PA. However, recent research using inclinometers and other technology that allow more precise quantifications of the time spent in sedentary pastimes suggests that the effects of excessive sedentary behavior, independent of PA levels, may play an important and unique role in the development of CVD and other noncommunicable diseases (NCDs) (Hamilton, Hamilton, and Zderic 2007).

Over the past 60 years, research has demonstrated the essential role of physical inactivity in the development of CVD and other noncommunicable chronic diseases (Archer and Blair 2011; Blair 2009; Blair et al. 1989). It is now unequivocal that physical inactivity leads to significant morbidity and early mortality (Beaglehole et al. 2011; Cecchini et al. 2010; Lee et al. 2012) and that sedentary lifestyles have severe consequences for all people. The risk factors for CVD and other NCDs begin early in life and increase with advancing age. As such, a lifetime of physical inactivity and excessive sedentary behavior hinders the development of a healthy cardiovascular system (Booth, Laye, and Roberts 2011; Charansonney 2011; Thijssen et al. 2010; Gidding et al. 2009; Kavey et al. 2003), muscle strength, and bone density (Booth, Laye, and Roberts 2011), while predisposing people to a host of morbidities in later life (Thorp et al. 2010; Thorp et al. 2011; Booth, Laye, and Roberts 2011) such as type 2 diabetes (Aman et al. 2009; LaMonte, Blair, and Church 2005), osteoporosis (Faulkner and Bailey 2007), sarcopenia (Pillard et al. 2011), frailty (Weiss 2011; Charansonney 2011), cancer (Kushi et al. 2012; Hu et al. 2005; Sui et al. 2010; Lagerros, Hsieh, and Hsieh 2004), and fatty liver disease (Nobili, Alisi, and Raponi 2009).

Numerous studies have demonstrated that the CVD risk factors associated with a sedentary lifestyle (e.g., dyslipidemia, hyperinsulinemia, obesity, and hypertension) are present in early childhood (Freedman et al. 1999). Findings from the Bogalusa study indicate that as the number of risk factors increases, so does the evidence for the early development of CVD (i.e., atherosclerotic processes in the aorta and coronary arteries) (Freedman et al. 1999). Although an early reduction in risk factors minimizes the risk of CVD in adulthood (Kavey et al. 2003), the sedentary lifestyles that significantly increase CVD risk are often initiated in very early childhood and continue into adulthood (Janz, Dawson, and Mahoney 2000). In 2003, the American Heart Association provided guidelines that explicitly stated that the primary prevention of CVD should begin in childhood and the success of this objective necessitates daily PA and reductions in sedentary behavior (Kavey et al. 2003). Nevertheless, many children and most adolescents and adults lead sedentary lives (Macera et al. 2005).

Research examining the effects of sedentary behavior may represent a different empirical paradigm than traditional investigations into the effects of PA or exercise. Recently, it has been suggested that sedentary behavior, independent of exercise or PA levels, may play a unique and important role in the development of CVD (Hamilton, Hamilton, and Zderic 2007). Furthermore, there is increasing evidence that excessive sedentary behavior at any age is associated with increased CVD risk factors (Nelson et al. 2005; Nissinen et al. 1989). As children have become more sedentary over the past few decades, the prevalence of CVD risk factors and the clinical manifestations of CVD have increased significantly in children. For example, work by Gidding and colleagues (1995) and Tuzcu and colleagues (2001) suggests an increasing trend in CVD risk factors, with >16% of adolescents having coronary atherosclerosis.

In 2012, the World Heart Federation, American Heart Association, American College of Cardiology Foundation, European Heart Network, and European Society of Cardiology collectively produced a report outlining a global strategy to reduce preventable deaths from CVD. The first and foremost proposed target was a 10% reduction in the prevalence of insufficient physical activity (Smith et al. 2012).

Mechanisms Linking Sedentary Behaviors and CVD

Sedentary behavior represents one of the lowest levels of energy expenditure that humans experience. Evidence exists that some forms of sedentary behavior (e.g., TV viewing) acutely decrease resting energy expenditure (REE) or metabolic rate below that of sleeping (Klesges, Shelton, and Klesges 1993). Evidence also exists that chronic sedentary activity may induce long-term decrements in REE in a dose–response manner. Cooper and colleagues found a significant dose–response relationship "in which REE decreased as average weekly hours of TV viewing increased" (2006, page 105). This significant reduction of energy expenditure is one of the primary mechanisms by which sedentary behavior increases the risk of atherosclerosis and manifest CVD. When a person is sitting or lying down, the contractile activation of the skeletal musculature of the entire body is diminished significantly. Because skeletal muscle energy demand is a function of contractile activity, inactive muscle cells have a reduced need to obtain nutritive energy molecules (e.g., glucose, triglycerides, and fatty acids) from the blood. This will lead to increasing concentrations in the blood (Leung et al. 2008; Yung et al. 2009) and an increased potential for pathological oxidative processes that lead to the production of reactive oxygen species, oxidative damage to the intima, and the initiation of atherosclerosis.

Sedentary behavior differs from low levels of PA in that it diminishes activity in all muscle fibers, inclusive of the highly oxidative postural muscles (which use relatively more lipids for energy) and the more glycolytic skeletal musculature (which use relatively more glucose and glycogen). By contrast, any nonsedentary activities (e.g., standing) activate the highly oxidative postural muscles, causing them to expend energy and remove lipids that would otherwise induce the formation of reactive oxygen species and cause oxidative damage (Corbi et al. 2012). On the molecular and cellular levels, sedentary behavior suppresses the activity of skeletal muscle lipoprotein lipase (LPL) as well as the muscle's sensitivity to insulin. LPL activity is necessary for the uptake (i.e., removal from the blood) of lipids (e.g., triglycerides), and any reduction in this activity leads to the storage of lipids in adipocytes (i.e., fat cells) and detrimental increases in visceral adiposity (Thyfault and Krogh-Madsen 2011). Insulin sensitivity is essential for the uptake of glucose, and reduced sensitivity leads to insulin resistance. Over many years, reduced insulin sensitivity may lead to type 2 diabetes (Olsen et al. 2008; Jensen et al. 2011). It is the inactivity-induced reduction in both insulin sensitivity and LPL activity that allows the nutritive energy molecules to increase in concentration and undergo the pathological oxidation or glycation processes that lead to injury of the endothelial cells of the vasculature. Any reduction in activity or increased sedentary behavior reduces the ability of the skeletal musculature to remove glucose and lipids from the blood (Olsen et al. 2008).

Television Viewing and CVD

Television viewing is one of the most ubiquitous behaviors of the modern world and one of the primary correlates of sedentary behavior (Grontved and Hu 2011). Recent governmental and industry research suggest that Europeans spend approximately 40% of their free time (i.e., ~4 hr/day) watching TV, while Australians and Americans spend more than 50%. Americans on average spend 5 hours per day sitting in front of their TVs (ABS 2008; Nielsen 2011), despite the fact that there is evidence that more than 2 hours of viewing per day promotes obesity (Davis et al. 2011), and multiple reviews have demonstrated that TV viewing (as a surrogate for sedentary behavior) is a strong independent predictor of CVD risk and mortality. A number of correlates of TV viewing exist, such as race/ethnicity and age. African-Americans have the highest rates of TV viewing, and Hispanic and African-American children are more likely to have a TV in their bedroom (Taveras et al. 2009; Sisson and Broyles 2012). Globally, older adults watch significantly more TV than younger adults (Touvier et al. 2010; Evenson et al. 2002), and obese people spend significantly more time in all sedentary activities, including watching TV, than their nonobese counterparts (Levine et al. 2005).

In 2011, Grontved and Hu performed a meta-analysis of prospective cohort studies to examine the association between TV viewing and the risk of NCDs such as type 2 diabetes, CVD, and all-cause mortality. When examining both fatal or nonfatal CVD on 34,253 people with 1,052 incident cases, the pooled relative risk per every 2-hour increase in TV viewing per day were 1.15 (95% CI, 1.06-1.23), and were even higher for type 2 diabetes at 1.20 (95% CI, 1.14-1.27). They estimated that the absolute risk difference was 38 cases of fatal CVD per 100,000 people per year, and concluded that TV viewing is a significant correlate of CVD.

TV viewing is the predominant leisure-time activity in Australia. In 2010, Dunstan and colleagues examined TV viewing in relation to subsequent CVD mortality with a median follow-up of 6.6 years among 8,800 adults 25 years of age or older in the Australian Diabetes, Obesity and Lifestyle Study (AusDiab). After 58,087 person-years of follow-up, there were 87 CVD deaths. After adjusting for numerous confounders such as age, sex, waist circumference, and exercise activity, the hazard ratios for CVD mortality for each 1-hour increase in TV viewing per day was 1.18 (95% CI, 1.03-1.35). When they compared people who watched <2 hours per day of TV to those who watched between 2 and 4 hours per day and those who watched >4 hours per day, the fully adjusted hazard ratios for CVD mortality were 1.19 (95% CI, 0.72-1.99) and 1.80 (95% CI, 1.00-3.25). They concluded that the prevention of NCDs should focus on reducing sedentary time and promoting physical activity and exercise.

In 2009, Katzmarzyk and colleagues prospectively examined daily sitting using a simple questionnaire at baseline that asked respondents if they sat "almost none of the time, one fourth of the time, half of the time, three fourths of the time and almost all of the time." After 12 years and 204,732 person-years of follow-up, there were 759 CVD deaths. After adjustment for potential confounders, there was a progressively higher risk of CVD mortality across increasing levels of sitting time (HR: 1.00, 1.01, 1.22, 1.47, 1.54; trend $p < 0.0001$). Comparable results were obtained when stratified by age, sex, smoking status, and body mass index. The age-adjusted all-cause mortality rates per 10,000 person-years of follow-up for physically inactive participants were 87, 86, 105, 130, and 161 (trend $p < 0.0001$) and for active participants were 75, 69, 76, 98, 105 (trend $p < 0.0001$) across sitting time categories (Katzmarzyk et al. 2009) These results suggest that there is a dose–response relationship for mortality related to both increased sitting time and inactivity. Perhaps more importantly, they suggest that excessive sedentary behavior (i.e., sitting time) is an independent risk factor for CVD, but that increments in PA can partially ameliorate the negative effects.

Warren and colleagues (2010) examined both TV viewing and the time spent sitting in a vehicle in 7,744 men (20-89 years old) initially without diagnosed CVD who returned a mailed survey during 1982 as part of the Aerobics Center Longitudinal Study. Data on mortality were acquired through the National Death Index. Cox regression analyses quantified the associations between each of the sedentary behaviors (hours per week) of watching TV and riding in a vehicle with CVD death, as well as the total time participating in these behaviors combined and CVD mortality rates. Over the 21-year follow-up, there were 377 CVD deaths. After adjusting for age, both the time spent in a vehicle and the combination of the time in a vehicle plus time watching TV were positively associated with CVD death (trend $p < 0.001$). Men who reported >10 hours per week riding in a vehicle or >23 hours per week combined sedentary behavior (i.e., TV and vehicle time) had 82% and 64% greater risk of dying from CVD than those who reported <4 or <11 hours per week, respectively. They concluded that these two strong correlates of total sedentary behavior were significant CVD mortality predictors. As with the Katzmarcyk and colleagues (2009) study, they found that high levels of PA or CRF partially ameliorated the effects of sedentary behavior on CVD. These authors suggested that health promotion efforts targeting physically inactive men should emphasize both reducing sedentary behavior and increasing levels of PA for optimizing cardiovascular health (Warren et al. 2010).

Summary

Cardiovascular diseases are the leading cause of death in the United States and throughout the developed and developing world (Go et al. 2013; Roger et al. 2012). Globally, CVD accounts for more than 10% of the total disease burden and approximately 30% of all deaths. Many of these deaths are early mortality (i.e., in people <60 years of age) and are thus preventable through reductions in physical inactivity, sedentary behavior, and smoking (Beaglehole et al. 2007). Nevertheless, over the past half century, there has been a large decrease in PA across the world in all domains of daily life (Church et al. 2011; Archer, Shook, et al. 2013; McDonald 2007). The increased use of passive transportation (driving rather than walking or biking) and spectator-based entertainment, as well as the development of technologies that save time and reduce the necessity of both occupational and household PA, have created an environment that is conducive to excessive sedentary behavior. Concomitant with this increase in sedentary behavior has been an increase in risk factors for CVD such as obesity, dyslipidemia, diabetes, and hypertension. More disheartening has been the dramatic increase in coronary calcification (Lee et al. 2009) and atherosclerosis (McGill et al. 2002) in children and adolescents. This suggests that the improvements in CVD mortality achieved in the United States in last decades may not be maintained.

The proportion of younger people (i.e., ≤18 years of age) who report engaging in no regular PA is high, and the proportion increases with age. Based on objective measurements, the vast majority of the U.S. population does not meet the Physical Activity Guidelines for Americans, and many adults report engaging in no aerobic leisure-time PA (Tucker, Welk, and Beyler 2011). Given that the pathological processes that lead to CVD begin in childhood and that PA interventions have been shown to reduce risk factors for CVD in children (Sallis et al. 1997), perhaps the most efficacious manner for reducing the future burden of CVD is initiating and implementing policies that increase PA while decreasing sedentary behavior in both children and adults.

KEY CONCEPTS

▸ **Atheroma (plaques):** The accumulation of macrophages, fatty acids, cholesterol, and fibrous tissue in arterial walls.

▸ **Atherosclerosis:** A pathological response to an injury of the endothelial cells of the vasculature that results in the development of atheromatous plaques. Atherosclerosis is the primary pathophysiologic process that underlies the majority of CVD deaths.

▸ **Cardiovascular diseases (CVD):** A group of chronic diseases of the heart or vasculature. CVDs are a major cause of morbidity and mortality. Physical inactivity and sedentary behavior are independent, major modifiable risk factors for CVD.

▸ **Endothelial function:** The ability of the lining of the vasculature (i.e., the endothelium) to respond to physical and chemical signals to regulate vascular tone, cellular adhesion, and vessel wall inflammation.

▸ **Myocardial infarction:** A reduction or interruption of blood flow (i.e., ischemia) to the myocardium that results in tissue damage; commonly known as a heart attack.

▸ **Oxidative injury:** Tissue damage from the excessive production of highly reactive molecules known as free radicals. Oxidative injury to the vascular intima is the first step in the atherosclerotic process. Smoking and the glycoxidation or glycation of nutritive energy molecules (e.g., glucose, lipids) are the primary sources of the reactive oxygen species that lead to intimal lesions. The progression from an intimal lesion to plaque rupture is exacerbated by inactivity-induced reductions in endothelial function.

▸ **Stroke:** Damage to the brain from a lack of blood flow (ischemic) or bleeding (hemorrhagic); also known as a cerebrovascular accident.

▸ **Thromboembolus:** A clot (i.e., a thrombus) in a blood vessel that travels from where it was originally formed to occlude blood flow in another part of the body.

▸ The associations among inactivity, sedentary behavior, and health have been known for many centuries.

▸ Sedentary behavior leads to reductions in the activation and consequent energy requirements of the skeletal musculature. This increases the substrate (i.e., nutritive energy molecules) available for glycation and the potential for oxidative injury to the intima.

▸ The time spent in sedentary behavior is an independent predictor of fatal and nonfatal CVD events, with a possible dose–response relationship.

▸ Exercise and high levels of PA can improve endothelial function through increases in fluid shear stress and thereby offset the pathological vascular remodeling of atherosclerotic processes.

▸ An increased frequency of breaks taken within episodes of sedentary behavior may diminish the deleterious effects of sedentary behavior.

▸ The number one leisure-time activity in the developed world is TV viewing.

▸ Obesity is a risk factor for CVD, and obese people spend significantly more time sitting and participating in sedentary behavior such as watching TV.

STUDY QUESTIONS

1. What are the major cardiovascular diseases?
2. What are the major modifiable and nonmodifiable risk factors for CVD?
3. What is the underlying pathophysiological mechanism in most CVDs?
4. How does sedentary behavior affect the activation of the skeletal musculature?
5. How does a decrease in skeletal muscle energy expenditure lead to an increased risk of atherosclerosis?
6. What is an atheroma?
7. What is a thromboembolus?
8. What precipitates a plaque rupture?
9. How does endothelial dysfunction predispose a person to atherosclerosis?
10. How can sedentary behavior and PA coexist in the same person?
11. How do exercise and high levels of PA improve endothelial function?

CHAPTER 10

SEDENTARY BEHAVIOR AND CANCER

Brigid M. Lynch, PhD; and Christine M. Friedenreich, PhD

The reader will gain an overview of sedentary behavior research within a cancer control context. By the end of this chapter, the reader should be able to do the following:

▶ Identify cancer sites for which there is evidence of an association with sedentary behavior
▶ Discuss health outcomes that have been associated with sedentary behavior in cancer survivors
▶ Define and discuss hypothesized biological mechanisms underlying the association between sedentary behavior and cancer
▶ Discuss the recommendations for future research

Sedentary behavior has been independently associated with chronic disease–related risk factors such as adiposity (Hu et al. 2003; Blanck et al. 2007; Wijndaele et al. 2010), insulin resistance (Balkau et al. 2008; Schmidt et al. 2008; Healy et al. 2011), and inflammation (Healy et al. 2011) in healthy adults. These factors are also hypothesized to be operative in the development and progression of some cancers. Hence, it is biologically plausible that sedentary behavior may be a contributing factor to some types of cancer, and there is increasing research interest in this potential association.

This chapter updates the review of the epidemiological studies regarding the association between sedentary behavior and cancer provided by Lynch (2010). Here, we provide an overview of the burden of disease attributable to cancer and describe the main established risk factors associated with the disease. We then provide a comprehensive review of the epidemiological literature related to associations of sedentary behavior with cancer risk and health outcomes for cancer survivors. Finally, we highlight the hypothesized biological mechanisms whereby sedentary behavior may influence cancer pathogenesis and progression.

Cancer Epidemiology

More than 100 different types of cancer exist that are identified by the site of disease and morphology. Cancer types can be grouped into five main categories: carcinoma, sarcomas, leukemia, lymphoma and myeloma, and central nervous system cancers. Cancers arise as a consequence of a lengthy (often decades long) multistep process involving the progressive accumulation of genetic and epigenetic changes that ultimately transform normal cells into neoplastic cells. Malignant cells are characterized by self-sufficiency, limitless replication potential, resistance to cell death, new and sustained angiogenesis, the ability to invade tissues, and a propensity to metastasize. Given the multitude of sites where cancers can originate, the resulting types of cancers are heterogeneous with respect to both their distributions by person, place, and time within populations and factors that are associated with their occurrence. The following sections provide an overview of the global burden of cancer with respect to incidence and mortality as well as a description of the major cancer risk factors.

In 2010, more than 13 million incident cases of cancer (excluding nonmelanoma skin cancers) were recorded worldwide and nearly 8 million cancer deaths occurred (Ferlay et al. 2010). By 2020, cancer incidence and mortality are projected to increase to more than 16 million new cases, with 10 million deaths (World Cancer Research Fund and American Institute for Cancer Research 2007). Cancer may soon surpass cardiovascular diseases to become the number one cause of mortality worldwide. Furthermore, by 2030, it is estimated that 70% of cancer deaths will occur in developing countries (World Cancer Research Fund and American Institute for Cancer Research 2007). Presently, nearly 30 million people are cancer survivors worldwide, and this number is expected to rise steadily given the trends of increasing cancer incidence and improved early diagnosis and cancer treatment.

This projected increase in cancer incidence and mortality is attributable to a combination of factors that include an increase in the global population, an aging world population, the increase in tobacco smoking prevalence in many countries, the increase in industrialization in many countries, a Westernization in dietary intake and lifestyle, and an increase in the prevalence of HIV and AIDS (World Cancer Research Fund and American Institute for Cancer Research 2007). A real age-adjusted, population-adjusted increase in cancer rates is projected (Ferlay et al. 2010). However, some cancer rates are decreasing in developed countries; large differences in incidence over time and absolute numbers of cancers demonstrate that a percentage of these cancers are, in principle, preventable (World Cancer Research Fund and American Institute for Cancer Research 2007).

The most commonly diagnosed cancers (excluding all types of skin cancer) are of the lung, colorectal, breast, stomach, and prostate. Clear geographical and socioeconomic differences exist for the most common cancers, with cancers associated with infectious agents more prevalent in developing countries and hormone-related cancers more common in developed countries.

Key Risk Factors

The etiology of cancer is complex and multifactorial, with the main causes broadly categorized into either genetic or host factors and environmental or lifestyle factors. The main host factors that have been identified are age, race, and family history of cancer. Age is the strongest determinant of cancer risk since it parallels the cumulative exposure to carcinogens over time and the accumulation of mutations needed for unregulated cell growth that is cancer. Race defines a constellation of genetic factors that relate to susceptibility to a given cancer. An underlying predisposition to cancer exists for people who are carriers of highly penetrant cancer susceptibility genes, which account for <5% for most cancers. Genetic susceptibility for cancer can also interact with environmental exposures to increase cancer risk within subsets of the population with this predisposition.

Several different types of environmental factors are established as cancer risk factors, including tobacco use, infectious agents, hormones, sunlight, ionizing radiation, industrial chemicals and exposures, dietary intake, physical inactivity, and obesity. The single most consistently established and strongest risk factor that has been associated with the most cancers is tobacco use and environmental tobacco smoke, which account for approximately one-third of cancers in the developed world (Secretan et al. 2009). Tobacco is an established initiator and promoter of carcinogenesis. Several viruses have been identified that strongly increase the risk of developing cancer, including human papillomaviruses (associated with cervical cancer), hepatitis B and hepatitis C (liver cancer), human T-cell leukemia or the lymphoma virus, human immunodeficiency virus (Kaposi sarcoma), Epstein–Barr virus (lymphoma), human herpesvirus 8 (Kaposi sarcoma), and Helicobacter pylori (stomach cancer) (Bouvard et al. 2009). Approximately one in four cancers in developing countries is estimated to be attributable to infection (World Cancer Research Fund and American Institute for Cancer Research 2007). Menopausal hormone therapy may increase breast cancer risk, and use of diethylstilbestrol during pregnancy is associated with increased risks of breast cancer in the mothers and cervical cancer in the daughters (Grosse et al. 2009). Ultraviolet radiation and ionizing radiation from radioactive fallout, radon gas, and X-rays increase the risk of several cancers (El Ghissassi et al. 2009). Numerous industrial chemicals and exposures have been classified by the International Agency for Research on Cancer (IARC) as sufficient causes of cancer. The main exposures classified as carcinogens in industrial settings are asbestos, benzene, cadmium, nickel, and vinyl chloride, but several thousand exposures have been classified as potentially increasing cancer risk (Baan et al. 2009).

The American Institute of Cancer Research has estimated that inappropriate diet, physical inactivity, and unhealthy body weight alone could together account for 30% to 40% of cancer incidence (World Cancer Research Fund and American Institute for Cancer Research 2007). Excessive alcohol intake has been related to the risk of specific cancers potentially accounting for 3% to 5% of the incidence of all cancers worldwide and is classified as a carcinogen by the IARC (Secretan et al. 2009). Being overweight or obese increases the risk of several cancers and accounts for 20% of all cancer cases (World Cancer Research Fund and American Institute for Cancer Research 2007). Physical activity reduces the risk of colon, breast, and endometrial cancers by 20% to 30% and for prostate, lung, and ovarian cancers by 10% to 30% (Courneya and Friedenreich 2011). Consistent and strong evidence now exists for an increased risk associated with red meat and processed meat for colorectal cancer and a probable decrease for several cancers for fruit and vegetable intake (World Cancer Research Fund and American Institute for Cancer Research 2007).

Sedentary Behavior and Cancer Research

In this section, we provide a summary of studies examining associations of sedentary behavior with cancer risk, published to June 2014. Where multiple publications from the same study (relating to the same cancer site) were found, the most recent publication was included for review. The risk ratios extracted from studies represent the highest versus lowest category of sedentary behavior. We define study results as null if the odds or hazard ratios fell between 0.9 and 1.1, inclusive. If the lower limit of the 95% confidence intervals was greater than 0.95, we consider the results to be of borderline significance.

To date, 21 published studies have assessed the association between self-reported *sedentary behavior* (where participants estimated their total sitting time, screen time, and occupational sitting time) and cancer risk. The main design features and results of these key studies are summarized in table 10.1. An additional 15 studies have compared participant self-reported *occupational activity* (categories generally include sitting, standing, some walking and light lifting, and heavy manual labor) and cancer risk, and these are also reviewed. Studies in which participants' activity levels were assigned based

Table 10.1 Associations of Sedentary Behavior and Cancer Risk

Breast cancer	
Study: Design and measure	Results
Rosenberg et al. 2014: Prospective cohort study, sitting time; 5+ vs. <1 hr/day	All women, TV: **RR** = 1.13 (95% CI: 0.91, 1.40) All women, occupational sitting: **RR** = 1.05 (95% CI: 0.90, 1.22) ER+, TV: **RR** = 0.94 (95% CI: 0.69, 1.28) ER+, occupational sitting: **RR** = 0.92 (95% CI: 0.74, 1.13) ER−, TV: **RR** = 1.39 (95% CI: 0.94, 2.07) ER−, occupational sitting: **RR** = 1.19 (95% CI: 0.90, 1.57)
Cohen et al. 2013: Nested case control study, sitting time; top vs. bottom quartile	All women: **OR** = 1.41 (95% CI: 1.01, 1.95) Black women: **OR** = 1.23 (95% CI: 0.82, 1.83) White women: **OR** = 1.94 (95% CI: 1.01, 3.70)
Hildebrand et al. 2013: Prospective cohort study, sitting time; top vs. bottom quartile	All women: **RR** = 1.10 (95% CI: 1.01, 1.21), p trend = 0.20
Lynch, Courneya, and Friedenreich 2013: Case control study, sitting time	Postmenopausal: **OR** = 0.71 (95% CI: 0.52, 0.97) Premenopausal: **OR** = 0.85 (95% CI: 0.58, 1.24)
George et al. 2010: Prospective cohort study, OA; standing or walking vs. sitting all day; total sitting or TV ≥9 vs <3 hr/day	Invasive: **RR** = 1.16 (95% CI: 1.02, 1.35) Invasive, TV: **RR** = 1.56 (95% CI: 0.89, 1.41) Invasive, sitting: **RR** = 1.08 (95% CI: 0.92, 1.27) In situ: **RR** = 0.90 (95% CI: 0.63, 1.28) In situ, TV: **RR** = 1.01 (95% CI: 0.56, 1.83) In situ, sitting: **RR** = 1.12 (95% CI: 0.78, 1.61)
Mathew et al. 2009: Case control study, sitting time; ≥180 vs. <60 min/day	No statistically significant associations between TV time and breast cancer in either pre- or postmenopausal women.
Lahmann et al. 2007: Prospective cohort study, OA; sedentary vs. standing	Premenopausal: **HR** = 0.98 (95% CI: 0.82, 1.16) Postmenopausal: **HR** = 1.09 (95% CI: 0.95, 1.23)
Levi et al. 1999: Case control study, OA; mainly sitting vs. standing	15-19 years: **OR** = 1.67 (95% CI: 1.10, 2.50) 30-39 years: **OR** = 2.22 (95% CI: 1.14, 4.76) 50-59 years: **OR** = 1.85 (95% CI: 0.98, 3.45)
Thune et al. 1997: Prospective cohort study, OA; sedentary vs. walking	Overall: **RR** = 1.19 (95% CI: 0.89, 1.59) Premenopausal: **RR** = 1.22 (95% CI: 0.75, 2.00) Postmenopausal: **RR** = 1.15 (95% CI: 0.81, 1.64)
Colorectal and colon cancer	
Study: Design and measure	Results
Howard et al. 2008: Prospective cohort study, sitting time; ≥9 vs. <3 hr/day	Men, TV: **RR** = 1.56 (95% CI: 1.11, 2.20) Men, total sitting: **RR** = 1.22 (95% CI: 0.96, 1.55) Women, TV: **RR** = 1.45 (95% CI: 0.99, 2.13) Women, total sitting: **RR** = 1.23 (95% CI: 0.89, 1.70)
Friedenreich et al. 2006: Prospective cohort study, OA; sedentary vs. standing	Colon: **HR** = 1.02 (95% CI: 0.84, 1.23) Rectal: **HR** = 0.90 (95% CI: 0.70, 1.18)
Colbert et al. 2001: Randomized controlled trial, OA; sitting vs. walking quite a lot	Colon: **RR** = 1.67 (95% CI: 0.96, 2.94) Rectal: **RR** = 1.41 (95% CI: 0.73, 2.78)
Steindorf et al. 2000: Case control study, sitting time; ≥2 vs. <1.14 hr/day	Colorectal: **OR** = 2.22 (95% CI: 1.19, 4.17)
Thune and Lund 1996: Prospective cohort study, OA; sedentary vs. walking	Men, colon: **RR** = 1.09 (95% CI: 0.78, 1.49) Men, rectal: **RR** = 1.11 (95% CI: 0.76, 1.64) Women, colon: **RR** = 1.22 (95% CI: 0.66, 2.27) Women, rectal: **RR** = 1.05 (95% CI: 0.44, 2.50)
Endometrial cancer	
Study: Design and measure	Results
Arem et al. 2011: Case control study, sitting time; ≥8 vs. <4 hr/day	**OR** = 1.52 (95% CI: 1.07, 2.16), p trend = 0.024
Friedenreich et al. 2010: Case control study, sitting time; hr/week/year increase	Each hr increase: **OR** = 1.02 (95% CI: 1.00, 1.04) 5 hr increase: **OR** = 1.11 (95% CI: 1.01, 1.22)
Moore et al. 2010*: Prospective cohort study, sitting time; ≥9 vs. <3 hr/day	**RR** = 1.15 (95% CI: 0.87, 1.53), p trend < 0.01
Patel et al. 2008: Prospective cohort study, sitting time	Not associated with statistically significant increased risk in fully adjusted model
Friberg, Mantzoros, and Wolk 2006: Prospective cohort study, sitting time; ≥5 vs. <5 hr/day	**RR** = 1.66 (95% CI: 1.05, 2.61)

(continued)

Table 10.1 *(continued)*

Kidney cancer	
Study: Design and measure	Results
George et al. 2011: Prospective cohort study, sitting time; ≥9 vs. <3 hr/day	TV: **HR** = 1.56 (95% CI: 0.89, 1.41) Total sitting: **HR** = 1.08 (95% CI: 0.92, 1.27)
Mahabir et al. 2004: Randomized controlled trial, OA; mainly sitting vs. walking quite a lot	**OR** = 0.73 (95% CI: 0.44, 1.22)
Lung cancer	
Study: Design and measure	Results
Ukawa et al. 2013: Prospective cohort study, sitting time; ≥4 vs. <2 hr/day	Men: **HR** = 1.36 (95% CI: 1.04, 1.80) Women: **HR** = 1.03 (95% CI: 0.67, 1.62)
Lam et al. 2013: Prospective cohort study, sitting time; ≥5 vs. <3 hr/day	TV: **HR** = 1.06 (95% CI: 0.77, 1.46) Total sitting: **HR** = 1.28 (95% CI: 0.96, 1.72)
Steindorf et al. 2006: Prospective cohort study, OA; sitting vs. standing	Men: **RR** = 0.74 (95% CI: 0.56, 0.98) Women: **RR** = 0.88 (95% CI: 0.64, 1.20)
Bak et al. 2005: Prospective cohort study, OA; sitting vs. standing	Men: **RR** = 0.60 (95% CI: 0.38, 0.94) Women: **RR** = 0.58 (95% CI: 0.37, 0.93)
Thune and Lund 1997: Prospective cohort study, OA; sedentary vs. walking	Men: **RR** = 0.87 (95% CI: 0.68, 1.11) Women: **RR** = 1.23 (95% CI: 0.57, 2.70)
Non-Hodgkin lymphoma	
Study: Design and measure	Results
Teras et al. 2012: Prospective cohort study, sitting time; ≥6 vs. <3 hr/day	Women: **HR** = 1.26, (95% CI: 1.01, 1.59), $p = 0.011$ No significant association among men
Ovarian cancer	
Study: Design and measure	Results
Xiao et al. 2013: Prospective cohort study, sitting time; ≥7 vs. <3 hr/day	TV: **RR** = 1.02 (95% CI: 0.67, 1.55) Total sitting: **RR** = 1.06 (95% CI: 0.81, 1.39)
Pan et al. 2005: Case control study, OA; sitting vs. light occupational activity	Averaged lifetime: **OR** = 0.86 (95% CI: 0.57, 1.33) Past 2 years: **OR** = 1.43 (95% CI: 0.96, 2.08)
Patel et al. 2006: Prospective cohort study, sitting time; ≥6 vs. <3 hr/day	**RR** = 1.55 (95% CI: 1.08, 2.22)
Zhang et al. 2004: Case control study, sitting time	TV: >4 vs. <2 hr/day, **OR** = 3.39 (95% CI: 1.0, 11.5) Total sitting: >10 vs. <4 hr/day, **OR** = 1.77 (95% CI: 1.0, 3.1) Work sitting: >6 vs. <2 hr/day, **OR** = 1.96 (95% CI: 1.2, 3.2)
Pancreatic cancer	
Study: Design and measure	Results
Stolzenberg-Solomon et al. 2002: Randomized controlled trial, OA; mainly sitting vs. walking quite a lot	**OR** = 1.30 (95% CI: 0.74, 2.22)
Prostate cancer	
Study: Design and measure	Results
Lynch et al. 2014: Prospective cohort study, sitting time; TV viewing ≥5 vs. <3 hr/day, total sitting ≥7 vs. <3 hr/day	All, TV: ≥7 vs. <1 hr/day, **HR** = 1.03 (95% CI: 0.92, 1.15) All, total sitting: ≥9 vs. <3 hr/day, **HR** = 0.98 (95% CI: 0.91, 1.05) Advanced, TV: **HR** = 0.93 (95% CI: 0.79, 1.09) Advanced, total sitting: **HR** = 0.91 (95% CI: 0.77, 1.08) Fatal, TV: **HR** = 1.07 (95% CI: 0.85, 1.33) Fatal, total sitting: **HR** = 1.07 (95% CI: 0.84, 1.35)
Orsini et al. 2009: Prospective cohort study, OA; mostly sitting vs. mostly standing	All: **OR** = 1.27 (95% CI: 1.10, 1.45) Localized: **OR** = 1.39 (95% CI: 1.11, 1.72)
Lacey et al. 2001: Case control study, OA; sitting vs. light labor	1998: **OR** = 0.59 (95% CI: 0.29, 1.25) Aged 40-49: **OR** = 0.37 (95% CI: 0.18, 0.77)
Thune and Lund 1994: Prospective cohort study, OA; sedentary vs. walking	**RR** = 1.30 (95% CI: 0.92, 1.85)
Testicular cancer	
Study: Design and measure	Results
Thune and Lund 1994: Prospective cohort study, OA; sedentary vs. walking	**RR** = 1.67 (95% CI: 0.64, 4.35)

*Updating Gierach et al. 2009; ER+ = estrogen receptor positive, ER– = estrogen receptor negative, CI = confidence intervals, OA = occupational activity, HR = hazard ratio, RR = relative risk, OR = odds ratio on job title (usually from industry and occupation codes) were not included in our review because of the likelihood of misclassification and measurement error of sedentary behavior.

Twelve (57%) of the 21 studies assessing self-reported sedentary behavior and cancer found a statistically significant risk increase when comparing the highest versus lowest category of sedentary behavior (Steindorf et al. 2000; Zhang et al. 2004; Friberg, Mantzoros, and Wolk 2006; Patel et al. 2006; Howard et al. 2008; Patel et al. 2008; Friedenreich et al. 2010; Arem et al. 2011; Teras et al. 2012; Cohen et al. 2013; Hildebrand et al. 2013; Ukawa et al. 2013). Three studies (14%) observed a statistically nonsignificant risk increase (Moore et al. 2010; Lam et al. 2013; Rosenberg et al. 2014), five studies (24%) produced null effects (Mathew et al. 2009; George et al. 2010; George et al. 2011; Xiao et al. 2013; Lynch, Courneya, and Friedenreich 2014), and one study (5%) reported a significant risk reduction (Lynch, Courneya, and Friedenreich 2013). Fifteen of the 21 studies examined the trend of the association between sedentary behavior and cancer risk in fully adjusted models, and six found evidence for a dose–response relation (Patel et al. 2006; Howard et al. 2008; Patel et al. 2008; Moore et al. 2010; Arem et al. 2011; Teras et al. 2012). Most studies presented results from models that had been adjusted for a range of sociodemographic, health, and lifestyle variables, with the exception of some of the older studies that adjusted for age, geographic region, and BMI (Thune and Lund 1994) or education and total energy intake (Steindorf et al. 2000). Figure 10.1 presents outcomes by cancer site.

Given the emerging nature of this field of research, further prospective cohort studies are needed to quantify the associations of sedentary behavior with cancer risk. Investigating associations between sedentary behavior and additional cancer sites for which a biologically plausible link exists, such as liver, esophageal, and pancreatic cancer, should be a research priority.

Eight prospective studies examined the association between self-reported sedentary behavior and overall cancer mortality (see table 10.2). Three studies reported a statistically significant risk increase (Patel et al. 2010; Matthews et al. 2012; Seguin et al. 2014). Each study adjusted models for a range of potentially confounding variables. It should be noted that one of these studies (the Women's Health Initiative) was comprised of women only (Seguin et al. 2014) and that the significant association

reported in one of the other studies (the American Cancer Society's Cancer Prevention Study II Nutrition Cohort) was among women only (Patel et al. 2010). Two studies observed nonsignificant risk increases (Dunstan et al. 2010; Wijndaele et al. 2011) and the remainder produced null effects (Katzmarzyk et al. 2009; Kim et al. 2013; Matthews et al. 2014), although there was a very small, nonsignificant risk increase among the black participants of the Southern Community Cohort Study (Matthews et al. 2014). Figure 10.2 presents a summary of the hazard ratios across studies for cancer-specific mortality.

Additionally, two studies have examined the association of sedentary behavior and site-specific mortality (see table 10.2). Postdiagnosis leisure-time sitting (≥6 versus <3 hr/day) was associated with colorectal cancer–specific mortality in the Cancer Prevention Study II Nutrition Cohort (RR = 1.62, 95% CI: 1.07, 2.44); the association for prediagnosis sitting was not statistically significant (RR = 1.33, 95% CI: 0.96, 1.84) (Campbell et al. 2013). Television viewing time was not significantly associated with liver cancer mortality in the Japanese Collaborative Cohort Study (HR ≥6 versus <3 hr/day = 1.20, 95% CI: 0.82, 1.77) (Ukawa et al. 2013).

Additional prospective studies are needed to determine the association of sedentary behavior with site-specific cancer mortality. Etiological pathways differ between cancer sites, and it is likely that sedentary behavior is a risk factor for some, but not all, cancers. Significant associations for specific sites are likely masked when cancer mortality is considered as a homogenous outcome.

Two of the 15 studies on occupational activity and cancer risk (13%) found a statistically significant risk increase associated with employment in jobs categorized as sitting versus standing (Levi et al. 1999; Orsini et al. 2009). An additional two studies (13%) demonstrated a risk increase of borderline significance (Colbert et al. 2001; Pan et al. 2005), and five studies (34%) observed a statistically nonsignificant risk increase (Thune and Lund 1994, 1996, 1997; Thune et al. 1997; Stolzenberg-Solomon et al. 2002). Two studies (13%) produced null effects (Friedenreich et al. 2006; Lahmann et al. 2007), and four studies (27%) found an inverse association between sedentary behavior or a sedentary occupation and cancer risk (Lacey et al. 2001; Mahabir et al. 2004; Bak et al. 2005; Steindorf et al. 2006). Figure 10.3 presents the associations of occupational activity category with site-specific risk.

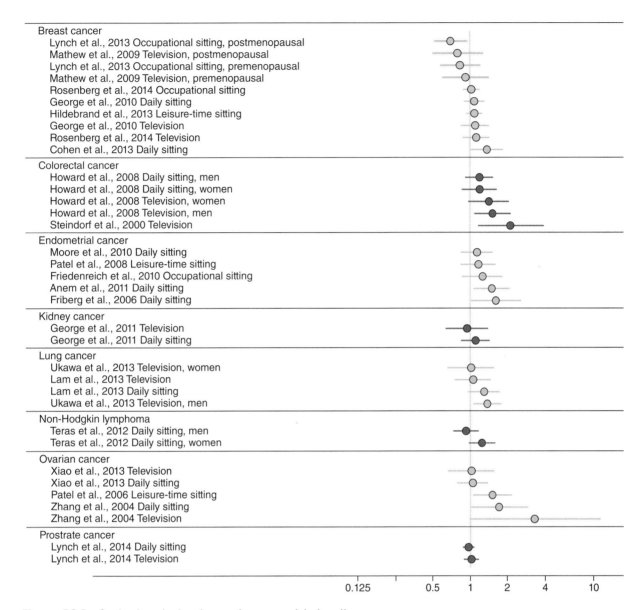

Figure 10.1 Sedentary behavior and cancer risk, by site.

Sedentary Behavior and Cancer Survivorship

Only 12 publications to date have considered the effect of sedentary behavior on health outcomes for cancer survivors (see table 10.3). Five of these studies utilized methods of objective activity monitoring to assess sedentary behavior (Lynch et al. 2010; Lynch, Dunstan, et al. 2011; George et al. 2014; Lowe et al. 2014; Vallance et al. 2014); seven studies relied on self-reported estimates (Wijndaele et al. 2009; Hawkes et al. 2011; Lynch, Cerin, et al. 2011; Rogers et al. 2011; Forsythe et al. 2013; George et al. 2013; Trinh et al. 2013). Each

study adjusted models for a range of potentially confounding variables.

Prospective cohorts of cancer survivors are needed to study the associations of sedentary behavior with disease prognosis and other health outcomes, including quality of life. Television viewing time has been shown to have deleterious effects on BMI, cardiovascular health, and quality of life for colorectal cancer survivors (Wijndaele et al. 2009; Hawkes et al. 2011; Lynch, Cerin, et al. 2011); however, the effect of sedentary behavior in other cancer survivor groups is largely unknown.

Two studies examined the cross-sectional associations between accelerometer-assessed sedentary

Table 10.2 Associations of Sedentary Behavior and Cancer Mortality

All cancer mortality	
Study: Design and measure	Results
Matthews et al. 2014: Prospective cohort study; sitting time, >12 vs. <5.76 hr/day	Blacks: **HR** = 1.12 (0.92, 1.36), p trend = 0.17 Whites: **HR** = 1.04 (0.74, 1.46), p trend = 0.29
Seguin et al. 2014: Prospective cohort study; sitting time ≥11 vs. <4 hr/day	**HR** = 1.21 (1.07, 1.37)
Kim et al. 2013: Prospective cohort study; sedentary behavior ≥10 vs. <5 hr/day	Men: **HR** = 0.97 (0.87, 1.07) Women: **HR** = 0.97 (0.87, 1.09)
Matthews et al. 2012: Prospective cohort study; watching TV ≥7 vs. <1 hr/day, total sitting ≥9 vs. <3 hr/day	TV: **HR** = 1.22 (1.06, 1.40) Sitting: **HR** = 1.12 (1.02, 1.24)
Wijndaele et al. 2011: Prospective cohort study; hr/day increase in TV viewing time	No association between TV viewing time and cancer mortality
Patel et al. 2010: Prospective cohort study; sitting ≥6 vs. <3 hr/day	Women: **RR** = 1.30 (95% CI: 1.16, 1.46), p = <0.0001 Men: no association
Dunstan et al. 2010: Prospective cohort study; hr/day increase in TV viewing time	No association between TV viewing time and cancer mortality
Katzmarzyk et al. 2009: Prospective cohort study; sitting almost all of the time vs. almost none of the time	No association between daily sitting time and cancer mortality
Site-specific mortality	
Study: Design and measure	Results
Campbell et al. 2013: Prospective cohort study; sitting ≥6 vs. <3 hr/day	Prediagnosis, all-cause: **RR** = 1.36 (1.10, 1.68) CRC specific: **RR** = 1.33 (0.96, 1.84) Postdiagnosis, all-cause: **RR** = 1.27 (0.99, 1.64) CRC specific: **RR** = 1.62 (1.07, 2.44)
Ukawa et al. 2013: Prospective cohort study; sitting ≥4 vs. <2 hr/day	All: **HR** = 1.20 (0.82, 1.77) Men: **HR** = 1.23 (0.76, 2.02) Women: **HR** = 1.13 (0.62, 2.13)

HR = hazard ratio, RR = relative risk, CRC = colorectal cancer

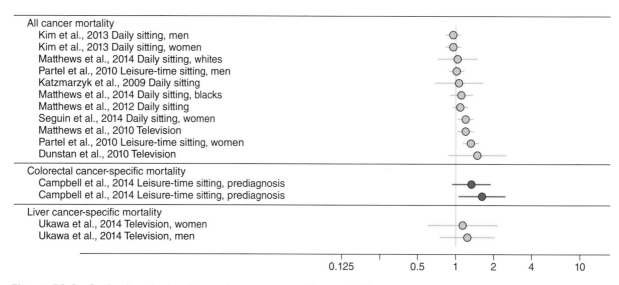

Figure 10.2 Sedentary behavior and cancer-specific mortality.

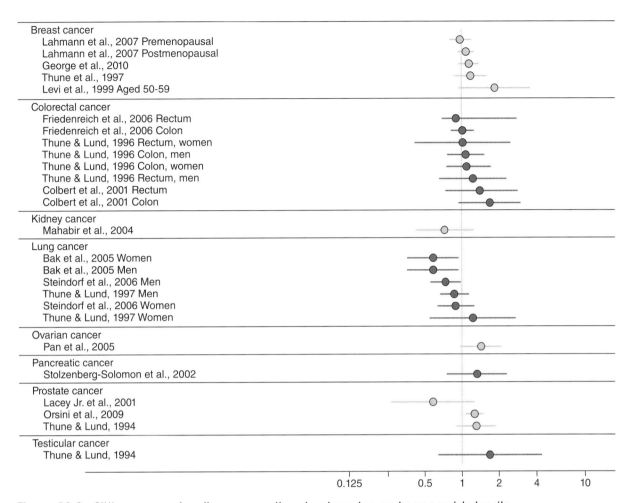

Figure 10.3 Sitting versus standing occupational categories and cancer risk, by site.

time and measures of adiposity in breast (n = 111) and prostate cancer survivors (n = 103) in the National Health and Nutrition Examination Survey. A cutoff of fewer than 100 counts per minute was used to define sedentary time. Sedentary time was not significantly associated with adiposity in fully adjusted models for survivors of either breast (Lynch et al. 2010) or prostate cancer (Lynch, Dunstan, et al. 2011). Three other cross-sectional accelerometer studies reported divergent findings relating to sedentary time and quality of life: Vallance and colleagues (2014) found no association in a sample of 178 stages I to III colon cancer survivors, George and colleagues (2014) demonstrated an inverse association between sitting time and physical functioning and general health among 54 cancer survivors with mixed diagnoses, and Lowe and colleagues (2014) found that greater volumes of time spent sitting or lying down were significantly associated with poorer psychosocial functioning but better

physical functioning in 31 cancer patients with brain metastases.

Three studies used data from the Colorectal Cancer and Quality of Life Study to examine the prospective effect of television viewing time on various health outcomes among nearly 2,000 colorectal cancer survivors (Wijndaele et al. 2009; Hawkes et al. 2011; Lynch, Cerin, et al. 2011). Watching 5 hours or more versus 2 hours or less of television per day was positively associated with a mean increase in BMI of 0.71 kg/m^2 over approximately 18 months (Wijndaele et al. 2009). Colorectal cancer survivors who watched 5 hours or more of television per day had a 16% lower total quality of life score than did participants reporting 2 hours or less per day. Deleterious associations were strongest for functional well-being (23% difference in quality of life scores between highest and lowest television viewing categories) and weakest for social well-being (6% difference) (Lynch, Cerin et al. 2011).

Table 10.3 Associations of Sedentary Behavior and Health Outcomes in Cancer Survivors

Breast cancer survivors	
Study: Design and measure	Results
Rogers et al. 2011: Case control study; weekday and weekend sitting; fatigue (FACT-F) and depressive symptoms (CES-D)	Adjusted mean fatigue scores significantly different across sitting categories: ≤120 min = 12.5; >120 to ≤360 min = 14.2; >360 min = 17.2, p = 0.0029. No significant association with depressive symptoms.
Lynch et al. 2010: Case control study; accelerometer-measured sedentary behavior (<100 counts/min; waist circumference and BMI	Sedentary time not associated with waist circumference (β = 2.687, 95% CI: −0.537, 5.910) or BMI (β = 0.412, 95% CI: −0.811, 1.636) in fully adjusted models.
Colorectal cancer survivors	
Study: Design and measure	Results
Lynch, Cerin, et al. 2011 : Prospective cohort study; TV time ≥5 vs. ≤2 hr/day; quality of life scores (FACT-C)	Watching TV associated with 16% lower total quality of life score. Participants who increased their TV viewing by one category had a proportional decrease of 6% in quality of life score.
Hawkes et al. 2011: Prospective cohort study; TV time ≥5 vs. ≤2 hr/day; concurrent and *de novo* cardiovascular disease and diabetes	TV, *de novo* ischemic heart disease: **OR** = 4.50 (95% CI: 1.73, 11.74) TV, nonsignificant risk increase for *de novo* diabetes: **OR** = 1.56 (0.87, 2.18)
Wijndaele et al. 2009: Prospective cohort study; TV time; BMI from baseline to 24 and 36 months post diagnosis	Watching TV ≥5 vs. ≤2 hr/day associated with increase in BMI at 24 months (0.72 kg/m^2, 95% CI: 0.31, 1.12, p < 0.001) and 36 months (0.61 kg/m^2, 95% CI: 0.14, 1.07, p < 0.01)
Prostate cancer survivors	
Study: Design and measure	Results
Lynch, Dunstan, et al. 2011 : Case control study; accelerometer-measured sedentary behavior (<100 counts/min); waist circumference	Sedentary time not associated with waist circumference (β = 0.678, 95% CI: −1.389, 2.745) in fully adjusted model

OR = odds ratio

Television viewing time was also associated with *de novo* ischemic heart disease among rectal cancer survivors (OR = 4.50, 95% CI: 1.73, 11.74) and with a nonsignificant risk increase for *de novo* diabetes in colon cancer survivors (OR = 1.56, 95% CI: 0.87, 2.18) (Hawkes et al. 2011).

Two reports were from the Health, Eating, Activity, and Lifestyle Study, a prospective study of women diagnosed with *in situ* to stage IIIa breast cancer. No significant association was found between self-reported television viewing time and health-related quality of life or fatigue (George et al. 2013), nor with pain (Forsythe et al. 2013). A cross-sectional study of 540 kidney cancer survivors found no association between self-reported sitting time and quality of life or fatigue, although stratified analyses showed a significant association among younger (<60 years) participants (Trinh et al. 2013). Finally, in a cross-sectional study of breast cancer survivors, adjusted mean fatigue scores were significantly different across categories of sitting time, but no significant differences in depressive symptoms were found (Rogers et al. 2011).

Proposed Biological Mechanisms

A number of biological pathways relating sedentary behavior to the development and progression of cancer have been proposed, but these are not well understood (Lynch 2010). An overview of the hypothesized pathways is illustrated in figure 10.4. It is likely that these proposed mechanisms are interrelated and that the relative contribution of each mechanism varies by cancer type.

Observational studies are needed for examining associations with biomarkers. How sedentary behavior may be associated with mechanisms operative in cancer pathogenesis has only begun to be explored, and there are numerous avenues for enquiry to be pursued. Sedentary behavior may plausibly be associated with sex hormones,

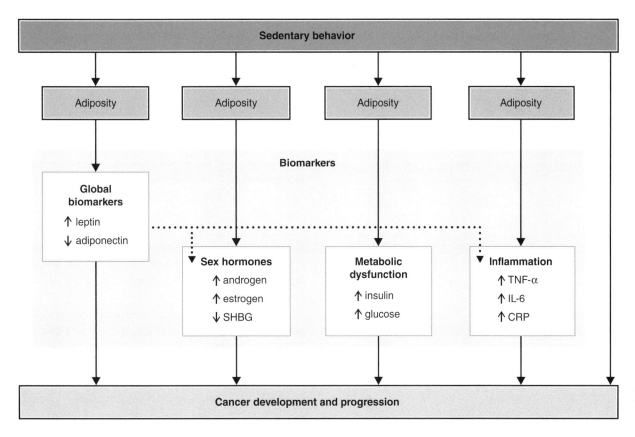

Figure 10.4 Biological model of hypothesized pathways from sedentary behavior to cancer.

Adapted, by permission, from B. M. Lynch, 2010, "Sedentary behavior and cancer: A systematic review of the literature and proposed biological mechanisms," *Cancer Epidemiology Biomarkers and Prevention* 19(11): 2691-2709.

metabolic hormones, and inflammatory peptides or cytokines. Future research should consider if and how the effect of physical activity on quality of life is mediated by other molecular pathways, genetic and epigenetic processes, immune response, the microbiome, and the tumor microenvironment. Mechanistic understanding could strengthen causal inferences from epidemiological data, provide insights into gene–environment interactions, and identify novel drug targets. The following sections summarize the sites for which there is evidence of an association.

Adiposity

Adiposity may facilitate carcinogenesis directly or through a number of pathways, including increased levels of sex and metabolic hormones, chronic inflammation, and altered secretion of adipokines (Neilson et al. 2009; van Kruijsdijk et al. 2009). Convincing evidence exists that adiposity increases risk of colon, postmenopausal breast, endome-

trial, kidney, and esophageal cancers and cancer-related mortality (Reeves et al. 2007; World Cancer Research Fund and American Institute for Cancer Research 2007; Renehan et al. 2008).

Sedentary behavior and adiposity are consistently associated in cross-sectional studies; however, results from prospective studies are mixed, with some evidence of bidirectionality (Lynch 2010). Review of the literature on sedentary behavior and health outcomes in adults concluded that time spent in sedentary behavior is associated prospectively with an increased risk of obesity and weight gain (Thorp et al. 2011). However, a systematic review conducted with a small number of studies meeting rigorous inclusion criteria concluded that there was insufficient evidence for the relationship between sedentary behavior and obesity or weight gain (Proper et al. 2011).

Nonetheless, there is a highly plausible and increasingly well-understood mechanism by which sedentary behavior contributes to adiposity. Time in sedentary behavior generally displaces time spent in light-intensity physical activity (Owen et al. 2010); such a shift reduces overall cumulative daily energy expenditure. Displacement of 2 hours per day of light-intensity activity (2.5 METs) by sedentary behavior (1.5 METs) would reduce activity energy expenditure by approximately 2 MET-hours per day. For a 70 kg (154 lb) male, this change in behavior would result in a decrease in daily energy expenditure equivalent to 140 kcal per day and potentially a 0.5 kg (1 lb) weight gain over 1 month. Unstructured movement and variation in posture have been shown to differ sufficiently between obese and lean people, explaining differences in weight independent of purposeful physical activity (Levine et al. 2005; Johannsen et al. 2007).

Sex Hormones

Exposure to biologically available sex hormones is a risk factor for hormone-related cancers, particularly breast, endometrial, and prostate cancers (Friedenreich and Orenstein 2002; McTiernan 2008). Sex hormone–binding globulin (SHBG) may also affect cancer risk by binding to sex hormones, rendering them biologically inactive (Friedenreich and Orenstein 2002; Neilson et al. 2009). Sedentary behavior may be associated with endogenous sex hormones through adiposity. In postmenopausal women, the main source of circulating estrogen is from conversion of androgens within adipose tissue (Lukanova and Kaaks 2005; Kendall, Folkerd, and Dowsett 2007); hence, adiposity directly influences levels of total and bioavailable estrogen (Cust 2011). Furthermore, visceral adipose tissue is important in the production of adipokines, which influence estrogen biosynthesis (Pou et al. 2007). Finally, sedentary behavior may increase blood insulin (see chapter 8), which is inversely associated with circulating SHBG.

The question of whether or not sedentary behavior directly affects sex hormone levels has not received much research attention. Only one study has considered the association: A cross-sectional study of 565 postmenopausal women examined associations of sitting time with various estrogens, androgens, and SHBG and found no statistically significant associations (Tworoger et al. 2007). A recent bed-rest study of 20 healthy men observed short-term increases in serum testosterone levels and sustained decreases in SHBG levels that were not fully explained by increases in body fat. Although the results of bed-rest studies may not extrapolate

to free-living humans, these findings suggest that the association between sedentary behavior and SHBG, in particular, warrants further investigation (Belavy et al. 2012).

Metabolic Dysfunction

Associations between insulin levels and colorectal, postmenopausal breast, pancreatic, and endometrial cancers have been demonstrated in epidemiological studies, and fasting glucose levels have been directly associated with pancreatic, kidney, liver, endometrial, biliary, and urinary tract cancers (Becker, Dossus, and Kaaks 2009). Neoplastic cells use glucose for proliferation; therefore, hyperglycemia may promote carcinogenesis by providing an amiable environment for tumor growth (Xue and Michels 2007).

High insulin levels increase bioavailable insulin-like growth factor-I, which is involved in cell differentiation, proliferation, and apoptosis (Nandeesha 2009). Decreasing blood insulin levels also results in increased hepatic synthesis of SHBG; hence, insulin indirectly increases bioavailability of endogenous sex hormones (Kaaks and Lukanova 2001).

Sedentary behavior could plausibly affect metabolic function through increased adiposity and decreased skeletal muscle mass. The sustained periods of muscular inactivity that occur during sedentary behavior may reduce glucose uptake through blunted translocation of GLUT-4 glucose transporters to the skeletal muscle surface (Hamilton, Hamilton, and Zderic 2007; Tremblay et al. 2010). Although cross-sectional studies mostly demonstrate significant associations between sedentary behavior and biomarkers of metabolic dysfunction, no clear evidence of an association has emerged from the limited prospective research to date (Proper et al. 2011; Thorp et al. 2011).

Adipokines and Inflammation

Chronic inflammation is acknowledged as a risk factor for most types of cancer (McTiernan 2008; Neilson et al. 2009). Inflammation may induce cell proliferation, microenvironmental changes, and oxidative stress, which in turn could deregulate normal cell growth and promote progression and malignant conversion (Coussens and Werb 2002). Obesity is considered a low-grade systematic inflammatory state (Lee and Pratley 2005). Adipose tissue is a complex metabolic and endocrine organ that secretes multiple biologically active polypeptides known collectively as *adipokines* (Kershaw and Flier 2004; Antuna-Puente et al. 2008), including leptin, adiponectin, tumor necrosis factor-α (TNF-α), and interleukin-6 (IL-6). C-reactive protein (CRP) is an acute phase protein produced in the liver in response to TNF-α and IL-6 levels; these factors are biomarkers of inflammation.

The release of adipokines may play a central role in the development of insulin resistance. Both leptin and adiponectin enhance insulin sensitivity through activation of AMP protein kinase (Antuna-Puente et al. 2008). Further, studies have demonstrated an interaction between cytokine receptors (such as the IL-6 receptor) and insulin signaling pathways that leads to decreased insulin signaling (Antuna-Puente et al. 2008). Elevated levels of adipokines might also increase cancer risk by affecting estrogen biosynthesis and estrogen activity (Pou et al. 2007).

Few epidemiological studies have linked sedentary behavior with biomarkers of inflammation. A prospective study examined the association of television viewing time with leptin and CRP in 468 men. A significant positive association between average television time (four assessments over 6 years) and leptin was observed; however, no association was seen with CRP (Fung et al. 2000). Similarly, change in television viewing time over a 5-year period was not associated with CRP in a sample of 1,001 female participants of the Australian Diabetes, Obesity and Lifestyle Study (Wiseman et al. 2014). In contrast, data from NHANES have demonstrated statistically significant cross-sectional associations between accelerometer-assessed sedentary time and CRP in postmenopausal women (Lynch, Friedenreich, et al. 2011) and in the broader adult population (Healy et al. 2011).

Summary

As the global burden of disease attributed to cancer continues to rise, identifying methods to reduce risk and enhance health post diagnosis will become increasingly important. Cancer represents a major burden of disease in both the developed and developing world; it is second only to cardiovascular disease in terms of cause of deaths. The majority of cancers could be prevented through avoiding tobacco products and smoke, maintaining a healthy body weight, eating a healthy diet, exercising regularly, and limiting alcohol intake. Sedentary behavior is hypothesized to be another modifiable cancer risk factor that will provide another intervention point for cancer control. Accumulating epidemiological evidence suggests that sedentary behavior may increase the risk of colorectal, endometrial, and lung cancers and possibly of breast and ovarian cancers. Sedentary behavior has also been implicated with poorer prognosis for colorectal cancer survivors. Additional research is needed to provide a clearer picture of the role that sedentary behavior plays in cancer development and progression and to establish whether reducing sedentary behavior is a viable new cancer control strategy.

MECHANISM QUESTIONS

How sedentary behavior may be associated with mechanisms operative in cancer pathogenesis has only begun to be explored. Findings from other scientific disciplines may provide avenues for inquiry to be pursued by epidemiological studies. For example, animal studies have identified genes in rat skeletal muscle whose expression is most sensitive to inactivity. These genes may be involved in the initial muscle adaptation to repeated episodes of sedentary behavior and in the etiology of diseases for which sedentary behavior is a risk factor (Bey et al. 2003). In another animal study, lifelong sedentary behavior in mice led to accelerated muscle mitochondrial dysfunction and increased levels of mitochondrial oxidative damage (Figueiredo et al. 2009). Molecular biologists have shown that mitochondrial dysfunction can lead to oxidative stress, resulting in significant damage to cell structures, including deoxyribonucleic acid (de Moura et al. 2010). Hence, mitochondrial function is hypothesized to contribute to neoplastic transformation and metastasis. Epigenetic modifications represent another plausible, but as yet unexamined, field of inquiry. A number of cross-sectional studies have demonstrated that methylation is a mediating factor between health behaviors, such as smoking and diet, and cancer risk (Lim and Song 2012; Shenker et al. 2013). Studies exploring the possible mediating role of methylation in the relationship between sedentary behavior and cancer are warranted.

KEY CONCEPTS

▶ **Adiposity:** The accumulation of adipose (fat) tissue. This term can be used to describe site-specific accumulation of fat (e.g., central adiposity) or for general body composition (e.g., high levels of adiposity).

▶ **Inflammation:** The response of body tissue to injury, infection, or irritation, characterized by redness or swelling. Acute inflammation provides protection against pathogens and stimulates tissue repair. Chronic inflammation may lead to disease, including cancer.

▶ **Metabolic dysfunction:** The disruption of normal metabolism (conversion of food to energy on a cellular level). The dysregulation of blood glucose, insulin resistance, hypertension, and cholesterol abnormalities are examples of metabolic dysfunction.

▶ **Sex hormones:** Steroid hormones (androgens, estrogens, progestogens) formed by testicular, ovarian, and adrenocortical tissue that affect the growth or function of the reproductive organs or the development of secondary sex characteristics.

STUDY QUESTIONS

1. What are the key limitations of the epidemiological research to date on sedentary behavior and cancer risk?

2. How might objective activity monitoring be incorporated into studies of cancer risk? What are some of the logistical issues that might limit the use of accelerometers in cohort studies?

3. Why might reducing sedentary behavior be a practical strategy for improving health outcomes in cancer survivors?

4. What other health outcomes might sedentary behavior contribute to in cancer survivors?

5. Name three potential biological mechanisms that may mediate the association between sedentary behavior and cancer risk.

The authors would like to thank Qinggang Wang for the production of the forest plots presented in this chapter.

CHAPTER 11

SEDENTARY BEHAVIOR AND LOWER BACK PAIN

Marco S. Boscolo, PhD; and Weimo Zhu, PhD

The reader will gain an overview of the scientific background of how sedentary behavior affects lower back pain. By the end of this chapter, the reader should be able to do the following:

▸ Discuss the association between sedentary behavior and lower back pain

▸ Understand and identify the mechanical causes of lower back pain

▸ Discuss the mechanisms by which sedentary behavior contributes to lower back pain

▸ Explain the mechanisms by which regular core muscle activation reduces the effects of sedentary behavior

▸ Review the financial costs associated with sedentary behavior and lower back pain

▸ Discuss the benefits of leisure-time physical activity as a modality for lower back pain prevention

Lower back health is an important consideration for overall health. Without good lower back health, it becomes increasingly difficult to accomplish many activities of daily living (e.g., rising from a chair, washing dishes, and dressing) and decreases the likelihood of participation in physical activity (PA) during leisure time (Heuch et al. 2013). Poor lower back health can also lead to poor functional ability and even disability. Lower back pain (LBP) is one of the most significant risk factors that causes millions of lost work days each year around the world (Ehrlich 2003) and contributes to more than 800,000 disability-adjusted life years lost annually (Punnett et al. 2005). How has this happened, and what is the role of prolonged sitting (or sedentary behavior and postures) in the LBP epidemic? As advances in technology have led to fewer jobs requiring moderate-to-vigorous intensity physical activity (Manson et al. 2004; Ng and Popkin 2012) and more sedentary jobs, such as deskbound work, continued increases in sedentary-related disabilities remain on the horizon. Human spines are not designed to sit for extended periods of time. Sedentary jobs (i.e., sitting jobs) are stagnant, and do not provide sufficient low-load muscle stimulation throughout the day to maintain a healthy spine and lower back. Sitting jobs require less core muscle activation (CMA) (i.e., muscle contraction) than standing, walking, or carrying objects. Sitting jobs also place the spine in a flexed posture that promotes issues such as bulging discs. This posture places more stress on the static (nonmuscular aspects) stability of the spine.

This chapter discusses the scope of the health hazards of sedentary behavior related to lower back health. It addresses the association between sedentary behavior and LBP, as well as the mechanical and psychological stresses involved with prolonged sitting. It also discusses the benefits of regular physical activity as a means to prevent LBP, and how to make people less likely to incur a lower back injury.

Lower Back Pain and Its Effects

Lower back pain refers to pain in the lower back due to either an acute or overuse injury or disease. Pain, which is the perception of discomfort, is caused by disruption of the nerve endings. Pain is either acute or chronic, and the perception of pain is very individualized (McCaffery and Pesero 1999). Pain warns us that something is injured or wrong in the body and reminds us to allow time to heal or to cease an action so as to avoid injury. Pain in the lower back,

and along the nerve roots leaving the lower back, is an indicator of a general lower back disorder (LBD) (i.e., mechanical disruption due to injury, disease, or genetic condition). Stuart McGill, a leading spine biomechanics researcher, defines LBDs as "disabling low back troubles" (2007, page 22). Specific LBDs typically have common mechanisms of injury. In general, LBP is produced when an LBD is sufficient enough to cause noxious nerve pressure. Lower back pain's origin then is due to a dysfunction of one or more of the following: lumbar sacral muscles, soft tissues (e.g., ligament, vertebral discs, and joint surfaces), or nervous tissue. To simplify the discussion in this chapter, *LBP* will be the term used unless the discussion is aided by the use of the term *LBD*.

LBP affects not only the lower back but also the functional ability of the individual. Lower back pain can make the simple act of walking difficult (Arendt-Nielsen et al. 1996; Vincent et al. 2013) and it alters whole-body stability (McGill et al. 2003), both of which contribute to making someone less physically active (Hendrick et al. 2013). A person with LBP is also less likely to be able to function at work (Maetzel and Li 2002) and to be physically active, which together could contribute to sedentary behavior (Hamilton et al. 2008). In general, anyone with poor lower back health will have difficulty functioning normally in daily life.

Annually, 34 million U.S. adults are affected by LBP (Hootman 2007). Eighty percent of people have suffered from LBP, and LBP is the fourth most common diagnosis at doctor visits (Chou 2014). The effects of poor lower back health place a huge burden on society (Becker et al. 2010), with the main consequences being days of lost work (Dagenais, Caro, and Haldeman 2008):

▶ LBP accounts for 40% of all workers' compensation claims (Lis et al. 2007), with a total of $56 billion workers' compensation paid in the United States in 2004 (Manchikanti et al. 2009).

▶ In the United States, 50 to 100 billion dollars are spent by employers for LBP-related disability every year (Frymoyer and Cats-Baril 1991; Stewart et al. 2003), and 50 billion dollars are spent by the public alone on LBP (National Institute of Neurological Disorders and Stroke 2015).

With sedentary behavior's increasing prevalence (Manson et al. 2004), coupled with higher medical care costs (Stern 2013) and a greater reporting of disability (Berecki-Gisolf et al. 2012), the future economic effects of LBP likely will increase.

Spine Anatomy

To fully understand LBP and its causes, a brief description of the anatomy of the spine and its stability is helpful. Specifically, an understanding of the anatomy of the spine will help understanding concerning the effects of sedentary behavior on LBP.

The spine is fundamental to the body's health. The spine permits the extremities to work, protects the central nervous system, allows for locomotion, and incorporates the musculoskeletal system in intricate patterns to produce torque, stability, and function. Ideally, the spine is relatively straight when viewed from behind (figure 11.1) and has three curved sections when viewed from the side. For a more complete understanding of spine anatomy and mechanics, the authors suggest reviewing a basic anatomy text and an advanced spine mechanics text (McGill 2007). Together the spine, rib cage, and pelvis form the foundational base for core of the body, which protects organs and nervous tissue. In between the bones of the spine (i.e., vertebra) sit intervertebral discs, which can be compressed with prolonged sitting in flexed spine posture. If these nerve roots become compressed through swelling, vertebral disc bulging, or bony compression, pain and dysfunction can result at the lower back and along the leg.

Spine Stability

For the purpose of understanding the effects of sedentary behavior on LBP, it is helpful to have a basic understanding of static (nonmuscular) and dynamic (muscular) spinal stability as they relate to LBP. *Static stability* refers to the support provided by the thick ligaments surrounding the spine, the vertebral discs, the facet joints, and the vertebral bones themselves. *Dynamic stability* refers to the neuromuscular control of the 20-plus muscles of the core (i.e., primarily the lower torso muscles). Without dynamic stability, the spine would quickly fail. Dynamic stability is a learned pattern that starts at birth. Infants' dexterity and stability are very limited, and their movement patterns look like those of a giant sea monster in classic seafaring movies attacking a boat with its tentacles in that their arms and legs are flailing everywhere. As the child develops, the body learns to maintain an

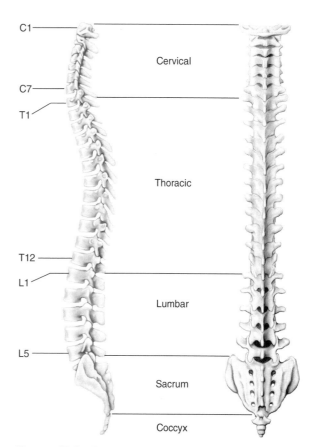

Figure 11.1 Bony anatomy and regions of the spine.

upright posture, to walk, and then to lift and move objects. These movements require complex coordination of the neuromuscular system and sufficient muscle strength.

Each of these movement patterns—walking, lifting a box, throwing a ball, rising from a chair, or pushing on an object—requires complex coordination of the core muscles. Without this coordination, spine stability can easily become compromised. The core muscles that encompass the spine act to provide stability during different body movement patterns. The core muscles do so dynamically by varying contraction patterns and contraction lengths as the body moves. The stiffness of the spine and core muscles can be thought of as forming a platform from which the body operates. The core muscle's function is similar to that of the support wires on masted sailing ships, which attach the hull of the ship to points along the mast, act to broaden the base of stability, and transfer force from the sails to the ship to provide directional movement. Similarly, the core muscles attach to the pelvis and the horizontal processes (e.g., the vertebral bodies' bony processes and ribs) to facilitate movement by more complex and intricate neuromuscular patterns. If one of the wires (or muscles) is not working properly, the mast (or spine) becomes less efficient and more prone to failure or injury.

The neutral spine—a spine with neither too much curvature anteriorly or posteriorly and very little rotation, flexion, or extension—is capable of bearing significant weight and resisting torque without injury (Cholewicki and McGill 1996). No one perfect spinal posture exists. Each person has their own ideal neutral spine. Whenever the weight or torque applied to the spine is too great, or if the spine is positioned outside its best neutral position, there is a greater risk for injury. Positions outside the neutral spine posture, as when the spine is rotated, reduce the spine's ability to bear weight by 50% (Aultman et al. 2004). Biering-Sørensen (1984) showed that risk indicators for lower back trouble were weak trunk muscles and increased spine mobility, also known as spine instability.

A good visual example of stability of the spine is the stout empty soda can. If the walls of the soda remain undamaged, it can bear a reasonable amount of downward force. But if one side becomes dented, the stability of the can is compromised and its ability to bear a downward force is decreased, and the soda can will be crushed. Although the human spine mechanically operates differently than a soda can, a similar principle applies. Decrease the stability of the spine by flexing, extending, or twisting the lumbar spine too far out from its margin of stability, and it becomes unstable and less capable to withstand downward force. It is the unstable spine that is more likely to become injured and lead to LBP. A common view about the mechanics of human joint stability is that with increased mobility comes an increased chance of injury. This is very true for the lower back static structures, which have a low margin of error before the probability of tissue failure increases (Cholewicki and McGill 1996; Tanaka et al. 2001). This potential for injury is compounded in sedentary people. Compromised lower back dynamic muscle support is found in the injured or people with insufficient core muscle strength. For normal daily activities like walking and sitting erect, only a moderate amount of CMA—actually only 10% of CMA (Escamilla et al. 2010)—is needed to stabilize the lumbar spine; higher demand activities require a much higher percentage of CMA.

Known Risk Factors of Lower Back Pain

Many factors have been found related to lower back pain, including aging, genetics, occupation, sedentary lifestyle, excess weight, poor posture, pregnancy, and smoking. These factors have been well described in systematic reviews or meta-analyses (Kwon et al. 2011; Ribeiro et al. 2012; Roffey et al. 2010; Taylor et al. 2014). Only a few selected factors are briefly described in this section.

Disuse and Deconditioning

Historically, humans had to move on a regular basis to survive and procure food, shelter, and safety. With modern conveniences, humans do not need to move as much; thus, muscles are used less (Owen et al. 2010). This leads to the situation where people can become deconditioned unless they actively engage the core muscles either through sufficient activities of daily living or purposeful exercise. LBP is further exacerbated in sedentary people with a compromised ventilatory system (McGill, Sharratt, and Seguin 1995); healthy ventilation is important to PA. People with compromised ventilatory systems fail to use their diaphragm efficiently, which results in their using their core muscles to help them breathe, especially the erector spinae muscles. Spinal extension helps facilitate inspiration. However, increased activation of the erector spinae muscles also increases compression of the intervertebral discs, leading to increased LBP and perpetuating the cycle of pain and disuse. What is needed is regular conditioning of core muscles through nonfatiguing activity.

Nonfatiguing activity relates to nonsedentary behavior such as walking, washing the dishes, vacuuming, carrying groceries, and gardening, or a combination of nonfatiguing activities done regularly throughout the day. Regular nonfatiguing activities help condition the muscles. This then helps increase dynamic stability, which makes people more resistant to injury. According to Handrakis and colleagues (2012), regular nonfatiguing activities help college-age students avoid LBP. They showed that core muscle endurance strength was lower in sedentary college students with LBP compared to college students who were more active. The key message here is that being more active leads to greater muscle conditioning and aids in the maintenance of dynamic stability.

Obesity and Body Mass

A higher body mass index (BMI) is associated with more sedentary behavior (Heuch et al. 2013), more disability, and more pain symptoms than in the nonobese (Fanuele et al. 2002), as well as a higher prevalence of LBP (O'Sullivan et al. 2011; Strine and Hootman 2007). The relationship between higher BMI and sedentary behavior is circular concerning LBP. Sedentary behavior associated with higher BMI leads to muscle disuse; with muscle disuse, dynamic lower back stability is likely to decrease. This decrease is from not only core muscle disuse but also the disuse of other transfer muscles in the lower extremity, such as those of the hip, thigh, leg, knee, ankle, and foot. Properly conditioned core muscles stiffen the spine to keep it in a neutral posture while the body moves. Strong hip extensors function to extend the hips, which keeps the trunk erect during functional activities. However, with greater body mass to move relative to muscle mass, the dynamic support system can become compromised.

Environment Effect

How someone moves or sits is directly related to the environment. When motorized means are used for transportation, there is an increase in sitting time as opposed to physically active transportation such as walking or biking. By doing more regular physically active tasks, we are able to condition the core muscles by practicing CMA in different neuromuscular patterns. Opening a door requires the body to generate torque. Walking with groceries in one hand requires us to maintain an upright posture and breathe from the diaphragm while counterbalancing the grocery bag's weight with the core muscles. Pushing a heavy cart in a factory requires the core muscles to brace the spine in order to apply force to the cart through the upper body. Less core activity is required for sedentary activities such as driving and sitting at a desk. Activities like walking, one of the easiest forms of PA, have been shown to be a factor in the prevention and treatment of LBP (Nutter 1988), and fast walking has been shown to increase core stiffness (Kubo et al. 2006) and be more therapeutic over slow walking (Callaghan, Patla, and McGill 1999).

Relationship Between Lower Back Pain and Sedentary Behavior

Sedentary behavior is defined as too much sitting; it is different from inactivity, which is a lack of moderate-to-vigorous intensity activity (Owen et al. 2010; see also chapter 1 of this book for more information). Prior to this new definition, sedentary behavior also included inactivity or little to no PA (Owen and Bauman 1992). Sedentary behavior and inactivity reflect specific metabolic values used to establish what type of PA a person is doing at any given time. According to Owen and colleagues (2010), metabolic equivalents for sedentary behavior fall in the area of approximately 1.0 to 1.5 METs and inactive behavior falls in the area of approximately 1.6 to 2.9 METs. Knowing the metabolic demands of sedentary behavior versus inactivity helps researchers identify behaviors that are related to metabolic disease. The new definition of sedentary behavior is more appropriate in that it reflects a public health need to reduce sitting time for general health reasons (Salmon et al. 2011), but it could underrepresent injurious sitting behaviors that lead to LBP. This is because knowing the metabolic demands of sedentary behavior and inactivity does little to help in the understanding of LBP. Instead, understanding the physical positions and environments people are in for extended periods is more important when studying LBP.

Increased Sitting Behavior

People today are sitting more and for longer durations than ever before. There are now many more opportunities and reasons to sit at home and at work, largely due to technology. Watching TV, cruising the Internet, and playing a video game are all sedentary activities in which the spine is usually not held in proper postures. The U.S. Department of Labor (2005), for example, estimates that 77 million people use a computer at work daily in 2003. Currently, 92% of Americans use computers, 81% use them at home and 68% at work, and 68% find computers essential to their work (Gilkey 2014). In the last 20 years, computer use in the home, which primarily requires sitting, has increased from approximately 8.2% to 75% (File 2013).

Prolonged Sitting and Health

Sitting, the most common sedentary behavior affecting lower back health, is a serious health hazard (Hamilton et al. 2008). The health risk of sitting was in fact noted more than 300 years ago by Bernardino Ramazzini, an Italian physician and the father of occupational medicine. Ramazzini (2001) identified prolonged sitting as bad for health because it causes the spine to permanently deform and produces LBP. He also indicated PA and good posture as medicine for sitting, or sedentary, behavior.

Sitting-related injuries of the lower back are thought to be the result of long-term passive tissue strain that is caused by prolonged sitting with a flexed spine. The flexed spine posture results in passive tissue creep (Jackson et al. 2001). As Ramazzini said in reference to prolonged sitting, "the outermost vertebral ligaments are kept pulled apart" (2001, 1380). Passive tissue creep is a result of mechanical stress placed on the spine's ligaments and discs that causes the ligaments to elongate and the discs to compress where they are stressed. Compressed spinal discs and joint surfaces lose their hydraulic support capability when they remain in a fixed position for an extended period of time. Prolonged sitting compromises the static stability of the lower back, decreases spine stability, and increases the risk for injury (McGill and Brown 1992). When people with an unstable spine, either due to injury or temporary spinal instability due to prolonged sitting in a flexed spine posture, are asked to perform tasks such as picking up a *light* object on the floor by bending the spine but not the hips or lifting a heavy object without good lifting mechanics, they are at an increased risk for injury to the ligaments and discs of the lower back (Little and Khalsa 2005; McGill and Brown 1992; Twomey and Taylor 1982). Mechanically, prolonged sitting and the back do not have a healthy relationship.

Another key factor to having a healthy lower back is to unload the spine with opposite loading activities. Opposite loading provides a release of compression on one side of the spine and tension on the other side. It reduces and helps ameliorate the tissue creep caused by sitting with a flexed spine posture. McGill (2007) provides a good example of how technology has led to an increase in LBD and why opposite loading activities are important for reducing the effects of sedentary behavior. Prior to the redesigning of a power plant, the control room where the engineers sat and monitored equipment, there was no history of reported LBP because the engineers needed to stand every 10 minutes to press a vigilance buzzer. After the control room received a technological upgrade, engineers no longer had to stand to push the vigilance buzzer during their 12-hour shifts. Subsequently, they started reporting lower back problems.

Two key points emerge from this example. The first is that the design of the old engineering control room forced the engineers into an opposite loading activity, which is important when considering overuse injury and spine stability. The engineers' need to stand brought their flexed spine into a neutral spine posture. They had to do this nonfatiguing activity, which provided more CMA than sitting at a computer, on a regular basis throughout the day. The second key point is that the nature of these engineers' work was sedentary, and these types of jobs typically have a larger proportion of people who are categorized as either overweight or obese. Given that the engineers in both the old and new control rooms were most likely in this category of worker and given their apparent waist girth (see figure 11.2), the key factors between having and not having a LBD could be directly attributed to the amount of regular nonfatiguing PA and opposite loading activities engaged in on a daily basis.

Other studies have shown that poor sitting posture can lead to LBP (Lis et al. 2007), disuse of core muscles (Nocera et al. 2011; Tomlinson et al. 2014), and tissue damage due to unequal vertebral disc pressure (McGill and Brown 1992; Tanaka et al. 2001). Recent inactivity physiology research also strongly suggests that sedentary behavior could lead to disability (Dunlop et al. 2014). Disability due to musculoskeletal disorders has increased 45% compared to an average increase of 33% for all other diseases combined and is largely attributed to an aging population, obesity, and lack of PA (Bone and Joint Decade 2012). Among the 291 conditions studied by Hoy and colleagues (2014), LBP was found to be the leading cause of disability. The prevalence of LBP was about 31% of the population worldwide. In older adults, it has been shown that for every hour spent sedentary, the risk for becoming disabled increases by 46% (Dunlop et al. 2014). Poor sitting posture, as discussed here, does not promote good lower back health.

It should be noted that up to this point, the empirical evidence on an association between LBP and prolonged sitting, collectively, has not been consistent. A systematic review by Chen and colleagues

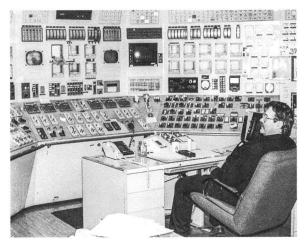

a

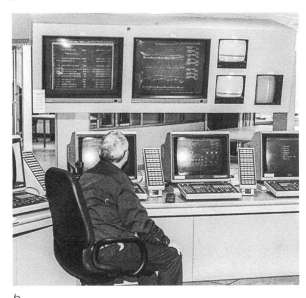

b

Figure 11.2 Comparison of work environments: noncomputerized and computerized.

Reprinted, by permission, from S. McGill, 2016, *Low back disorders: Evidence-based prevention and rehabilitation* (Champaign, IL: Human Kinetics), 207.

(2009) could not find any systematic evidence showing that prolonged sitting was associated with LBP. The authors suggested that a potential reason for this lack of association is that the included studies (*n* = 15) lacked a good measurement of cumulative load over one's lifetime. That is, the cumulative load from sitting may reach a threshold at which injury occurs, and the current evidence does not identify this exposure. A systematic review by Proper and colleagues (2011) also found no association between LBP and prolonged sitting. These authors also questioned the ability of the studies included in their systematic review to capture the causal

relationship between sedentary behavior and LBP. However, ample justification exists for the continued study of the association between sedentary behavior and LBP. Because work is becoming increasingly sedentary, it can have a negative effect on health. Mechanically, it has been shown that the stability of the lumbar spine is compromised during prolonged sitting, thus contributing to compromised core stability (Howarth et al. 2013).

Sedentary Behavior and Inactivity

It should be pointed out that sedentary behavior and inactivity could also promote body positions and environments that can lead to LBD and LBP. These positions and environments include lying down, sitting, sitting in vibratory environments (such as a car), and standing. For the purpose of referencing standardized positions and environments, the *Physical Activity Compendium* (Ainsworth et al. 2011) lists several PA categories, their accompanying MET values, and a description of the activity. Several of the compendium activities that fall in either the sedentary behavior or inactive MET categories, as outlined by Owen and colleagues (2010), describe lying down, sitting, and standing activities. The lying-down activities (typically around 1 MET) do not lead directly to LBDs except for lack of CMA in these positions, which can lead to core muscle disuse and deconditioning. The latter two activities, if prolonged, can contribute to decreased spine stability. The sitting activities typically range in MET values from 1.3 ("sitting quietly and watching television") to 2.5 ("mowing lawn, riding mower"). Sedentary-related behaviors in occupations such police work (i.e., driving a squad car) have a MET value of 2.5. Only a few standing activities in occupations fall below the inactivity threshold of 2.9 METs. These include a police officer directing traffic (2.5 METs) and road construction worker directing traffic (2.0 METs). Standing itself does not typically lead to lower back pain unless the person stands with a stooped posture for an extended period or has lingering LBP from a prior injury that is aggravated by standing. Standing with bad posture can increase contraction of erector spinae muscles (i.e., the erector spinae muscles attach along the sacrum and posterior spine). When contracted, this muscle group extends the spine. This contraction prevents forward slippage of one vertebra onto another and pulls together adjacent vertebrae to increase spinal stiffness, which consequently also increases intervertebral disc pressure, provoking nerve pain. The key here is use regular and varied movement to combat the static postures of sedentary behavior.

Prevention of Lower Back Pain

In theory, preventing most spinal injuries is easy. Use correct mechanics when moving and lifting (i.e., maintain a neutral spine) and always engage the correct muscles while lifting. Note here that other lifting postures, such as allowing the spine to flex while lifting an object from the floor or stooped lifting, are also viable lifting techniques; however, the stooped lifting technique can lead to dramatic vertebral shearing forces (see McGill 2007 for further discussion). Considering that LBP is the leading cause of referral to a physician's office (Debono, Hoeksema, and Hobbs 2013), perfect back use is obviously not occurring in the context of everyday life, and no injury can be prevented entirely. Many jobs demand us to work while in specific postures and repeatedly use our bodies for specific duties throughout the workday. In sitting jobs, often there is no choice but to sit, such as a bus driver who must sit and drive. According to the U.S. Department of Health and Human Services (2008), reducing sitting time helps reduce metabolic diseases such as heart disease, diabetes, and stroke. The real solution to reducing the incidence of LBP is to stand more and be more active throughout the day. As mentioned earlier, standing every 10 minutes was sufficient to alleviate the effects of prolonged flexed spine posture; moving every 20 or 30 minutes may suffice.

Sitting can lead to the shortening of the hamstring and hip flexor muscles (McGill and Brown 1992). Tight hamstrings and hip flexors, however, are not the cause of LBP (Johnson and Thomas 2010; Koley and Likhi 2011; Nourbakhsh and Arab 2002), although they may be present in people with LBP. Rather, it is a person's activities and habits that lead to LBP unless other diseases are present, such as osteoporosis (Hoozemans et al. 2012; Jones, Pandit, and Lavy 2014) or cancer. Normal body mechanics include standing and sitting with good posture and lifting an object from a low elevation (such as knee level). Picking an object up off the floor with a neutral spine requires a higher degree of hip range of motion (ROM), which is limited by genetics and age. Hip ROM lessens with age. Recognizing their reduction in ROM, older adults are then more likely to use static support of the spine and hamstrings to pick an object up from the floor and rise from a

chair. Activities like regular gardening, moderate manual labor, walking, and carrying weights (e.g., grocery bags) can help influence normal muscle length and good posture as long as a person becomes self-aware of posture, develops sufficient core endurance muscle strength, and uses good lifting habits.

In addition, the benefits of regular CMA also translate to a stronger and more stable core. A stronger core aids in preventing future LBD (Steele, Bruce-Low, and Smith 2014) and enhances distal limb (i.e., hip, knee, and ankle) stability (Pfile et al. 2014). This added distal limb stability helps prevent fall-related injury and aids in general functional ability. With increased ability and stability in the aging population, greater independence can be maintained further into the life span.

Habits

Several strategies can help alleviate possible LBP, such as standing and contracting the posture muscles regularly throughout the day (i.e., standing in a "champion" posture with hands over the head and contracting the posterior muscles), consciously practicing better posture, sitting in a neutral spine position, rising from a chair properly, and using correct lifting technique. The final strategy includes lifting the body correctly when transitioning from sitting to standing and moving or lifting a heavy box correctly using the hip extensor muscles (e.g., gluteus maximus) instead of the back extensors and hamstrings as the primary movers. Often people transition from sitting to standing by pitching their upper torso forward over their knees and then contracting their spinal extensors and hamstrings in order to achieve an upright posture. This repeated pitching forward motion is challenging for older adults (Bohannon 2012) due to age-related loss in muscle mass and for obese people (Galli et al. 2000) because of extra upper-body mass. Instead they use a transition strategy with flexed spine posture that causes the lumbar curve to flex into a flattened posture, causing anterior compression of the lumbar vertebral discs, which forces the fluid material of the disc to push posterior. Movement of fluid then predisposes them for a posterior bulge injury. A better strategy is to transition to standing by holding the trunk upright while engaging the hip extensors and assuming a wide base with the feet.

The best way to sit and what to sit on remain a matter of debate (see chapters 4 and 26); however, many experts will agree that the best sitting posture is the next one (O'Sullivan et al. 2012). This means adjusting your sitting posture often throughout the time spent sitting. The body will not tolerate being stagnant for extended periods of time. The human body is homeostatic. It thrives on frequent and varied movement. Without movement, the body tissues would not receive intra- and extracellular fluid, nutrients, and blood flow with which to replenish energy. Most lower back injuries are believed to occur as a result of long-term poor body mechanics that eventually lead to tissue failure (Callaghan and McGill 2001). Additional causes, however, include traumatic events (e.g., falling or car accidents). Conversely, practicing good body mechanics on a daily basis leads to a healthier lower back (O'Sullivan et al. 2011).

Occupational Sedentariness

Sedentariness has increased in the workplace and contributes to unhealthy behavior and obesity (Luckhaupt et al. 2014). Occupational-related LBP occurs not just in sedentary professions, but also in positions that require repetitious or prolonged activity (Walsh et al. 1989) in spine-compromising postures or movement patterns. Sedentary jobs place the worker in a seated posture for extended periods of time (McGill 1997; Videman, Nurminen, and Troup 1990). More bulged disk–type injuries are found in sitting jobs (Lis et al. 2007). Prolonged sedentariness in itself can contribute to age-related sarcopenia and obesity (Nocera et al. 2011). Conversely, active heavy jobs can also have a variety of occupational stresses, including prolonged or repeated bending over, heavy lifting, and heavy pushing or pulling at odd angles and under heavy loads. An active heavy job that requires flexion and extension, or prolonged disc compression, can predispose workers to vertebral shear injury and disc compression injury.

Sedentary types of jobs have been shown to play a role in shortening the time to the first episode of LBP and increasing one's risk for obtaining a LBD. A good example, as first demonstrated in McGill's 2007 book, is the comparison between two large occupational epidemiology studies. These studies showed that nurses reported fewer lower back injuries (53.3%) compared to police officers (59.5%), even though their job is more demanding throughout the day and requires a variety of physical activities (Burton et al. 1996; Burton et al. 1997). Irish police officers, the focus of one of the studies, who wore an 8.4 kg (18.5 lb) body armor vest (thus placing a larger load on their upper body) and sat in a vibratory environment more often had a shorter time period before first reporting of LBP (Burton et al. 1996). Burton and colleagues (1996) also showed that English police officers who did not wear body armor vests had a longer time period until their first report of LBP. An association could be made that the higher load borne by the Irish police officers was similar to the increased load borne by overweight and obese people. Also, the physical position in which police officers worked for extended periods (i.e., sitting) and the environment (i.e., in a vibrating vehicle) might be the mechanisms leading to an injury compared to a nurse, whose job is more upright in physical position, variable throughout the day, and less sedentary.

Keep in mind that LBP is not entirely a sedentary issue. Overuse or injury of the lower back can also lead to LBP, which can lead to sedentary behavior after being injured. For example, a roofer and a desk worker can both have LBP after a long career. The roofer has a job that is classified as very heavy and the desk worker most likely has a job classified as sedentary to light (Matheson 2003). As mentioned previously, the nature of the job has a heavy influence on the type of LBD—spinal stenosis, disc bulge, or vertebra fracture. Finding the optimal balance between regular use of the core muscles and using the right back or movement mechanics, while not overstressing the spine, is key for maintaining optimal lower back health throughout the life span.

Leisure-Time Physical Activity

Leisure-time physical activity (LTPA) appears to have a positive influence on making people more resistant to LBP (Cady et al. 1979; Leino 1993; McQuade, Turner, and Buchner 1998), although it has the potential for causing musculoskeletal injury (Hootman et al. 2002). LTPA appears to facilitate a cross-training effect. For example, Stevenson and colleagues (2001) found that factory and construction workers who partook in personal fitness were less likely to incur LBP. Pinto and colleagues (2014) found that high- to vigorous intensity LTPA had a positive effect on a group of LBP sufferers in reducing the rate of reported pain and disability compared to a sedentary group. The likely lower back protective mechanism from LTPA is that it helps facilitate muscle activation patterns that are different from the movement patterns imposed by work, thus bringing the stability of the spine back into balance. How much PA is needed to provide a protective mechanism is not yet clearly understood. A dose–response relationship of the ideal amount of LTPA relative to someone's work may be apparent from jobs classified as both sedentary and heavy labor.

Care, however, must be taken when transitioning from a sedentary to an active lifestyle. An inappropriate increase in PA can not only lead to LBP, but it might also exacerbate current LBP symptoms in those using PA as a means to reduce LBP symptoms (Hootman et al. 2002). Many sedentary people show up at their doctor's office with orthopedic injuries due to doing too much PA too soon in their attempt to transition from a sedentary to an active lifestyle. Some have tried commercialized fitness programs like P90X or CrossFit, which are high impact, high intensity, and accelerated routines designed for already active people. Sedentary people who use these kinds of programs can more easily become injured because their bodies are not ready for such demanding PA programs. People characterized as sedentary, especially older adults, initially may find decreasing time spent in sedentary behavior to be a more attainable goal than increasing moderate-to-vigorous intensity PA right away (Dunlop et al. 2014; Hootman et al. 2002).

Summary

The recent history of LBP largely reflects the sedentary behavior of sitting. Prolonged sitting in static postures leads to lumbar instability through muscle disuse and ligamentous tissue creep. This instability sets people up for increased LBDs and LBP, which can result in disability. The epidemiological evidence has yet to show a strong causal relationship between LBP and sedentary behavior, but ample biomechanical studies and exercise studies show the benefit of regular PA and good spine mechanics concerning LBP. The selection of exercises for PA addressing LBP should be based on sound biomechanical evidence of the tissue stresses being placed on the spine during various body postures and exercise activities. Selection of the correct exercises for LBP interventions or LBP and injury prevention programs are crucial for successful outcomes and for the safety of the participants.

WORKPLACE PHYSICAL ACTIVITY PROGRAMS

Sitting is a serious health hazard (Hamilton et al. 2008), yet its prevalence in society appears to be increasing. Although a strong relationship between sedentary behavior and LBP has not yet been demonstrated, people in sedentary jobs continue to experience LBP from sitting too much. If sedentariness-related LBP is to be reduced in the future, workers and those who manage work environments need to place greater emphasis on practicing regular PA that unloads the spine and taking ample breaks from sitting that encourage nonfatiguing CMA.

When designing PA programs for those transitioning from a sedentary to active lifestyle, proper selection of exercises should include exercises for the lower back that are solid, evidence based, and biomechanically sound (McGill 1998). A variety of general transitioning programs exist for people moving to an active lifestyle, but we still do not know the exact dose–response of how much initial PA is too much PA or the exact amount of opposite loading activities required for achieving optimal lower back health (McGill 2007). Dose–response studies with humans are difficult to conduct due to the cost associated with studying the many combinations of factors typically found in these studies and because human variability influences study consistency, thus inflating the number of participants needed. Boscolo (2013) provided a design of experiment solution for human-based optimization studies that explored just a fraction of the possible factor combinations required in order to reduce study cost and resources, yet still effectively estimated the optimal outcome, making this once seemingly impossible study possible.

KEY CONCEPTS

▸ **Core muscle activation:** The contraction of the core muscles to support spine stiffness.

▸ **Lower back disorder:** Any dysfunction in the lower back that produces lower back pain and disability.

▸ **Opposite loading activities:** Any activity that unloads prolonged tension on human tissue; flexed spine posture is best relieved by assuming an opposite posture of standing erect.

▸ **Optimal loading:** The amount of regular physical activity required for maintaining lower back health; regular nonfatiguing core muscle activation.

STUDY QUESTIONS

1. How does regular core muscle activation help stabilize the spine?

2. What positions are the lower back and spine typically placed in while sedentary?

3. What type of activities help prevent lower back disorders and pain?

4. Describe the mechanism by which posterior disk pressure is ameliorated while transitioning from sitting to standing.

5. How does sedentary behavior increase the odds of someone incurring lower back pain?

6. In what position is the spine most stable?

7. What is the recommended progression for a sedentary person to become more active?

CHAPTER 12

SEDENTARY BEHAVIOR AND PSYCHOLOGICAL WELL-BEING

Stuart J.H. Biddle, PhD; and Stephan Bandelow, PhD

The reader will gain an overview of the evidence for associations between sedentary behavior and psychological well-being. By the end of this chapter, the reader should be able to do the following:

▸ Appraise the evidence for associations between sedentary behavior and various psychological indicators of well-being, including depression, health-related quality of life, and cognitive functioning

▸ Discuss how different types of sedentary behavior may be differentially associated with psychological well-being

▸ Discuss possible explanations for any associations between sedentary behavior and psychological well-being

▸ Understand how reverse causality may be in operation for some or all of these associations

Psychological well-being can be seen in the context of both the treatment of mental ill-health and the enhancement of normal states of well-being into higher levels of mental health. It is also multidimensional, with aspects of mental health comprising generalized mood states, emotions, and core affect (see Ekkekakis 2013a), as well as specific conditions such as depression, anxiety and stress, and self-esteem. In addition, more functional aspects of our mental health are evident through cognitive performance and cognitive decline.

Although we all seek good mental health and higher states of well-being, it has been poor mental health that has been the focus of a great deal of research and, indeed, public health concern. Mental illness is widespread. The World Health Organization has estimated that unipolar depression will be the second most prominent cause of disease burden across the world by 2020 (Murray and Lopez 1997). An analysis of the public health effects of chronic disease in 60 countries concluded that depression produces the greatest decrement of health, ahead of angina, arthritis, asthma, and diabetes (Moussavi et al. 2007). The prevalence of mental illness in the UK is 230 per 1,000 referrals to primary care services, and 1 in 6 adults living in the UK reports some kind of neurotic disorder such as depression, anxiety, or a phobia.

The prevalence of cognitive impairment is rapidly increasing as the population ages. About 820,000 people in the UK have dementia, and 98% of those are over the age of 65 years. In high-income countries, Alzheimer and other dementias are predicted to be the seventh leading cause of death and the third leading cause of morbidity (disability-adjusted life years) by 2030 (Mathers and Loncar 2006). Mental illness is as common as high blood pressure and much more common than heart attacks and strokes. Its treatment requires 17% of all health care expenditure, and mental and behavioral disorders now account for more incapacity benefit claims than musculoskeletal problems such as lower back pain (Henderson, Glozier, and Elliot 2005). Large economic costs are associated with mental illness, and mental health conditions are also an important cause of absence from work.

Mental health, therefore, is not a trivial issue. It is a key part of public health, and many forms of prevention and treatment have been studied. For centuries, humans have reported positive psychological effects of being physically active. Over the past few decades, there has been an explosion of research investigating many aspects of physical activity and mental health (Ekkekakis 2013b). Despite challenging methodological issues, evidence clearly points to an association between higher levels of physical activity and lower depression and anxiety (Mutrie 2000; Rethorst, Wipfli, and Landers 2009; Wipfli, Rethorst, and Landers 2008); more positive feelings of self-esteem (Spence, McGannon, and Poon 2005), especially physical self-worth (Fox 2000); higher perceptions of quality of life (Rejeski, Brawley, and Shumaker 1996); and better cognitive functioning (Colcombe and Kramer 2003; Hamer and Chida 2009). The majority of studies have been conducted with adults, but evidence is also available showing similar effects in young people (Biddle and Asare 2011).

As is clear from the burgeoning literature on sedentary behavior, and this book of course, sedentary behavior encompasses a set of behaviors that involve sitting or reclining and low energy expenditure (Newton et al. 2013; Sedentary Behaviour Research Network 2012). Sedentary behavior is not the same as low levels of physical activity; this is defined as being physically inactive. This begs the key question: Do mental health effects exist that stem from high levels of sedentary behavior? In this chapter, we summarize evidence concerning sedentary behavior and psychological well-being. We attempt to focus on sedentary behavior, but because the study of sedentary behavior and mental health is new, we will sometimes need to refer to studies that focus primarily on physical activity. However, this is not a chapter on physical activity and mental health—there are many of those (see Ekkekakis 2013b). We focus on studies where the exposure variable of interest is sedentary behavior and the outcomes are facets of psychological well-being. We address the outcomes of depression, cognitive functioning, and other domains of psychological well-being, such as quality of life. It is important to state before we review evidence that sedentary behavior research in the mental health domain is quite new, and is still testing associations using primarily observational (cross-sectional) studies. It is clear that such designs cannot conclude about causality. Indeed, they are open to the interpretation that where sedentary behavior is associated with better or worse mental health, this may be explained through the notion of *reverse causality*—that is, for example, where those with poor mental health choose to be more sedentary.

Sedentary Behavior and Depression

Teychenne, Ball, and Salmon (2008) conducted a systematic review on depression and sedentary behavior in adults. Seven observational (5 cross-sectional and 2 longitudinal) and four intervention studies were included. Of the observational studies, 6 of 7 showed a positive association between sedentary behavior and depression; that is, higher sedentary behavior was associated with greater depression. The other study also showed this for time spent surfing the Internet, but reported negative associations for depression with hours spent e-mailing and using chat rooms. This suggests that the type of sedentary behavior may be an important moderator of any association between sedentary behavior and depression. More is said on this subject later in the chapter.

The four intervention studies reviewed by Teychenne et al. (2008) showed mixed results: one study showed no effect and one showed an increase in depression after the introduction of free computer and Internet use, while two showed that the risk of depression was reduced during the intervention. One provided extra computer and Internet use while the other used extra chat sessions. The latter may have boosted well-being through social interaction. It is important to note that the authors of the review concluded that at the time, no interventions had attempted to reduce sedentary behavior in an effort to assess changes in depression.

Since the review by Teychenne et al. (2008), there have been several large-scale epidemiological studies published on this topic. Vallance and colleagues (2011) analyzed data from 2,862 adults from the National Health and Nutrition Examination Survey (NHANES) for 2005-2006. This is a national survey of U.S. adults that, for this time period, assessed physical activity and sedentary behavior objectively using accelerometers. Depression was assessed using the Patient Health Questionnaire-9.

Results showed that in comparison to the least sedentary quartile (the reference group), there was a trend for a greater risk of depression for those with higher levels of sedentary behavior. This was most clearly shown in the most sedentary quartile. This is shown in figure 12.1 for data from model 1 (odds ratios adjusted for gender, ethnicity, and age) and for model 2 with additional adjustment for other sociodemographic factors, health status, and moderate- to vigorous-intensity physical activity (MVPA). Although model 2 shows some attenuation of the odds for depression, the same trend is evident, and the most sedentary group has a twofold elevated risk of depression over those in the lowest sedentary quartile.

In a cross-sectional study of 3,645 Australian women from disadvantaged neighborhoods (Teychenne, Ball, and Salmon 2010a), four types of

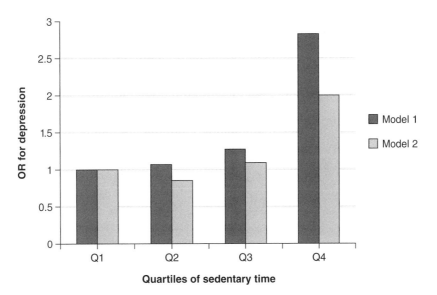

Figure 12.1 Odds ratios (OR) for depression across quartiles of objectively assessed sedentary time from the NHANES study. Model 1 is the least adjusted model and model 2 is the most adjusted.

Data from Vallance et al. 2011.

self-reported sedentary behavior (use of computer, watching TV, total screen time, and total sitting time) were shown to be associated with higher levels of depression. Figure 12.2 illustrates results for the most adjusted model and shows that the women in the highest sedentary tertile had higher odds of depression, although not all tertile differences were significant.

In a 10-year prospective follow-up of women initially free of depression in the Nurses' Health Study (Lucas et al. 2011), the risk of depression was shown to increase with additional time spent watching television (see figure 12.3). Although the temporal trend is significant, the relative risk in each quintile is not. The authors concluded that "increased television watching was associated with a trend toward an elevated risk (of depression)" (page 1022).

Most of the studies investigating links between sedentary behavior and mental health in children and adolescents focus on outcomes other than

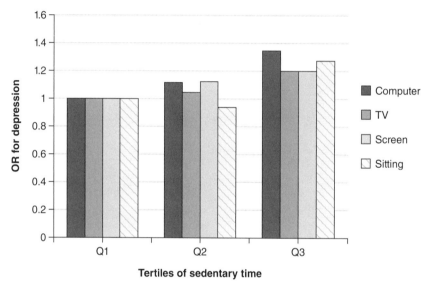

Figure 12.2 Odds ratios (OR) for depression across tertiles of four types of self-reported assessed sedentary behavior for Australian women.

Data from Teychenne, Ball, and Salmon 2010a.

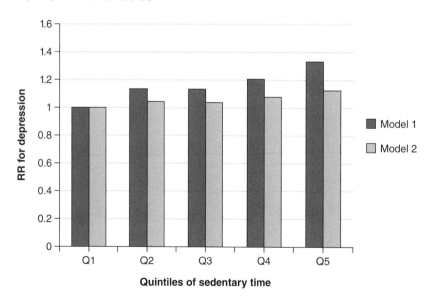

Figure 12.3 Odds of depression across quintiles of TV viewing time over a 10-year follow-up from the Nurses' Health Study. Model 1 is age adjusted relative risk (RR) and model 2 is the most adjusted model.

Data from Vallance et al. 2011.

depression (Biddle and Asare 2011). However, Primack and colleagues (2009) conducted an analysis of the National Longitudinal Survey of Adolescent Health to study the association between sedentary behavior in the form of electronic media use and depression over a period of 7 years. The sample comprised just over 4,000 adolescents who were not depressed at baseline. Depression at 7-year follow-up was associated with greater use of electronic media at baseline. When individual sedentary behavior using electronic media was analyzed, this trend was mirrored by levels of TV viewing, but not by video viewing, playing computer games, or listening to the radio. Effects were greater in males.

A new meta-analysis by Zhai, Zhang, and Zhang (2015) confirms an association between sedentary behavior and depression. However, it is noteworthy that although relative risk (RR) ratios were significant, they were smaller for longitudinal (RR = 1.14) compared with cross-sectional (RR = 1.31) studies and for studies controlling for physical activity (RR = 1.12) compared to those that did not (RR = 1.34). Interestingly, the association was slightly higher for computer and Internet use (RR = 1.22) than TV viewing (RR = 1.13).

In summary, higher levels of depression are associated with greater sedentary behavior in adults and young people. However, this research field is still quite new, and relatively few studies exist. We cannot rule out reverse causality, and this reverse direction of effect is certainly plausible for depression. Moreover, not all studies control for the effects of MVPA. It also may be the case that only some types of sedentary behavior are associated with depression. Data suggest that depression may be associated most obviously with TV viewing. This could be due to indiscriminant watching of TV with little cognitive engagement and, of course, no physical activity. Similarly, lethargy may also be exacerbated by poor diet, such as snacking (Pearson and Biddle 2011). More cognitively engaging behaviors, such as social networking and video games, may not have the same association with depression. Indeed, as we have reviewed, there may even be some psychological benefits, notwithstanding the likely physical ill-effects of prolonged sitting from such behaviors (Wilmot et al. 2012). There is a danger, therefore, in analyzing data for only either total sedentary time or composite behaviors, such as screen time. Although such measures can be informative, it might also be important to provide a breakdown by specific behaviors.

Sedentary Behavior and Cognitive Functioning

Numerous studies have demonstrated the benefits of regular exercise at or above recommended levels for cognitive function. For example, consistent improvements, especially in executive function, were found in older adults in a meta-analysis of 18 exercise intervention studies published between 1966 and 2001 (Colcombe and Kramer 2003). Across these studies, women appear to benefit more strongly from exercise than men, which has also been found for older adults with mild cognitive impairment (Clifford et al. 2009). Given such gender-specific effects on cognition, it seems likely that sedentary behavior may also have different effects on cognitive function in men and women.

A consistent overlap exists between risk factors for cardiovascular disease and cognitive decline, such as lack of physical activity (Hogervorst et al. 2012). However, beyond merely a lack of physical activity, the effects of sedentary behavior on cognitive function are considerably more complex and less well researched. Such effects seem to depend on age, the specifics of the sedentary behaviors and cognitive functions in question, and the cognitive testing methodology, which varies widely across studies. Before turning to specific age groups, it is important to appreciate the considerable range of assessment methods that are grouped together under the heading of cognitive function tests, since they are crucial in determining the results of studies.

Cognitive science has traditionally sought to categorize mental functions into larger domains such as attention, memory, and executive functions (including planning, goal-directed behavior, and response monitoring). Although the underlying assumption is that functions in these domains can operate and change with at least some degree of independence, a wide range of theoretical models with different groupings of specific functions indicates that there is little general agreement on the grouping of cognitive functions into broader domains. Even more problematic is that individual tests that are supposed to measure the same function can often yield quite different results. It is thus difficult to generalize effects on overall cognitive function, and the specific cognitive tests used have a significant role in producing each set of results.

Another approach to cognitive function assessment, more frequently used in child research, is to measure far more global functions such as intelligence, school achievement, and reading scores. Such compound measures are a complex mix of individual cognitive functions and learned knowledge. Although they may have more ecological validity and functional relevance, it is often difficult to delineate how the effects of physical activity or specific behaviors on such global outcomes may be mediated. For example, IQ scores or school achievement could be improved through general improvements in attention and the ability to concentrate or by more time spent on studying task-relevant materials. The task-specific nature of mental practice suggests that more time spent in specific behaviors is likely to result in better performance on cognitive tests that include the relevant ability, but not necessarily wider improvements across cognitive functions. Conversely, improvements in less closely related tasks are more likely to result from general improvements in cognition, often hypothesized to result from better executive function. Research is therefore required on how different measures of cognitive functioning might be associated with variations in sedentary behavior, since the literature has primarily focused on physical activity.

Infants

Early (prelingual) motor development has long been hypothesized to be an important precursor of later cognitive development, and baby and toddler sports and activity courses are becoming increasingly popular. Some evidence supports this notion. For example, one study found a significant linear relationship between age of learning to stand without support and adult (age 33-35) categorization skills, a measure of executive function (Murray et al. 2006). The same study also looked at other cognitive functions, including visuospatial memory, verbal learning, and visual object learning, but there were no significant associations for these cognitive domains. Nevertheless, if the association holds true for at least executive function, then conversely it would be likely that excessive sedentary behavior during infancy, to a degree that negatively affects motor development, may also negatively affect later executive function.

However, the idea of an early motor-cognition correlation remains controversial. Correlation does not mean causation; hence, an alternative explanation for the preceding results might be that an underlying factor, such as birth weight, nutritional factors, or parent's socioeconomic status, drives both motor and cognitive development (Jefferis, Power, and Hertzman 2002; Richards et al. 2001). Furthermore, other studies fail to find similar results. For example, Capute and colleagues (1985) collected early motor data on 213 children, including ages of rolling supine to prone, sitting alone, crawling, and walking, and compared these to Stanford-Binet IQ at 3 years of age. Significant but small correlations were driven by participants with high or low outlier IQ scores, and no correlation remained when these were removed. Numerous studies also document subtle motor abnormalities, especially in fine motor control, in developmental psychological disorders such as autism, schizophrenia, and dyslexia. Hence, an effect of early motor development on later-life measures of cognitive function may be driven by people with low motor and cognitive function due to underlying factors such as developmental disorders or low birth weight.

Young Children

The amount of time spent watching television and other screen-based activities has become a subject of considerable debate and concern regarding preschool toddlers and young school children. In a sample of more than 1,200 children from the U.S.-based National Longitudinal Survey of Youth, hours spent watching television at ages 1 and 3 were associated with attentional problems (hyperactivity) at age 7 (Christakis et al. 2004). Even after controlling for factors such as maternal education and IQ, hours of daily TV watching before age 3 had significant negative correlations with reading recognition and comprehension scores, as well as with working memory (digit span) at ages 6 to 7 (Zimmerman and Christakis 2005). These children watched an average of 2.2 hours per day at ages 1 to 3, which is probably not uncommon across developed countries. This large survey did not differentiate between different types of television programs, which may have differential effects on cognitive outcomes.

A recent systematic review of 23 published studies covering more than 22,000 participants that included sedentary behavior measures, health outcomes, and cognitive development in children up to 4 years of age confirms the trend for a negative association between television watching and cognitive development in the wider literature (LeBlanc et al. 2012). There was no evidence of any benefits of television watching for cognitive development. Several studies reported a dose–response effect where more time spent watching television was correlated with poorer cognitive development, similar to the study by Zimmerman and Christakis (2005). The evidence for potential negative effects of television watching on cognitive development in very young children appears to be relatively consistent, therefore, especially when TV-watching time exceeds 2 hours per day.

One problem inherent in these observational studies is the fact that many predictors of sedentary behavior are also predictors of poorer cognitive development. The observed correlations could be driven by underlying factors. Many of the studies make attempts to correct for such factors statistically, but this correction can only be as good as the quality, range, and relevance of the covariates. Accordingly, an important aspect of the debate is to consider these factors.

No intervention studies with cognitive function outcomes were found for this age group, so it remains unclear to what extent specific types of sedentary behavior may directly affect cognitive development in infants and young children. However, the idea that excessive television watching may directly cause attentional deficits and other problems with executive function is theoretically plausible because information in this medium is received quite passively, with little of the attention-driven seeking of specific information that would occur in more interactive settings where the child actively explores the environment or takes part in interpersonal interactions.

School-Age Children and Adults

Extensive brain development is still taking place well into the onset of puberty, lending plausibility to lasting effects on cognitive function. Independent of physical activity levels, more sedentary time confers increased risk of cardiovascular disease (CVD) and psychological measures including self-esteem, prosocial behaviors, and academic achievement in school-age children (Tremblay et al. 2011). These findings are from a large systematic review that included 232 studies with more than 980,000 participants aged 5 to 17 years. Time spent watching TV was the most common measure of sedentary behavior, with more than 2 hours per day again being associated with worse performance on all psychological outcomes, lower fitness, and unfavorable body composition. Although not all these effects

are found consistently across studies, none showed a benefit from more sedentary time.

Obesity is also associated with cognitive deficits, especially in executive function, in children, adolescents, and adults (Smith et al. 2011). Accordingly, sedentary behavior, which is linked to higher BMI (van Uffelen et al. 2010) and obesity risk independently of physical activity (Thorp et al. 2011), may influence cognitive function through this link. It is often difficult to distinguish whether obesity is a cause or a consequence of cognitive deficits, and a bidirectional relationship seems the most likely scenario (Smith et al. 2011). Plausible pathways for obesity to affect the brain include systemic inflammation, elevated lipids, and insulin resistance. Cognitive deficits can, in turn, affect eating behavior; reduced executive function has been hypothesized to lead to weight gain (Joseph et al. 2011).

Besides this route of adverse body composition and other cardiovascular risk factors mediating the effect of sedentary behavior on cognitive function, there also appear to be direct effects on cognition independently of physiological health indicators. This could be, at least in part, caused by underlying conditions such as depression (e.g., depression-reduction hypothesis), arthritis, and CVD, which affect both sedentary behavior and cognitive function (Teychenne, Ball, and Salmon 2010b). However, it is also plausible that nonsedentary social activities could directly stimulate cognitive function (social stimulation hypothesis), and excessive time spent in sedentary behavior may indicate a lack of participation in such activities. The depression-reduction hypothesis and social-stimulation hypothesis were compared directly in one study of 158 community-dwelling elders that included measures of sedentary behavior and cognitive function, and a partial role for both theories was confirmed (Vance et al. 2005). This needs testing in other ages. It is thus highly likely that several routes mediate the relationship between sedentary behavior and cognitive function: a link through body composition and related chronic conditions (e.g., CVD, diabetes mellitus), a link by which underlying chronic conditions such as depression affect both, and decreased social and other cognitive stimulation that results from increasing time spent on sedentary (nonstimulating) behaviors instead.

However, it is plausible that in contrast to the quite consistent negative effects of time spent watching television, other types of sedentary behavior may also be beneficial for cognitive outcomes similar to social stimulation, for example, time spent reading or on mathematical puzzles (Uchida and Kawashima 2008). It may be beneficial, especially for those with chronic conditions that limit physical activity, and this becomes even more relevant for the older age group, discussed in the following section, to readjust sedentary time away from passive pursuits like TV toward other sedentary behaviors with cognitive benefits as well as toward active pursuits, of course. Identifying such activities is difficult due to a lack of research with detailed measures of different types of sedentary behavior and cognitive outcomes, and most studies look at either young children or the elderly.

One approach that seems to have good face value and popularity is to undertake brain-training activities, supported by the "use it or lose it" view, which essentially posits that cognitive functions can be trained. Significant but modest effects have been reported in some studies of older adults (Papp, Walsh, and Snyder 2009; Smith et al. 2009) and preschool children (Thorell et al. 2009), but because of overlap between intervention and outcome measures, it is unclear if any such benefits transfer to untrained tasks or possibly a more general improvement in cognitive functioning. One large online study of brain training methods included 11,430 participants across all ages and asked participants to train in cognitive tasks designed to improve reasoning, memory, planning, visuospatial skills, and attention once a day for 6 weeks (Owen et al. 2010). The authors documented significant improvements on each of the trained cognitive tasks, but found no evidence for benefits on untrained tasks, even on closely related cognitive tests in the same domains. Hence, at present there is little consistent evidence for wider benefits of brain training in healthy adults, so it remains a challenge to find evidence for specific cognitively beneficial sedentary behaviors.

Older Adults

In contrast to the relatively consistent results in younger age groups, the relationship between obesity and cognition is uncertain in the elderly, as is illustrated by contradictory results (Smith et al. 2011). This may be partly due to the inadequacies of body mass index as a measure of adiposity with aging, as well as the rapid weight loss that often accompanies severe health conditions that also affect cognitive function in the elderly (e.g., cancer and advanced dementia). However, just as in

younger age groups, maintaining a healthy weight and physical activity (Zhao, Tranovich, and Wright 2013) are still beneficial to cognitive function in healthy elderly people and in those with mild cognitive impairment and dementia (Clifford et al. 2009; Hogervorst et al. 2012). Interestingly, new research by Arnardottir and colleagues (2016) has shown that both physical activity and sedentary behavior in older adults, when measured by accelerometers, are associated with measures of brain atrophy and that change over time is associated with both behaviors in the expected directions. This contributes to the argument concerning biological plausibility of connections between sedentary behavior and cognitive functioning. Moreover, Hamer and Stamatakis (2014) furthered the argument that sedentary behavior has direct effects on mental health and cognition independent of body composition and fitness. High TV viewing (≥6 hr/day versus <2 hr/day) in the English Longitudinal Study of Ageing cohort measured in 2008-2009 predicted higher depressive symptoms and poorer global cognitive function after a 2-year follow-up, when participants were on average 65 years old. Internet use resulted in the opposite effects. These remained significant after correction for BMI, socioeconomic status, and a host of other variables.

The confounding variable with underlying conditions that affect both sedentary behavior and cognitive function is also much more pronounced in older people because of the higher frequency and severity of chronic disease and acute events such as falls. As life expectancy continues to increase, dementia has become an ever-growing concern. The concept of cognitive reserve (Stern 2002) suggests that a drop in cognitive function below a certain threshold leads to dementia. This means that improving cognitive function in midlife people and healthy elderly people is likely to reduce the risk for dementia. A lifetime effect of cognitive resources on late-onset (after 65 years of age) dementia risk has been well documented, with even childhood measures of mental ability having significant negative correlations with dementia risk (Whalley et al. 2000).

Hence, just as in the younger age groups, sedentary behavior is likely to affect cognition through body composition and cardiovascular health effects, mental health conditions such as depression, and the effects of sedentary behavior on the amount of cognitive stimulation for key mental skills. Cognitive stimulation and brain training research have been conducted much more extensively in the elderly. For example, there appears to be an effect of premorbid reading activity on the rapidness of cognitive decline in Alzheimer's disease patients even after controlling for baseline cognitive function and education (Wilson et al. 2000), suggesting that time spent reading may have a different cognitive influence than other sedentary behaviors. Some cognitive intervention studies report positive results on cognitive function in healthy elderly people, such as for general cognitive training (Ball et al. 2002) or more specific working memory training (Buschkuehl et al. 2008).

However, larger reviews have found no consistent effects of cognitive interventions on dementia risk (Papp, Walsh, and Snyder 2009), largely due to methodological problems such as inconsistent interventions, follow-up times, and outcome measures across studies, and the frequent lack of well-matched control groups. Nevertheless, even in elderly participants with dementia, there are reports of positive effects of cognitive stimulation therapy interventions, even on global cognitive function (mini-mental status exam) and Alzheimer's disease cognitive scales (Spector et al. 2003). A meta-analysis of clinical trials concluded that cognitive stimulation programs benefit cognition in people with mild to moderate dementia (Woods et al. 2012), and another review also supports the utility of cognitive training in healthy elderly people and those with significant cognitive decline (Gates and Valenzuela 2010), despite also finding many methodological issues in the published work in the area.

Sedentary Behavior and Health-Related Quality of Life

In addition to the study of depression, researchers are now investigating associations between sedentary behavior and other indices of psychological well-being. Typically, these include generic measures of well-being, such as health-related quality of life.

Data from nearly 4,000 participants in the Scottish Health Survey were analyzed by Hamer, Stamatakis, and Mishra (2010). Sedentary behavior in leisure time was reflected in a measure of time spent on television and screen-based entertainment (TVSE). Mental health was assessed using the General Health Questionnaire (GHQ-12), which measures happiness, depression, anxiety, and sleep disturbance. The mental health component of the SF-12 was also used. Scores on the GHQ-12 were significantly higher (reflecting worse mental health) with more than 4 hours per day of TVSE. However, when confounders were included in the analysis, including physical activity and physical function, this was substantially attenuated, although the association remained significant.

Another cross-sectional study was reported by Davies and colleagues (2012) with data from just under 3,500 Australian adults. Measures were taken of health-related quality of life (HRQL), physical activity, and screen time (TV and computer use in leisure time and at work). Results were analyzed by looking at the joint associations for physical activity and screen time. In men, HRQL was worse for those with no physical activity and high screen time separately. In addition, the odds for one measure of HRQL (14 or more unhealthy days in the past 30) for those with no physical activity and high screen time in combination were 4.52 when compared to the reference group, who had sufficient physical activity and low screen time. However, the trends were not so evident for women.

A large-scale study in Spain on more than 10,000 university students, with 6-year follow-up, was reported by Sanchez-Villegas and colleagues (2008). The authors computed a sedentary index from self-reported screen time and assessed mental health through depression, bipolar disorder, anxiety, and stress. From data on just over 8,000 participants, it was shown that the group with the highest sedentary index score (>42 hr/week screen time) had increased odds of a mental disorder (OR = 1.31) compared with those spending fewer than 10.5 hours per week sitting. The trend across quintiles of the sedentary index was significant even in the most adjusted model, although adjustment for physical activity was not reported.

A prospective cohort study was conducted by Balboa-Castillo and colleagues (2011). Also conducted in Spain, this study assessed more than 1,000 adults aged 62 years and older in 2003 for leisure-time physical activity and the number of hours they spent sitting each week. Six years later, they were assessed for HRQL using the SF-36. This measure of HRQL reflects physical health and mental health, with four subscales assessing the latter (vitality, social functioning, emotional role, and mental health). Example items from these four subscales reflect the following:

▸ Vitality: energy, worn out
▸ Social functioning: extent and time

▶ Emotional role: accomplishing less

▶ Mental health: nervous, peaceful, happy

In the study by Balboa-Castillo and colleagues, self-reported weekly hours of sitting predicted HRQL 6 years later independent of typical confounders, including physical activity (see figure 12.4). All four mental health subscales showed significant linear trends from the reference group (least amount of sitting) to the highest quartile for sitting. Trends for vitality and mental health appear most clearly for those in the highest group, whereas social functioning and emotional role have more of an obvious linear trend.

Interestingly, an 8-year follow-up of just over 1,000 older adults in Taiwan showed positive associations on subjective well-being for both physical activity and some types of sedentary behavior (Ku, Fox, and Chen 2015). These included TV viewing, social chatting, and reading. This suggests that some social sedentary behavior, unsurprisingly, may be beneficial for well-being, and other forms may provide cognitive engagement. This requires further investigation.

Biddle and Asare (2011) conducted a review of reviews concerning physical activity and mental health in children and adolescents. In this paper, they provided the first brief review of the associations between sedentary behavior and mental health for this age group. Nine studies were reported, and these led the authors to conclude that higher levels

of sedentary behavior, primarily in the form of screen viewing, were associated with poorer mental health. One of these studies, from Primack and colleagues (2009), is discussed earlier in this chapter (see the section Sedentary Behavior and Depression). The other studies assessed various types of sedentary behavior, such as TV viewing, computer use, use of a phone, listening to the radio, self-reported sedentary behavior by diary or log, and total sedentary time using an accelerometer. Mental health outcome measures included HRQL, psychological well-being, body image, happiness, self-esteem, and quality of relationships. All studies showed at least one analysis reflecting higher scores on sedentary behavior being associated with worse mental health. Although this was most clearly shown for screen time, this measure was also assessed in some form or another in all studies, while some forms of sedentary behavior (e.g., phone, radio) were not assessed in more than a couple of studies. Only half of the studies analyzed physical activity as a confounder.

Tremblay and colleagues (2011) reported a comprehensive systematic review of health outcomes of sedentary behavior. It was unclear why only self-esteem was selected as the key psychosocial indicator rather than HRQL or depression (although there were also analyses of prosocial behavior and academic achievement). Studies reviewed on self-esteem suggested that higher levels of sedentary behavior were associated with lower levels of self-esteem. However, a more comprehensive systematic review has now

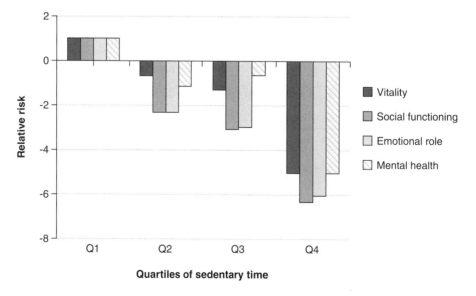

Figure 12.4 Odds (relative risk) of four domains of HRQL from self-reported weekly hours of sitting over 6-year follow-up with 1,097 persons aged 62 years and over.

Data from Balboa-Castillo et al. 2011.

THREE KEY SEDENTARY BEHAVIOR AND PSYCHOLOGICAL WELL-BEING RESEARCH ISSUES

1. **The exposure**: measurement of sedentary behavior. A key issue in the study of sedentary behavior, and in particular for research on mental health outcomes, is to identify the nature and context of the sedentary behavior. For the study of mental health outcomes, it may not be enough to quantify total sedentary (sitting) time, but rather the nature of sedentary behavior, such as TV viewing, computer use, and car travel, and then to identify the context, such as whether there is social interaction, low cognitive involvement, and so on. Such variability may account for why some studies are showing that TV viewing—often a largely passive behavior with minimal cognitive involvement or social interaction—shows associations with worse mental health, yet other types of sedentary behavior may have no effect or even beneficial effects. The latter might include sedentary socializing and cognitively challenging computer tasks.

2. **The outcome**: types of mental health outcomes. Measures of mental well-being have been assessed through multiple or generic domains of mental health. It is plausible for associations with sedentary behavior, if they exist, to be complex and dependent on the nature of the outcome variable. It is plausible for associations to exist between TV and depression, but maybe not for self-esteem.

3. **Reverse causality**: It is plausible that poor mental health precedes sedentary behavior, hence reflecting reverse causality. Cross-sectional designs are insufficient, and more experimental designs are required. In addition, longitudinal and prospective designs, some of which exist (Primack et al. 2009), are also required. Large data sets are now being used to test some of the assumptions in this field, and this should help resolve whether sedentary behavior can precede or predict future mental well-being.

reported an indeterminate association between sedentary behavior and self-esteem for young people (Suchert, Hanewinkel, and Isensee 2015).

Summary

In addition to the burgeoning evidence concerning the adverse physical health effects of high levels of sedentary behavior, there is a case that mental health may also be affected. However, this area is complex because of the varying nature and contexts of different forms of sedentary behavior and the question of whether some mental health outcomes will be more affected than others.

This chapter shows that at least there are cross-sectional associations between sedentary behavior, and in particular TV viewing, and indicators of poor psychological well-being. Whether these are the product of reverse causality is not known. That said, there is some evidence of prospective and longitudinal associations but little experimental evidence. Associations between sedentary behavior and cognitive functioning exist across all age groups. Physical activity has consistent positive effects, and excessive sedentary behavior may negatively affect cognitive

function through reduced physical activity and increased risk for obesity and unhealthy body composition, which have consistent negative effects on cognitive function. However, at least part of the association with sedentary behavior may also be driven by underlying health conditions that affect both. Finally, it seems that specific types of sedentary behavior (e.g., watching television) may negatively affect cognitive function, while cognitively stimulating activities and social interaction appear to be beneficial for cognitive function. More research is needed, especially in this last area, on specific activities and behaviors that may benefit cognitive function.

The evidence reviewed in this chapter concerns mental health outcomes of sedentary behavior and complements the literature on physical outcomes. Overall, it is possible to conclude that greater exposure to some sedentary behaviors is associated with poorer mental health. However, the quality of evidence is quite low, and several important issues require more discussion to put such a conclusion in proper context and offer a cautionary note. Three key issues exist: the measurement of the exposure of sedentary behavior, the mental health outcome of interest, and the issue of reverse causality.

KEY CONCEPTS

▸ **Health-related quality of life:** Multidimensional construct involving perceptions of physical, psychological, and social functioning, including subjective well-being.

▸ **Mental health:** A generic term referring to positive and negative mental states and tendencies.

▸ **Reverse causality:** Where a plausible explanation for the direction of association (e.g., between sedentary behavior and a mental health outcome) could be in the reverse direction.

▸ Sedentary behavior appears to be a significant cluster of behaviors associated with poor physical health. Less is known about psychological outcomes.

▸ Sedentary behavior, and in particular TV viewing, is associated with poor mental health.

▸ This association could reflect reverse causality, where people with poorer mental health choose to sit more.

STUDY QUESTIONS

1. Why might some types of sedentary behavior be associated with low levels of psychological well-being?

2. The strongest associations appear to be for TV viewing. Why might this be?

3. Why might some forms of sedentary behavior be beneficial for cognitive functioning?

4. How much sedentary behavior might be detrimental for mental well-being?

5. Might breaking up sitting time be important for mental health rather than just reducing total sitting time?

6. What is reverse causality and why might this be an explanation for some associations between sedentary behavior and psychological well-being?

PART III

MEASURING AND ANALYZING SEDENTARY BEHAVIOR

For research on sedentary behavior and health, high-quality measures are essential. Thus, the five chapters in part III, taken together, address measuring and analyzing sedentary behavior comprehensively. Both conventional approaches in measuring sedentary behavior and future possibilities are covered.

In chapter 13, Barbara E. Ainsworth and colleagues deal with the assessment of sedentary behavior using questionnaires. The majority of epidemiological evidence on sedentary behavior and health—as addressed in the preceding chapters in part II—comes from studies in which the relevant sedentary behavior exposures have been assessed using questionnaire methods.

Following Ainsworth's account of established measurement fundamentals in Chapter 13, we have three chapters that deal with the cutting edge of development in measurement technologies relevant to sedentary behavior, none of which—as the authors would readily acknowledge—in any way negate the importance of the self-report methodologies described in chapter 13. Self-reporting remains the mainstay of capturing behavior in context and allows important aspects of behaviors to be characterized and taken into account. In understanding the determinants of sedentary behavior and in develop-

ing interventions, high-quality self-report–derived data remain crucial aspects of the research agenda. Understanding the contexts, purposes, and functions of sedentary behavior is particularly important in the development and evaluation of interventions, as is addressed subsequently in the chapters that make up part V.

New and emerging measurement technologies provide exciting opportunities for sedentary behavior research. In chapter 14, Kong Y. Chen and Richard P. Troiano address the assessment of sedentary behavior using motion sensors, providing fascinating insights into the technology involved and the potential of small-scale powerful unobtrusive devices for capturing huge volumes of data in population-based studies in assessing the outcomes of intervention and for a plethora of other research purposes. In chapter 15, David Bassett and Dinesh John provide a comprehensive overview of assessing sedentary behavior using physiological sensing devices; this chapter illustrates the large number of behavioral, biological, and functional dimensions that can now be characterized through the use of new and rapidly evolving device-based capacities. Dinesh John goes further down this captivating new technology-capacities track with Stephen Intille in chapter 16, dealing with the assessment of sedentary behavior using new technology. Small-scale devices with impressively functional sensing, data-storage, and data-transmission capacities provide numerous opportunities for innovative research to characterize sedentary behavior, behavioral change, and relationships with important health outcomes.

Part III provides compelling illustrations of the technology-driven sensing, data-acquisition, storage, and transmission capacities that are now available for sedentary behavior research. However, all data must eventually become information. In chapter 17, Weimo Zhu addresses psychometric issues in analyzing data on sedentary behavior. He provides strong guidance for students and researchers, highlighting the importance of reflection on the meanings to be extracted from data and the new methods being developed for doing so.

CHAPTER 13

ASSESSING SEDENTARY BEHAVIOR USING QUESTIONNAIRES

Barbara E. Ainsworth, PhD, MPH; Alberto Flórez Pregonero, MEd; and Fabien Rivière, MS

The reader will gain an overview of how to measure sedentary behavior with questionnaires used in research and practice. By the end of this chapter, the reader should be able to do the following:

- ▶ Identify the purpose of questionnaires for assessing sedentary behavior
- ▶ List the key components of questionnaires
- ▶ Identify types of validity and define reliability for questionnaires
- ▶ List skills needed for administering questionnaires
- ▶ Evaluate gaps in existing questionnaires used for assessing sedentary behavior

As the name implies, questionnaires are survey instruments that consist of a set of questions selected and arranged to identify information about a person or what a person thinks about a topic. Most large-scale research studies and opinion surveys use questionnaires to obtain information. At the largest scale, every 10 years, the U.S. Census mails a questionnaire to households to identify demographic characteristics of people who live in homes and apartments. They ask residents to identify their age, sex, race and ethnicity, marital status, household income, educational attainment, and occupation, as well as the number of people living in the household (U.S. Department of Commerce 2010). Other government agencies administer surveys annually that contain questionnaires arranged into the topics called modules. The Behavioral Risk Factor Surveillance System (BRFSS) has modules to identify topics such as fruit and vegetable intake, exercise and physical activity, risky driving, and cancer screening practices, and others to identify behavioral risk factors that can place adults at risk for premature accidents, injuries, and chronic diseases (U.S. Centers for Disease Control and Prevention 2014).

Questionnaires come in various types and lengths. Physical activity and sedentary behavior questionnaires may contain simple questions with respondents answering yes or no to questions such as, "Did you watch television yesterday?" Others require detailed arithmetic calculations to derive an answer. For example, a questionnaire may ask the respondent to recall the hours spent watching television during the past week, which requires knowing the number of days one watched television and the average hours per day spent watching television. The time frame for information recall may be as current as yesterday or as distant as the past year or a lifetime. The length of questionnaires also may vary from 2 to 300 questions. Ideally, a questionnaire should be as short as needed to obtain the desired information. The delivery mode for questionnaires has evolved over the years, shifting from writing answers to questions on paper with the responses hand scored and entered into data storage, to filling in bubbles on a form for scanning into machine data readers, to now using computers or mobile applications to administer questionnaires on touch screens with answers fed directly into a web database.

The types of questionnaires used to identify sedentary behavior are varied. Some questionnaires focus on time spent sitting during occupational (Clark et al. 2011; Yore et al. 2006) and nonoccupational settings, such as time spent watching television, using a computer, and traveling by car, truck, bus, plane, or train (Gardiner et al. 2011; Rosenberg et al. 2010). Questionnaires also assess multiple types of sedentary behavior in the past day or week (Clark et al. 2013; Rosenberg et al. 2008). This chapter focuses on the characteristics of questionnaires, important measurement qualities to consider when selecting a questionnaire, and dos and don'ts for administering questionnaires. It also provides some examples of questionnaires used to study sedentary behavior and the associated health outcomes.

Key Components of Questionnaires

Most questionnaires used to assess sedentary behavior rely on a person's ability to recall the frequency, duration, and types of sedentary behavior performed during a period in the past. Since sedentary behavior is regarded as low intensity, it is unnecessary to identify the intensity of the behavior in the questionnaires. Sedentary behavior is expressed as time spent sitting or reclining. Types of activities include watching television, working on a computer, riding in a car or on public transport, listening to music, talking, and reading. Summary scores for sedentary questionnaires include the units of minutes or hours per day or per week or a combination of an intensity score referred to as the metabolic equivalent (METs) and the multiplication of intensity and time in minutes or hours expressed as MET-minutes and MET-hours, respectively. The administration style may be self- or interviewer administered. The following sections explain the essential components of questionnaires. Examples of the essential components of selected sedentary behavior questionnaires are presented in table 13.1.

Recall Frame

The recall frame for questionnaires is varied. As shown in table 13.1, the Sedentary Behavior Questionnaire (SBQ) (Rosenberg et al. 2010) uses a typical weekday and a typical weekend day recall frame to assess time spent in sedentary behavior, while the International Physical Activity Questionnaire (IPAQ) (Craig et al. 2003) uses a single day in a typical weekday recall frame. A common recall

Table 13.1. Characteristics of Sedentary Behavior Questionnaires

Recall frame	Frequency	Duration	Mode	Domains
International Physical Activity Questionnaire Short Form (Rosenberg et al. 2008; Craig et al. 2003)				
Typical weekday		Open ended: hr or min/day	Time sitting in general and physical activity	Purpose, environment, posture, and time
Workplace Sitting Time Questionnaire (Clark et al. 2011)				
Average workday during last week	Number of breaks during 1 hr at work	Open ended: hr or min/day; Categorical: number of breaks	Time sitting	Purpose, environment, posture, and time
Self-Reported Sedentary Time Questionnaire (Gardiner et al. 2011)				
Past week		Open ended: hr or min/week	Time sitting or reclining during leisure	Purpose, posture, social, and type
Past-Day Adults' Sedentary Time Questionnaire (Clark et al. 2013)				
Past day		Open ended: hr or min/day	Time sitting and reclining in various types of activity	Purpose, environment, posture, time, and type
Sedentary Behavior Questionnaire (Rosenberg et al. 2010)				
Typical weekday, weekend		Categorical: hr/week	Time sitting at home and work	Purpose, posture, and type
Sedentary Time and Activity Reporting Questionnaire (Neilson et al. 2013; Csizmadi et al. 2014)				
Average day during the last 4 weeks	Number of days during past 4 weeks	Open ended: hr or min/day	Total 24 hr physical activity, sedentary behavior, and sleep	Purpose, environment, posture, status, time, and type
Yale Physical Activity Survey (DiPietro et al. 1993)				
Average day over the last month		Categorical: hr/day	Overall sitting time and physical activity	Posture and time
Adolescent Sedentary Activity Questionnaire (Hardy, Booth, and Okely 2007)				
Each day of a normal school week	Number of days during the week	Open-ended: hr or min-day	Time siting in various types	Purpose, environment, posture, time, and type
Youth Risk Behavior Survey (Schmitz et al. 2004)				
Average school day		Categorical: hr/day	Overall sitting time	Posture, time, and type
Self-Administered Physical Activity Checklist (Sallis et al. 1996)				
Yesterday before and after school		Open-ended: hr or min/day	Physical activity and screen time	Time and type
SIT-Q-7d (Wijndaele et al. 2014)				
Average week and weekend day during the last 7 days	Number of breaks during the day	Categorical: hr or min/day, number of breaks	Sedentary and sleeping time	Purpose, posture, social, associated behaviors, time, and type

frame for many questionnaires is one week because it is difficult to recall information during long periods in the past, and one day may not reflect usual behaviors (Healy et al. 2011).

Frequency

Frequency refers to the number of times one performs a behavior in terms of days, weeks, months, or years. On the Self-Reported Sedentary Time Questionnaire, respondents recall how many days in the past week they watched television (Gardiner et al. 2011). On the other hand, the Past-Day Adults' Sedentary Time Questionnaire (Clark et al. 2013) has respondents recall the number of times they watched television in a single day. Often, it is difficult to recall information from a prior week. On the other hand, recalling information about television watching during a single day may underestimate the time spent watching television during other days of the week.

Duration

Duration refers to the hours or minutes spent in a sedentary behavior. The IPAQ has only one question about the duration of hours and minutes per day of sitting on a typical weekday. Although most questionnaires ask respondents to recall the duration of their sedentary behavior in hours and minutes, the 2009 BRFSS included an occupational question that asked respondents to indicate if they spent most of their time at work sitting, standing and walking, or engaged in labor activities (U.S. Centers for Disease Control and Prevention 2009).

Mode

The types of sedentary behavior performed are also referred to as the mode of behavior. By and large, television watching is the most common type of activity used as an indicator of sedentary behavior. Most questionnaires developed identify multiple types of sedentary behavior, such as watching television, working, watching children, doing homework, transportation, or other leisure-time pursuits (Healy et al. 2011). For example, the SBQ (Rosenberg et al. 2010) identifies the time spent in nine types of sedentary behavior (TV, computer games, listening to music, talking on the telephone, office and paper work, reading, playing a musical instrument, arts and crafts, and driving in a car). Asking respondents to identify their posture (reclining, sitting, and

standing) during these activities allows for a finer understanding of sedentary behavior.

The types of sedentary behavior included in a questionnaire and the nature of information obtained for frequency, duration, and recall frame should be specific to the study or survey objective. If a goal is to identify how many people watch television five or more days a week, then asking about the duration is unimportant. Instead, the question could be written as, "How many days per week do you watch television?" However, if a goal of a study is to determine the dose–response relationship between the hours of television watched per week and a health condition (i.e., watching fewer hours of television is better for health), then asking respondents to recall the number of days and the hours per day they watched television is important.

Domains

Considering which characteristics of sedentary behavior need to be measured is an important step in the process of selecting a questionnaire. Based on a consensus taxonomy of sedentary behavior (Chastin, Schwarz, and Skelton 2013), nine main domains describing the following attributes might be distinguished: the purpose (why), the environment (where), the posture, the social context (with whom), the measurement (instruments and quantification issues), the associated behaviors (what else), the status (mental and functional states of the person), the time (when the behavior take place), and the type of behavior (what). Each domain is composed of many subcategories; for example, the domain of *posture* is composed of the subcategories *sitting*, *lying*, and *other*. Important differences in the characteristics of sedentary behavior measured by the questionnaires are observed. For example, most of the sedentary behavior questionnaires measure sitting time spent watching TV during a day, but only two questionnaires measure the associated behaviors such as snacking: the Sit-Q-7d (Wijndaele et al. 2014) and the SIT-Q-12m (Lynch et al. 2014). When developing or selecting a questionnaire, one should determine which characteristics of sedentary behavior are of interest depending on the population and purpose of the study.

Global questionnaires aim to provide a general categorization of a person's sedentary behavior level; thus, they don't need to measure as many sedentary behavior characteristics as more comprehensive questionnaires. Global questionnaires are short enough (1-3 items) to be used in population health surveys where the number of items is limited by space constraints. For example, a questionnaire designed to evaluate potential questions for use in surveillance activities evaluated a single item assessing time spent watching TV as a proxy of total sitting time (Pettee et al. 2009). In the opposite direction, some questionnaires have been developed to obtain more comprehensive measurement of sedentary behavior. These questionnaires purport to characterize the patterns of sedentary behavior during daily life by measuring subcategories within most of the domains identified in the taxonomy. The SIT-Q-7d is one of the more comprehensive sedentary behavior questionnaires. It has 68 items and measures time spent in different sedentary activities for work, transportation, domestic, education, and social eating and caregiving behaviors, during both a weekday and a weekend day. A systematic review of the content of sedentary behavior questionnaires has identified and compared the characteristics of sedentary behavior measured by each questionnaire and may help investigators or practitioners select the most appropriate questionnaire (Rivière et al. 2015).

Measurement Principles of Questionnaires

When selecting a questionnaire to collect information about sedentary behavior, one should ask several questions. First, is the questionnaire valid? That is, is the respondent able to recall the types of sedentary behavior listed on the questionnaire (Thomas, Nelson, and Silverman 2010)? Also, does it measure the types of sedentary behavior I seek to assess?

Validity has several forms. *Logical validity* is when a questionnaire addresses the types of information an investigator seeks to identify. For example, if one wants to get a general idea if a respondent mostly sits, stands, or walks while at work, then the question used in the 2009 BRFSS, "In general, which best describes what you do at work? (a) mostly sit; (b) mostly sit and stand; (c) mostly walk," would have logical validity because it involves a straightforward question about the types of behavior desired.

Another form of validity is *content validity*. As the name implies, content validity assures that the questionnaire contains sufficient content for assessing a behavioral domain. The questionnaire used to measure sedentary behavior in the Australian Longitudinal Study on Women's Health (Marshall

et al. 2010) aims to identify different settings when one may be sedentary, such as during transportation (e.g., car, bus), while working (e.g., sitting at a desk), in the home (e.g., sitting or reclining during television and computer use), during leisure-time activities (e.g., power boating, fishing). The content validity is deemed acceptable if the questionnaire is reviewed by experts who agree that the questionnaire includes the desired domain behaviors.

Construct validity relates to how well a questionnaire fits into a definition, or the construct of sedentary behavior. For example, assume sedentary behavior is defined as nonmovement or light-intensity movement with a metabolic energy cost (MET) of ≤1.5 times the resting energy expenditure. This would classify activities such as sleeping (0.95 METs), sitting quietly (1.3 METs), and standing (1.3 METs) as sedentary behavior (Ainsworth et al. 2011). A questionnaire that addresses participation in activities within this MET value range would have acceptable construct validity.

In research settings, investigators often want to assure that the questionnaire is measuring sedentary behavior as intended. They do this by comparing a questionnaire against some criterion, often an objective measure of sedentary behavior or another questionnaire. This is called *criterion validity*. Two types of criterion validity are used to evaluate sedentary behavior questionnaires: *concurrent validity* and *predictive validity*. Concurrent validity is measured most often by correlating responses from the sedentary behavior questionnaire with outputs from wearable activity monitors (i.e., accelerometer or inclinometer) or with another previously validated questionnaire used to assess sedentary behavior. To validate the past-day recall questionnaire, Clark and colleagues (2013) compared the scores from the questionnaire with those obtained by two criterion measures: an accelerometer (ActiGraph model GT3X+) that detects the intensity and duration of movement and nonmovement and an inclinometer (activPAL) that detects reclining, sitting, and standing postures and ambulatory movements. Another way concurrent validity is assessed is to compare the sedentary behavior questionnaire with a previously validated questionnaire that has a similar content. Rosenberg and colleagues (2010) validated the SBQ by comparing responses with an accelerometer and the IPAQ. Significant associations ($p < 0.00$) were observed between the SBQ sedentary score and hours per day of sitting time obtained from the IPAQ, which contributed to the concurrent validity of the SBQ.

Researchers who use questionnaires to predict the risks of sedentary behavior for a future event, such as the development of obesity, diabetes, or cardiovascular disease, are concerned with the *predictive validity* of the questionnaire. As the name implies, predictive validity involves using information about a person's behaviors and demographic information (such as age, weight, and sex) to develop equations that predict one's risk for a future event. Prediction equations using sedentary behavior data have not been reported; however, Hu and colleagues (2003) observed that among women enrolled in the prospective Nurses' Health Study, each increment of 2 hours per day of television watching was associated with a 17% to 30% increase in obesity and a 5% to 23% increase in the risk for diabetes. These relationships are discussed in chapters 7 and 8.

The second question one must ask before using a sedentary behavior questionnaire is, Is it reliable over repeat administrations? Reliability, also referred to as repeatability, refers to the consistency of a questionnaire to produce the same results when administered to the same person multiple times under similar conditions (Thomas, Nelson, and Silverman 2010). A common way to measure reliability is to administer the questionnaire two times one week or one month apart. A similar score reflects higher reliability. The reliability of a questionnaire is important in intervention studies where the goal is to reduce sedentary behavior. If a questionnaire is not reliable between one administration and another, the researcher has no confidence that the study goals are producing the desired result. A questionnaire with high reliability ($r = >0.70$) will provide a consistent measure of the behavior reported as long as the questionnaire is valid and avoids other sources of error. The validity and reliability of a sample of sedentary behavior questionnaires are presented in table 13.2.

The third question to ask before using a sedentary behavior questionnaire is, What are the sources of error that could influence the results of the questionnaire? Two sources of error are common in questionnaires: random error and systematic error. Random error results from unreliable reporting of sedentary behavior related to the respondents and the testing conditions and unrelated to the questionnaire itself. Sources of random error can be minimized by standardizing the testing conditions to prevent participant fatigue and enhance motivation

to recall information and by using a questionnaire administration style that fits the respondent, such as using in-person, web-based, and interviewer- or self-administered delivery styles. If a questionnaire is used in a research setting to assess sedentary behavior, there must be enough participants in a study so that one person's score does not distort the group averages.

Systematic errors relate to the properties of a questionnaire and can change the intent of the questionnaire to present falsely high or low scores. Conditions that promote systematic errors include mismatching the type of questionnaire used and the respondent's ability to understand and complete the questionnaire; using a questionnaire with content that does not measure the behaviors sought; using a questionnaire that is too long or wordy, or that requires numeral skills to compute an answer in people with low literacy skills; and using a questionnaire that has a complex scoring protocol and is hard to follow without the use of sophisticated computer programming. Systematic errors also can be minimized by assuring that the questionnaire is valid and has good reliability.

Practical Guidelines

As with all questionnaires, sedentary behavior questionnaires that identify the frequency, duration, and types of sedentary behavior need to have ongoing examination of the validity and reliability in diverse populations. Too often, small convenience samples with defined demographic characteristics such as college students or worksite employees are used to examine a questionnaire's validity and reliability. Once deemed valid and reliable, the questionnaire is used in different populations where it may operate with different validity and reliability. Since the validity and reliability of a questionnaire are specific only to the population for which it is tested, questionnaires need to be examined for their validity and reliability prior to use in targeted populations. For example, Neilson and colleagues (2013) performed several one-on-one cognitive interviews with adults to assess understanding of the Sedentary Time and Activity Reporting Questionnaire developed to estimate adults' activity energy expenditure and sedentary behavior. From the interviews, they identified problems with ambiguous wording and terms for selected questions, inability of the respondents to recall information as asked on the questionnaire, and average time spent across multiple activities.

Table 13.2. Measurement Qualities of a Sample of Sedentary Behavior Questionnaires

Study	Validity		Reliability	
	Criterion measure	Coefficient	Test–retest recall frame	Coefficient
International Physical Activity Questionnaire Short Form (Rosenberg et al. 2008; Craig et al. 2003)	ActiGraph CSA 7164 worn for 7 days	Spearman's r = 0.34[a]	3 to 7 days	Spearman's r = 0.81[a]
Workplace Sitting Time Questionnaire (Clark et al. 2011)	ActiGraph GT1M worn for 7 days	Total sitting time, Spearman's r = 0.29, 95% CI (0.22, 0.53); Breaks in sitting, Pearson's r = 0.26, 95% CI (0.11, 0.44)	Not measured	Not measured
Self-Reported Sedentary Time Questionnaire (Gardiner et al. 2011)	ActiGraph GT1M worn for 7 days	Total sitting time, Spearman's r = 0.30, 95% CI (0.02, 0.54)	1 week	Spearman's r = 0.56, 95% CI[b] (0.33, 0.73)
Past-Day Adults' Sedentary Time Questionnaire (Clark et al. 2013)	activPAL version 3 and ActiGraph GT3X+ worn for 7 days, counts < 100	activPAL total, Pearson's r = 0.58, 95% CI (0.40, 0.72); ActiGraph < 100 counts, Pearson's r = 0.51, 95% CI (0.29, 0.68)	6 months	ICC = 0.50, 95% CI (0.32, 0.64)
Sedentary Behavior Questionnaire (Rosenberg et al. 2010)	ActiGraph 7164 worn for 7 days, counts < 100; IPAQ total sitting time	ActiGraph < 100 counts, Males, r = −0.01 (p = 0.81), Females, r = 0.10, (p = 0.07); IPAQ total sitting, Males, r = 0.31 (p = 0.00), Females, r = 0.28 (p = 0.00)	2 weeks	Weekday Spearman's r = 0.79, 95% CI (0.58, 0.85); Weekend Spearman's r = 0.74, 95% CI (0.65, 0.78)
Sedentary Time and Activity Reporting Questionnaire (Neilson et al. 2013; Csizmadi et al. 2014)	Not reported	Not reported	3 months	Sedentary time, ICC = 0.53, 95% CI (0.37, 0.66)
Yale Physical Activity Survey (Dipietro et al. 1993)	Not reported	Not reported	2 weeks	Spearman's r = 0.42-0.65
Adolescent Sedentary Activity Questionnaire (Hardy, Booth, and Okely 2007)	Not reported	Not reported	2 weeks	ICC = 0.57, 95% CI: 0.25, 0.76
Youth Risk Behavior Survey (Schmitz et al. 2004)	245 middle school students filled out a log	Spearman's r = 0.46, mean difference = −0.04 hr	1 week	Spearman's r = 0.68
Self-Administered Physical Activity Checklist (Sallis et al. 1996)	Caltrac accelerometer worn for 1 school day	Pearson's r = 0.30, (n = 97)	Not reported	Not reported
SIT-Q-7d (Wijndaele et al. 2014)	activPAL3 worn for 6 days	Spearman's r = 0.37, (n = 402)	Median = 3.3 weeks	ICC (95%) = 0.53 (0.44-0.62)

[a]Standard deviation or confidence interval not reported; [b]CI = confidence interval

171

Respondents also placed activities into the wrong categories listed and were unable to differentiate between types of self-care activities. The investigators revised the questionnaire to reduce the problem areas before using it in a study setting.

Questionnaires used to assess sedentary behavior in children, adults with low reading and numeral literacy, and older adults with cognitive impairments may limit the information asked to the frequency of a behavior only. The recall frame also is shorter, limiting recall to the past 72 hours (Clark et al. 2013). These modifications are made due to the difficulties in recalling information and performing mathematic calculations required to average time spent in various behaviors over multiple days and activities (Ainsworth et al. 2012). For example, the 3-Day Physical Activity Recall (Pate et al. 2003) is a 24-hour recall questionnaire for youth that has respondents check a box if they performed one of nine listed activities every half hour. In this case, respondents avoid recalling the exact duration of the behavior. The ARIC-Baecke questionnaire for adults presents the duration in a range from "not at all" to "most of the day" to avoid issues with numeral literacy (Richardson et al. 1995).

The following six steps can be used when planning questionnaires for assessing sedentary behavior (Ainsworth et al. 2012):

1. *Identifying need.* Prior to use, an investigator should determine the purpose for conducting a survey. Is it to measure sedentary behavior at one point in time, track sedentary behavior over time, or correlate sedentary behavior with a disease and health outcome?

2. *Selecting a questionnaire.* The questionnaire must match the respondent's cognitive abilities, culture, and literacy capabilities. The questionnaire also should have documented and acceptable validity and reliability evidence and measure the types of behaviors sought for the study. Avoid tinkering with the questionnaire by deleting or adding questions or changing the wording, since this will negate the established validity and reliability. It is the task of the survey administrator and people administering the questionnaire to select the appropriate questionnaire for the intended purpose.

3. *Collecting data.* Respondents must understand the wording and intent of a questionnaire in terms of the types of behaviors assessed and the time frame of recall. Data collectors should be trained in procedures used to administer the questionnaire and how to prompt respondents to recall information if the questionnaire is interviewer administered. Interviewers also should give the same instructions to each respondent when completing the questionnaire and avoid giving suggestions for answers. Providing respondents with a calendar that has salient information, such as holidays or work schedules, may be a useful prompt for recalling information.

4. *Analyzing data.* Questionnaires should always be checked for accuracy in the presence of the respondent for missing data, items with hours or minutes that are unrealistically high or low, and unacceptable responses, such as a question mark if one does not recall an answer. For investigators with statistical support, statisti-

CULTURAL TRANSLATION

An important concern when using questionnaires with non-English speaking people is the comprehension of the instrument after it has been translated into a new language. Prior to use, questionnaires should go through both linguistic and cultural translation processes with groups of people similar to the population who will receive the survey. The linguistic translation involves a word-for-word translation of the questionnaire. A cultural transla-

tion involves modifying the types of words used and examples of behaviors listed in the questionnaire to reflect how a target population understands the subject matter. A cultural translation can be done by having focus groups or people from the respondent survey group critique the questionnaire following the linguistic translation. Arredondo and colleagues (2012) provide guidelines for the cultural translation of questionnaires.

cal procedures can be applied to account for random error that may occur as a result of the questionnaire administration process.

5. *Creating a summary score.* Always apply the scoring protocol that is provided for the questionnaire. Changing the scoring protocol will render the questionnaire's results useless for comparison with other studies using the same questionnaire. The summary score should be checked for unrealistic scores that could result from errors in applying the scoring protocol and corrected before reporting the results of the survey.

6. *Data interpretation.* The person managing the questionnaire should have a thorough understanding of the prevalence of sedentary behavior and the typical responses for the populations surveyed. If the questionnaire results are statistically compared with other physical activities, health behaviors, or health and disease conditions, investigators should know how their results should compare with similar studies having the same purpose.

Summary

Questionnaires are useful when assessing the types and estimated duration of sedentary behavior in targeted populations. Questionnaires must be valid and reliable for the populations where they are used. Additionally, questionnaires used in sedentary behavior intervention studies should demonstrate acceptable responsiveness to assessing changes in sedentary behavior.

First and foremost, those planning to assess sedentary behavior should avoid the desire to create a new questionnaire. Instead, they should select a questionnaire that has been validated and deemed reliable in a population similar to the proposed sample in age, race and ethnicity, and other demographic characteristics. Healy and colleagues (2011) have compiled a list of sedentary behavior questionnaires with their validity and reliability coefficients for use in adult populations. If a survey has not been evaluated for validity and reliability evidence in a targeted population, then an examination of validity and reliability is needed prior to use in a research study.

Further research is needed to validate and examine the reliability of questionnaires in diverse populations to include people of all ages, races and ethnicities, and educational levels, and those living in urban or rural settings. Since most questionnaires have been developed for use in English-speaking populations, translating questionnaires using a linguistic translation only may result in the use of phrases and words that have little meaning without a cultural context. Cultural translations also are needed if questionnaires are to be used in non-English speaking populations. Research is also needed to examine the ability of sedentary behavior questionnaires to detect changes in behaviors arising from intervention studies. Aside from requiring a questionnaire to have acceptable validity and reliability, questionnaires used to assess behavior changes must be responsive to the behaviors undergoing change. Clark and colleagues (2013) provide an example of how to evaluate a questionnaire for responsiveness in their examination of the past-day recall of sedentary time in a sample of breast cancer survivors.

KEY CONCEPTS

▸ **Domains of sedentary behavior:** 9 main domains describing sedentary behavior have been identified: the purpose (why), the environment (where), the posture, the social context (with whom), the measurement (instruments and quantification issues), the associated behaviors (what else), the status (mental and functional states of the person), the time (when the behavior take place), and the type of behavior (what).

▸ **Duration:** One of the key components of a questionnaire that specifies the amount of time expressed in hours or minutes spent in a sedentary behavior.

▸ **Frequency:** One of the key components of a questionnaire indicating the recurrence at which a sedentary behavior occurs or is repeated over a particular period of time (i.e., days per week).

▸ **Mode:** One of the key components of a questionnaire describing the types of sedentary behavior performed (i.e., watching television, or driving a car).

▸ **Questionnaires:** Survey instruments that consist of a set of questions selected and arranged to identify information about a person or what a person thinks about a topic.

▸ **Recall frame:** One of the key components of a questionnaire referred to the period of time a person is asked to recall events from the past (i.e., a day, or a week).

▸ **Reliability:** The degree to which a questionnaire yields stable and consistent results over time. For example, a questionnaire is reliable if in a 1-month period the test–retest survey produces similar results.

▸ **Validity:** Quality of the questionnaire indicating that it is measuring what we want to measure. Different types of validity include logical, content, construct, and criterion.

STUDY QUESTIONS

1. Go to the IPAQ website (www.ipaq.ki.se) and download one of the questionnaires. Identify which question is asking for sedentary behavior and identify what types of activities the respondent may be considering as sedentary.

2. You are looking for a questionnaire to identify sedentary behavior in pregnant women, and there are no published questionnaires on this topic available in the literature. How can you identify a suitable questionnaire for assessing sedentary behavior in pregnant women?

3. You have to choose one sedentary behavior questionnaire for a study. You have found two sedentary behavior questionnaires that are suitable for your population characteristics. One of the questionnaires has good reliability ($r = 0.90$) but does not mention anything about its validity; however, it seems to have questions sufficient for assessing the behaviors you need to measure. The second questionnaire has lower reliability ($r = 0.70$) but mentions that its validity was assessed by a panel of experts. Which one would you select? Provide the rationale for your choice.

4. For an epidemiological study, you need to determine the MET-intensity dose of sedentary behavior related with health outcomes. What types of questions would you include in your questionnaire?

5. In a questionnaire, what qualities are necessary for measuring decreases in sedentary behavior during an intervention focused on reducing sitting time in office workers?

CHAPTER 14

ASSESSING SEDENTARY BEHAVIOR USING MOTION SENSORS

Kong Y. Chen, PhD, MSCI; and Richard P. Troiano, PhD

The reader will gain technical and applied knowledge of how motion sensors are used for sedentary behavior monitoring, and how to integrate them into field applications. By the end of this chapter, the reader should be able to do the following:

▸ Understand what motion sensors are

▸ Explore how motion sensors work in principle and in practice

▸ Compare different types of motion sensors and their potential for assessing sedentary behavior

▸ Discuss future needs and developments

By definition, motion sensors measure or detect movements. The rationale of assessing motion as a way to quantify human activity is based on the physical principle that a change of motion requires forces that are typically provided by the person. To generate such forces requires energy output, or energy expenditure (EE). Therefore, measurement of motion can be, in theory, directly linked to estimations of activity-associated EE. However, this is not trivial in practice because multiple factors influence the presence and degree of measurement and modeling errors.

The history of using motion sensors to assess biomechanics of human movement dates back as early as the 15th century, when Leonardo da Vinci drafted a design of a mechanical step counter (pedometer) for military applications (MacCurdy 1938). More recently, in the 1960s, a triaxial accelerometer was constructed by mounting strain gauges on three steel plates at perpendicular orientations to each other (Cavagna, Saibene, and Margaria 1961). Each plate was fixed at two ends with a weight at the center. When this sensor was firmly applied to the subject, it was able to measure dynamic movements such as walking, running, jumping, and throwing. Soon, this type of sensor found its way into medical research for movement disorders such as Parkinsonism (Brody 1992), artificial limbs (Lanyon 1971), and gait analysis (Morris 1972, 1973). Montoye and colleagues (1983; see also Wong et al. 1981) were among the earliest researchers to show that accelerometers could provide continuous movement outputs that were significantly correlated with EE, thus paving the way for motion sensors to be used for objective physical activity measurements in laboratories. Field studies soon followed and flourished.

Welk (2002) thoroughly reviewed the use of accelerometer-based activity monitors for assessing physical activity. However, with the evolving research and public health focus on sedentary behavior, we hereby reexamine the use of motion sensors for assessing sedentariness. As with any sensor-based measure, in order to apply motion sensors appropriately in assessing sedentary behavior, one has to understand the characteristics of the behavior itself. In chapter 1, the definition of sedentary behavior includes meeting all three of the following criteria: (1) waking behavior characterized by (2) an energy expenditure ≤ 1.5 METs (3) while in a sitting or reclining posture. This chapter addresses the use of motion sensors for these three criteria specifically and how we could improve the

accuracy, precision, and reliability for measuring sedentary behavior in the future.

Key Components of Motion Sensors

Several types of motion sensors exist. The most commonly recognized motion sensors or detectors are used in security alarms, light switches, and other similar qualitative functions. These are typically called *active* sensors—they send out a beam (e.g., infrared, microwave) and detect its return back to the receiver (figure 14.1). When the return signal is perturbed, either in timing or amplitude over a certain predetermined threshold, it is judged that motion is detected, which triggers a downstream action. We use this method in closely controlled laboratories such as a respiration chamber, where motion and EE (through the determinations of oxygen consumption and carbon dioxide production rates) are measured simultaneously. The measurement of motion is typically used to gauge a minimal level of activity that indicates resting or sleeping status, and EE during these periods is calculated with decreased activity artifacts or noise. A similar concept is applied in animal calorimeters using uniformly placed laser or infrared beams across the chamber.

In the context of measuring motion in free-living humans, we generally use sensors that are attached to the subject's body to objectively measure the type and intensity of movements. In contrast to the active sensors, these are a class of *passive* sensors where no waves or beams are sent out or received. Instead, these sensors measure motion based on electromechanical properties within their sensing elements or transducers (they transfer one form of energy to another, i.e., from motion to electrical signals) (Chen et al. 2012).

Measurement Principles of Motion Transducers

A wide variety of motion transducers can be used singly or in combinations to assess human movements. These include pedometers, tilt sensors, electronic load transducers, foot contact monitors, global positioning systems, barometers, gyroscopes, and cameras. A traditional pedometer typically consists of a simple mechanical movement counter that is clipped onto a belt at the waist or worn on the

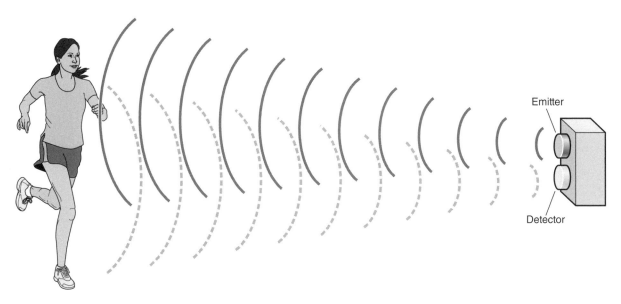

Figure 14.1 A schematic plot of an active motion sensor.

ankle. As a small, portable, affordable, and simple device, it operates by counting steps during walking and running. Thus, pedometers are popular tools for exercise prescription, weight-loss interventions, and general health promotion. However, several different earlier types of mechanical pedometers have been reported to underestimate distances walked at slower speeds and overestimate distances during fast walking or running (Washburn, Chin, and Montoye 1980; Bassey et al. 1987). Recently developed electronic pedometers allow better step detection and can be attached to the shoelaces, carried in a pocket, and even placed in a backpack. These devices for step counting and distance traveled have been reported to be accurate within ±4.0% (Giannaki-dou et al. 2012). However, as a tool for monitoring sedentary behavior, pedometers are limited because they measure only steps or locomotive movement.

A tilt sensor, such as the large-scale integrated (LSI) motor activity monitor, is a simple device that uses a mercury switch sensitive to angular position (i.e., a tilt) in a single axis (shown in figure 14.2). LSI monitors were used in one study to distinguish between groups of adults who grossly differed in PA status (Cauley et al. 1987). Although LSI readings correlate poorly with estimated energy expenditure (or oxygen consumption) levels during walking, running, and bicycle riding (Montoye et al. 1983), this type of sensor could be modified to measure posture if it could overcome being a switch sensor with only on or off qualitative output.

Electronic load transducers and foot contact monitors are available that can be inserted into the heels of shoes to monitor loads held, lifted, or carried and walking activity (Barber et al. 1973). For example, the ambulatory foot contact monitor can estimate metabolic cost of human locomotion from body weight and foot contact time during each stride (Hoyt et al. 1994). Due to technical and practical limitations such as transducer drift and discomfort, these devices (i.e., in-shoe step counters, foot contact time monitors) have not been used widely in epidemiological research, and little information is currently available on their accuracy in assessing habitual PA status and daily EE (Hoyt et al. 1994). However, this technology could be used to detect standing versus sitting due to the pressure differences at the foot.

Other sensors, including global positioning systems, barometers, gyroscopes, and cameras, can be used to detect motion as a primary device or as a secondary device in a multisensor arrangement. They are included here for the sake of completeness, but their capacity to contribute to the measurement of sedentary behavior might be limited. The Global Positioning System (GPS) is a satellite-based navigation system that provides location and time information using specialized satellite networks. It requires unobstructed line of sight to four or more GPS satellites and a receiver. A GPS receiver calculates its position by precisely timing the signals sent by GPS satellites high above

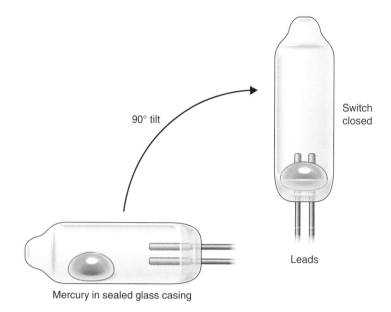

90° tilt

Switch
closed

Leads

Mercury in sealed glass casing

Figure 14.2 A mercury tilt sensor moves from an *off* or an open position to an *on* or a closed position with the mercury switch.

the Earth. Each satellite continually transmits message signals that include the time when the message was transmitted and the satellite position at time of message transmission. The receiver uses the messages it receives to determine the transit time of each message and computes the distance to each satellite based on the speed of light. These distances and the satellite locations are used to compute the location of the receiver using geometric triangulation to resolve the latitude and longitude and even elevation. Since the receiver sends and receives transmissions continuously, any change in these three parameters represents a motion. However, commonly used commercial GPS receivers are fairly imprecise (2-3 m of error range or ambiguity), which makes it hard to differentiate minor movements from staying still. Recent developments in what is called Carrier-Phase Enhancement GPS can potentially improve the precision by about 100-fold (3 cm ambiguity).

A change in altitude or elevation can be measured with a barometer by detecting changes in atmospheric pressure. Barometers have been used in conjunction with other sensors, such as accelerometers and GPS devices, to provide or refine measures of elevation change. The elevation data can allow distinctions between walking on the flat and walking on an incline, stairs, or hills. However, the major limitation of these sensors is that ambient changes of atmospheric pressure and temperature

require the barometer to be frequently calibrated. The sensitivity to detect small changes is also limited by most marketed portable barometers.

Positional tilt and rotation can be measured by a gyroscope, which is a sensor that measures the angular movement around one or more axes. Gyroscopes quantify angular position and yield continuous measures of angular velocity and acceleration. These outputs contrast with mercury switches that output only *on* and *off* positions and with accelerometers (to be covered in later sections) that measure linear acceleration. The main limitations of gyroscope sensors are their larger size, greater cost, and relatively high power consumption, which are all critical issues for a portable monitor that needs to operate over several days in a small and inexpensive unit.

Wearable cameras record the context in which behaviors occur by taking images automatically every fraction of a minute to provide measures of physical activity and sedentary behavior. For example, if the photo shows a steering wheel and view through a windshield, we know the wearer is sitting while driving a car. If a series of photos shows bicycle handlebars and changing scenery, the wearer is riding a bike. Although some wearable cameras have a privacy feature to prompt the camera to stop taking pictures during inopportune times, privacy for people photographed remains a concern with the use of wearable cameras.

Accelerometers

In the past two or three decades, accelerometer-based sensors have represented the predominant sources for detecting human motion as a primary device or as a secondary device in a multisensor arrangement. Their application and contribution to the measurement of sedentary behavior has been documented in numerous cross-sectional and longitudinal studies (Atkin et al. 2012; Matthews et al. 2008; Colley et al. 2011; Arnardottir et al. 2012; Bankoski et al. 2011).

By strict definition, an accelerometer measures what is called proper or true acceleration, which is defined as the acceleration relative to free fall. So an accelerometer at rest relative to the Earth's surface will measure approximately 1 G (9.8 m/s²) upward.

However, depending on the type of the transducer, this has not always been the case.

Beginning with accelerometers devised in the 1980s (Klesges et al. 1985) and used widely until a few years ago, most sensing elements of accelerometers were piezoelectric transducers configured in cantilever beams (figure 14.3a) or compressive plates (figure 14.3b) with seismic masses (Chen and Bassett 2005). Although such devices are capable of measuring the dynamic changes in acceleration (change of velocity) over a range of several Gs, the nature of these transducers does not allow them to measure static loads, meaning that when they are at rest, their output is zero. This is due to the phenomenon known as leakage (Togowa, Tamura, and Oberg 1998). Although some earlier versions of the transducers were piezoresistive, and used

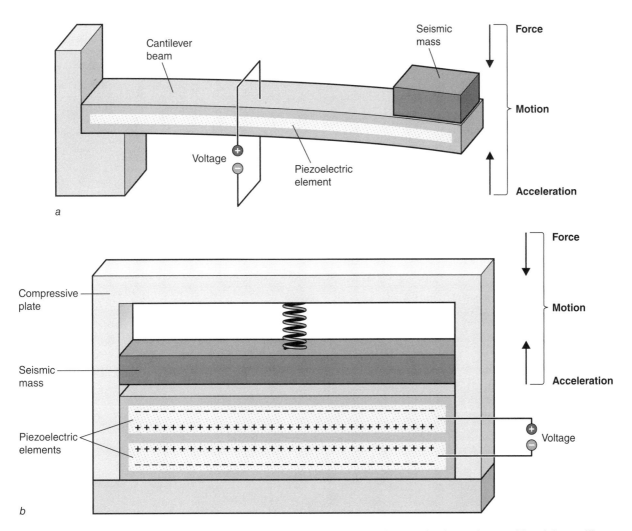

Figure 14.3 Two common configurations of piezoelectric accelerometer transducers. The (*a*) cantilever beam accelerometer and (*b*) piezoelectric compressive plate accelerometer.

Adapted from Chen and Bassett 2005.

Wheatstone bridges to detect both static and dynamic components of acceleration (Montoye et al. 1983), temperature-sensitive drift and limited dynamic range significantly hindered the capabilities of this type of sensor.

Technological advance has allowed transducers to be developed and manufactured to evolve from the piezoelectric cantilever beam and piezoelectric or piezoresistive compressive integrated chips to differential capacitance accelerometers. Most of these newer transducers are true accelerometers that measure resting gravitational inertia (1 G). They are now micromachined within or on the surfaces of a polysilicon structure. In such a device, called a microelectromechanical system (MEMS), a differential or variable capacitance sensor is typically constructed with plates attached to a moving mass and fixed plates, and the capacitance between these plates is dependent on the distances between the plates as an acceleration is applied to the moving mass (figure 14.4). The piezoresistive and differential capacitance accelerometer are sensitive to both motion-induced accelerations and gravitational acceleration. Moreover, they can be used to measure tilt angle based on the measured signal in the y-axis (ay)—at a tilted angle, Θ is equal to $1\ \mathrm{G} \times \cos(\Theta)$. Conversely, the angle Θ can be solved when a static signal is measured (figure 14.4).

This unique property of capacitance sensors has allowed a new class of accelerometers to emerge and function as tilt sensors similar to gyroscopes. A good example of this application is the activPAL (PAL Technologies, Glasgow, Scotland), an accelerometer-based monitor worn on the top surface of the thigh that can differentiate sitting or lying from standing postures and indicate locomotive activities based on the dynamic components of acceleration (Ryan et al. 2006).

Accelerometer Counts

A common output of accelerometers that has historically been used for physical activity and sedentary behavior research is counts. However, substantial confusion is still associated with this nomenclature. It is believed that the origins of the term *count* can be traced to early generation activity monitors that had little or no solid-state capacity to quantify multiple levels of activity, such as in a pedometer, where motion that caused the acceleration signal to exceed the threshold was counted as activity; anything below this threshold was ignored. At the end of the measurement period, the number of activity counts would be recorded. More recently, the output of the accelerometer has been put through analog-to-digital (A/D) conversion to generate a continuous measure, but many manufacturers retained the nomenclature of output units as *counts* without using a threshold crossing counter.

For example, the ActiGraph 7164 accelerometer transducer has a maximum range of ±2.13 G. The A/D is an 8-bit device yielding 2^8 levels (256 counts) to cover the entire range of acceleration, in this case, 4.26 G. This resulted in 1 count representing 4.26 G/256 quantization levels; because acceleration is being sampled 10 times a second, the result is 0.001664 G/bit (or 0.001664 G/count). Since the lowest resolution is 1 second, this becomes 0.01664 $\mathrm{G \cdot count^{-1} \cdot second^{-1}}$ on the ActiGraph 7164 device.

However, counts can mean different quantities when comparing outputs from one type of accelerometer to another due to differences in sensor ranges, linearity, A/D types, sampling rates, and integration algorithms (Chen and Bassett 2005; Welk, McClain, and Ainsworth 2012), and not all manufacturers release their specific description of this critical measure. The analytical process of calculating counts has been previously described in detail (Chen and Bassett 2005), including a discussion of the pros and cons of the process.

Translating Counts Into Energy Expenditure

Although the accelerometer counts are arbitrary in nature and vary greatly between monitor manufacturers, they provide objective and continuous measures that represent the intensity of the movements of the subjects. Many researchers have taken the counts from accelerometers and modeled them into energy expenditure (EE) metrics, particularly activity-associated EE, labeled as activity energy expenditure (AEE), energy expenditure of activity, or physical activity energy expenditure (Butte, Ekelund, and Westerterp 2012).

Multiple modeling approaches exist for estimating EE from the accelerometer counts. By far the most commonly used approach has been linear regression, owing to historical evidence of a high correlation coefficient between counts assessed at the hip and certain locomotive activities such as walking. However, although walking is a common form of physical activity in the free-living condition, the generalization of a simple linear regression result

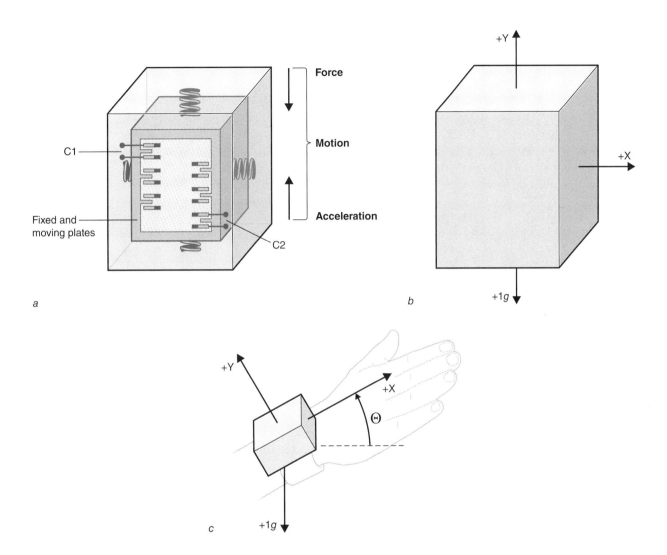

Figure 14.4 A capacitive accelerometer that can detect static (tilt) and dynamic signals. The internal structure of the capacitance-based microelectromechanical system (MEMS) triaxial accelerometer (*a*). C1 and C2 represent capacitors for the upper and lower surfaces, which change their capacitances with the moving seismic mass in the middle. The differential signals (*b, c*) from different axes (x and y) can be used to calculate the angle (Θ) at which the sensor is positioned in relation to the gravitational axis (+1 G).

Adapted from Chen et al. 2012.

to all activities can lead to errors for activity type identification and total EE prediction (as measured by doubly labeled water) (Plasqui, Bonomi, and Westerterp 2013; Plasqui and Westerterp 2007; Staudenmayer, Zhu, and Catellier 2012). Several causes exist for this error. One is that the linear relationship assumption between AEE and counts was established during steady-state conditions of intensity within a few specific activities, while free-living activities consist of multiple activity types and intensity levels as well as transitions between different activities and postures. Another error source is that the baseline EE, which is used to determine METs, was not always carefully measured in calibration studies. Classically, resting metabolic rate (RMR) or resting EE is measured while the subject maintains a comfortable and quiet supine posture in a thermally comfortable and low ambient noise room, after having been fasted and well rested for at least 8 hours. Without accurate measurements of this baseline, calculations of METs or AEE can be skewed.

Other models and approaches have been applied to counts in attempts to improve AEE prediction over a wide range of activity types and intensities, such as nonlinear regressions (Chen and Sun 1997; Chen et al. 2003; Puyau et al. 2004; Campbell, Crocker, and McKenzie 2002), multivariate regressions including terms such as *lags* (time points prior to the direct one-to-one matched counts) (Butte et al. 2010; Zakeri et al. 2010; Choi et al. 2010), and two-regression models based on variability over adjoining time samples (Crouter, Clowers, and Bassett 2006). Regardless of the specific modeling approach, the goals of developing calibration equations have traditionally been oriented toward obtaining certain thresholds or cut points to categorize daily physical activities into different intensities (e.g., moderate-intensity or vigorous-intensity activity), or the multiplier of resting EE (often measured in METs). A common intensity categorization metric for adults is sedentary (≤1.5 METs), light (1.5-2.99 METs), moderate (3-5.99 METs), and vigorous (≥6 METs), and thus the corresponding count values can be derived from these models and used for field studies.

Assessing Sedentary Behavior by Counts Threshold

As use of accelerometers increased, researchers extended the aspects of physical activity behavior measured by the devices from moderate- or vigorous-intensity activity to lower-intensity activity and even sedentary behavior. A threshold of 100 counts per minute (cpm) is frequently used to distinguish sedentary behavior from light-intensity activity. This threshold derives from methodological research done in conjunction with the Trial of Activity in Adolescent Girls (TAAG) study (Treuth et al. 2004). The TAAG investigators found that a threshold of 100 cpm (actually 50 counts/30 seconds) had no false positives or false negatives for identifying light-intensity activity in their calibration study. Therefore, counts of less than 100 cpm were classified as sedentary behavior.

Higher ActiGraph count thresholds have been proposed, with values as high as 800 (Puyau et al. 2002) and 1,100 cpm (Jackson et al. 2003). The threshold of 800 cpm was based on a linear regression of counts against activity energy expenditure, which may have influenced the sedentary estimate, since sedentary-defined activities within this study generated counts between 14 and approximately 300 cpm. The value of 1,100 cpm may have been influenced by the age of participants, which was limited to ages 3 to 4 years (Jackson et al. 2003). A study that examined thresholds of 50, 100, 150, and 200 cpm determined that 150 cpm provided a better estimate of sedentary behavior than 100 cpm, but the increase in precision was small (Kozey-Keadle

FREE-LIVING CONDITIONS AND ACCELEROMETER MEASURES

Because the development of accelerometer hardware and its application in the past two to three decades was focused on physical activity, establishment of counts-METs models focused on activity intensity of 2 METs or greater. As a result, sedentary behavior, which is defined as less than 1.5 METs in intensity, has often been defined as periods during which subjects are not active by deduction rather than by direct measurement. This is likely due to two major factors. First, obtaining accurate and precise reference measures of EE during sedentary and light-intensity activities is a challenge because the signal-to-noise ratio is low at these low levels of expenditure. Second, the traditional accelerometer placement on the hip or waist does not measure the movements of the limbs that occur while being sedentary. Another potential factor is that some model developers measure AEE during multiple activity types or intensities, but often include only one or two sedentary behaviors. When each activity is treated as a single data point and an overall minimum error in estimation is optimized (e.g., least sum of squares), this assumes that there is an equal probability of one type of sedentary behavior (e.g., sitting) relative to one type of activity (running). However, in the free-living condition, the proportions of time spent active or sedentary are likely to be vastly different, with sedentary behavior encompassing a larger proportion of the day (Matthews et al. 2008). As a result, some laboratory accelerometer models developed for predicting EE do poorly under free-living conditions (Plasqui and Westerterp 2007).

et al. 2011). These higher values have not had wide application, especially in research on adults.

The 100 cpm threshold was further supported by its application in the report of population estimates of sedentary behavior from NHANES 2003-2004 (Matthews et al. 2008). The use in this study was supported by a validation study in adults that compared postural and motion data measured by the Intelligent Device for Energy Expenditure and Activity (IDEEA) monitor to ActiGraph count data. Although the validation study is unpublished, the methods and results were described by Matthews and colleagues (2008).

A lower threshold of 50 cpm has also been proposed (Crouter, Clowers, and Bassett 2006). In an evaluation of several objective measures of sedentary behavior, Hart, McClain, and Tudor-Locke (2011) compared the ActiGraph, activPAL, and IDEEA monitors. They found that an ActiGraph threshold of 50 cpm had good agreement with the postural measures of combined sitting and lying time, while a higher threshold of 259 cpm agreed well with measures of combined lying, sitting, and standing. This study points out an important issue for use of accelerometer-based devices to measure sedentary behavior. As typically worn on the waist, or more recently the wrist, an accelerometer can detect motion, but distinguishing postural position is a challenge because, for example, the orientation of the waist while sitting up straight may be the same as while standing. ActivPAL addressed this challenge by locating the device on the thigh, but the orientation of the thigh is similar while sitting or lying down.

Practical Guidelines

A challenge when using accelerometers to measure sedentary behavior relates to the first criterion in its definition, that the behavior occurs during wakefulness. This requires the ability to detect sleep. A related issue when considering sleep, which is a quite inactive state, is to be able to distinguish sleep from times that the accelerometer is not being worn.

Determining Accelerometer Nonwear

The first step in any analysis of accelerometer data will usually be to distinguish time that the device was worn from when it was not worn. This step is required for evaluating whether sufficient data are available for a given day or participant to be included in the analysis as well as to exclude nonwear periods from subsequent calculations. In practice, the critical aspect is defining and identifying nonwear periods. This identification is typically based on periods of continuous zero counts under the assumption that an accelerometer that is not worn will not be moving.

Investigators have defined accelerometer nonwear as periods of 10, 15, 20, 30, and 60 minutes (Evenson and Terry 2009) and some have even proposed 90 minutes as a criterion (Choi et al. 2011). Initially, fixed windows of time were used, such that a decision of wear or nonwear based on presence of any zero-count epochs (usually minutes) was made for minutes 1 through 20, then for minutes 21 through 40, and so on. Later procedures incorporated a moving window approach to evaluate wear or nonwear (Troiano et al. 2008).

The choice of nonwear definition is not likely to affect estimates of physical activity of moderate or vigorous intensity, except by affecting the inclusion or exclusion of a given day's data. However, the classification of sedentary behavior is very sensitive to the nonwear definition because a low or sensitive threshold for identifying nonwear is more likely to classify sedentary periods as nonwear. For example, when comparing 20- and 60-minute nonwear criteria for initial analysis of a subset of the accelerometer data from the 2003-2004 National Health and Nutrition Examination Survey, a criterion of 20 minutes of zeroes led to 21% of the sample having more than five wear to nonwear transitions per day, with 50% of older adults having more than five transitions. These values seemed implausible, so the 60-minute criterion was selected. Note that the extent of misclassification will vary by population. Although many older adults may have legitimate periods of low activity that could be misclassified as nonwear, studies with children may be able to use shorter periods for nonwear definition. The effect of different nonwear criteria on the determination of sedentary behavior among a sedentary adult population was explored (Oliver et al. 2011). Based on both sensitivity and specificity, they concluded that at least 60 minutes of continuous zero counts should be used to determine nonwear in an adult population with primarily sedentary occupation and further suggested that in particularly sedentary populations, a period of 180 minutes of continuous zeroes should be considered.

Technological advances have improved the ability to correctly classify accelerometer nonwear. Some multisensor devices, such as the GENEActiv (Activinsights Ltd., Kimbolton, England) or Body-Media arm bands (BodyMedia, Inc., Pittsburgh, PA), incorporate temperature sensors that can detect when the device is being worn. Furthermore, as increasing device memory has facilitated shorter measurement epochs (time-integrated) and even raw data (typically referred as acceleration signals not integrated over time and usually in higher frequency, 30-100 Hz), the sensitivity for detecting nonwear is improved.

Determining Sleep

Accelerometers have been used in sleep research for nearly as long as in activity research. Sleep researchers used a wrist-mounted piezoelectric accelerometer in a group of hospital-bound inpatients and outpatients and found that the wrist data could distinguish sleep from wakefulness with greater than 94.5% accuracy compared to the standard clinical polysomnographic scoring (Mullaney, Kripke, and Messin 1980). Other researchers soon followed this discovery by developing and validating automated algorithms (decision tree with thresholds) to utilize nonobstructive accelerometer measurements from the wrist to identify sleep and wakefulness (Cole et al. 1992; Tracy et al. 2014; Webster et al. 1982). Wrist-worn accelerometer-based sleep watches continue to be used today as an accepted in-home sleep monitoring tool to study insomnia, circadian sleep and wake disturbances, and other sleep disorders (Broughton, Fleming, and Fleetham 1996). Intriguingly, a hip-worn accelerometer was also shown to measure sleep duration in adolescents as reliably as wrist actigraphy (Weiss et al. 2010). Collectively, the use of accelerometers to efficiently and accurately distinguish sleep from wakefulness is established.

Potential of Raw Accelerometer Data

Owing to the challenges of predicting the intensity and the types of physical activity using only counts, the physical activity field has encouraged device manufacturers to move away from counts, and researchers have started to explore the raw accelerometer data with the goal of improving the accuracy and precision of assessing physical activity. The rationale is that the counts represent only one dimension of the movement captured by the accelerometer, which is a product of the activity intensity and time (epoch). Other components or features of the raw data, which are lost after integration and filtering, may actually be useful for distinguishing different types of activities and the small differences between or within individuals that cause a divergence in EE.

Unlike the regression approaches that were frequently used to model counts to EE, modeling AEE and activity types using large amounts of raw data or multiple features of the raw data requires more sophisticated approaches, such as hierarchical decision trees (Kiani, Snijders, and Gelsema 1997; Mathie et al. 2004), k-nearest-neighbor classification (Bussmann et al. 1998), support vector machines (Lau, Tong, and Zhu 2009), naive Bayes classifier (Long, Yin, and Aarts 2009), Gaussian mixture model (Allen et al. 2006), hidden Markov model (Pober et al. 2006; Mannini and Sabatini 2010), artificial neural networks (Kiani, Snijders, and Gelsema 1998: Rothney et al. 2007; Staudenmayer et al. 2009), and other machine learning techniques (Liu, Gao, and Freedson 2012). Although many of these approaches demonstrated substantial improvements (>50% reduction in root mean square error of METs) compared to simple linear regression estimates of a variety of activity types and intensities, the focus was not on sedentary behavior.

However, the great potential to use different features (time domain, frequency domain, and heuristic) (Preece et al. 2009; Troiano et al. 2014) to simultaneously quantify postures (sitting vs. standing), intensity (EE ≤1.5 METs), and sleep from the raw accelerometer signals provides a promising way forward for sedentary behavior (Rowlands et al. 2014; Rowlands et al. 2016). Future research regarding raw data should address the following issues:

1. Focus on model development in a variety of sedentary behaviors, or include more sedentary behaviors with active components, and use appropriate weighing factors to adjust for probability distribution of sedentary versus active components in the free-living condition.

2. Test multiple locations of sensor attachments for posture detection that could yield sensitive measurements of sitting versus lying down versus standing and locomotion, as well as for EE estimations (summarized in table 14.1).

3. Determine the minimum number of sensors and locations for optimizing the balance of measurement accuracy and precision with subject convenience and acceptability as well as model complexity.

Summary

With increasing interest in examining the role of sedentary behavior in chronic disease morbidity and mortality, high-quality assessments of sedentary behavior in population-based settings are becoming increasingly important (Atkin et al. 2012). Motion sensors are commonly used for objective measurements of physical activity, particularly for locomotive body movements such as walking and jogging. Motion sensors have also been used to estimate the time of sedentariness if the intensity fails to reach a threshold associated with light-intensity physical activity. The enhanced definition of sedentary behavior requires three criteria: wakefulness, energy expenditure < 1.5 times resting metabolic rate, and a sitting or reclining posture. Currently, no activity monitor can accurately and precisely quantify all three criteria simultaneously. Although several different kinds of motion or movement sensors exist, accelerometers are the most widely used sensors because the differential capacitive transducers are sensitive to both dynamic changes (active linear movements) and static changes (postures). To improve the objective assessment of sedentary behavior, future research should take advantage of devices with advanced sensor technology, either independently or in combinations with other sensors, and consider applying devices to more than one body location. The raw accelerometer data or derived features should be analyzed with modern sophisticated modeling approaches and appropriate model development and validation considerations.

Table 14.1 Ability to Measure Sedentary Behavior Characteristics at Common Body Locations

Body location	Wakefulness	≤1.5 METs	Sitting or reclining
Waist, hip, back	Possible by motion profile	Yes, by regression calibration or thresholds	Not easy to distinguish sitting vs. standing
Chest, sternum	Possible by motion profile	Yes	Not easy to distinguish sitting vs. standing
Thigh	Possible by motion profile	Possibly, based on stepping frequency	Possible by motion profile
Ankle	No, because of restless leg syndrome	Possibly, based on stepping frequency	No
Foot (load cell)	No	Possibly, based on stepping frequency and load	Yes
Upper arm	Yes	Yes, by regression calibration or thresholds	No
Wrist	Yes	Yes, by regression calibration or thresholds	Possible by motion profile

KEY CONCEPTS

▸ **Accelerometers:** A single piezoelectric sensor, commonly used in activity monitors before 2009, cannot measure static (postural) changes in positions or angles. Current accelerometers are generally capacitive based, multiaxial, and constructed as microelectromechanical systems (MEMS) that can measure both static and dynamic signals. The output of accelerometers originates from m/s² or proportions of the Earth's surface gravitational constant (G) but is quite frequently expressed in counts, which are generated by devices internally or by software processing.

▸ **Basic needs of motion sensors for measuring sedentary behavior:** In addition to the common requirements of physical activity monitors, the ideal motion sensor will be able to differentiate wakefulness from sleeping states and sitting or reclining from standing postures and ambulation and to quantify the intensity of physical activity levels.

▸ **Different types of motion sensors:** Active sensors (e.g., radar sensors) are useful in confined spaces (laboratories); passive sensors are suited for free-living applications. Pedometers are not well suited for measuring nonambulatory movements. Tilt sensors do not measure intensity of activity. Among new technologies, GPS, barometer, gyroscopes, and wearable cameras all have unique features that need to be optimized for assessing sedentary behavior. Accelerometers have been used broadly for estimating physical activity intensities (activity energy expenditure) for the last two+ decades. Now with enhanced abilities to estimate body segment angles (postures), they have been developed and used for quantifying sedentary behavior.

▸ **Nonwear and sleep detections:** Accelerometer counts for nonwear and sleep may be very similar to sedentary behavior if using simple threshold methods. Improving this area could include using more sophisticated algorithms from raw multiaxial data and incorporating temperature or conductance sensors to detect if the device is being worn next to the body. Sleep detection using wrist-worn accelerometers has been established.

▸ **Predicting activity intensity levels using counts and counts thresholds:** Activity energy expenditure can be modeled from accelerometry signals by regression approaches. However, sedentary behavior types vary greatly. Measuring energy expenditure using criterion measure at or below 1.5 METs is challenging. Typical studies for energy expenditure model development and calibration are not focused on sedentary behavior. All of these factors cause errors in current accelerometer methods for estimating sedentary behavior. A threshold of 100 cpm (using hip-worn ActiGraph accelerometers) is frequently used to distinguish sedentary behavior from light-intensity activity. Wrist-worn accelerometers can improve subject compliance (increase wear time) and estimate sleep, but predicting activity intensity using counts alone seems to be challenging.

▸ **Raw-data accelerometry:** Compared to counts, raw-data accelerometry offers great potential for enabling use of different features (time domain, frequency domain, and heuristic) to detect sleep, differentiate among postures (sitting vs. standing), and quantify intensity (EE ≤ 1.5 METs) simultaneously from the raw accelerometer signals.

STUDY QUESTIONS

1. What characteristics define sedentary behavior?

2. What are the principles of motion sensors?

3. How can we use motion sensors to measure physical activity intensity?

4. How can a capacitance-based accelerometer detect sensor positions (i.e., body segmental angles)?

5. How can we optimize different motion sensors, alone or in combinations, to measure sedentary behavior, considering its three-pronged definition?

6. What can cause errors when estimating energy expenditure using accelerometry counts in low-intensity activities, including sedentary behavior?

7. What alternative approaches have been (can be) used to improve the quantification of sedentary behavior from raw-data accelerometers?

8. In the future, what types of motion sensors should be considered to improve the measurement of sedentary behavior, alone or in combination?

K.Y.C. is supported by the National Institute of Diabetes and Digestive and Kidney Diseases Intramural Research Program (Z01 DK071013 and Z01 DK071014).

CHAPTER 15

ASSESSING SEDENTARY BEHAVIOR USING PHYSIOLOGICAL SENSORS

David R. Bassett, PhD; and Dinesh John, PhD

The reader will gain an overview of the inner workings of various devices used to assess sedentary behavior that contain physiological sensors. By the end of this chapter, the reader should be able to do the following:

▸ Describe the importance of combining physiological sensors with motion sensors to accurately measure sedentary behavior

▸ List three reasons why it is important to accurately measure sedentary behavior in research studies

▸ Describe the various types of physiological responses that can be used to improve measurement of sedentary behavior

▸ Describe the key components of physiological sensors

▸ Describe the measurement principles of physiological sensors

▸ Provide practical guidelines on how to assess sedentary behavior with physiological sensors

---

Two components exist for measuring sedentary behavior:

1. Posture (i.e., sitting or reclining)
2. Energy expenditure of 1.0 to 1.5 METs

One MET, or metabolic equivalent, is equivalent to the average resting oxygen uptake of a healthy normal-weight adult, i.e., 3.5 ml·kg^{-1}·min^{-1} (Ainsworth et al. 2011). The previous chapter describes how motion sensors are used to directly measure body postures (e.g., lying, sitting, standing). However, these technologies do not provide the most accurate method of addressing the second component of this definition (i.e., energy expenditure).

If a researcher is using a single motion sensor (e.g., ActiGraph or Actical), sedentary behavior can be misclassified. For instance, if a person performs limb movements while sitting in a kayak, on an assembly line, or on a recumbent bicycle, energy expenditure may exceed 1.5 METs. A waist-worn device would classify these activities as sedentary when in fact they are not. Multisensor systems that combine physiological and motion sensors, or multiple motion sensors on different limbs, can minimize this problem.

Another limitation of single motion sensors is that they tend to group sitting and lying down together. Studies measuring sedentary behavior over a 24-hour period need to distinguish between these two body postures. Importantly, sedentary behavior is distinct from sleep (which is almost always performed lying down). Sleep has restorative powers on mental and physical function and adequate sleep is important for maintaining a healthy body weight (Owen et al. 2012). Use of physiological sensors in combination with motion sensors, or multiple motion sensors, can overcome this problem.

Why are more accurate measurements of sedentary desirable? Currently, sedentary behavior research is in its infancy. Most of the early evidence regarding the health hazards of prolonged sedentary behavior comes from epidemiological cohort studies of people with active or sedentary occupations (Morris et al. 1953a, 1953b; Paffenbarger et al. 1970). Subsequent studies of more diverse adult populations have confirmed that prolonged sedentary behavior is associated with an increased risk of death from all causes and cardiovascular disease (Dunstan et al. 2010; Katzmarzyk et al. 2000; Owen et al. 2010; Warren et al. 2010) and with reduced life expectancy (Katzmarzyk and Lee 2012). These studies have shown that people who accumulate more time in sitting and those who fail to break up prolonged sitting with bouts of physical activity exhibit unfavorable cardiometabolic profiles and are at increased risk of death from all causes, cardiovascular disease, and cancer (Katzmarzyk et al. 2000). Some short-term investigations have been done on the physiological effects of sedentary behavior in humans, a field that is becoming known as inactivity physiology (Bey and Hamilton 2003; Hamilton, Hamilton, and Zderic 2007; Howard et al. 2013; Stephens et al. 2011; Zderic and Hamilton 2006). A few pilot longitudinal intervention studies have also been done to reduce sedentary behavior (John, Thompson, et al. 2011; Steeves et al. 2012; Tucker et al. 2011), and larger randomized clinical trials are currently ongoing (Salmon et al. 2011). However, improved measures of sedentary behavior are needed to clarify the relationships of sedentary behavior and health outcomes and measure the efficacy of sedentary behavior interventions.

Physiological sensors are wearable devices used to assess and visualize physiological function in research and clinical practice. These devices detect responses to stressors that perturb the system, such as physical activity, diet, psychological stress, and environmental exposures to pathogens. Some examples of physiological variables that can be used to improve sedentary behavior assessment are body temperature, heart rate, oxygen saturation, respiration, heat flux, galvanic skin responses, and surface electromyography (EMG).

Motion sensors detect only posture, and physiological sensors can be used to document the level of energy expenditure. Combining these two will allow the distinction between true sedentary behavior (sitting or reclining with EE = 1.0–1.5 METs) and bouts where person is sitting but engaging in upper-body physical activity that elevates energy expenditure above 1.5 METs. In addition, these physiological measurements can provide unique insights into mechanisms underlying the health risks of prolonged sedentary behavior.

Key Components of Physiological Sensors

The key components (see figure 15.1) of devices used to sense physiological responses to particular behaviors are as follows:

▶ Power source
▶ Physiological sensor

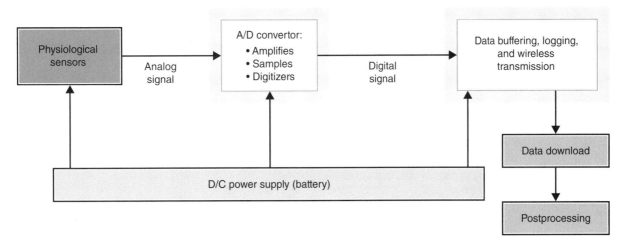

Figure 15.1 The key components of devices used to sense physiological variables during particular human behaviors.

▶ Data logger or wireless transmitter

▶ Post-processing software to make the data usable

When considering the power source, battery life and size are two major factors that can limit the wearability and recording of data over prolonged durations. However, recent advances in battery technology (e.g., lithium ion) enhance miniaturization of the device, rapid recharging, and prolonged data collection.

Physiological sensors are the miniature electronics that form the core of the sensing device. Typically, the sensor is sensitive to an external physical property that is converted to an electrical signal. The electrical signal is then processed (using an internal or external computer) and displayed in a format that is usable, and represents the changes in physiological variable of interest in the body.

Up until recently, limited onboard memory did not allow researchers to collect data over prolonged durations. This limitation has been overcome through current microcontroller and solid-state memory data-logger technology, which allow the procurement and recording of data for periods ranging between 1 week and 1 year. However, keep in mind that storage capacity also depends on the preset sampling rate or epoch in which one chooses to collect data. In addition, low-cost, low-power-consumption wireless transmission platforms are available (BlueTooth v.4.0, ZigBee, and ANT+ protocols). These allow users to wirelessly download data from the data logger to a handheld or stationary computer when they are in close proximity.

Once data have been downloaded, post-processing is done with computer software. This essentially converts the electrical signal into a physiological measurement that has meaning and can be interpreted by researchers. For example, the electrical signal that corresponds to voltage changes made through the use of skin (surface) electrodes (as shown on an electrocardiograph machine) can be converted to heart rate. Heart rate is an example of a physiological variable that has meaning to researchers. Measurements of heart rate can then be used to estimate other variables such as energy expenditure.

Measurement Principles of Physiological Sensors

Physiological sensors have been designed that measure a number of different variables, including oxygen uptake, heart rate, heat flux between the skin and environment, sweating, electrical activity of skeletal muscles, and respiration (breathing). All of these physiological variables tend to increase as the rate of energy expenditure increases.

Oxygen Uptake

Oxygen uptake represents a gold standard for measurement of energy expenditure. Indirect calorimetry refers to the indirect measurement of body heat production through measurements of respiratory gas exchange. If the rates of O_2 uptake and CO_2 production are known, the rate of caloric expenditure (or kJ/min) can be precisely computed. However, from an exercise physiologist's perspective, energy expenditure is often quantified simply by expressing oxygen uptake ($\dot{V}O_2$) adjusted for body mass in units of ml·kg^{-1}·min^{-1}.

In lab research, there may be some instances where a very accurate measure of oxygen consumption is desirable for establishing whether a person falls within the 1.0 to 1.5 METs range. Under these circumstances, a researcher could quantify the energy cost of an activity by either portable indirect calorimetry or room calorimetry. Both of these methods make use of open-circuit spirometry and the respiratory Fick principle, which holds that the rate of oxygen consumption is equal to the ventilation rate multiplied by the difference in partial pressures of gases upstream and downstream of the individual.

With a portable calorimeter, a face mask is placed over the subject's nose and mouth, and ventilation is assessed using turbines that spin on jeweled bearings. An infrared beam detects the number of revolutions of the turbine and uses this to assess the minute ventilation rate (V_E in L/min). A gas-sampling port next to the turbine samples the inspired and expired gas fractions, and the rate at which oxygen is consumed by the body is determined on breath-by-breath basis. An advantage of this technique is that the subject does not need to be confined to a room or tethered to a metabolic cart and can perform a wide range of activities inside and outside of the laboratory.

With a room calorimeter, outside air is pulled through a specially constructed chamber, and the subject is free to move about within the tightly enclosed space. The rate of airflow is measured, as well as the gas fractions of air on the upstream and downstream sides. The gas analyzers must be highly accurate, since the extraction of O_2 and CO_2 is extremely small due to the high rates of airflow. Corrections for air temperature must also be made, since these affect the measurements.

$\dot{V}O_2$ measurements are used to quantify the energy costs of lying, sitting, standing, and walking. For instance, the 2011 Compendium of Physical Activities (Ainsworth et al. 2011) gives the energy cost of these activities and corresponding studies on which the values are based. Table 15.1 shows a sample of physical activities from the compendium, with each activity represented by a different 5-digit code. The authors of the compendium found 11 studies that quantified the energy cost of lying quietly and 27 studies that quantified the energy cost of sitting quietly. The values shown in the METs column

Table 15.1 Energy Cost (METs) of Common Activities, Based on a Number of Studies

Activity	Activity code	Number of studies	METs
Sleeping	07030	2	0.95
Lying quietly	07010	11	1.0
Sitting quietly, general	07021	27	1.3
Reclining, reading	07070	1	1.3
Standing quietly (standing in a line)	07040	21	1.3
Standing, fidgeting	07041	1	1.6
Walking, 3.2 kmph (2.0 mph), level ground, firm surface	17152	7	2.8
Walking, 4 kmph (2.5 mph), level ground, firm surface	17170	9	3.0
Walking, 2.9-5.1 kmph (1.8-3.2 mph), level ground, firm surface	17190	17	3.5

Data from Compendium of Physical Activities. Available: https://sites.google.com/site/compendiumofphysicalactivities.

represent the average of those original investigations. Interestingly, the oxygen costs of sitting and standing are the same (1.3 METs). Hence, from an energy expenditure standpoint, these two activities are identical, and only with the initiation of walking is there an increase in metabolic rate.

Heart Rate

Heart rate (HR) is a physiological variable that correlates with oxygen uptake over a wide range of exercise intensities. Heart rate can be detected through the use of skin electrodes placed on the torso that measure the potential difference between positive and negative electrodes in response to depolarization of the heart muscle. The number of R waves generated within a given time period can be used to determine heart rate. Heart rate information can be either stored in a data logger or transmitted to a wristwatch-style receiver, where it is stored until later downloaded.

Heart rate is not the most sensitive method for detecting changes in body posture and small changes in energy expenditure. The signal–noise ratio is less than with other methods, and heart rate has a tendency to increase with excitement or anxiety. Hence, heart rate may not be the method of choice for documenting when someone is in the range of 1.0 to 1.5 METs. That said, the flex HR method relies on measurement of HR during the supine, seated, and standing conditions and during light activity (Janz 2002). The heart rate versus oxygen uptake response is graphed, and the inflection point (often 70-90 beats/min) is used to denote the heart rate value above which the linear relationship between HR and oxygen uptake is used to estimate energy expenditure. Below flex HR, the subject is credited with an energy expenditure of 1 MET.

Nevertheless, heart rate has been used in determining how much time is spent in sedentary behavior. Helmerhorst and colleagues (2009) used a heart rate monitor to determine the amount of time spent in sedentary behavior in 376 adults. The ratio between time spent below an individually determined threshold (designated as flex HR) and the total wear time was used to measure sedentary time. In this study, they found that the amount of sedentary time was significantly related to the fasting plasma insulin independent of the amount of MVPA performed.

Various studies have also examined the use of a simultaneous heart rate–motion sensor method for estimating energy expenditure (Haskell et al. 1993; Strath et al. 2002; Strath, Bassett, and Thompson 2001). For instance, Strath and colleagues (2002) had 10 adults perform physical tasks in a field setting, while heart rate, oxygen uptake, and acceleration data were collected on a near-continuous basis for 6 hours. Arm and leg accelerometers were used to detect upper- and lower-body movements, and oxygen uptake was predicted from individual heart rate–oxygen uptake calibration curves. The authors compared predicted METs with measured METs obtained using a portable metabolic measurement system as the criterion. The simultaneous motion sensor–heart rate method closely tracked the gold standard, which was energy expenditure as measured by indirect calorimetry.

Heat Flux and Galvanic Skin Response

Devices that use a combination of physiological and motion sensors are now commercially available. For instance, the SenseWear armband (BodyMedia, Pittsburg, PA) is a device that has an accelerometer and physiological sensors that measure near-body temperature and ambient temperature, heat flux,

and galvanic skin response. These variables serve as input for manufacturer-specific equations for estimating energy expenditure. This device is worn on the bare arm over the triceps and is secured with an elastic armband with Velcro closure.

The validity of the SenseWear armband has been tested in numerous studies, and the device and accompanying software have been modified over time to improve energy expenditure estimation. New versions of the device use machine-learning algorithms to convert the signals from these sensors into energy expenditure. Although early versions of the armband examined mainly walking, running, and cycling (Fruin and Rankin 2004; Jakicic et al. 2004), more recent studies have examined the ability of the armband to accurately measure EE over a wide range of activities (Colbert et al. 2011; Drenowatz and Eisenmann 2011; Dudley et al. 2012; King et al. 2004; Wadsworth et al. 2005; Welk et al. 2007).

Dudley and colleagues (2012) examined the SenseWear Pro 3 against indirect calorimetry in 19 activities. The device was quite accurate for identifying the energy cost of four sedentary activities (seated rest, driving a golf cart, seated television viewing, and reading a book while sitting) (figure 15.2). Output variables included minutes of physical activity, time spent in sleep, sedentary behavior (<3.0 METs), moderate activity (3.1-6.0 METs), vigorous activity (6.1-9.0 METs), very vigorous activity (>9.0 METs), and total daily energy expenditure (kcal). Obviously, the BodyMedia company's definition of sedentary behavior is not the same as that used in this chapter, but researchers can determine when an individual is in a range of 1.0 to 1.5 METs by using the energy expenditure data.

Surface Electromyography

Surface electromyography (SEMG) is a technique used to measure the electrical activity of skeletal muscle. SEMG devices consist of two or three electrodes (positive, negative, and ground) that are adhered to the surface of the skin above the muscle of interest. The electrodes detect the electric activity of muscle cells at rest (–90 MV) and during depolarization (action potential +30 MV) and transmit an electric signal proportional to the detected electrical activity. This signal is then amplified and stored onboard for later analyses.

SEMG technology has undergone rapid advancements. Traditionally, SEMG measurements involved wired electrodes connected to a desktop data-logging

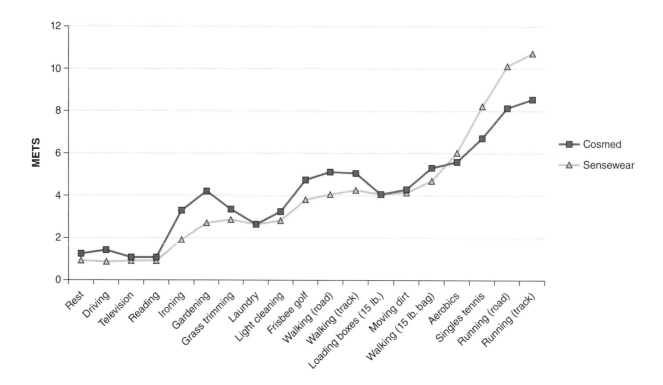

Figure 15.2 Validity of the Sensewear Pro 3 armband for estimating energy expenditure in adults (*N* = 68). The armband was reasonably accurate at detecting sedentary behaviors. In this study, indirect calorimetry (Cosmed K4b^2, a portable metabolic system) served as the criterion.

and processing unit. New developments have miniaturized the electronics required for logging and transmitting SEMG data. SEMG manufacturers now provide the small recording units that can be worn on the surface of the skin for prolonged periods of time while simultaneously recording EMG activity of the muscle.

Theoretically, combining SEMG data with motion data could provide supplementary information to reduce misclassification of sedentary behavior. A relevant example is misclassification of standing as sedentary behavior when using hip-worn activity monitors like the ActiGraph. Most standing activities are classified as sedentary when using the ActiGraph sedentary behavior cut point of <100 counts per minute because there is no vertical movement of the hip while standing. However, static muscular contractions of muscles in the back and legs are increased greatly to support standing posture compared to the seated position (Nag et al. 1986; Soames and Atha 1981). SEMG monitors can be used to detect the electrical activity of postural muscles (Suzuki et al. 2010;

Watanabe et al. 2006). Combining SEMG output with ActiGraph output will help to correctly distinguish those standing bouts that may have been incorrectly classified as sedentary behavior when using the ActiGraph alone. Researchers can also use the EMG data to refine existing advanced pattern recognition techniques that estimate sedentary behavior from a single motion sensor. Time-stamped SEMG output can be synchronized with motion sensor data to identify those periods that were misclassified as sedentary behavior by the motion sensor output. Misclassified acceleration outputs could be used to train the pattern recognition technique to correctly identify sedentary behavior.

Some drawbacks of SEMG are as follows:

1. High cost (The technology is still developing and is relatively expensive.)

2. Inappropriate for long-term investigations (High sampling rates of three channels of data limit battery life to about 1 day.)

MULTIPLE MOTION SENSORS

In addition to using physiological sensors, using two or more motion sensors can improve the classification accuracy of sedentary behavior. The activPAL is an accelerometer-based monitor that is typically worn on the thigh and classifies daily human behavior into sitting or lying, standing, or ambulation. The monitor detects orientation of the thigh and discriminates between sitting or lying and upright posture, and it has been validated for measurement of sedentary behaviors (Kozey-Keadle et al. 2011).

Four distinct behaviors (lying down, sitting, standing, and ambulation) can be correctly classified by using the activPAL. Until recently, this could be achieved using two devices, one on the thigh and one on the chest or torso. In one study (Bassett et al. 2013), participants wore one device on the

right thigh and another on the torso. Both monitors were synchronized and initialized to record data in 15-second epochs. Participants performed a choreographed routine of activities for 3 minutes each. If both activPAL monitors recorded "sitting or lying," the body position was classified as lying down. If the activPAL on the chest recorded "standing" and the one on the thigh recorded "sitting or lying," the body position was classified as sitting.

The use of a triaxial sensor in more recent iterations of the ActivPal allowed a method to be developed that distinguishes lying from sitting using a single thigh-worn sensor (Lyden et al 2016). This method computes changes in the angle of the y-axis (perpendicular to the long axis of the femur) of the sensor when people roll from side to side when lying, and it classifies those events as lying.

---

3. High user burden (Depending on the muscle being examined, one or more SEMG monitors may be required to obtain valid measures of muscular activity.)

Respiration

Respiration can be measured using strain gauges to measure chest wall expansion. For example, an integrated measurement system (IMS) was developed as part of the National Institutes of Health Genes, Environment, and Health Initiative (John, Liu, et al. 2011). This device contains a triaxial capacitive MEMS accelerometer, a respiration sensor, and an ultraviolet selective thin-film light sensor. The output from these sensors was analyzed using a pattern recognition method in order to predict physical activity and sedentary behaviors. The accuracy of the IMS device was high for sedentary activity (89% correctly identified), household activities (94%), walking at a moderate pace (83%), and vigorous activities (87%). The overall accuracy for predicting activity type and intensity improved after including the respiratory sensor.

Practical Guidelines

When choosing a technique for measuring sedentary behaviors, researchers must be cognizant of the strengths and limitations of the device. For large-scale population studies that examine relationships

between sedentary behavior and health, single motion sensors like the activPAL and ActiGraph are sufficient. Multiple motion sensors (i.e., the two-activPAL method described previously) can provide a more accurate measure of sedentary behavior and should be used as a criterion variable to validate other measures of sitting. For example, a questionnaire that aims to determine the amount of time spent sitting during the course of a 24-hour period must be validated against a gold standard. The most accurate method for determining sedentary behavior is to directly observe posture and measure energy expenditure using indirect calorimetry. These combined measures should be used in short-term lab-based studies of the physiological responses to sedentary behaviors.

Summary

Sedentary behavior is defined by both body posture (i.e., sitting or reclining) and a low rate of energy expenditure (1.0-1.5 METs). Physiological sensors are wearable devices used to assess and visualize physiological function. They can be used in conjunction with motion sensors to improve the accuracy of measuring sedentary behaviors. Physiological signals of interest include oxygen uptake, heart rate, heat flux and galvanic skin response, surface EMG, and respiration. In addition, use of multiple motion sensors placed on different locations of the body can provide more detailed information on body posture and the rate of energy expenditure. The field of sedentary behavior measurement is evolving, and future technological advancements will yield improvements in our knowledge of the health effects of sedentary behaviors.

Future research should strive to improve the accuracy, reliability, and wearability of wearable monitors. Transdisciplinary collaborations among physiologists, engineers, computer programmers,

and behavioral scientists are needed to move the field forward. The ideal location of sensors on the body should be determined, as well as the types of sensors utilized. In addition to motion sensors and physiological sensors, another area that holds promise is the use of flexible pressure-sensing pads. More sophisticated methods of data processing are needed, including pattern recognition. Nanotechnologies, manufacturing advances, and cost reduction will make the wearable sensors of the future more practical and affordable.

KEY CONCEPTS

- **Compendium of Physical Activities**: A valuable resource for obtaining rough estimates of the energy cost of various physical activities.
- **Physiological monitoring devices**: Examples include portable calorimeters, heart rate monitors, surface EMG devices, heat flux monitors, and respiration monitors.
- **Physiological sensors**: Particularly useful in obtaining closer estimates of oxygen uptake and energy expenditure and more accurate than those available from wearable movement sensors.
- **Sedentary behavior:** The Sedentary Behaviour Research Network (2012) defines this as any behavior during waking hours that is characterized by energy expenditure less than or equal to 1.5 METs while in a sitting or reclining posture. One MET, or metabolic equivalent, is equivalent to the average resting oxygen uptake of a healthy normal-weight adult, i.e., 3.5 $ml \cdot kg^{-1} \cdot min^{-1}$.
- **Wearable devices that measure physiological variables** include the following key elements: power source, physiological sensor, data logger or wireless transmitter, and post-processing software.

STUDY QUESTIONS

1. In considering the definition of sedentary behavior provided by the Sedentary Behavior Research Network (2012), why might it be important to use physiological sensors to assess sedentary behavior?
2. A healthy adult who is exercising at an oxygen uptake of 14.0 $ml \cdot kg^{-1} \cdot min^{-1}$ is said to be exercising at how many METs?
3. Identify the MET level that is considered to be the threshold (or low end of the range) for light-intensity physical activity.
4. Identify the range of MET levels for moderate-intensity physical activity.
5. List the key elements that make up a wearable device that measures physiological variables.
6. List some physiological variables that can be readily measured using wearable devices.
7. What is meant by the technique known as indirect calorimetry, and how is it measured?
8. What special types of physiological sensors does the SenseWear armband use that most other wearable devices do not?
9. What type of physiological sensor can detect the recruitment of skeletal muscle fibers during physical activity?
10. How does the use of two activPAL devices (one on the thigh and one on the torso) help to discriminate between sitting and lying postures?

CHAPTER 16

ASSESSING SEDENTARY BEHAVIOR USING NEW TECHNOLOGY

Dinesh John, PhD; and Stephen Intille, PhD

The reader will learn about existing techniques for measuring sedentary behavior. By the end of this chapter, the reader should be able to do the following:

▶ Describe key measurement areas that provide an improved understanding of sedentary behavior and its determinants

▶ Describe various emerging technologies to measure sedentary behavior and its determinants

▶ Understand how new technologies will help to meet expectations of study participants and researchers to maximize the quantity and quality of usable data

---

The prevailing modern environment signifi-cantly promotes sedentary behavior, which has detrimental effects on cardiometabolic indicators of health (Healy et al. 2007; Healy, Dunstan, Salmon, Cerin, et al. 2008; Healy, Dunstan, Salmon, Shaw, et al. 2008; Katzmarzyk et al. 2009). Sedentary behavior is a complex construct influenced by one or multiple determinants, and it typically translates to a measurable behavior: sitting (Owen et al. 2011). Social and physical environmental determinants interact with and influence sedentary behavior. For instance, Kirchengast (1998) demonstrated that switching from a rural lifestyle involving active commuting and occupation to a more sedentary urban lifestyle with passive commuting in automobiles and seated desk jobs promotes weight gain—a known risk factor for diabetes and other negative health outcomes (Abasolo et al. 2011; Bankoski et al. 2011; Brownson, Boehmer, and Luke 2005; Dunstan et al. 2010; Healy et al. 2007). Modernization has greatly contributed to increasing sedentary behavior and associated health risks.

Novel interventions targeting social and physical environments may counteract the strong environmental cues that promote sedentary behavior in modern society. An example of an integrated socio-physical environmental intervention is establishment of a workplace culture promoting standing meetings (Marsiglia 2009). Moreover, technology, which contributes to increasing sedentary behavior, may itself be used to create new interventions to reduce sedentary time. For instance, modifying the physical workplace environment using innovative treadmill and sit-to-stand workstations decreases sedentary behavior while allowing users to simultaneously perform work (Healy et al. 2013; John, Thompson, et al. 2011). New video games using motion sensors transform sedentary video game playing into a more active experience (Peng, Lin, and Sun 2011). Applications of such technologies in interventions may be required to counteract other environmental and societal cues that promote sedentary behavior.

Current motion-sensing technology has greatly improved the measurement of sedentary behavior. A new generation of measurement tools based on emerging technologies is likely to provide researchers with enhanced capability to measure both sedentary behavior and its determinants, and thus allow a much richer understanding of the purported independent relationship between sedentary behavior and health. These new tools will also support innovative research methodologies and novel computer-assisted interventions that may help measure and curtail the harmful effects of sedentary behavior on health.

Existing Technology for Measuring Sedentary Behavior

Prior to the early 2000s, sedentary behavior (sitting) was not a key variable measured in health behavior and physical activity research. Few subjective assessment techniques collected information on sitting behavior (Kriska and Caspersen 1997). However, reports of objectively measured sitting time can be traced back to as early as 1967 in a study by Bloom and Eidex. These scientists developed a wearable monitor with a normal wind-up watch worn above the knee with a gravity-sensing switch that stopped the watch when the person was sitting and worked only when the person was upright. Upright time was subtracted from total wear time to derive sitting time. This device was used to measure postural allocation in obese and lean people for up to 35 days (Bloom and Eidex 1967). Technology has since advanced, and chapters 14 and 15 describe miniaturized wearable sensors used to measure two key components of the sedentary behavior definition: posture and energy expenditure.

Emerging evidence on the negative effects of sedentary behavior on health also prompted large surveillance studies such as the United States National Health and Nutrition Examination Survey (2003-2006) (Matthews et al. 2008) and the UK Biobank study to estimate sedentary behavior using electronic hip-worn accelerometers. Both of these studies are now using advanced wrist-worn sensors that save detailed data about limb motion to estimate population-level physical activity and sedentary behavior (Troiano and McClain 2012). Advanced modeling techniques may be used to distinguish among activity type and postures (e.g., sitting versus standing), but additional research is required to improve estimates of sedentary behavior from wrist- and hip-worn sensors (Mannini et al. 2013).

While few subjective techniques measure sedentary behavior (Barwais et al. 2013; Matthews et al. 2013), most sedentary behavior studies use a single sensor to quantify postural allocation. The activPAL (PAL Technologies, Glasgow, Scotland) monitor is a commonly used device in sedentary behavior research, and measures time spent sedentary (sitting or lying down), standing, and stepping, breaks from being sedentary, total number of steps, and total MET-hours. The device provides highly valid (Lyden et al. 2012; Kozey-Keadle et al. 2011) yet simple and interpretable output to the user. The validity of the activPAL in providing accurate estimates of sedentary behavior (sitting) is attributable to the location of recommended wear, the midline of the thigh. The activPAL uses a triaxial capacitive acceleration sensor to detect changes in static and dynamic acceleration. However, the device is fundamentally similar to that invented by Bloom and Eidex (1967)—both devices determine thigh orientation to distinguish among postures. This location is powerful for distinguishing typical sitting from standing and other physical activities. However, defining sitting as a horizontal position of the thigh does not eliminate the possibility that a person is lying down, sitting upright in a recliner chair, or excessively sleeping.

Sedentary Behavior Measurement Goals

Most objective methods for measuring sedentary behavior are used for one week and rarely for longer durations. These techniques usually estimate postural allocation and energy expenditure. Sedentary behavior determinants like location, context, and the type of behavior are seldom detected. New technologies will also permit longitudinal tracking of behavior change. This allows flexibility of measurement duration that will change depending on the type of positive behavior used to replace sedentary behavior, health outcomes of interest, and the rate at which the positive behavior improves these outcomes. For example, behavior change tracking for a longer duration may be required when targeting simple postural changes like replacing sitting with standing because such interventions may take a longer time to affect cardiometabolic variables as compared to interventions aimed at replacing sitting time with low-intensity activity. Long-term tracking will also facilitate timely interventions in case of relapse and permit measurement of the sustainability of behavior change using technology-driven interventions beyond the *novelty* period of the devices. Thus, there is a need for tools that can be practically deployed for longer periods than the current standard of 3 to 7 days of measurement. Additionally, the use of adhesive-based techniques to adhere thigh sensors to the skin may aggravate the skin, which typically limits long-term measure-

ment. New technologies may be useful in developing more comfortable systems that do not require thigh placement and allow continuous, longitudinal tracking of both sedentary and overall human behavior. Emerging technologies may also be used to extend the capabilities of existing measurement devices. This may improve the capability of researchers to accurately quantify and distinguish healthy behaviors like regular physical activity and sufficient sleep from harmful behaviors like prolonged sitting.

Measuring various determinants of behavior and their characteristics may be necessary for differentiating between modifiable and unmodifiable sedentary behaviors. For instance, a CEO of an organization may be able to stand and break sedentary behavior using a sit-to-stand table in his office. However, it may not be feasible to stand during a board meeting. Such contextual information may be useful, or even necessary to design and implement influential and sustainable interventions. Thus, measurement tools that detect when, where, and why a person sits may inform the development of multifaceted interventions effective in modifying sedentary behavior and sustaining the behavior change (Stratton et al. 2012; van Dantzig, Geleijnse, and van Halteren 2011).

Emerging sensor technology may also reduce some of the logistical and statistical challenges of analyzing data. Larger-scale studies may be able to exploit consumer technologies that study participants may already own, such as mobile phones, thereby reducing the need to purchase expensive hardware. These consumer technologies may be able to not only measure behavior, but also deliver real-time interventions responsive to ongoing behavior. Furthermore, combining more than one type of miniaturized wireless sensor with a data processing and storage platform (i.e., phones) that can be conveniently carried by the user may facilitate the capture of most aspects of sedentary behavior.

Figure 16.1 highlights influential determinants and their characteristics. Measurement and detection of all or some of these determinants may provide researchers with a richer model of sedentary behavior and lead to improved sedentary behavior interventions. Thus, an ideal objective monitor for sedentary behavior research must be able to *detect* and *measure* more than what is obtained from currently used monitors, including the following:

▶ Whether the person is sitting or lying down
▶ Whether the person is awake or asleep

▸ Whether energy expenditure is less than 1.5 METs

▸ Sedentary and physical activity type

▸ Transitions between sedentary and physical activity behavior

▸ Contextual characteristics when the behavior occurs

▸ Nonwear of the measurement technology

In addition, the monitor should have the following features:

▸ Practical to use for prolonged durations with minimal subject and researcher burden

▸ Capable of providing real-time data to researchers and real-time and retrospective feedback to end users

▸ Affordable

This wish list for sedentary behavior monitoring also includes information about physical activity and sleep behavior because these may significantly influence sedentary behavior.

Based on the complexities of behavior and its determinants illustrated in figure 16.1, we have identified five key measurement goals. Although these are being addressed in varying degrees by existing monitoring solutions, some areas need to be addressed by new technologies.

Goal 1: Reliably Distinguish Between Sleep and Wake States

Sleep is an integral part of the working sedentary behavior definition and in proper amounts, sleep is beneficial to health (Chaput, Klingenberg, and Sjodin 2010). Information on sleep is commonly measured using wrist actigraphy. This technique uses an acceleration sensor at the wrist to detect motion or the lack thereof when a person is asleep. Researchers have developed algorithms to infer whether short movements are true waking periods or if they are due to change in lying posture while asleep (Ancoli-Israel et al. 2003; Pollak et al. 2001). Actigraphy is limited in providing comprehensive information on sleep quality, which may be important to understand the relationship between sleep and sedentary behavior patterns throughout the day. Newer methods involve instrumenting the bed with sensors that detect changes in pressure, ambient light, and gross body movements using passive infrared imaging (Peng, Lin, and Crouse 2006).

Like actigraphy, these sensors detect a change in body position and rely on algorithms to distinguish between wake and sleep, but the algorithms may be prone to error during wake–sleep transitions and vice versa. The third technique for measuring sleep is to use physiological sensors such as portable EEG measurement (Huang et al. 2013) to obtain detailed information about sleep and wake and sleep stage and quality. However, existing systems are too cumbersome and impractical for long-term and free-living studies.

Most of these techniques may be most effective in detecting sleep duration, especially those episodes that are prolonged (e.g., sleeping at night). Although practical long-term measurement of sleep quality and stage remains a challenge, existing techniques could be augmented using additional environmental or phone-based sensors. When combined with wrist actigraphy, a simple audio sensor that automatically detects and analyzes change in ambient noise may greatly improve estimates of sleep duration and quality. Self-reported time in and out of bed may be improved using just-in-time phone-based momentary assessment. For example, the audio sensor in a participant's phone, when combined with its internal clock and acceleration sensor, can detect changing noise and motion between nighttime and morning and prompt timely questions when a person wakes up in the morning. These questions can be designed to confirm events such as inferred bedtime or gather additional contextual information such as the source of any notable audio disturbances and how it influenced sleep.

Goal 2: Identify Sitting or Lying When Energy Expenditure Is Greater or Less Than 1.5 METs

A caveat of using a single thigh sensor is that it will not accurately measure METs if someone is engaging in only upper-body motion (e.g., seated resistance training, specialized seated jobs requiring substantial upper-body movement). Thus, a more accurate estimation of both energy expenditure and sitting or lying behavior will likely require multiple sensors used simultaneously to capture upper-, whole-, and lower-body motion and thereby infer additional information that improves energy expenditure estimation (John, Liu, et al. 2011; Tapia et al. 2007). Multisensor monitoring may also improve the measurement of physical activity behavior (John, Liu, et

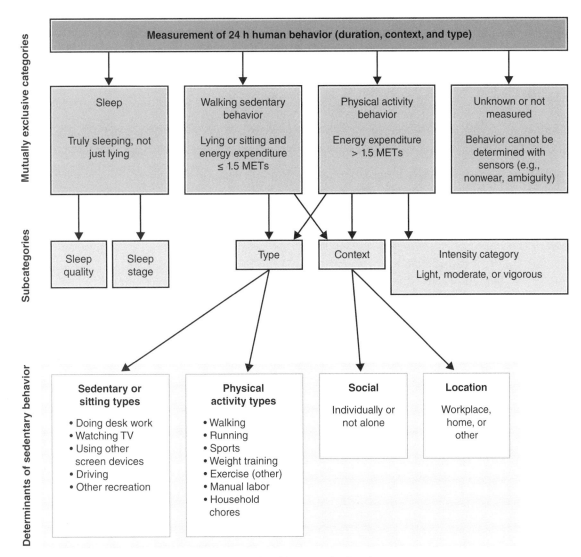

Figure 16.1 Measurement of various aspects of human behavior.

al. 2011). Chapter 15 provides a detailed discussion on sensors that may improve the measurement of energy expenditure.

Goal 3: Measure Physical Activity Behavior Above 1.5 METs

The quality of estimating METs and activity-type highly depends on sensor location. Although thigh-accelerometry is good for distinguishing between sitting or lying down from standing and estimating lower-body activity, it is a poor location for capturing any upper-body motion. A single acceleration sensor at the hip or the wrist is commonly used to measure physical activity. Information from a single sensor may be insufficient to obtain a complete pic-

ture of activity behavior. Using machine-learning techniques to model triaxial acceleration from the hip may improve free-living estimates of sedentary behavior and physical activity (Lyden et al. 2014). However, advances in the measurement of physical activity are likely to be improved to a greater extent through new systems that use multimodal sensor fusion. These systems will combine data from several types of sensors located on different parts of the body or embedded in the environment using pattern recognition algorithms to infer precise second-by-second details about physical activity type, amount, and location. Pattern recognition algorithms compute features that encode information about the raw data collected from one or more sensors. A simple example is the encoding of features that determine if a particular sensor is moving in a periodic or rhythmic way using frequency domain analysis, such as Fourier transforms. Typically, pattern recognition models are developed using data collected on a subset of people performing a set routine of physical activities while wearing a variety of sensors. The data are labeled, and then machine-learning algorithms look for clusters of features that allow one type of activity to be clearly differentiated from other types of activity. For example, an algorithm might learn that during bicycling, a motion sensor on the wrist is vibrating (is not still) and a motion sensor on the ankle moves in a periodic way within a certain range of frequencies common when someone is pedaling. The same algorithm may be incapable of reliably detecting bicycling from a single sensor at the hip because the minimal motion may appear similar to other activities where the hip moves or shifts slightly.

More field-based studies with large numbers of participants are required to develop and validate such complex algorithms using multisensor monitoring systems. Feasibility concerns about multisensor systems will diminish as sensors continue to be miniaturized and, as discussed later, new opportunities are created for real-time feedback using real-time activity detection systems. Work in activity recognition using multiple sensors tends to be consistent: more sensors usually improve recognition because capturing movements of different parts of the body yield enriched information on the unique properties of particular activities of interest (John, Liu, et al. 2011; Tapia et al. 2007).

Goal 4: Identify Social and Environmental Contexts That May Influence Sedentary Behavior

Accurate identification of behavior context will create new opportunities for the development of tailored interventions. Interventions tailored to a person's environment are more likely to be effective and sustainable. One way to gather information about the social and environmental characteristics influencing sedentary behavior is to detect location and then use databases that tag locations with relevant information. These databases may be tied either to the general geographical region (e.g., whether a particular longitude or latitude is a park or business district), or to the person (whether a location is a home, workplace, or some other frequently visited site). GPS devices detect

longitude and latitude, and they are typically effective outdoors. The advent of smartphones has enabled both indoor and outdoor position finding using wireless networks. Smartphones can also combine location data with available databases and facilitate instant onboard processing and interpretation of the data. Technologies such as active or passive radio-frequency identification (RFID) technology will further improve location detection systems, including the detection of location within buildings (Koch et al. 2007). With RFID systems, users typically wear small thin tags that are detected by small tag readers placed in the location of interest. These readers can be programmed to record the exact times a tag enters and leaves a preset radius.

Detecting social context and whether a behavior was performed alone or in the presence of others may be important when designing sedentary behavior interventions. Since smartphone use is becoming increasingly widespread, wireless proximity sensing using Bluetooth radios in phones can be used to determine if someone is alone or with other users (Eagle and Pentland 2004). However, since individual sensors typically capture information on only one characteristic of the context in which an activity is occurring, a challenge with contextual sensing is the combination of information from multiple sensors to provide accurate contextual information. For instance, a Bluetooth proximity sensor in a phone might detect other phones belonging to family members and estimate that the person is at home. However, it is possible that the person may not be at home and forgot to carry the phone with them. Combining acceleration data from the phone, which detects absolutely no movement, may be useful for determining that the phone is not with the owner and is sitting on a table at home. This may further be refined by the use of a miniature wearable wireless sensor that informs the phone that the person is not within a certain radius of the phone. Thus, context may be best detected using a combination of motion, location, and proximity sensing.

Goal 5: Detect Wear Time of Sensors

Existing technology can be redesigned to facilitate the detection of wear time. For instance, wearable activity monitors that include motion sensors can be optimized to detect very small movements, and this will help to distinguish whether a sensor is completely motionless while on the table or attached to someone's body during sleep. A complementary strategy is to use temperature, touch, or proximity sensors to detect if the sensor is in contact with the skin. Additionally, wear–nonwear algorithms developed using the primary sensor (e.g., acceleration) could be improved using data from other sensors. Another valuable solution for identifying wear–nonwear problems will be the use of just-in-time experience sampling. Such systems may use phones to communicate with participants and will be based on variability in sensor signals. When a particular signal pattern is detected, the phone will prompt a question asking the participant about whether the sensors are or were being worn as expected.

Improvements and Emerging Technology for Measuring Sedentary Behavior

Sedentary behavior researchers can expect to see improvements in the quality and types of sensors available to measure sedentary behavior. Rapidly evolving technology will incrementally enhance the achievement of measurement goals from the previous section through increased efficiency and accuracy of existing sensors and supplementation with new sensors that have not been explored in the context of sedentary behavior.

Accelerometers

Current devices use microelectromechanical systems (MEMS) sensors that typically detect acceleration up to ±6 or 8 G and store raw data. Advancing manufacturing and signal processing technology is resulting in improved noise reduction, decreased power consumption, and lower costs. Thus, it is increasingly viable to develop devices that are highly sensitive to small movements and allow the measurement of typical human motions (±6 G) and also high-impact forces (±12 G) without any signal distortion. These advances will improve sleep–wake detection without sacrificing overall MET or activity-type detection. Battery size is a major contributing factor to the weight and dimension of an activity monitor. Improved power management will also enable manufacturers to use smaller batteries and thereby decrease the size of the device. New technologies may also result in smaller self-powered devices that use motion or miniaturized solar cells to power devices. However, such small devices may have limited or no ability to transmit data wirelessly. In addition to these hardware improvements, a new direction for standardization of data from different accelerometers is to have complete transparency of all specifications on signal acquisition and filtering performed prior to data storage (Intille et al. 2012).

Researchers should expect current measurement methods that are stand-alone data logging devices (e.g., ActiGraph and activPAL monitors) to evolve into networks of devices with a central data receiving and processing hub (e.g., mobile phone). This strategy permits further miniaturization of the sensors by exploiting the massive computational and storage capacity of the mobile phone. The systems can also exploit the desire of end users to keep their devices with them and create further opportunities for multisensor data fusion to capture information on sedentary behavior and its various determinants.

Gyroscopes

Unlike accelerometers, these devices measure spatial orientation and can provide information on 3-D positioning based on a calibrated starting point. Gyroscopes may be useful for obtaining information on overall limb motion and the specific pattern of movement in 3-D space (Mayagoitia, Nene, and Veltink 2002). This may improve automatic detection of certain activity types that have specific patterns of limb movement in 3-D space that are undetectable when only using characteristics like movement frequency or intensity.

Audio Sensors

Audio sensors may prove valuable for detecting the context of behavior. For example, audio sensors can be used to detect if someone is in a social situation by detecting human voice and sounds (Smith, Ma, and Ryan 2006). Audio analysis can also be used to improve activity recognition, because some activities involve distinct sounds that can be identified by algorithms similar to those used to process accelerometer data. Audio sensors in conjunction with movement sensors can be used to detect events that may cause sleep disturbances and thus help to better infer sleep–wake states. Audio may also help to identify environmental context. For instance, audio sensors in mobile phones could also be used to detect whether a person is at work if the workplace has distinct sounds.

Point-of-View Camera Sensors

These devices will provide sedentary behavior researchers with a powerful measurement tool because point-of-view images can be used to validate other sensors and to characterize the type of behavior and its environment and social context. Researchers are now developing algorithms to automatically cluster point-of-view images and perform efficient semiautomatic classification of several days of data (Kerr et al. 2013). The Revue (Vicon Motion Systems Ltd., Oxford, England) (formerly the SenseCam) is a camera worn on a lanyard around the neck that is used to measure physical activity and sedentary behavior (Kerr et al. 2013). Head-mounted point-of-view cameras (with associated head-mounted displays) that connect to mobile phones, such as Google Glass (Google, Inc., Mountain View, CA), will permit real-time analysis of images and create new intervention opportunities. Even when these types of systems are not used as the primary sensor, the ability to review point-of-view image data from participants can resolve data ambiguity (Nam, Rho, and Lee 2013).

Other Modes of Location Sensing

Stand-alone GPS monitors may be limited in detecting indoor locations. Mobile phones that combine GPS with other location-finding strategies, such as detecting Wi-Fi and cell tower signals, can continuously determine approximate indoor and outdoor location with minimal effect on the phone's battery (Chon and Cha 2011). Algorithms that process this data can also infer mode of transportation, such as walking or riding in a car and even riding on public transportation versus riding in a car (Mun et al. 2008; Thiagarajan et al. 2010). Positioning systems are now being developed to identify indoor locations using a combination of audio sensing and radio frequency signal detection (Azizyan, Constandache, and Choudhury 2009; Kim et al. 2009). Some systems require calibration to specific environments, while other systems require inserting beacon technologies into an environment (Azizyan, Constandache, and Choudhury 2009; Kim et al. 2009).

Supplemental Environmental Sensors

Future sedentary measurement systems are likely to combine wearable and environmental sensors. Simple environmental sensors include object usage sensors that can be stuck on devices within a home or office. These are triggered when device use is commenced and completed then wirelessly transmit an ID to a computing platform like the phone (Tapia, Intille, and Larson 2007). Object usage sensors can be put on television sets and remote controls, tablet computers, beds, exercise equipment, and other devices related to sedentary behavior. These data can be combined with data from wearable sensors to better understand the environmental determinants of sedentary behavior. The same sensors can also be used to improve indoor location sensing. Other often-used environmental sensors are infrared motion detectors that are placed in environments to determine location of people or movement in areas of particular interest (Intille et al. 2005; Makonin and Popowich 2011).

New sensing opportunities are not limited to passive sensors. Ecological momentary assessment (EMA) uses a computing device that prompts a person to provide feedback about the present moment in time (or some recent moment in time) to gather data on physical activity, sedentary behavior, and their determinants (Shiffman, Stone, and Hufford 2008). EMA is particularly useful for gathering information regarding the context in which behavior occurs. EMA can be deployed easily and cost-effectively among people who already have mobile phone devices by simply downloading new software onto the phone. Based on sensor data, context-sensitive EMA (Intille 2007) can be used to time prompts with activity, resolve ambiguity with self-report, or gather additional contextual information that cannot be sensed directly. For example, context-sensitive EMA (CS-EMA) and context-sensitive ecological momentary interventions (CS-EMI) executed on a platform such as mobile phones can instantly analyze data from sensors and present tailored or timely just-in-time questions or feedback to the participant. For example, consider the difference between these two clarifying questions: "Were you sitting between 10:05 and 10:25 earlier today?" and "Are you sitting right now?" The second question is much easier to answer. Improper sensor positioning or nonwear of the system detected by the sensors can prompt immediate and possibly engaging feedback that helps the participant use the system as intended. In some cases, participants can be incentivized to properly wear or maintain (e.g., charge) the technology. CS-EMA may be the most efficient and least burdensome way to gather contextual information about sedentary behavior or the behavior itself. Further, it can be used selectively

DEVELOPING INDIVIDUAL MODELS OF SEDENTARY BEHAVIOR

No single sensor provides definitive answers about behavior in most circumstances, but a combination of multiple sensors, either the same or different types, can dramatically reduce uncertainty. Eventually, systems that combine passive sensing with active participation from the person wearing the sensor system may provide researchers with detailed information about behavior and its determinants throughout the course of their day. Algorithms that use statistical models to combine data from multiple sensors may be able to infer what someone is doing, what that person may do next, and even

possibly whether that person is receptive to information that might change what he or she may do next. These models will output soft decisions that include certainty, or likelihood, information. Ideally these models would not depend on a specific sensor type being available at any given time, but rather use whatever information is available to make the best decision possible at that time. These models are likely to resolve ambiguity by using data from multiple sensors gathered over long durations of time on the same person. Longer-term measurement will incrementally lead to higher fidelity models.

when the system detects passive data collection failure. Thus, CS-EMA can be used to fill in the gaps in missing sensor data. For instance, if the system detects a 2-hour nonwear of the system prior to commencement of data reception, a question could appear on the participant's mobile phone asking about what happened for those 2 hours.

Data Collection, Storage, and Open Source Processing

Emerging technologies for measurement will advance the field only by meeting the expectations of both study participants and researchers. Participants will adhere to long-term measurement technology only if it is easy to use and comfortable to wear. Participant compliance will also depend on how much the measurement system will change normal routines. Participants may not be receptive to measurement tools that are invasive due to bulky or wired sensing and data storage modules. Such systems will increase participant discomfort, affect normal behavior, and result in decreased wear time. Getting study participants to wear a single sensor can be difficult at times. Thus, compliance may be a challenge when using multisensor systems that do not provide continuous feedback. Multisensor fusion combined with mobile data processing enables instant feedback and has the potential to make wearing the sensor system a stimulating and engaging experience. On the other hand, researchers expect technology to yield simple modes to process complex data using advanced data processing platforms and have high usability and the ability to remotely monitor data and prompt behavior modification.

Usability

Application of innovative technologies holds promise to yield a richer model of the multifaceted sedentary behavior construct. Researchers will prefer that regardless of the underlying sensing and algorithmic complexity, the measurement tools are valid for free-living measurement of behavior. To facilitate long-term and iterative refinement of research findings without dependence on particular technologies or manufacturers, all algorithms and electronics used for multisensor fusion must be fully described and reproducible. Relying on black box proprietary devices that may be changed or superseded in the future will slow scientific progress. At the same time, highly capable systems that are difficult to understand and deploy, with output data that are hard to interpret, will in all likelihood not be used by the research community. Tools are required to simplify the process of collecting and interpreting data, even as the complexity of the underlying sensing increases.

It is becoming increasingly common for electronic sensors to provide raw, high-frequency digitized representations of a physical attribute like movement acceleration or geographical location coordinates. A researcher may not know how to derive usable information from these raw signals. The end user is typically interested in ready-to-use valid and reliable objective monitoring systems that yield simplified and standardized summary information on the different aspects of physical activity and sedentary behavior. The popularity of the single-sensor activPAL monitor in sedentary behavior research is a good example of meeting end-user expectation. Scientists use this device to continuously record acceleration data up to 14 days and then use proprietary software to obtain simple output in the form of hourly and daily estimates of time spent sitting or lying down, standing, and walking.

End users of multisensor monitoring systems will expect similar point-select-click solutions for obtaining summary estimates of sedentary behavior and its determinants. In an ideal scenario, the scientist must be able to download data from a multisensor monitoring system, select those sensors of interest to the study on a computer screen, choose the time frame of measurement, and define the level of data processing to be performed (dictated by the desired outcome of study). Depending on the sensors selected by the researcher, the measurement system must also be able to inform the user how uncertainty is propagated throughout the system. For example, determining location from a GPS sensor alone may provide estimates of location that are correct only 80% of the time. Conversely, determining location using a phone's internal location sensor (without GPS) may provide an estimate that is correct only 70% of the time. However, combining information from both sensors might provide estimates that are correct 90% of the time. Software is needed that interactively explains these trade-offs as researchers set up a study and analyze data later.

Data Processing Platforms

Simplifying multisensor data fusion and processing requires large data storage capacity and advanced processing platforms for executing both simple and complex prediction algorithms. A single ActiGraph accelerometer collecting uncompressed raw data at 80 Hz for 7 days roughly requires 250 MB of memory. Processing this data using a typical computer takes approximately 1 hour and 20 minutes per subject (Mannini et al. 2013). Thus, storing and analyzing accelerometer data from multiple subjects collected over long durations would require a high availability of computing resources. The need for additional storage and computing resources increases greatly as more sensors and channels of data are added to a study. Cloud computing is becoming increasingly popular to store, process, and share data among research groups. Projects like SPADES (Albinali 2013) and MoveeCloud (Hiden et al. 2013) enable end users to seamlessly scale, store, and visualize large volumes of raw sensor data stored on remote computers on the Internet and use web interfaces to visualize and then process these to obtain usable

output. Such cloud-based platforms may support combining data sets from various researchers and using open algorithm sharing and comparison on the same data sets. This will permit incremental improvement of estimation models for sedentary behavior on increasingly complex data sets, using an expanding set of underlying sensor technology. These systems may enable sensor manufacturers and engineers to collaboratively build and improve measurement systems that are not dependent on a single proprietary device.

Cloud-based computing will also provide users with flexibility on how their data should be analyzed. Researchers will have the option of choosing processing algorithms developed with and for samples representative of the population being studied. In addition, new algorithms can be developed for specific situations when standardized thresholds and techniques may not be appropriate. For instance, the sit-to-stand threshold of 20° in the activPAL may lead to misclassification of sitting as standing when sitting on elevated chairs where the knee does not bend as much as when sitting in a conventional chair. Using this threshold for a person who is sitting in a pub on a barstool for around 3 hours may lead to a misclassification of standing by the activPAL. In well-defined cloud-based data sharing systems, the raw thigh orientation data would be in the system, permitting advanced algorithms to detect and minimize such errors using secondary data sources as appropriate. For instance, an advanced algorithm might use data from a secondary sensor on the wrist or location information (proximity to a bar) to flag ambiguous standing data for additional scrutiny. Cloud-based tools can also facilitate collaborative improvement of the data sets. Researchers studying a data set and using the cloud-based multisensor data visualization systems who notice abnormal postural allocation detected in conjunction with other environmental sensors (e.g., audio feedback to identify a social setting) can modify algorithm selection for specific periods of time to obtain accurate estimates of sedentary behavior. They might also add additional labels to existing data sets that may be used in future tool validation studies.

Remote Data Monitoring

The application of new technologies may also improve the quality of data by minimizing missing data. Missing data may lead to inaccurate conclusions about the effects of sedentary behavior, physical activity, and sleep on health. A research team can use advancing cellular and server technology to remotely monitor participant compliance to the measurement system on a daily basis (Intille et al. 2012). Data can be transferred from wireless sensors to a remote server through smartphones. Daily remote monitoring will allow researchers to contact participants as soon as noncompliance is detected, address the potential problems that cause noncompliance, and apply improvements to the data collection process for all participants. Remote monitoring will also help researchers detect problems like malfunctioning sensors yielding abnormal data, replace them quickly, and thereby reduce lost data (Intille et al. 2012). Incremental transfer of data from a measurement system to a server also helps researchers to regularly clean and analyze incoming data faster. This will allow faster dissemination of findings and the identification and implementation of necessary changes in the data collection process or intervention (Intille et al. 2012). Remote data monitoring may be especially useful in large cohort research studies. For example, remote data collection and compliance monitoring using mobile phones that people already own will not only be economically feasible, but also enables large-scale data mining for new discoveries and trends (Intille et al. 2012).

Expanding Opportunities for Intervention

The bulk of this chapter discusses the use of emerging technology to improve sedentary behavior measurement, but the same technologies may support novel sedentary behavior change strategies enabled by real-time monitoring and feedback. The sensor-fusion algorithms discussed previously can often be implemented directly on mobile devices such as phones, allowing real-time detection of sedentary behavior and context. Further, if the devices have wireless data connections, detected information can be sent to cloud-based servers, which allows immediate monitoring by interventionists.

Vibrotactile feedback is currently used in commercial monitors as a form of real-time feedback to break sedentary behavior. However, these monitors are not sensitive to situational and environmental context and do not consider the feasibility of breaking sedentary time when providing a vibrotactile cue. Untimely cues may lead to decreased adherence to the measurement system and compromise study or intervention design and findings. Real-time monitoring will enable an interventionist to prompt

behavior modification with feedback when appropriate, that can be triggered automatically based on sensor data or initiated manually based on analysis of a person's data by a human observer using the cloud-based data visualization tools. Phones provide flexibility in feedback type (vibrotactile, auditory, or intelligent text and visual messaging) and end-user tailoring opportunities—characteristics that may be harnessed to enhance contextual sensitivity and feasibility of novel sedentary behavior interventions. Eighty-five percent of American adults use cell phones (Fox and Duggan 2012) and two out of three users have a smartphone (Nielsen Company 2013). This ubiquity creates new opportunities for longitudinal measurement and monitoring of behavior that are only just beginning to be explored. Increasing use, availability of multiple sensors, and data processing capability of smartphones may propel these devices as stand-alone platforms for measuring sedentary behavior and delivering tailored interventions to modify behavior.

Summary

The first sensor for sedentary behavior measurement was introduced in 1967, but the use of similar devices for research has only recently become popular. Current devices primarily consist of a single accelerometer placed at one point on the body and are sometimes augmented with self-report or another stand-alone sensor, such as a GPS. Next-generation technology will use multiple sensors and multisensor data fusion algorithms that will aim to provide improved measurement of sedentary behavior and context and gather a more complete daily, weekly, and longer-term picture of a person's behavior, context, and corresponding decision-making that is absent in current monitors. The algorithms used by these systems should be less dependent on single proprietary devices and more dependent on a variety of wearable and in-environment sensing (including, in some cases, participant self-report) to build a rich model of sedentary behavior. These systems will not only improve measurement capabilities, but create opportunities for just-in-time computer and human-driven interventions. By exploiting consumer technologies such as mobile phones, new studies will be possible with thousands, and perhaps tens of thousands, of participants.

New cloud-based tools will support the massive amounts of data collected and the subsequent computational analysis, hopefully providing a simplified interface for researchers while at the same time ensuring that all algorithms and hardware used to the collect the data are fully described and reproducible by others.

Sedentary behavior has now been identified as an autonomous health hazard. Modernization has contributed to the problem, but new technologies will advance our understanding of the health effects of sedentary behavior. Mobile and other pervasive technologies will also help in the development of behavior modification strategies that can be implemented at a population level and improve overall health. Successful development and application of these tools will require collaborative efforts of scientists from multiple fields of study.

KEY CONCEPTS

▸ **Individual models of sedentary behavior:** Wearable multisensor systems combining passive sensing with active participation from the user may allow researchers to infer what people are doing and build individual models that predict what they may do next. These individual models can be used to provide timely and appropriate feedback to change what the user may do next.

▸ **Measurement goals:** Five goals must be targeted when measuring human behavior using sensors: (1) reliably distinguish between sleep and the waking state, (2) identify sitting or lying when energy expenditure is greater than or less than 1.5 METs, (3) measure physical activity behavior above 1.5 METs, (4) identify characteristics of the social and environmental context that may influence sedentary behavior, and (5) detect wear time of body-worn sensors and ambiguous situations. Achieving these goals will provide a refined and clear understanding of physical activity and sedentary behavior and their determinants.

▸ **User expectations from sensor-based measurement systems:** Maximizing the potential of sensor technology depends on meeting expectations of both the person wearing the sensors and the researcher interested in measuring behavior. Adherence to a measurement system is a primary concern that researchers face. Adherence may be maximized if the system enables instant feedback with the potential to make sensor wear a stimulating and engaging experience. Conversely, researchers are looking for ready-to-use valid and reliable objective monitoring systems that output simplified and standardized summary information on the different aspects of physical activity and sedentary behavior. New technologies may allow researchers to simplify the process of storing, analyzing, and sharing large data sets. Researchers may be able to remotely and regularly monitor data quality and expand opportunities to intervene in real time when the likelihood of behavior modification is high.

STUDY QUESTIONS

1. Describe the five goals of measuring sedentary behavior.
2. Name some types of sensors that can be used to detect sleep, limb position in 3-D space, environmental context, and location.
3. Describe the types of expectations researchers may have when using a multisensor measurement system in research.
4. You are an interventionist who wants to continuously measure and change sedentary behavior in a group of sedentary office workers. You have access to unlimited resources to design a comprehensive sensor-based measurement system based on various aspects of sedentary behavior and its determinants. Describe your system design by creating a flowchart that identifies the behavior and determinant you want to capture, the sensor that you will use to do so, and how you will process, store, and analyze the information.

Dr. Dinesh John's research related to this chapter is funded by the Centers for Disease Control and Prevention/ National Institutes for Occupational Safety and Health (1R21OH010564) and the Harvard School of Public Health (G00004015). Dr. Stephen Intille's contribution to this work was made possible by the National Heart, Lung and Blood Institute, National Institutes of Health award #5UO1HL091737 (Stephen Intille, PI).

CHAPTER 17

CRITICAL MEASUREMENT AND RESEARCH ISSUES IN ANALYZING SEDENTARY BEHAVIOR

Weimo Zhu, PhD

The reader will gain an overview of the critical measurement and research issues in analyzing sedentary behavior data. By the end of this chapter, the reader should be able to do the following:

▶ Understand key characteristics of sedentary behavior data
▶ Identify common problems, inappropriate practices, and challenges in analyzing sedentary behavior data
▶ Identify correct methods for addressing problems and challenges based on the data structure and related research questions

The preceding chapters in part III have addressed ways to measure sedentary behavior. After the relevant data have been collected, the next set of questions naturally will be as follows:

1. How should the data be analyzed so that accurate and meaningful information can be generated?

2. Can conventional statistical methods, such as correlation, *t*-test, and ANOVA, be applied directly to the data?

3. How can the results of the data analysis be correctly and appropriately interpreted?

This chapter addresses these questions. After a review of the characteristics of sedentary behavior data, this chapter describes the challenges in analyzing sedentary behavior data. Specifically, the limitations of conventional statistical methods in analyzing these data and inconsistencies in defining sedentary behavior are outlined and described. New and appropriate statistical methods are then introduced. Thereafter, some practical suggestions on how to analyze and report sedentary behavior data are explained.

Sedentary Behavior Data Characteristics

Understanding the characteristics of a data set is essential in any data analysis procedure. Without knowing the specific aspects of a data set, statistical methods for the data analysis may not be appropriately selected. As a result, the information generated will likely be inaccurate or even misleading. What then are the characteristics of sedentary behavior data?

One of the features of sedentary behavior data is that the data belong to a class of compositional data, which is defined as data with relative portions summing up to 1% or 100%. Compositional data are not unfamiliar to us in our daily life: Proportion of allocated times of a day, proportion of energy we get from different meals, and percentages of students from different geographical areas are just a few examples. Physical activity (PA) data are compositional data, in which total PA, depending on how operationally defined, may be seen to consist of light, moderate, and vigorous PA. This same principle also applies to sedentary behavior data, which can be further broken down

as TV, reading, computer, and video game times. Please note that current physical activity research literature often considers sedentary behavior to be on the physical activity continuum. To distinguish *sedentary behavior* from *physical activity* (see chapter 1 for more details), sedentary behavior is intentionally not placed on the continuum in this chapter. For future research including sedentary behavior on such a continuum, the continuum would be better called the *physical- and sedentary-activity continuum*.

According to van den Boogaart and Tolosana-Delgado (2013), each part of a compositional construct is called a *component*, which has an amount representing its contribution to the total. The amount could be presented in its original measurement units (e.g., time, amount, size) or as the proportion or percentage, which can be determined by the component amount divided by the total. Depending on the units or interest chosen for the composite measure, the actual portions of the parts in a total can be varied. For example, percentages of time spent on different types of PA or sedentary behavior could be different from the percentages of energy spent in different behaviors during the same period. A portion can be further broken down into subportions. For example, sedentary behavior is a proportion of the total of the actions performed during waking hours and itself can be further broken down into different types of sedentary behaviors (e.g., watching TV, playing video games, using a computer, driving, and reading).

The second known characteristic of sedentary behavior data is that the data are often collected, especially for device-derived data (as described, for example, in chapter 14), in continuous time-stamped series for each person. As a result, large and rich time-series data are generated. A time series is a sequence of observations that is ordered by time of occurrence. Although most sedentary data are continuous, they can also be discrete (e.g., if a specific behavior, such as playing video games, happens in a specific time interval). There are two ways to look at time-series data from the data structure point of view.

First, according to Cattell's well-known data box (1952, 1988), time-series data integrate three primary dimensions—persons, variables (e.g., PA and sedentary behavior time), and occasions (see figure 17.1)—from which at least six different structural relationships can be utilized to address specific research questions:

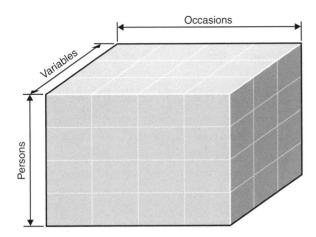

Figure 17.1 Illustration of Cattell's data box.

1. Variables over persons, fixed occasion
2. Persons over variables, fixed occasion
3. Persons over occasions, fixed variables
4. Occasions over persons, fixed variables
5. Variables over occasions, fixed persons
6. Occasions over variables, fixed persons

Second, time-series data can also be considered a multilevel data structure, with occasion-related variables at the within-person level and persons demographics or group membership at the person level (Bolger and Laurenceau 2013, 27-39; Zhu 1997). An example may be helpful for explaining this structure. Table 17.1 presents a hypothetical time-series data with four time points and n persons, where ID is the identification of the individual person, O is the occasion or time points (it is common to use a code 0 for the first observation), X is an independent variable (e.g., physical activity and sedentary behavior), Y is a dependent variable (e.g., heart rate or energy expenditure), and W is a predictor variable that varies between persons only (e.g., sex, exercise intervention versus control). Thus, the X and Y variables belong to the within-person level variables and W belongs to the between-persons variables.

In addition, several other specific features are related to time-series data. First, there is usually a trend component in the time-series data that is often represented by the changes in a dependent variable (DV) over time in relation to an independent variable (IV), individually or jointly with other IVs. The changes further include the underlying direction (e.g., an upward or downward movement) and rate of the change. Second, there is often a cyclical com-

Table 17.1 Time-Series Data

ID_j	O_i	X_{ij}	Y_{ij}	W_j
1	0	x_{11}	y_{11}	w_1
1	1	x_{21}	y_{21}	w_1
1	2	x_{31}	y_{31}	w_1
1	3	x_{41}	y_{41}	w_1
2	0	x_{12}	y_{12}	w_2
2	1	x_{22}	y_{22}	w_2
2	2	x_{32}	y_{32}	w_2
2	3	x_{42}	y_{42}	w_2
n	0	x_{1n}	y_{1n}	w_n
n	1	x_{2n}	y_{2n}	w_n
n	2	x_{3n}	y_{3n}	w_n
n	3	x_{4n}	y_{4n}	w_n

ponent that describes the DV's regular fluctuations or cycle in relation to the IV. Weekday and weekend PA is a recognizable cycle that is a good example of this component. Third, there could be a seasonal component that indicates that the variations in the time-series data are related to the time of year. An increase or decrease in outdoor physical activities or indoor sedentary behaviors across seasons is a good example of this component. Conceptually, the seasonal component can be considered a special case of the cyclical component since the former is the cycle related only to seasons, while the latter is related to any cycles in the data. Finally, the last component in studying time-series data is called the *irregular component*. Known also as *noise*, this component is the variation in the data left after taking into account other components.

The third characteristic is related to the variation of the data. Although this characteristic has not been well studied, and many PA and sedentary behavior researchers are not aware of it, we learned from our PA and sedentary data analysis experiences that both low-intensity PA data and sedentary behavior data may have a larger variation than moderate- and vigorous-intensity data, which is true for both total PA time or total minutes and the proportion of the total time (see table 17.2). This table presents the statistical results of the 2005-2006 NHANES study for all participants (48.22% male), adults (47.77% male), and children (49.05% male). As we all have learned, when running statistical analysis, a large

Table 17.2 Descriptive Statistics of Physical Activity and Sedentary Behavior in the 2005-2006 NHANES Data

Activity type and ratio	N	Mean	SD	Maximum	Minimum
Total					
Sedentary min per day	6,344	459.20	125.72	1,044.86	67.50
Light PA min per day	6,344	344.73	100.30	769.43	16.00
Moderate PA min per day	6,344	25.53	22.90	307.00	0.00
Vigorous PA min per day	6,344	5.04	9.96	115.00	0.00
MVPA min per day	6,344	30.57	28.61	331.00	0.00
Sedentary min per day/total	6,344	0.55	0.13	0.98	0.10
Light PA min per day/total	6,344	0.41	0.11	0.79	0.02
Moderate PA min per day/total	6,344	0.03	0.03	0.32	0.00
Vigorous PA min per day/total	6,344	0.01	0.01	0.15	0.00
MVPA mins per day/total	6,344	0.04	0.03	0.39	0.00
Adults ≥ 18 years old					
Sedentary min per day	4,130	478.29	124.97	1,044.86	67.50
Light PA min per day	4,130	333.65	105.19	769.43	16.00
Moderate PA min per day	4,130	22.97	24.71	307.00	0.00
Vigorous PA min per day	4,130	0.98	3.53	53.00	0.00
MVPA min per day	4,130	23.95	26.23	331.00	0.00
Sedentary min per day/total	4,130	0.57	0.13	0.98	0.10
Light PA min per day/total	4,130	0.40	0.12	0.79	0.02
Moderate PA min per day/total	4,130	0.03	0.03	0.32	0.00
Vigorous PA min per day/total	4,130	0.00	0.00	0.08	0.00
MVPA min per day/total	4,130	0.03	0.03	0.39	0.00
Children and youth < 18 years old					
Sedentary min per day	2,214	423.61	119.25	965.20	110.71
Light PA min per day	2,214	365.40	86.78	639.43	22.50
Moderate PA min per day	2,214	30.30	18.13	159.14	0.00
Vigorous PA min per day	2,214	12.61	13.14	115.00	0.00
MVPA min per day	2,214	42.91	28.78	252.14	0.00
Sedentary min per day/total	2,214	0.51	0.12	0.97	0.14
Light PA min per day/total	2,214	0.44	0.10	0.74	0.03
Moderate PA min per day/total	2,214	0.04	0.02	0.21	0.00
Vigorous PA min per day/total	2,214	0.02	0.02	0.15	0.00
MVPA min per day/total	2,214	0.05	0.03	0.33	0.00

MVPA = moderate- to vigorous-intensity physical activity

variation (e.g., expressed in standard deviation) has often led to a nonsignificant result or a smaller effect size even if there is an obvious difference between groups. This characteristic means that even if an intervention has already resulted in a reduction in sedentary time, our statistical analysis may not be able to detect it.

In addition to all the preceding characteristics, another critical issue in analyzing sedentary data is related to its operational definition. Although sedentary behavior itself has been well described and defined in the literature (Owen et al. 2010; Pate, O'Neill, and Lobelo 2008; see chapter 1 for more details), how to measure it using a specific device is operationally defined and can be done so inconsistently. As described by Cain and colleagues (2013), for the youth population alone, there are already 11 sedentary behavior cutoff scores for the ActiGraph accelerometer, the most popular accelerometry device being used for PA and sedentary behavior research. It is to be expected that more cutoff scores are coming! In addition, not all sitting is alike in terms of health effects (e.g., sitting to view TV versus Zen meditation sitting, which differ greatly in terms of the use of postural muscles), and most of the current measures of sedentary behavior have ignored the distinctive natures of different types of sitting and were not able to distinguish them from each other.

Challenges and Solutions in the Analysis of Sedentary Behavior Data

Currently, most sedentary behavior data have been analyzed using conventional parametric statistics, such as correlation, regression, t-test, ANOVA, and MNOVA. Unfortunately, due to the structure and characteristics of the sedentary behavior data as described previously, these statistics are sometimes not appropriate, or do not take full advantage of what the data could provide. This is because one of the fundamental assumptions of all of these conventional statistics is that the data should be independent of each other. Sedentary behavior and PA data belong to compositional or subcompositional data, which means the data can be correlated to each other. In addition, these conventional statistical methods assume normal distributions for estimates and estimation errors,

which conflicts with the bounded frequency distributions of composition data. Therefore, simply applying conventional statistical methods to compositional data may not be appropriate and could lead to problems such as spurious correlation, constant sum, negative bias, null correlation, and difficulties with closure (Aitchison, Barcelo-Vidal, and Pawlowsky-Glahn 2002).

Another common inappropriate practice in analyzing sedentary behavior data is to ignore the rich information embedded in continuous data that can be derived, for example, from accelerometers. Too often, only the daily average of sedentary time has been computed and analyzed in reported research studies. In contrast, recent research on PA and sedentary behavior indicates that examining patterns of physically active and sedentary behavior can be more informative and can identify attributes that other critical to heath. According to Owen and colleagues (2010), for example, being both physically active, but also highly sedentary and moving often could be as important as moving more. That is., a "breaker," or person who has more breaks from prolonged sitting, will likely be healthier than a "prolonger," who takes fewer breaks (Dunstan et al. 2010, Healy et al. 2008; Healy et al. 2011). Accordingly, the traditional way of analyzing PA data, in which only a specific type of activity (e.g., moderate and vigorous PA or sedentary behavior time) is analyzed individually, clearly cannot take advantage of the rich information embedded within PA and sedentary behavior time-series data.

In addition, as pointed out earlier, inconsistencies in setting cutoff scores is a concern. Although a great deal of attention has been devoted on how to set cutoff scores for accelerometers or similar devices (most often, these correlate with signals generated from the devices with an intensity measure, such as $\dot{V}O_2$ consumption, % of $\dot{V}O_2$max, and % maximal heart rate), there remains the need to further validate the developed cutoffs.

Finally, an ongoing problem in all areas of research: Statistical findings in PA and sedentary behavior research have often been interpreted based on p-values only; therefore, the data were incorrectly interpreted. As an example, when validating a PA measure, many low correlations were called significant simply because p-value of less than 0.05 was achieved. Fortunately, methods and solutions are already available to address the problems and challenges described previously. These are briefly addressed in this section. More specific details can be found in the cited references.

Matching Data Structure, Research Questions, and Methods

With a theoretical framework and understanding of a specific data structure, statistical methods can be appropriately selected for specific research questions. As an illustration, under the framework of Cattell's data box (Cattell 1952, 1988), R-technique (e.g., a commonly used approach to factor analysis) can be used for the data dimension of "variables over persons, fixed occasion," Q-technique (e.g., cluster analysis for subgroups of persons) for the dimension of "persons over variables, fixed occasion," S-technique (e.g., persons clustering based on growth patterns) for the dimension of "persons over occasions, fixed variables," T-technique (e.g., time-dependent clusters based on persons) for the dimension of "occasions over persons, fixed variables," O-technique (e.g., time-dependent [historical] clusters) for the dimension of "variables over occasions, fixed persons," and P-technique (e.g., intra-individual time-series analyses) for the dimension of "occasions over variables, fixed persons." In fact, many modern statistical methods are either derived from these techniques (e.g., dynamic P-technique, which is useful in examining relationships among dynamic constructs in a single person or a small group of people over time) (Engle and Watson 1981) or interpreted under the framework of Cattell's data box (e.g., growth curve modeling and longitudinal factor analysis) (Ram and Grimm 2015).

The multilevel structure of time-series data provides another useful aspect for selecting the appropriate statistical method for analysis. For example, if the research interest is to determine if there is a change or pattern at within-person level variables (X, Y, or the relations between X and Y) and, if there is, whether the change or pattern is caused by between-person variables. In this case multilevel statistical methods, such as the hierarchical linear models (Raudenbush and Bryk 2002; Zhu and Erbaugh 1997), can be employed for the data analysis. If the interest is for when the Y variable varies at both levels or whether X-to-Y relations exist at both levels, time as a third variable, or in the random effects (i.e., between-subjects heterogeneity) and autocorrelated errors, a set of intensive longitudinal methods are available (Bolger and Laurenceau 2013).

Compositional Data Analysis

That problems occur when applying conventional statistical methods to composition data is not new information. In fact, Karl Pearson (1897) pointed out such problems in his well-known paper on spurious correlations more than 100 years ago! The geologist Felix Chayes (1960) took up the problem and warned against the application of standard multivariate analysis to compositional data. But it was Aitchison, whose works in the 1980s (1981, 1982, 1983, 1984, and 1986) made compositional data analysis a subdiscipline in statistical data analysis, who proved that log ratios are easier to handle mathematically than ratios and that after the log-ratio translations, standard unconstrained multivariate statistics can be applied to the transformed data and statistical inferences can be made thereafter. Around 2000, a new set of statistical methods based on the principle of working in coordinates were further developed and applied (e.g., Billheimer, Guttorp, and Fagan 2001; Pawlowsky-Glahn and Egozcue 2001; for more information of the development of the compositional data analysis, see a nice summary by Pawlowsky-Glahn, Egozcue, and Tolosana-Delgado 2015). In addition, a number of text books on the compositional data analysis have been published:

- *The Statistical Analysis of Compositional Data* by J. Aitchison (2004)
- *Compositional Data Analysis in the Geosciences: From Theory to Practice* by A. Buccianti, G. Mateu-Figueras, and V. Pawlowsky-Glahn (2006)
- *Compositional Data Analysis: Theory and Applications* by Vera Pawlowsky-Glahn and Antonella Buccianti (2011)
- *Modeling and Analysis of Compositional Data (Statistics in Practice)* by Vera Pawlowsky-Glahn, Juan José Egozcue, and Raimon Tolosana-Delgado (2015)

Finally, R-based computational analytical procedures have been developed for compositional data analysis. A book titled *Analyzing Compositional Data With R* by van den Boogaart and Tolosana-Delgado (2013) has been published on this subject.

Error-Grid Analysis for Real-Time Monitoring

With a few exceptions (e.g., a reminder to people when sitting too long), most PA and sedentary behavior monitors currently are employed to provide summary information (e.g., the minutes of MVPA time), although long-term, real-time PA and sedentary behavior wearable devices are already widely used in practice. For effective training, intervention, or rehabilitation, the ability to control exercise intensity or behavior within a targeted zone is extremely important and valuable. For similar purposes, a set of variability control methods has been developed in diabetes care for the purpose of glucose monitoring. Among them, Clarke's error-grid analysis (EGA) (Clarke et al. 1987) is mostly studied and applied. EGA breaks down a scatter plot of a reference glucose monitor and an evaluated glucose meter into five areas (see figure 17.2):

a. Where the values are within 20% of the reference sensor

b. Where the values are outside of 20%, but would not lead to inappropriate treatment

c. Where the values could lead to unnecessary treatment

d. Where the values indicate a potentially dangerous failure to detect hypoglycemia or hyperglycemia

e. Where the values could confuse treatment of hypoglycemia for hyperglycemia and vice versa

Many new methods and useful information have been generated since then (see e.g., Breton and

Kovatchev 2008; Gilliam and Hirsch 2009; Rice and Coursin 2012; Wentholt, Hoeskstra, and DeVries 2006). PA and sedentary behavior research and practice would benefit from taking greater advantage of these methods and the novel information that they can generate.

Validating Cutoff Scores

Because the differences in samples and the criterion measures employed in validation and so on, it is expected that inconsistency in the setting of cutoff scores for PA and sedentary behavior data derived from accelerometers and related devices will continue. Meanwhile, a systematic effort should be made after a cutoff score is set up so that additional validity evidences can be accumulated and the credibility of the cutoff scores can be further evaluated. When validating a cutoff score or standard, Kane (1994, 2001) proposed collecting four kinds of validity evidences, including (1) the conceptual coherence of the standard setting process (e.g., if the standard-setting method and related assessment procedure are consistent with the conception of achievement underlying the decision procedure, such as if a new device can correctly distinguish sitting that involves purposeful task performance from more passive forms of sitting such as television viewing), (2) procedural evidence for the descriptive and policy assumptions (e.g., if the standards were set up in a reasonable way by people who are knowledgeable about the purpose of the standards and familiar with the standard setting procedure), (3) internal consistency evidence (e.g., if the presumed relationship can be confirmed between a cutoff score and a performance standard, which could be very important in real-time, long-term monitoring), and (4) the agreement with external criteria (e.g., if the decision made is consistent with other assessment-based decision procedures or outcome variables). One should expect some differences when different health outcome variables (say cardiovascular health versus bone health) are employed to examine the external validity (Zhu et al. 2011). In addition, the role of consequences in standard setting and associated arbitrariness in standards must be examined (see also Zhu 2013 for a discussion from kinesiology's view on standard and cutoff score setting).

p-Value Abuse

Although the interpretation of statistical finding based only on p-values has long been criticized

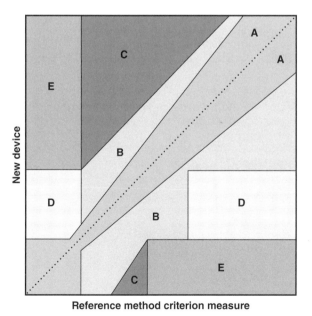

Figure 17.2 Illustration of Clarke's error-grid analysis (EGA).

(Cohen 1994), the practice still continues in the field of PA and sedentary behavior research (Zhu 2012; 2016). For correlational and regression-like research, statistical interpretation should be based on either absolute criteria or the variance percentages explained by the predictors; for inferential statistical findings, the interpretation should be based on the effect size or confidence intervals (Zhu 2012; 2016). In addition, true meaning of the statistics and practical significance of the outcome variables should be studied (e.g., for a special age and sex group, how many sedentary minutes should be reduced to result in a meaningful change in health?). For real-time, long-term monitoring, rich baseline information should be taken into consideration so that real or meaningful individual change can be determined from a person's baseline information.

Summary

With the increased awareness of the adverse effects of sedentary behavior on health and the availability and greater use of wearable PA monitoring devices, the big data era for PA and sedentary behavior research is already here. Yet, the field of PA and sedentary behavior research and practice has not taken full advantage of the new statistical methods and practices that can better analyze PA and sedentary data. In fact, some current practices are either inappropriate (e.g., using the wrong methods to analyze the compositional data) or incorrect (e.g., interpretation of statistical findings are based only on p-values, which are biased by the sample size).

To address these problems, the structure of real-time, long-term PA and sedentary behavior data was introduced. This chapter describes how to select the appropriate statistical method based on the data structure and research interests. It also introduces a number of new statistical methods that could address these problems. The applications of these methods will increase our understanding of PA and sedentary behavior as the data are correctly analyzed.

KEY CONCEPTS

▶ **Cattell's data box:** A way Cattell (1952, 1988) developed to describe the data structure by integrating three primary dimensions of persons, variables, and occasions.

▶ **Composition data:** Data with relative portions summing to 1% or to 100%.

▶ **Composition data analysis:** Statistical methods for analyzing composition data.

▶ **Cutoffs:** Data values for classification.

▶ **Data characteristics:** Data are a set of values of qualitative or quantitative variables. Their characteristics reflect how they were measured, collected, and stored and have a direct effect on how they should be analyzed and reported.

▶ **Error-grid analysis:** A method and illustration developed initially by Clarke and colleagues (1987) to quantify the accuracy of a monitor by comparing measured (true) and estimated values.

▶ **Multilevel data:** Data are organized based on relationship among subjects and contexts.

▶ **p-value abuse:** Making a statistical inference based only on p-value, which is unfortunately biased by the sample size.

▶ **Techniques of Cattell's data box:** These data analysis techniques include R-, Q-, S-, T-, Q-, and P-techniques.

▶ **Validating cutoff scores:** Collecting related evidence to validate the cutoff scores set up.

STUDY QUESTIONS

1. What are the key data characteristics of sedentary behavior?

2. What is composition data?

3. What is Cattell's data box? Describe sedentary behavior data using Cattell's data box.

4. What is a multilevel data structure? Describe sedentary behavior data using the multilevel data structure.

5. Why could the large variation of sedentary behavior data be a challenge in sedentary behavior research?

6. What are the problems related to setting cutoff scores in the measurement of sedentary behavior?

7. What are common problems in the analysis of sedentary behavior data?

8. List techniques based on Cattell's data box and describe how they are related to statistical methods and how they should be used in data analysis.

9. What is the composition analysis? Understand its concept, history, major statistical methods, and related software.

10. What is error-grid analysis? How can it be used in sedentary behavior monitoring?

11. Describe the key evidences and steps in validating cutoff scores.

12. Why can the p-value–based statistical inference be a problem in reporting scientific inquiry?

PART IV

SEDENTARY BEHAVIOR AND SUBPOPULATIONS

To design effective policies and programs for reducing the major health effects of sedentary behavior, which are illustrated so compellingly through the immediately preceding chapters in part III, we need to better understand characteristics of particular subpopulations' sedentary behavior. Part IV has four chapters that address this need.

In chapter 18, Gregory J. Welk and Youngwon Kim address the evidence available on the sedentary behavior of children, illustrating issues that are particular to young people and that highlight broader concerns for understanding and influencing prolonged sitting time in young people. In chapter 19, Wendy J. Brown deals with job-related sedentary behavior among working adults. Working adults spend a high proportion of their waking hours in the occupational environment; for many occupations, the majority of this time is spent in often unavoidable sitting. Brown's chapter thus addresses one of the major concerns for sedentary behavior and health and provides invaluable information on a particularly high-risk group. Sedentary behavior of older adults is addressed in chapter 20. Jorge A. Banda, Sandra J. Winter, and Abby C. King provide

a highly comprehensive—almost encyclopedic—account of the plethora of health implications of sedentary behavior for older adults. In chapter 21, Melicia C. Whitt-Glover and Tyrone G. Ceaser consider the evidence available on the sedentary behavior of racial/ethnic minorities. They make clear that for some minority groups (and in subsets of those groups), aspects of social disadvantage can be manifested through prolonged periods of time spent sedentary.

Of course, part IV does not consider all subpopulations in which sedentary behavior may be a significant health risk. Sedentary behavior is a key issue for people with disabilities, who have specific sedentary behavior–related issues. Variation in sedentary behavior and health consequences by gender—addressed in part through other chapters of this book—is another key subpopulation issue. Other subgroups could be identified, for example, by area of residence and by the nature of the environments in which they live: urban versus rural, suburban versus urban, or those living in urban areas where there are significant variations in access to services and neighborhood amenities.

CHAPTER 18

SEDENTARY BEHAVIOR IN CHILDREN

Gregory J. Welk, PhD; and Youngwon Kim, PhD

The reader will gain an overview of the unique behavioral and health implications of sedentary behavior in children as well as an understanding of the associated effects on assessing sedentary behavior. By the end of this chapter, the reader should be able to do the following:

▸ Understand issues associated with assessing youth sedentary behavior using various types of measurement tools

▸ Summarize adverse effects of excessive time spent sedentary on a variety of health indicators and outcomes in youth

▸ Document prevalence rates and temporal trends of youth sedentary behavior and their variation across different populations

▸ Characterize the context, nature, and underlying patterns of sedentary behavior in youth

▸ Discuss limitations of research on youth sedentary behavior

▸ Suggest future research directions and priorities

Humans are meant to move, but labor-saving devices and technologies have dramatically and permanently changed our society and our lifestyles. Children are the most active segment of society, but there are concerns that elements of our society are causing youth to become less active, more sedentary, more overweight, and less healthy. A frequently cited prognostication suggests that the current generation will be the first to have a shorter life span than their parents (Olshansky et al. 2005).

The concerns about sedentary behavior (SB) in youth evolved from studies showing that excess television viewing was a likely contributor to the increasing epidemic of childhood obesity. Interest in youth SB research was further sparked by studies documenting that SB affects health independent of physical activity (PA) behavior in adults (Healy et al. 2008). The evidence has led to a clear paradigm shift in public health research, but measures and methods are still evolving to study SB in youth.

One complicating factor in SB research is the ever-changing technology landscape. Although common forms of PA have remained largely consistent over the years, this is not the case with SB. TV viewing and computer games have been emphasized in early research and public health guidelines (American Academy of Pediatrics 2001), but it is now possible that youth spend more time on their cell phones or on handheld and tablet devices than with TV. The array of new media choices has also made it increasingly more difficult to distinguish and characterize SB. TV, for example, can now be watched on computers and the Internet can now be browsed on TV. Computers also come in an array of sizes, with the clear trend moving toward smartphone or tablet access as applications replace programs and games. The blurring of technology makes it difficult to characterize SB. Another complicating factor is that time spent in SB may include desirable behaviors such as homework, reading, or music, so it is important to distinguish discretionary or recreational SB from required or desired forms of SB.

Although research is still in its infancy, there is clear consensus that SB is distinct from PA behavior in youth and that a lack of PA cannot be inferred to reflect high SB (Biddle et al. 2004; Marshall et al. 2004; Pate et al. 2011). Similarly, high levels of PA cannot be assumed to reflect low SB because it is possible for youth to be both active and sedentary. These conclusions are based on consistently weak or null associations between indicators of PA and SB (Feldman et al. 2003; Marshall et al. 2002). The independence of these behaviors is also evident in studies demonstrating that boys tend to have higher levels of both PA and SB than girls (Fairclough et al. 2009). Some have assumed that SB would take time away from PA (often referred to as the *displacement hypothesis*), but this does not appear to be the case (Pearson et al. 2014). There appear to be sufficient opportunities for both PA and SB, and boys likely prioritize both to a greater extent than girls do. Interestingly, Feldman and colleagues (2003) reported that PA was associated with productive forms of SB, suggesting that students who regulate and manage their SB may be more likely to also be active.

This chapter further explores the issues and challenges of studying SB in youth. A number of comprehensive reviews have been conducted on correlates (Pate et al. 2011), health outcomes (Tremblay et al. 2011), and interventions (van Grieken et al. 2012), and readers are encouraged to read these reports to get updates on research in these specific areas. The focus in this chapter is to integrate the findings and provide insights about next steps in research. To facilitate integration, this chapter adopts a behavioral epidemiology framework to distinguish distinct types of research needed to study SB (Welk 2002). The categories are generally similar to other behavioral epidemiology models (Owen et al. 2010; Sallis, Owen, and Fotheringham 2000), but an advantage of the present model is that it shows how the different types of research relate to each other in a sequential or integrative way. As shown in the model (see figure 18.1), evidence about health risks associated with SB is used by public health officials to establish guidelines and recommendations. Guidelines, in turn, drive the underlying priorities for surveillance research, which seeks to evaluate patterns and trends in segments of the population. Theory and correlates research seeks to explain the underlying patterns in behavior and determine appropriate strategies for interventions aimed at changing SB. Another advantage of this framework is that it shows the centrality of accurate measurement techniques for advancing research on health outcomes, surveillance, correlates, and the effectiveness of interventions. Issues with the measurement of SB are described first, followed by summaries of each of the specific types of epidemiology research.

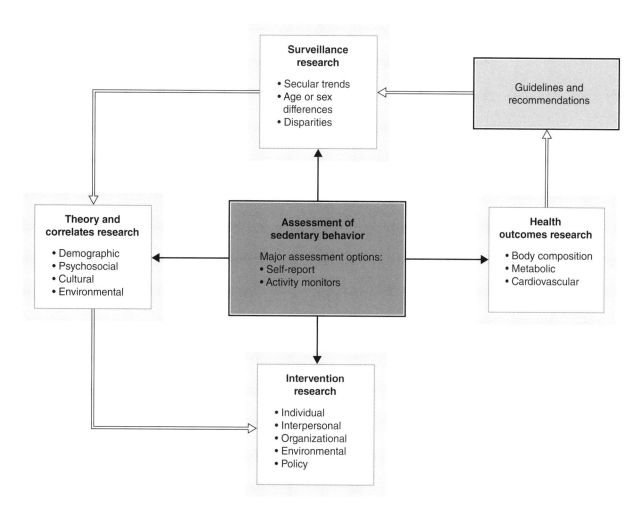

Figure 18.1 Behavioral epidemiology framework showing types of sedentary research and centrality of accurate measurements of sedentary behavior.

Adapted from G.J. Welk, 2002, Introduction to physical activity research. In *Physical activity assessments in health related research*, edited by G.J. Welk (Champaign, IL: Human Kinetics), 3-18.

Measures of Sedentary Behavior in Youth

Accurate measures of SB are critical for advancing research on the health implications of SB as well as evaluating correlates and interventions that influence SB. The implicit challenges of assessing SB are described in other sections of the book, but brief consideration is given here to the unique issues involved in assessing youth SB. Similar to PA assessments in youth (Welk 2002), the wide variability in body sizes, lifestyles, and cognitions with age makes it particularly challenging to assess SB in youth. Several review articles have described the advantages and disadvantages of approaches for assessing SB in youth (Hardy et al. 2013; Lubans et al. 2011; Sternfeld and Goldman-Rosas 2012), so

only brief comments are provided here about the specific methods and related issues. Emphasis is placed on the relative advantages and disadvantages of report-based measures (e.g., self-report) and monitor-based measures (e.g., accelerometers, inclinometers) as well as on the effect of measurement decisions on the ability to answer questions about SB in youth. The distinctions between report-based and monitor-based methods is important for evaluating and interpreting research on SB in youth.

Report-Based Approaches

Self-report measures are the most commonly used tool for examining SB, but there are challenges in using these tools with youth. An advantage of self-report measures is that they can provide information about the type and context of SB (e.g., location, purpose, and surrounding environment or setting)—details that cannot currently be obtained from typical objective measures. A key disadvantage is the difficulty in accurately characterizing and quantifying SB. Although objective monitoring offers some advantages, there has been increasing public health interest in improving the utility of self-report measures (Bowles 2012). Matthews and colleagues (2012) highlighted specific issues with measures of SB and described how bias and error in these measures may distort associations between SB and health indicators. They suggested the following three ways of improving the use of self-report methods:

1. Use of calibration studies and measurement error models to correct measurement errors

2. Use of objective indicators (assessed with objective instruments) of SB to remove reporting bias

3. Use of self-report instruments requiring recalls over a relatively shorter period of course (i.e., 24 hr) to minimize recall bias

Another report (Troiano et al. 2012) clarified the unique value of self-report tools and encouraged researchers to consider a multimethod approach that enables outcomes to be triangulated. Specific guidelines have also been proposed to assist researchers in choosing appropriate self-report instruments for SB assessment (Sternfeld and Goldman-Rosas 2012). The guidelines were composed of 10 questions that help researchers think through adopting an appropriate self-report method and an associated database structure for summarizing underlying features of self-report instruments.

Two previous comprehensive systematic review studies (Foley et al. 2012; Lubans et al. 2011) provided detailed insights on the validity and reliability of self-report measures for youth as well as limitations and future directions. Foley and colleagues evaluated the validity and reliability of use-of-time survey tools for assessing PA and SB for youth. Their summary of 16 articles revealed relatively low validity for standard time-use methods with correlation coefficients ranging from 0.30 to 0.40. Lubans and others reported similar conclusions regarding validity of self-report measures for children and adolescents (i.e., correlations of approximately 0.30). Both reviews indicated that there were few self-report tools specific for assessment of youth SB and that

self-report measures were evaluated against other methods of unknown validity. This limitation may partially explain the weak findings for both validity and reliability. Since youth SB is considered a construct independent of PA (Pate et al. 2011), key research priorities would be to develop self-report tools specifically for youth SB and validate them with appropriate reference measures.

Monitor-Based Approaches

The documented limitations of self-report measures have led to an increasing emphasis on more objective measurement techniques in public health research. Accelerometry-based measures have been widely accepted for assessing PA behavior and procedures have been proposed to enable these tools to assess SB. Accelerometry-based devices have considerable advantages in assessing SB. For example, they can provide information about breaks and bouts of SB in addition to relatively accurate estimates of total time spent sedentary. However, they also have some important limitations. Objective techniques, for instance, cannot distinguish specific types of SB or provide contextual information about SB.

On the surface, it is somewhat paradoxical to expect accelerometry-based monitors to quantify SB since they are designed to quantify movement. The logic is that the accumulation of little or no movement over a certain time interval could occur only if a person were sedentary; however, the fundamental challenge is to establish an appropriate cut point that identifies SB without capturing sleep or light-intensity PA. This is an important distinction since a relatively high cutoff threshold would result in higher estimates of SB time, and vice versa (Hislop et al. 2012). Since activity counts cannot be directly compared, cut points have to be developed specifically for each monitor and each population.

The most commonly used monitor is the ActiGraph, and there has been a convergence toward a default value of 100 counts per minute (cpm) (Evenson et al. 2008; Treuth et al. 2004). The 100 cpm value has been used in surveillance studies (Chinapaw et al. 2012; Matthews et al. 2008; Nilsson, Anderssen, et al. 2009; Ortega et al. 2013; Ruiz et al. 2011; Steele et al. 2010; Troiano et al. 2008) and in health outcome studies (Celis-Morales et al. 2012). However, other cut-point values have also been proposed or tested: 200 cpm (King et al. 2011; Trost et al. 2012; van Sluijs et al. 2010), 300 cpm (Stone, Rowlands, and Eston 2009), 500 cpm (Eaton et al. 2012), 800 cpm (Cliff et al. 2013; Janz, Burns, and Levy 2005; Pate et al. 2006; Puyau et al. 2002), and 1,100 cpm (Guinhouya et al. 2007; King et al. 2011; Reilly et al. 2003).

The classification accuracy of the default 100 cpm has been empirically tested by two previous validation studies (Fischer et al. 2012; Kim et al. 2014). Kim and colleagues compared six different commonly used sedentary cut points (i.e., 100 cpm, 200 cpm, 300 cpm, 500 cpm, 800 cpm, and 1,100 cpm) for hip-worn versus wrist-worn ActiGraph monitors relative to directly observed intensity categorization in a sample of 125 children. They asked each participant to perform a series of 12 activities (randomly selected from a pool of 24 activities) for 5 minutes each in a strictly controlled laboratory setting. Of the six cut points for hip-worn ActiGraphs, the 100 cpm had the highest classification accuracy in identifying sedentary activities with a kappa statistic of 0.81. However, classification accuracy was poor when the six cut points were applied to data from wrist-worn ActiGraphs: kappa statistics ranging from 0.44 to 0.67. Fischer and colleagues compared four different sedentary cut points (100 cpm, 300 cpm, 800 cpm, and 1,100 cpm) and found the 100 cpm to be the most accurate cut point for classifying four types of SB (i.e., playing computer games, playing non-electronic sedentary games, watching TV, playing outdoors) in a sample of 29 children ages 5 to 11. Convergent findings from the two studies support the continued use of the traditional sedentary cut-point value of 100 cpm for youth. However, more comprehensive validation studies that test larger samples of more representative children under more real-world conditions are needed for both hip-worn and wrist-worn ActiGraph monitors.

Another consideration with objective accelerometer-based measures is handling issues with wear time. Studies of PA often set minimum wear-time durations (e.g., 10-12 hr) to ensure that the available time for PA is captured. The minutes of nonwear time are a minor issue when quantifying PA since it is generally assumed these periods would not contribute PA minutes unless otherwise indicated in some type of log. However, isolating nonwear minutes has more relevance in research on SB since periods of nonwear time would be more likely to be during SB. A previous study (Tudor-Locke, Johnson, and Katzmarzyk 2011) demonstrated that failure to account for nonwear time can lead to considerable bias in estimates of SB. Another study (Winkler et al. 2012) also demonstrated that estimates of SB greatly varied depending on selection of different nonwear time algorithms.

Although these are pervasive challenges with most devices, some technologies circumvent the use of cut points and nonwear issues by directly classifying SB. The SenseWear armband monitor, for example, can directly detect wear time. It also discriminates sleeping and lying time using proprietary pattern recognition methods. The SenseWear uses pattern recognition technology to detect different movements and then provides energy expenditure (EE) estimates for the observed behavior. Therefore, the EE thresholds serve as the primary method for distinguishing SB from light-, moderate-, and vigorous-intensity PA. Similarly, the activPAL (a thigh-worn inclinometer) distinguishes time spent sitting or lying, standing, and stepping, thereby providing a way to directly distinguish posture and the detection of SB (i.e., sitting or lying). The activPAL has been used in studies with adults

UNIQUE MEASUREMENT ISSUES IN YOUTH

Some unique measurement issues come into play when quantifying measures of PA and SB in youth. One key distinction relevant to this paper is how to operationalize SB in terms of METs. The traditional MET-based threshold of SB (<1.5 METs) has been proposed as a universal definition by the Sedentary Behavior Research Network, but this value is not necessarily appropriate for youth. Youth have higher resting EE (REE) values, so researchers studying youth PA behavior have widely accepted that a higher threshold of 4 METs is more appropriate for quanti-

fying PA in youth (Trost et al. 2011). Therefore, it is logical for the threshold distinguishing SB from light activity to also be higher. In adults, the threshold of MVPA (i.e., 3 METs) is two times higher than the threshold for light activity (i.e., 1.5 METs). To preserve this ratio in youth, the corresponding MET threshold for youth would be 2.0 METs. A recent study (Saint-Maurice et al. 2015) confirmed that a value of 2 METs yields better agreement and classification accuracy of SB than 1.5 METs, so this value merits broader consideration for research on SB in youth.

(Clark et al. 2013; Dall et al. 2013; Hart, Ainsworth, and Tudor-Locke 2011; Sellers et al. 2012) but has not been widely used to study youth SB. However, a number of validation studies have been carried out to validate the accuracy of the activPAL for assessing SB in this population. Two studies (Aminian and Hinckson 2012; Davies et al. 2012) supported the classification accuracy of the activPAL using direct observation and video analyses as the criterion. However, another recent study (Van Cauwenberghe, Wooller, et al. 2012) found low agreement (kappa = 0.46) between the activPAL and an accelerometry-based activity monitor (i.e., Actical). The activPAL provides the best option for calculating sitting time but it is not able to distinguish lying time from sleep. Thus, there are advantages and disadvantages of different objective techniques for evaluating SB.

Health Effects of Sedentary Behavior in Youth

Research has documented significant health consequences associated with SB in adults (Dunstan et al. 2012; Owen et al. 2010) but the effects are somewhat less clear in youth. This is most likely due to the longer time course of chronic diseases—children may be at risk for future health problems, but the effects may not manifest themselves until later in life. Because of the latency issue, research in this area has generally focused on outcomes that are directly observable in youth such as obesity and the more immediate consequences of obesity in youth like metabolic syndrome. In general, the literature suggests that SB has small or negligible effects on obesity or health risks after taking participation in PA into account. The potent health benefits of MVPA appear to overpower the immediate health risks associated with SB in generally healthy kids, but risks may persist in overweight and obese youth or those already potentially at risk. The specific types of sedentary activities (i.e., TV viewing, screen time) appear to have unique detrimental effects on cardiovascular and metabolic health in youth. Therefore, it is important to explore further the interplay of different types of sedentary activities and their interacting effects on obesity and other health indicators in youth.

Effects on Obesity

Early research on SB indicated that excess TV viewing and game playing were likely contributors to overweight and obesity in youth (Andersen et al. 1998; Dietz and Gortmaker 1985; Ekelund et al. 2006; Gortmaker et al. 1996). These prominent papers and several high-profile interventions (Robinson 1999) increased attention on SB in youth. Several comprehensive reviews of studies from 1995 to 2005 (Academy of Nutrition and Dietetics 2006; Must and Tybor 2005) concluded that increased PA and reduced SB were both protective against excess weight (i.e., fat) gain during childhood and adolescence. The reviews both noted mixed findings and small overall effects, but the equivocal findings were attributed to measurement challenges and design issues. A meta-analysis conducted around the same time frame (Marshall et al. 2004) provided a more quantitative indicator of these effects. Sample-weighted effect sizes for studies evaluating links between SB and body fatness were small for both TV (0.07) and video game use (0.13). Although these links are statistically significant, the authors concluded that the effects were likely too small to be of much clinical significance.

A number of studies have revisited these findings and generally come to different conclusions. Fulton and colleagues (2009) used longitudinal data from Project Heartbeat to evaluate the influence of PA and SB on various body composition indicators. The results revealed no association between SB and indicators of body composition, but it is possible that these null findings could have been caused by the use of only a single 24-hour recall to estimate PA and SB. However, other studies have come to similar conclusions (Chaput et al. 2012; Mitchell et al. 2009; Must et al. 2007). An interesting finding was noted in a study by Byun, Liu, and Pate (2013) that examined associations of objectively measured SB with BMI z-scores in two samples of preschoolers (total N = 418). The authors found no associations between objectively measured (ActiGraph) SB and BMI z-scores, after controlling for MVPA time. These findings suggest that sedentary youth are not more likely to be overweight if they are physically active.

The equivocal nature of the literature makes it hard to draw definitive conclusions (Tanaka, Reilly, and Huang 2014). Newer studies have statistically controlled for participation in MVPA and have tended to use more advanced analytical methods. Kwon and colleagues (2013), for example, used growth models to evaluate the independent contributions of PA and SB on adiposity in a longitudinal sample of youth. Consistent with other studies, the time spent in MVPA was found to be associated with low fat mass (after controlling for SB and other variables), but sedentary time was not associated with fat mass after controlling for MVPA (Kwon et al. 2013). However, another well-designed study (Mitchell et al. 2013) showed an association between SB and weight outcomes using longitudinal data. Thus, the issue remains somewhat unresolved.

A challenge in interpreting this literature is that SB has been operationalized and studied in a number of different ways. Early research tended to rely on self-report measures such as time spent watching TV; later studies have tended to emphasize objective measures. A shift to objective measures has clear advantages, but, as mentioned previously, these measures may lack specificity to capture distinctions among types of SB. Therefore, conclusions still should be viewed with caution. It is possible, for example, that associations are blunted when total SB time is used instead of time spent in specific behaviors such as TV viewing. A review (Tremblay et al. 2011) specifically concluded that excess TV viewing (more than 2 hr) was associated with increased BMI in youth ages 5 to 17, so it may be that TV viewing confers a more specific risk for becoming overweight. A longitudinal study (Fuller-Tyszkiewicz et al. 2012) identified a bidirectional relationship between TV viewing and obesity—that is, children watching TV were more likely to gain weight and obese children were more likely to watch TV. Future research is clearly warranted to determine the direction of causal pathways between TV viewing and obesity in youth.

Effects on Metabolic Health and Health Risks

A number of studies have examined the direct effects of SB on chronic disease risk factors and indicators of metabolic health such as metabolic syndrome. The review by Tremblay and colleagues (2011) concluded that hours of SB were associated with increased metabolic syndrome risk (in a dose–response manner). However, a quantitative review (Ekelund et al. 2012) using pooled data from 14 accelerometer-based studies determined that SB in youth was not associated with chronic disease risk factors after controlling for MVPA. Colley and colleagues (2013) used primary data and more refined accelerometer-processing techniques that accounted for breaks in SB and they reported similar conclusions as the Ekelund study.

The findings showing little or no effects of SB on health are similar to the general conclusions reached earlier regarding BMI; however, there are also some exceptions and discrepant findings that merit attention. A cross-sectional study by Saunders and colleagues (2013) found that higher sedentary breaks and bouts were significantly associated with adverse cardiometabolic risk scores. However, since the study population was a group of children with a family history of obesity, it is possible that genetic factors predisposing the parents toward obesity might have influenced the relationships. Another study (Cliff et al. 2013) reported that SB remained significantly associated with HDL cholesterol after controlling for PA in a sample of overweight and obese youth. This same conclusion has been reached in other studies (Kriska 2013; Mitchell et al. 2013), so it is likely that the health effects of SB become more apparent or manifested in participants who are already somewhat at risk. This possibility is further supported by the detailed meta-analyses of Ekelund and colleagues (2012), since larger effects were observed in the most sedentary group. Thus, there may be a compounding of risk in people who are both inactive (i.e., low levels of MVPA) and sedentary (i.e., large amounts of sitting-related behaviors). The complexities of these relationships were summarized in a systematic review study by Saunders and colleagues (2014).

A factor contributing to the variability in findings is the lack of clarity about the ideal cut point for detecting SB with accelerometers. Atkin and colleagues (2013) used a meta-analytic approach to evaluate the effect of different SB cut points on metabolic risk indicators in the European Youth Heart Study. The association was moderated by cut-point value, with stronger associations observed for higher cut-point values (Atkin et al. 2013). A related study reached a similar conclusion (Bailey et al. 2013), so it is important to consider the possibility that cut points that best capture SB may not be the best thresholds for detecting risk. It is also possible that current measures from objective devices may not be sensitive enough to capture the potentially negative effects from specific types of SB. Support for this possibility is found in previous research (Hsu et al. 2011) that showed that self-reported estimates of SB were independently related to higher odds of metabolic syndrome after controlling for accelerometer-derived estimates of time in MVPA. The inability of accelerometers to detect the type of SB may obscure differential effects from specific

SB. It is possible, for example, that TV viewing may represent a distinct behavior that has different risk profiles than SB in general. This possibility is even more directly supported by a clinical investigation (Martinez-Gomez et al. 2012) where the authors reported that objectively measured sedentary time was not associated with cardiometabolic markers after controlling for confounders (e.g., PA); in contrast, subjectively reported TV viewing remained positively correlated with a number of risk markers. A similar relevant finding was noted in a cross-sectional study by Chaput and colleagues (2012) that examined combined effects of MVPA and SB on cardiometabolic health using both subjective and objective methods. The authors found that subjectively reported screen time was significantly associated with three of the six individual cardiometabolic risk factors, even after adjusting for MVPA time; however, total sedentary time (assessed with an accelerometer) was not associated with any of the six risk factors. Another study (Chinapaw et al. 2012) reported that neither objectively (i.e., total sedentary time) nor subjectively measured SB (TV time and PC time, separately) was significantly associated with individual metabolic risk factors. However, a large well-designed cross-sectional study by Stamatakis and colleagues (2013) reported that TV viewing was associated with cardiovascular risk factors but that computer use and electronic gaming were not. These findings indicate that the subtle aspects of SB may not be captured with objective techniques and that relationships of screen time with cardiovascular health may not be completely understood with a single screen-based activity indicator. Similar to results with obesity, the unique associations of TV and health risk may be due to the fact that TV viewing is also associated with unhealthy diets and habits (Pearson and Biddle 2011).

The use of alternative outcome measures (e.g., cardiorespiratory fitness, or CRF) has also shown potential for elucidating potential health effects of SB. Mitchell, Pate, and Blair (2012), for example, reported that screen time was associated with lower levels of CRF, independent of participation in vigorous PA and also after controlling for socioeconomic status (SES). The findings of their study were similar to another study that also controlled for PA behavior (Hardy et al. 2009). These studies show that SB may have direct effects on CRF that may then influence PA behavior or carry over into adulthood. The study by Mitchell, Pate, and Blair (2012) reported that the effect varied across the range of CRF values, with smaller effects observed at the lower end of the CRF distribution. A contradicting finding was identified from a study by Denton and colleagues (2013) that sedentary time was not associated with CRF, whereas vigorous PA was. Additional research is clearly warranted to better understand the specific mechanisms through which excessive youth SB has harmful effects on health.

Surveillance of Sedentary Behavior in Youth

It is difficult to find any definitive reports on the prevalence of SB in youth. This is partly because it varies greatly by age and also because it is assessed with a variety of measures. Another challenge is that there are no standardized guidelines that specify recommended amounts (maximums) of SB for youth. The American Academy of Pediatrics has recommended fewer than 2 hours per day of TV but surveillance tracking in the United States has used a threshold of fewer than 3 hours of TV per day and less than 1 hour of leisure computer use. A study by Lowry and colleagues (2013) reported on patterns of SB in the United States by summarizing recent findings from the National Youth Physical Activity and Nutrition Study. The authors found that approximately 28% of youth exceed the recommended levels for TV viewing (>3 hr per day) and 24% exceed the recommended level for computer use (>1 hr per day). Another well-designed study based on data from the 2009-2010 NHANES (Fakhouri et al. 2013) estimated prevalence rates of PA and screen time (i.e., a sum of computer use, video gaming, and TV viewing), as well as combinations of both indicators. Overall, about 70% and 50% of American youth met the guidelines for PA (i.e., 60 min of MVPA per day or more) and screen time (i.e., 2 hr per day or less), respectively (Fakhouri et al. 2013), but less than 40% met both of the guidelines. The difficulty in capturing the prevalence of SB is best captured in a comprehensive review conducted by Pate and colleagues (2011). They reviewed 76 studies that investigated prevalence and correlates of SB and concluded that daily SB time in youth ranged from 3.6 to 8.1 hours, depending on the population and how SB time was assessed.

Secular trends are even more difficult to confirm. The general perception among many people is that youth today spend more time being sedentary than previous generations, but it is difficult to find data to document these perceptions. Secular trends from a longitudinal study (Nelson et al. 2006) indicated substantial increases in computer use among adolescents, but this may be due to increased access to computers and not to SB, per se. Nationally representative data (Iannotti and Wang 2013) provide some indicator of how levels of SB in youth change over time. In that study (Iannotti and Wang 2013), time spent on three sedentary activities (i.e., TV viewing, video gaming, and computer use) was estimated using the Behavior in School-Aged Children survey at three distinct measurement cycles: (1) 2001-2002 (*n* = 14,607), (2) 2005-2006 (*n* = 9,150), and (3) 2009-2010 (*n* = 10,808). Of the three sedentary behaviors measured, only TV viewing time significantly decreased over time from 3.06 hours per day to 2.38 hours per day; however, PA time (assessed in the same survey) was somewhat static over the same period of time (Iannotti and Wang 2013). A similar pattern of findings was observed from a study by Li, Treuth, and Wang (2010) that used data from the Youth Risk Behavioral Survey (YRBS) to evaluate trends in PA and SB among high school youth from 1999 through 2007. Interestingly, the prevalence of youth reporting more than 3 hours per day of TV viewing declined from 42.8% to 35.4%. Neither of the studies reported secular trends in screen time, but the data do indicate increasing use of other forms of screen time. Plots showing more recent patterns from the YRBS are provided in figure 18.2 for both TV (top) and screen time (bottom). As is apparent, the prevalence of TV watching has continued to decrease, but the overall percentage of youth reporting 3 or more hours of screen time has increased. Thus, declines in TV viewing have been more than offset by increases in other sources of screen time.

Differences in Sedentary Behavior by Age and Gender

A major public health concern in society is the age-related decline in PA and the apparent increase in SB with age. Although the concerns are justifiable, it is somewhat unrealistic for youth to follow any other path. Studies show age-related declines in PA with all animal species, so the transition is largely a biological phenomenon (Rowlands 2009). As PA declines, it is logical to expect corresponding increases in SB. However, changes with age appear to be considerably dependent on types of instruments used to assess SB, specific types of sedentary activities investigated, and study populations included.

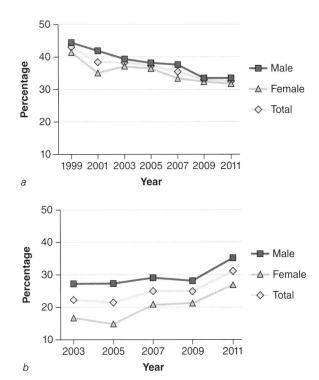

Figure 18.2 Secular trends of percentages of youth who watched TV (*a*) and used computer (*b*) for 3 or more hours by gender.

Data from YRBS. Available: www.cdc.gov/healthyyouth/data/yrbs/index.htm.

To be specific, data from objective assessment tools (i.e., accelerometers) clearly indicate that sedentary time increases with increases in age. For example, in a study by Whitt-Glover and colleagues (2009), objectively measured data from NHANES clearly indicated that total daily sedentary time substantially increased by more than 2 hours per day across the three age groups (i.e., 6-11 years, 12-15 years, and 16-19 years). This age effect was evident in all subcomparison groups by gender, ethnicity, SES background, and weight status. Moreover, cross-cultural comparisons of age-related patterns were provided by van Sluijs and colleagues (2010) using objective data from the European Youth Heart Study. The results of the study revealed very consistent age-related increases (cross-sectional data) in four countries. The estimates of SB ranged from approximately 190 to 230 minutes per day for 3rd graders and from 300 to 370 minutes for 9th graders.

In contrast to the clear, convergent findings with objective measurement tools, subjectively measured data provide disparate patterns of changes in SB across ages. For example, a longitudinal study using survey methods reported no significant changes in TV and video viewing time from early to late adolescence but significant increases in computer use time (from about 8 to 15 hr/week) over the same time frame (Nelson et al. 2006). In contrast, the detailed data from the YRBS (Li, Treuth, and Wang 2010) show that the prevalence of both TV viewing and screen time declines with age during the high school years (see figure 18.3). Somewhat contradictory findings were reported by Sisson and colleagues (2009) using NHANES data. They reported that older youth (i.e., 6-11 years and 12-15 years) exhibited higher proportions of spending 2 hours per day or more on all three types of sedentary activities studied (i.e., TV and video viewing, computer use, and total screen time) compared to younger youth (i.e., 2-5 years).

Regardless of the trend, a more fundamental question for behavioral researchers is to understand the contributing social and environmental factors and the decision-making processes that underlie choices youth make regarding SB. Using growth curve models, Mitchell and colleagues (2012) examined the longitudinal patterns of SB in a large sample of youth from the Avon Longitudinal Study of Parents and Children. They determined that the increases in SB closely matched the decrease in light PA. A similar conclusion was reached in another study (Treuth et al. 2009) using longitudinal data from the Trial of Activity in Adolescent Girls. The fact that sedentary time does not appear to be coming directly at the expense of time spent in MVPA reinforces the general perception that

SB is independent from PA. However, it is overly simplistic to generalize youth patterns based on changes in group-level distributions. It is possible (and likely) that dynamic shifts occur between the allocations (on an individual level) that cannot be detected with traditional group-level analyses. Time that is no longer spent in MVPA clearly has to appear in either the light or the sedentary category, but additional work is needed to understand these shifts and how they vary among people. Based on the available evidence, it does appear that light activity buffers the relative changes between MVPA and SB with age, but the effects may vary by the type of SB assessed (and the methods used to capture it).

Social and Cultural Differences in Sedentary Behavior in Youth

A key goal in public health is to reduce health disparities in the population. Obesity and chronic disease rates tend to be higher among minorities and lower SES groups, and prevalence rates for SB in youth mirror some of these patterns. Based on the analyses by Li and colleagues (2010), nearly 70% of black youth exceeded the daily TV viewing standard of 3 hours compared to around 30% of Caucasian youth. Prevalence rates for more than 3 hours of screen time (video, computer games, or nonschool computer use) were approximately 25%. These rates were also higher for black youth, followed by Hispanic and Caucasian subjects. Fulton and colleagues (2009) reported similar disparities

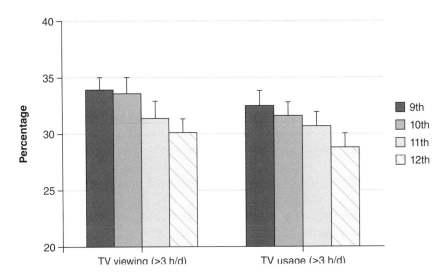

Figure 18.3 Percentages of youth who watched TV and used computer for 3 or more hours by grade.

Data from YRBS. Available: www.cdc.gov/healthyyouth/data/yrbs/index.htm.

in the prevalence of self-reported TV viewing and computer use in children evaluated in NHANES. For example, the prevalence of youth meeting the established pediatric guideline of ≤2 hours per day of TV viewing (American Academy of Pediatrics 2001) was about 50% in black youth, 63% for Hispanic subjects, and nearly 70% for Caucasian subjects (Fulton et al. 2009). However, another NHANES study (Sisson et al. 2009) reported that the proportions spending excess time with TV or video watching, computer use, and total screen time were considerably higher for African-American youth than for both Mexican-American and European-American youth. A more recent NHANES study by Fakhouri and colleagues (2013) reported that Hispanic children were even more likely than non-Hispanic white children to meet recommended levels of total screen time. An explanation for these disparate findings is that there may be differences in patterns depending on the type of screen time reported or evaluated. To examine this in more detail, the reported patterns of TV viewing were directly compared with other screen time behaviors using the most recent YRBS data (see figure 18.4). As is apparent, the distribution of screen time behaviors varies considerably for different racial and ethnic groups.

Differences by race often receive more attention in the literature, but it is likely that the patterns are more directly influenced by socioeconomic status than ethnicity. Clear disparities by income were evident in the study by Fakhouri and colleagues (2013), so more complex models with interaction terms may be needed to fully explicate the nature of health disparities. Another factor that must be considered when interpreting this literature is the type of assessment used in the study. Whitt-Glover and colleagues (2009) used objectively measured data (i.e., accelerometer) from NHANES to examine disparities in PA and SB in youth. Contrary to the findings from subjectively measured data, their study reported no differences in total sedentary time across SES and ethnic groups. Thus, it remains unclear whether the observed disparities in SB are real or artifact that arises due to measurement bias.

Sociodemographic patterns have also been reported in other countries. A study by Brodersen and colleagues (2007) reported that minority students and students from lower SES background in the UK tended to be more sedentary. These patterns were found to match the underlying patterns observed for obesity and chronic disease in society, prompting the authors to point out that "ethnic and SES differences are observed in PA and SB that anticipate adult variations in adiposity and cardiovascular disease risk" (page 140). This statement, although not directly testable, points out the potential effect that youth SB may have on adult health profiles. As previously described, SB may

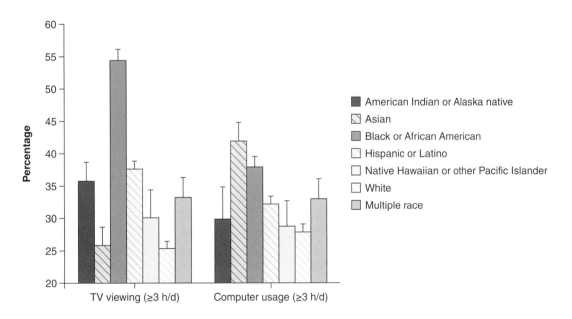

Figure 18.4 Percentages of youth who watched TV and used computer for 3 or more hours by ethnicity.

Data from YRBS. Available: www.cdc.gov/healthyyouth/data/yrbs/index.htm.

have independent effects on health, but it is also important to consider the possibility that SB may contribute to (or reflect) an overall unhealthy lifestyle profile that precipitates future risk. Continued surveillance using geospatial analyses may help to identify the underlying social and cultural factors that contribute to these patterns. The use of more complex system-science models may also prove useful in explicating the relative contributions of social, cultural, and economic factors that contribute to the social disparities in youth SB.

Considerable efforts have clearly been made to investigate prevalence rates and disparities of youth SB; however, the results are not consistent across studies. Similar to previous comments, this is mainly attributable to differences in types of SB as well as the various types of measurement tools used to assess these behaviors. It is important to note that subjective tools have been broadly used for large-scale epidemiological surveillance studies to assess and track prevalence rates and can provide detailed information about types and context of youth SB. However, a single type of SB (e.g., TV viewing or computer use) cannot be fully reflective of the wide spectrum of SB in youth (Biddle et al. 2004; Biddle, Gorely, and Marshall 2009; Olds et al. 2010). Therefore, a wider variety of sedentary activities should be examined to better understand underlying patterns and disparities of SB in children and adolescents. Moreover, future research is needed to accumulate more objectively measured longitudinal data in order to investigate temporal trends of youth SB.

Correlates of Youth Sedentary Behavior

A key step in behavioral epidemiology is to understand the correlates that underlie or explain a specific behavior—in this case, SB. The seminal paper by Owen and colleagues (2010) documented that SB is independent from PA behavior, and deserves to be studied independently of PA. Interestingly, the majority of papers examining correlates of SB have typically examined both SB and PA behavior together (Dolinsky et al. 2011; Lowry et al. 2013; Rusby et al. 2013; Van Der Horst et al. 2007). Although these comparisons have proven informative, a limitation of this approach is that, as noted in a previous study (Nilsson, Andersen, et al. 2009), correlates shown to relate to MVPA typically have little relation to SB. However, a detailed review of 76 studies (Pate

et al. 2011) determined that demographic profiles of SB seem to parallel profiles associated with low PA. For example, children who are older, nonwhite, or in a lower SES group were likely to spend more SB time compared to their counterparts.

A study of correlates was published by Lowry and colleagues (2013) using representative data from the National Youth Physical Activity and Nutrition Study. The battery of correlates emphasized constructs that would be expected to be related to PA. The correlates would not necessarily be expected to be associated with SB, but in adjusted logistic regression models, significant associations were observed for attitudes to PA (TV viewing and computer use), parent support for PA (computer use), and sports equipment (TV viewing). The authors, however, noted that these results suggest that correlates of PA may still have predictive utility on SB. An interesting observation from study by Lowry and colleagues is that it is likely that the predictive utility of PA correlates could be due to common underlying variables (e.g., parenting practices). However, the authors also noted that the effect of positive PA attitudes was evident only among youth who perceived that they lived in safe environments. Violence appears to be an important barrier to PA and it may also lead youth to spend more time indoors performing SB. This may explain the common observation of lower PA and higher SB in lower SES groups (Fairclough et al. 2009).

Some unique insights about SB have been reported in studies that have specifically examined correlates of SB. A prior study (Babey, Hastert, and Wolstein 2013), for example, determined that correlates of TV viewing are different from those influencing leisure-time computer use, so these may reflect clearly different behaviors. However, another review study (Hinkley et al. 2010) noted that parent rules about TV viewing appear to transfer to use of electronic games and computer use. Similarly, Jago and colleagues (2008) concluded that youth who have more autonomy over their own behavior are at greater risk of watching more than 2 hours of TV and playing more than 1 hour of computer games per day. Collectively, these findings support the importance of parental monitoring and rules for moderating and curtailing excess SB in youth. Teaching youth to regulate SB appears to be important, which is consistent with studies that support the general advantages of more authoritative parenting styles. Authoritative parenting styles, for example, have been shown to be associated with less obesogenic home environments (Johnson et al. 2012).

From an environmental perspective, studies have generally observed that SB is correlated with the number of TV sets in the home or the presence of a TV in a child's bedroom (Delmas et al. 2007; Jago et al. 2008); however, van Sluijs and colleagues (2010) observed that patterns were not consistent across countries. These indicators, however, may have less relevance in future studies of SB because TV time and access may not capture time spent on a cell phone or with a tablet or MP3 player.

To better understand SB, it is important to better understand patterns of SB in youth. A comprehensive review and meta-analysis by Pearson and colleagues (2014) concluded that there was a negative but minimal association between SB and PA in children and adolescents. This indicates that the absence of SB cannot be equated with presence of PA, and vice versa. However, it is still difficult to generalize any particular patterns of SB (and PA) in young people. Some interesting contextual information was obtained by Hardy and colleagues (2006), who examined patterns of small-screen recreation (SSR; defined as TV, computer, video, and DVD use) in a large sample of Australian adolescents (n = 2,750). This study documented that boys reported more time of SSR use in comparison with girls and that a prevalence of excessive SSR use (>2 hr/day) greatly differed by urbanization (urban versus rural), SES backgrounds (higher versus lower), and weight status (overweight versus normal weight). Two previous studies (Herman et al. 2014; Olds et al. 2011) indicated that overweight or obese youth were shown to spend more time being sedentary than normal weight youth. However, no contextual information of SB has been fully characterized or examined by weight status. Another large study by Biddle and colleagues (2009) described temporal and environmental patterns of TV viewing and computer use within a day in 1,500 adolescents aged 13 to 16 years. This study demonstrated that the adolescents watched TV and used computer most likely during the middle-to-late evening and that TV viewing was the most commonly occurring activity during weekend days. Other detailed hour-by-hour analyses by Van Cauwenberghe, Jones, and colleagues (2012) and Hesketh and colleagues (2014) revealed that preschoolers had relatively higher levels of SB (and lower levels of MVPA) in the mornings and on weekdays. Moreover, levels of SB and MVPA varied substantially by demographic and temporal factors during segmented hours of week versus weekend days.

A promising analytical approach in this area of research is the use of cluster analyses, which allow underlying patterns to be empirically derived and examined. Zabinski and colleagues (2007), for example, used cluster analyses to examine patterns in estimates of time spent performing six different SBs (TV, telephone, computer, music, homework, and reading). They classified four distinct subgroups of the sedentary cluster by the degree of sedentariness of the participants and demonstrated that time spent in all six SBs increased from the lowest sedentary group to the highest sedentary group. Several other studies have used similar cluster analyses to create distinct behavioral clusters that characterize behavioral typologies of SB (Boone-Heinonen, Gordon-Larsen, and Adair 2008; Trilk et al. 2012). Boone-Heinonen and colleagues identified seven and six discrete clusters for boys and girls, respectively. Their study specifically reported that girls in the sedentary cluster were more likely to be obese in relation to the referent group (i.e., the club and sports cluster), but this relationship was not observed for boys. In another study that employed cluster analyses, Trilk and colleagues (2013) identified six clusters (educational sedentary, sports and play, active transport and chores, electronic media, sleep, and organized sports teams, classes, or lessons in past year). This study reported that time spent in SB increased transitioning from 6th to 8th grade in 957 girls. These studies have helped to highlight the inherent complexity of youth SB. Straker and colleagues (2013) identified three clusters based on screen-based media use for adolescents: instrumental computer users (high e-mail use, general computer use), multimodal e-gamers (both high console and computer game use), and computer e-gamers (high computer game use only). High TV viewing time and substantial differences in steps taken and MVPA accumulated were observed among the three clusters (Straker et al. 2013).

Intervention Approaches for Sedentary Behavior in Youth

In the behavioral epidemiology framework, theory-based information about correlates of SB can be applied in intervention studies to test methods for reducing SB in youth. Progress has been made, but the variability in outcomes and approaches makes it difficult to draw conclusions about the effectiveness of behavioral interventions for SB. A study by Steeves and colleagues (2012) reviewed 18 studies focused on reducing SB (9 specific for SB and 9 targeting multiple behaviors). The authors reported that the majority of the studies directly targeted screen-based sedentary behaviors and most used one or more behavior modification approaches such as goal setting (78%) and self-monitoring (67%). Half of the interventions were found to yield statistically significant changes in SB, with effects ranging from −0.44 to −3.1 hours per day. The most successful interventions were those that used electronic monitoring devices or made TV viewing contingent on other behaviors. Using TV as a reward for PA was viewed as a counterproductive strategy since it would indirectly make the TV a more valuable activity. The authors recommended the need for additional research in different age ranges (e.g., preschool and adolescent) and different settings (e.g., pediatrician office, schools) since most of the studies were done with limited age ranges and through research environments rather than in community-based settings. The authors also noted that the overwhelming majority of the studies (89%) relied on self-report measures for evaluating outcomes, so it is possible that effects would be different if objective measures were used.

A meta-analysis (van Grieken et al. 2012) evaluated 34 randomized controlled trials on SB over the past 20 years. The mean differences were small but significant for both reductions in SB (mean difference of 18 min/day) and BMI (mean difference of 0.25 kg/m^2). A systematic review and meta-analysis (Kamath et al. 2008) described and evaluated randomized controlled trials intended to prevent childhood obesity through reductions in SB. They reviewed a total of 14 comparisons with 3,003 youth and obtained a pooled effect size of −0.29 (95% CI = −0.35, −0.22; I^2 = 63%), which indicates that intervention groups had reductions in SB compared to control groups. Another recent meta-analysis by Liao and colleagues (2014) reviewed a total of 24 randomized-controlled trials aimed at reducing BMI through reductions in SB in children and revealed that reductions in SB resulted in declines in BMI levels, with pooled effect sizes ranging from −0.060 to −0.089. DeMattia, Lemont, and Meurer (2007) carried out another comprehensive review of intervention studies aimed at decreasing SB in

youth. A total of 12 studies were retrieved for review: 6 of them were intervention programs targeting clinical populations (i.e., overweight or at-or-risk of overweight), while the other 6 studies were prevention programs targeting average populations in childhood. The authors reported that all the 12 intervention studies reviewed resulted in reductions in SB and improvements in weight status. Leung and colleagues (2012) found a similar finding from a systematic review of 12 randomized controlled trials aimed at reducing SB in school-aged children. They concluded that interventions targeted at decreasing SB were effective in reducing sedentary time and improving indicators of childhood obesity. The consistent evidence of declines in BMI is noteworthy, considering the fairly consistent findings (reviewed previously) that SB is not associated with BMI after taking PA into account. This suggests that interventions targeting SB (as a construct independent of PA) can have positive effects on reducing BMI.

Summary

This chapter covers findings on health outcomes, surveillance, correlates, and intervention approaches. A key aspect of the behavioral epidemiology framework used in this review (see figure 18.1) is that the assessment of SB plays a key role in better understanding each area of research. The importance of measurement issues is evident in the different outcomes observed for findings reached with subjective versus objective assessment tools.

Although considerable work has been done, it is difficult to concisely summarize and characterize SB in youth. This is due, in part, to the small number and short history of research on youth SB. All previously mentioned studies have contributed to identifying patterns of youth SB, but more studies are warranted in order to fully understand the underlying characteristics of SB in children. To date, the majority of studies on youth SB have emphasized screen-based activities, such as TV, computers, and video games. It is clear that these are common forms of SB in children, but little is known about the patterns of other forms of SB (e.g., sitting, standing, chatting, studying) in youth. Moreover, given that limited evidence exists in terms of location and purpose of youth SB, it is essential to examine contextual information of SB in youth.

KEY CONCEPTS

▸ **Findings from subjective assessments may differ from objective assessments:** The outcomes from various epidemiology studies tend to vary depending on the type of assessment being used. It is common to assume that the objective measures are more accurate than subjective ones, but this is an overly simplistic conclusion. Limitations are associated with both forms of measurement. Improvements and refinements in both assessment methods are needed to advance research on SB.

▸ **Health disparities are complex:** Many studies have examined disparities in SB and health using various sociocultural correlates and indicators. Research using single variables tends to obscure the complexities of these evaluations since many of the variables are intertwined. Measures used to evaluate SB may have differential forms of bias in different populations, so it is important to not overinterpret findings. More complex models and analytic techniques are needed to better understand these issues.

▸ **Not all forms of SB are equal:** Many studies have examined SB using composite indicators of screen time, but evidence exists that the associations may vary by type of SB. More consistent health risks are evident in studies examining TV viewing, but this may be due to stronger indicators of this behavior as well as to other related behaviors taking place while watching TV (e.g., eating). More systematic evaluations of types of SB are needed to understand the behaviors and the health implications of these behaviors.

▸ **Youth are not little adults:** Public health researchers have a tendency to assume that patterns and findings from adult research will hold true for youth. However, this is often not the case. With regard to youth, the evidence does not support the general observations in adults that SB has independent health risks after taking into account levels of MVPA. It is possible that the deleterious effects take longer to have an influence or that other factors affect health status more directly in youth.

STUDY QUESTIONS

1. What unique measurement issues need to be taken into account when studying youth SB?

2. Why might health implications of SB be different between adults and children?

3. What factors contribute to observed disparities in SB in youth?

4. What are unique measurement considerations for conducting different types of research on SB (e.g., health outcomes research, surveillance research, correlates research, and intervention research)?

CHAPTER 19

OCCUPATIONAL SEDENTARY BEHAVIOR IN ADULTS

Wendy J. Brown, PhD, FASMF, FACSM, FAAKPE

The reader will gain an overview of the research on occupational sitting, including how patterns of sitting at work have evolved over the course of time, and will consider the health effects of these patterns. By the end of this chapter, the reader should be able to do the following:

▶ Consider the changing nature of work over time

▶ Identify the broad occupational groups most at risk of high occupational sitting

▶ Illustrate different ways of measuring occupational sitting time

▶ Describe typical durations and patterns of accrual of occupational sitting

▶ Understand the health effects of occupational sitting and the strength of the evidence underlying these claims

It is generally agreed that since Paleolithic times, and more so over the last 50 years, there has been a decrease in population levels of physical activity (Ng and Popkin 2012). Although leisure-time physical activity has increased, occupational activity has declined, reflecting the 20th century transition from a reliance on human power for agricultural and industrial tasks to the widespread mechanization and computerization of work. With this change, there has been an enormous increase in the amount of time spent sitting at work.

The Changing Nature of Work

Changes in the overall energy expenditure of work are exemplified by the findings of a study of Old Order Amish people in the United States, who shun the use of petrol-powered transport and electricity in their everyday lives, including work activities (Bassett, Schneider, and Huntington 2004). Amish men and women were found to have daily energy expenditures of 299 and 207 MET hours per week, respectively. This can be compared with estimates from people in the then 15 member states of the European Union who achieved a median value of 24 MET hours per week (95% CI: 23.6, 24.8) using the same short form IPAQ measure (Rütten and Abu-Omar 2004). Others have shown that since the 1960s in the United States, there has been a progressive decrease in the proportion of people employed in agricultural and production jobs (which typically involve at least moderate-intensity activity) and an increase in sedentary and light-intensity service jobs (which typically involve long hours of sitting) (Church et al. 2011).

These declining levels of overall and occupational energy expenditure are illustrated in an analysis of time-use data from the United States, UK, China, Brazil, and India in the domains of sleep, leisure, occupation, transportation, and home-based activities over various periods from 1960 to 2005 (Ng and Popkin 2012). The data show an annualized decrease in occupational activity of 0.8 (India) to 9.0 (China) MET-hours per week, which accounts for almost all the decline in overall energy expenditure in these countries over 5 and 18 years, respectively. Occupational activity fell by 35% in the UK and by 41% in the United States, with estimates of annualized decreases of 1.5 and 1.8 MET-hours per week over this period.

Although most studies of declining energy expenditure do not explicitly measure occupational sitting time, Ng and Popkin (2012) provided estimates of occupational activity and overall sedentary time, which are inversely related. They show that overall sedentary time increased by 32% over 18 years in China and by 47% over 34 years in the UK. We now know that in Western developed countries, the majority of this sedentary time is accrued through *sitting at work* (the phrase used in this chapter to conceptualize occupational sedentary behavior). Reflecting changes in the nature of work, both small- and large-scale studies show that many working adults now spend more than half their working day sitting (Brown, Miller, and Miller 2003; Jans, Proper, and Hildebrandt 2007; McCrady and Levine 2009). These data are considered in the following sections.

At-Risk Occupational Groups

In the second half of the 20th century, most of the epidemiological studies in the field of occupational activity focused on a lack of physical activity. Although the landmark work of Jeremy Morris drew attention to the ill effects of work characterized by sitting (for example, in bus drivers, postal sorting workers, and civil servants), the emphasis was on lack of physical activity (Paffenbarger, Blair, and Lee 2001). Actual measures of occupational sedentary behavior, or sitting time, did not start to appear in the literature until the turn of the century (Brown, Bauman, and Owen 2009).

Early studies of time spent sitting at work conceptualized occupations in terms of broad categories, such as managerial and professional (e.g., executives, lawyers, doctors, and teachers), white-collar (e.g., technical, administrative, and clerical workers), and blue-collar (e.g., trades people, transport workers), but the descriptors and the occupations included in each study vary from country to country.

Some of the first occupational sitting time studies, which came from Queensland, Australia, relied on self-reported sitting time and used pedometer measures to indicate lack of movement. One study showed that managerial and professional workers in an Australian health facility reported more sitting and recorded fewer pedometer step counts than technical and blue-collar workers (Miller and Brown 2004). Another early study that did not measure sitting time confirmed, however, that average daily steps are markedly higher in blue-collar workers (8,757 steps/day) than in professional (2,835 steps/day) and white-collar (3,616 steps/day) workers in a regional Queensland University, implying that those with low steps spent more time sitting (Steele and Mummery 2003).

Other studies with self-report measures of sitting confirm that there is a gradient of sitting time, with professional workers sitting most and blue-collar workers sitting least, but these studies also note age and sex differences in sitting time, even within broad occupational categories (Brown, Miller, and Miller 2003; Duncan, Badland, and Mummery 2010; Mummery et al. 2005). These studies find a tendency for occupational sitting time to increase with age and job status and note that professional men report more sitting than professional women (Mummery et al. 2005). These gender differences may reflect the (unsurprising) fact that full-time workers, who were mostly men in these early studies, sit more at work than part-time workers, who were mostly women (Brown, Miller, and Miller 2003). Women who work at home in an unpaid capacity (usually caring for young children) have the lowest sitting times. Interestingly, these studies show that compared with mothers of young children, full-time workers spend not only four times longer sitting at work, but also twice the amount of time sitting for transport (Brown, Miller, and Miller 2003).

These early descriptions of significant variations in work-related sitting among broad occupational groups are confirmed by population-based studies. A significant study from the Netherlands involving a very large representative sample of Dutch workers shows that occupational groups described as legislators, senior managers, clerks, and those in scientific and artistic professions sit more than those in commercial, trade, transport, service, and agricultural occupations (Jans et al. 2007). When assessed by sector, workers in computerized jobs, commercial services, transportation, banking, and government sit most at work, and those in the welfare, retail, health, agriculture, other service, and catering sectors sit least (Jans et al. 2007). Similarly, an analysis of Australian National Health Survey data from 2007 to 2008 confirmed that professional and clerical or administrative workers are most likely to spend a large proportion of their working day sitting (Chau et al. 2012).

Overall, these studies shed light on the broad occupational groups that are most at risk of spending long hours sitting at work. It must be emphasized, however, that the amount of time spent sitting at work—even in similar occupational groups—is likely to vary according to specific job roles. Moreover, since most of these studies were conducted

in developed countries, there is little information with which to identify the groups most at risk in developing countries. It is clear that blue-collar workers generally sit less than their professional and white-collar colleagues in developed countries, but it is conceivable that production workers (who would be described as blue-collar) in developing countries may spend a large proportion of their working day sitting. For example, increasing numbers of workers in the large-scale clothing production and electronics industries may explain the very large overall decrease in occupational activity and increase in time spent sedentary in countries like China since 1991.

Patterns of Occupational Sitting

At the time of writing this chapter, most of the work on measuring occupational sitting time focused on office and administrative workers in Western developed countries. However, interest is growing in other sedentary occupations, including drivers. As indicated previously, the early Australian and Dutch studies of occupational sitting time relied on self-reported measures of sitting time. More recent studies have used objective methods of measuring time spent sitting. But unless there is a way to flag time at work using a log or diary, these studies often report *overall* sitting time in working populations, which includes time spent sitting at work, during transport, and in leisure time (including screen time and other leisure-time sitting activities).

Self-Reported Estimates

The large Dutch study, which included 7,720 full-time workers in a wide range of occupations, reports that between 2000 and 2007, average *overall* daily sitting time in the Netherlands was 7 hours per day, one-third of which was sitting at work. The longest occupational sitting time was 3 hours per day for legislators and senior managers and the shortest was less than 1 hour per day for service workers. Importantly, this study found that Dutch workers who sit for long periods at work do not compensate by sitting less in leisure time (Jans et al. 2007).

Data from the Australian National Health Survey indicate higher sitting times. On average, full-time workers sit for 3.8 (SD 3.0) hours per day at work, and those who identify as having jobs that involve mostly sitting sit for 6.3 hours per day at work (Chau et al. 2012). In contrast with the findings from the Dutch study, this Australian study found that workers with mostly sitting jobs were about 10% more likely to meet physical activity guidelines (based on walking for transport and leisure-time activities) than workers in more active jobs (Chau et al. 2012).

Australian data also show that occupational sitting times vary by sociodemographic characteristics. As might be expected from the at-risk occupational groups, people with higher levels of education and income tend to sit most (de Cocker et al. 2014). In the earlier regional Queensland sample, average sitting time at work was 20 minutes higher in men than women and 30 minutes higher in older (>50 years) than younger (18-30 years) workers (Mummery et al. 2005). The study of full-time and part-time workers found that full-time working men sat on average for 4.9 hours per day and full-time working women sat for 3.9 hours per day. Part-time workers sat for only 1.3 hours per day (Brown, Miller, and Miller 2003). However, these gender differences are influenced by the tendency, at least in Australia, for there to be more men working in professional roles and more women in technical or trade and clerical or administrative roles (Chau et al. 2012).

Objective Measures

Since the introduction of accelerometers to the field of PA epidemiology, several researchers have used these instruments to assess lack of movement, also described as *sedentary time*, although accelerometers do not easily distinguish time spent standing still from that spent sitting or lying down. Several researchers have combined accelerometer data with diary information to ascertain how much time is spent sitting (or with lack of movement) while at work.

An Australian study that used accelerometer and diary data to describe workplace sitting in office, customer service, and call center workers shows that 56% of waking time is spent at work. Of this work time, employees spend an average of 6.6 hours per day (77% of their time at work) in sedentary time (<100 cpm on the ActiGraph GT1M) (Thorp et al. 2012). This study found little variation in sedentary time across work groups (95% CI: 6.56–6.67 hr/day) but discovered that call center workers tend to be the most sedentary and customer service workers the least sedentary. This estimate of 6.6 hours per day of sedentary time at work is similar to the Australian self-reported sitting time estimate of workers who

identify as being in mostly sitting jobs (6.3 hr/day; Chau et al. 2012).

A Scottish study that used the activPAL inclinometer to assess sitting time reported slightly lower estimates of workday sitting time (Ryan et al. 2011). This could reflect the different occupational groups (lecturers, researchers, technicians, and administrators) in this study or differences in the way that accelerometers and inclinometers measure sitting time (Lyden et al. 2012; Ryde et al. 2012). For example, standing (still) at a counter serving a customer could be categorized as sitting instead of standing when using an accelerometer. The Scottish study used the activPAL to assess time spent in a sitting posture and reported that participants were seated at work for 5.3 (SD 1.0) hours per day ($N = 83$), or 66% of their time at work (Ryan et al. 2011).

In contrast with these two studies that focused on people in high-sitting occupations, an innovative Australian study compared sitting times in 65 young adult women (aged 18-36), half of whom had jobs in which they sat all day and half of whom had jobs that required them to be on their feet all day (Wane 2012). Using merged data from detailed diaries, the activPAL, and the ActiGraph GT1M, average time at work was around 8 hours per day in both groups. Women in the "I sit all day" group spent just over 6 hours per day, or 77% of their time, sitting. Women in the "I'm on my feet all day" group sat for 4.55 hours per day, or 56% of their time at work. Although there was wide variation in sitting time in both groups, overall, the average difference in workday sitting time between the two groups was only 93 minutes per day (95% CI: 66.7, 121.0). Even in *nonwork* time, more than half the time in both groups (average 3.7 hr, or 52% of nonwork time) was spent sitting (see figure 19.1).

Another innovative study of sitting at work was conducted using a sitting pad to measure the time office employees spend sitting at their own desk, with inclinometer, accelerometer, and diary data used to measure time spent sitting elsewhere and activity while at work (e.g., at lunch or in meetings away from the usual desk). This novel measure of occupational sitting uses a chair-based pressure sensor to provide detailed information about patterns of sitting time, including the total time spent sitting and the number of times that sitting at the desk is interrupted and for how long (Ryde et al. 2012).

The results of this study provide insight into how full-time office workers spend their time each day (asleep, at work, not at work) and how this time is divided among sitting, light activity, and activity at or above moderate level (Brown et al. 2013; Ryde et al. 2014). The 108 office workers (age 19-63 years) were, on average, out of bed for 16.3 hours per day.

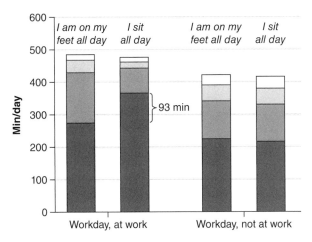

Figure 19.1 Proportion of time spent sedentary (dark bars); in very light (gray), light (pale gray), and moderate-vigorous (white) intensity activity; while at work (left) and in nonwork time (right) on workdays, in women who "are on their feet all day (*N* = 32) and who "sit all day" (*N* = 32). *p* < 0.05 for difference between groups.

Adapted, by permission, from S.L. Wane, 2012, *Young women and weight gain: What is the role of patterns of physical activity and sedentary behaviour?* PHD diss., The University of Queensland, Australia.

Of this, 8.7 hours were spent at work, of which 5.8 hours (67%) were spent sitting at the usual desk and another 0.4 hours were spent sitting elsewhere. As in the study of young adult women, these workers also spent about half of their nonwork time sitting. On average, they spent 44 minutes per day in at least moderate-intensity PA, of which 17 minutes were during work hours. A summary of the data from this study is provided in figure 19.2.

Data from the sitting pad also show that on average, Australian government office workers interrupt their desk-based sitting three times per hour or 29 times per day. Sitting for more than 1 hour occurred rarely in this group. This is important because there is accumulating evidence that the adverse health effects of too much sitting may depend not only on total daily sitting time, but also on the pattern of interruptions to sitting time (see chapter 3 for more detail). Although total desk-based sitting time may be high in office workers, people in the same office may have different sitting patterns, which also vary from day to day in individual employees, as shown in figure 19.3. For this person, over 4 days, desk-based sitting time ranged from 5.2 to 6.5 hours per day and the number of interruptions ranged from 45 to 97 per day. The figure shows few consistent patterns throughout the week, except a distinct interruption in desk-based sitting at lunch time (around 12-1 p.m.) every day (Ryde et al. 2014).

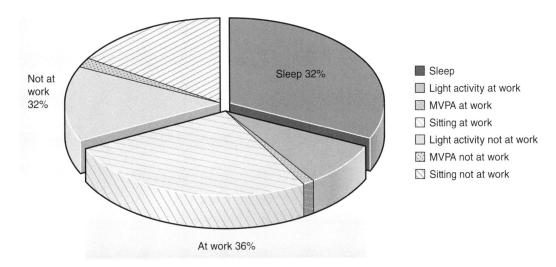

Figure 19.2 Average time spent per day sleeping, at work, and not at work. Data from objective (sit pad, accelerometer, inclinometer, and diary) measures of 105 Australian office workers. Dark = time asleep; medium gray = time in light-intensity activity at work (hatched area = sitting, spheres = moderate- to-vigorous intensity physical activity); pale gray = time in light-intensity activity not at work (hatched = sitting, spheres = moderate-to-vigorous intensity physical activity).

Data from Brown et al. 2013; Ryde et al. 2014.

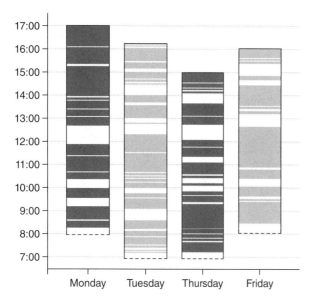

Figure 19.3 Desk-based sitting patterns of an office employee whose total sitting time at work was 5.9 hours per day on average. Black areas are time spent sitting at the employee's own desk, white areas are time away from the desk, and dashed lines indicate when the employee started work each day.

Reprinted, by permission, from G.C. Ryde et al., 2014, "Are we chained to our desks? Describing desk-based sitting using a novel measure of occupational sitting," *Journal of Physical Activity & Health* 11(7): 1318-1323.

The activPAL study of Scottish University employees also found that in an average working day, 5.3 hours of sitting were accumulated in 27 different bouts. However, notwithstanding the high number of interruptions, 25% to 67% of sitting time in that study was accumulated in bouts longer than 20 minutes (Ryan et al. 2011). In contrast, a recent study of occupational sitting and activity patterns in Swedish call center workers found that employees sat for 4.4 hours per day and interrupted their sitting time approximately five times per hour. Even in this occupational group, whose members are perceived to be extremely sedentary, the average duration of each sitting bout was only 11.2 minutes and, in this Scandinavian context, sitting for more than 60 minutes at a time was rare (Toomingas et al. 2012).

Similarly, patterns of sitting are highly variable in non-office or blue-collar workers. In this occupational group, U.S. NHANES data show very low sitting times in waiters and waitresses, sales representatives, and teachers (Steeves et al. 2015). Data from Denmark show that sitting times are lowest

in garbage collectors and cleaners and highest in mobile plant operators (Hallman et al. 2015).

Recent studies have also shown that sitting times are high in bus and truck drivers, but that there is also considerable variability within these groups. For example, one study has shown that bus drivers from a single regional bus depot in Queensland, Australia, sit for only 44% of their working day. This is because the drivers work split shifts and were supported to use a nearby gym during their breaks (Wong et al. 2014). In contrast, UK researchers have reported that bus drivers sit for 85% of their working day (Varela-Mato et al. 2015). Data from a sample of 44 Australian truck drivers show some of the longest occupational sitting times reported to date, with an average sitting time of 9.1 hours per day (Gilson et al. 2015).

In conclusion, studies using a variety of different measures indicate that full-time workers spend about one-third of their day at work. Between one-half and two-thirds of this time (or more in the case of drivers) is spent sitting, depending on job roles, which vary by occupation, sex, and age. Typical occupational sitting time in Australian office workers is around 6 hours per day. This time may, however, be accumulated in many short bouts, with patterns of interruption varying according to occupational roles. Long sitting hours are not confined to office jobs. Even people who describe themselves as being on their feet all day sit for long hours at work. Overall, there is consensus that more time is spent sitting at work than for transport or leisure (Parry and Straker 2013), but there is conflicting evidence on whether those who say they sit all day are less active in leisure time than their more active working counterparts.

Health Effects of Occupational Sitting

One of the earliest references to the ill effects of sitting at work is in Bernadino Ramazzini's *De Morbis Artificum Diatriba* (Diseases of Workers), which was first published in 1713 in the Italian city of Padua. In his book, Ramazzini, who is now known as the father of occupational medicine, covers illnesses experienced by workers in every imaginable profession of the time (for example miners, metalworkers, cleaners, bakers, millers, brewers, farmers, cobblers, tailors, seamstresses, scribes, clerks, and even "learned men").

Ramazzini stated that "those who sit at their work, and are therefore called chair workers, suffer from their own particular diseases." He described the many symptoms and conditions he observed among sedentary workers. These included damage to the vertebral ligaments (especially among those whose heads were bent over their books), compression injuries o the stomach, indigestion, obstruction of the viscera, checks on the flow of pancreatic juices (speculated now to be diabetes), nephritis, lumbago, numbness of the legs, hindrance of blood circulation, arthritis, lameness and sciatica (especially among tailors who sit "with one leg back against the thigh"), and "unhealthy habit." He observed that "women who do needlework in their homes day and night. . . suffer from the itch, are a bad color, and in poor condition."

Ramazzini noted that those who sit, but at the same time exercise their arms and feet, like potters and weavers, were less likely to develop symptoms, "as the impurities in their blood were more easily dispersed." Without exercise, he noted, the "blood becomes tainted, its waste matter lodges in the skin, and the condition of the whole body deteriorates."

Moving forward from Ramazzini's 18th-century treatise, the focus of several early studies of occupational epidemiology, such as those conducted by Jeremy Morris in London in the 1950s and 1960s, was on groups of employees who spent long hours sitting at work (Paffenbarger et al. 2001). These studies, which were among the first to demonstrate the health benefits of physical activity, also showed that those who sat for long periods of work, such as bus drivers and mail sorters, were more at risk of adverse cardiovascular risk factors than their work group colleagues who did not sit, such as bus conductors and mail delivery men.

Through the second half of the twentieth century, occupational epidemiology focused largely on the effects of lack of physical activity at work. As interest in sedentary behavior emerged, research started to focus on the health effects of too much sitting (see Brown et al. 2009). To date, most of this research has focused on outcomes associated with high levels of *total* sitting time, because it is difficult to isolate the long-term effects of sitting in a specific domain, such as at work or while watching television. It is clear, however, that for most people a large proportion of daily sitting is accumulated while at work (Parry and Straker 2013). Relationships between *occupational* sitting time and health outcomes are discussed in this section, beginning with a consideration of the effects of workplace sitting on weight and weight gain. This is important, as weight gain underlies many of today's most common chronic health problems.

Occupational Sitting and Weight Gain

Several of the early Australian sitting studies described previously noted a relationship between occupational sitting time and BMI. For example, the study of workers and mothers with different patterns of paid work reported an association between sitting time and BMI (those sitting for >7.4 hr/day were most likely to be overweight or obese) and reported that full-time working men were twice as likely as either full- or part-time working women to be overweight or obese (Brown, Miller, and Miller 2003). The study of full-time workers in regional Queensland also found that occupational sitting time was associated with overweight and obesity in men, but not in women. The odds of having a BMI > 25 were almost twice as high in men who sat at work for >6 hours per day compared with those who sat <45 minutes per day (after adjusting for age, occupation, and physical activity) (Mummery et al. 2005). Gender differences in overweight and obesity by occupational group are confirmed by secondary analyses of data from the 2005 Australian National Health Survey (Allman-Farinelli et al. 2010). It is important to note, however, that these cross-sectional studies do not tell us anything about the direction of the relationship between sitting and weight. It is plausible that overweight and obese people may choose more sedentary occupations, which may explain the findings of some of these early observational studies.

Data from the Australian Longitudinal Study on Women's Health (ALSWH) also shed light on the relationships among sitting, weight, and weight gain. Although this work does not focus specifically on occupational sitting, 80% of the women in the large ALSWH cohorts of young and middle-aged women are employed, so at least some of their sitting time is accrued through their work. Early prospective analyses of the ALSWH young cohort (age 18-23 at baseline; N = 8,726) data found that women in the lowest tertile of sitting time were least likely to gain weight over 4 years (Ball, Brown, and Crawford 2002). In middle-aged women (age 45-55 at baseline,

N = 8,071), those in the top quintile of sitting time were more likely to gain weight over 5 years (Brown et al. 2005). Analysis of data from these cohorts is complex because sitting time often reflects work status (full-time, part-time) and occupational roles, and it changes over time. In the middle-age cohort, each additional hour of sitting time in 2001 was associated with 110 g (0.22 lbs) and 260 g (0.57 lbs) more weight in overweight (N = 2,712) and obese (N = 1,896) women, respectively. Sitting time was also positively associated with weight change from 2001 to 2007, but only in normal-weight women (N = 3,625) (van Uffelen, Watson, et al. 2010). As with the earlier cross-sectional studies, these concurrent changes in weight and sitting time could also be interpreted as showing that as women gain weight, they tend to choose work that involves more sitting time.

The issue of whether long hours spent sitting at work cause weight gain is complex because those who work long hours may spend less time in other energy-expending activities, such as unpaid household tasks and leisure-time activities. Another analysis of ALSWH data (N = 5,164) showed that young adult women who remain in stable full-time work are more likely to gain weight than part-time workers and that if women move from full-time to part-time work, they are significantly more likely to lose weight. This is one of few papers to demonstrate that working fewer hours reduces the odds of weight gain, but the authors did not consider sitting time in their analyses (Au and Hollingsworth 2011).

It is very difficult to disentangle the effects of sitting from those of other energy-related variables in the weight gain literature. In their 2012 cross-sectional analysis of occupational and leisure-time sitting and obesity in 10,785 adults, Chau and colleagues (2012) found that workers with mostly sitting jobs were more likely to be active in leisure time than those with standing, walking, or heavy labor jobs. Nonetheless, those in high-sitting jobs had higher rates of overweight and obesity than those whose work involved mostly standing. These researchers concluded that leisure-time sitting may be more strongly associated with obesity than occupational sitting.

Occupational Sitting and Other Health Risk Outcomes

In 2010, a systematic review of the effects of self-reported sitting at work and health outcomes assessed the findings of 43 studies with a variety of different designs (21% cross-sectional, 14% case control, 65% prospective) (van Uffelen, Wong, et al. 2010). The outcomes assessed were BMI (12 studies), cancer (17), cardiovascular disease (8), diabetes (4) and mortality (6). In line with the evidence from studies of total sedentary time, sitting time at work was shown to be positively associated with mortality. (Of six prospective studies, four showed a positive association and one reported no relationship. One study found that the more people sat, the lower the chance of death.) Studies of sitting and diabetes were less convincing, although one of the earliest analyses estimated a 5% to 7% increased risk of obesity and diabetes with each 2-hour increment in occupational sitting time (Hu et al. 2003). There was a moderate association between occupational sitting and diabetes in one cross-sectional and one additional prospective study, but another prospective study found no associations. Three prospective studies and five cross-sectional studies also showed a relationship between occupational sitting with CVD, while four cross-sectional studies showed associations with cancer. The possibility of reverse causation cannot be ruled out in these studies.

The authors of this review noted that all the included studies used self-reported measures of occupational sitting (van Uffelen, Wong, et al. 2010). They also observed that most of the studies that assessed BMI as an outcome asked people to report how active they were at work, rather than asking specifically about time spent sitting. Many studies asked about sitting during a usual working day, which may have included leisure-time sitting that occurs in the evening on a work day and not specifically sitting during work hours. Because of the limitations of these types of questions and the heterogeneity of the study designs and exposure measures, the researchers could not make definitive conclusions about the health effects of sitting at work.

Since the publication of that systematic review in 2010, the evidence base has grown, but studies are still plagued by the challenges of measuring occupational sitting and accounting for numerous potential confounders, including what people do when they are not at work. Several large cohort studies are now using more objective measures of occupational sitting, but more years of data collection will be needed before the relationships between occupational sitting and illness can be confirmed with objective data.

One of the earliest prospective studies to introduce objective measures is the AusDiab study, which

WORKPLACE ACTIVITY AND PRESENTEEISM

In recent years, there has been emerging interest in relationships between workplace activity patterns (both physical activity and sitting time) and productivity, absenteeism, and presenteeism. Productivity is most easily assessed in manufacturing industries where the main focus is on creation of merchandise, but to date very little research has examined the relationships between sitting and productivity or between sitting and absenteeism. In contrast, *presenteeism* (defined as the extent to which physical or psychosocial conditions adversely affect the work productivity of people who choose to remain at work even when unwell; Chapman 2005) is gaining the attention of sedentary behavior researchers. However, measurement of presenteeism is in its infancy, making the examination of relationships between sitting time and presenteeism challenging.

A recent study examined detailed activity patterns at work and used scores on the Work Limitations Questionnaire (WLQ) to indicate aspects of presenteeism. The researchers did not demonstrate any relationship between occupational sitting time (measured with accelerometers and diaries) and work limitations, but found that sedentary time before and after work was associated with WLQ index scores (Brown et al. 2013). Difficulties with time management contributed most to this relationship. One hypothesis is that spending long periods of time sitting in transit to and from work may negatively affect perceived limitations at work, which are also potentially enhanced through perceptions of lack of time for unpaid caring and domestic responsibilities.

is tracking the development of diabetes in a large cohort of Australian adults. Although the researchers have not specifically focused on occupational sitting, seminal work from this study has shown that objectively measured total daily sedentary time in working adults is detrimentally associated with cardiometabolic risk markers (see chapters 7, 8, and 9). Importantly, the AusDiab researchers have also shown that interruptions to sedentary time (or breaks in sitting of >1 min) are beneficially associated with these risk markers (Dunstan et al. 2012; Healy et al. 2008). Those who sit for long periods have worse risk factor profiles than those with equivalent sitting time whose sitting time is regularly interrupted.

Although relationships between occupational sitting and back pain have been the subject of a great deal of research in the occupational health and rehabilitation fields, there is currently some debate about whether sitting causes back pain. A 2007 review found that sitting by itself does not cause back pain. However, when sitting is combined with whole-body vibration or awkward posture, the likelihood of back pain increases (Lis et al. 2007). A more recent systematic review did not find high-quality studies that met the criteria for causation in relationships between occupational sitting and lower back pain (Roffey et al. 2010). The evidence on sitting and back pain is presented in more detail in Chapter 11.

Changing Sitting at Work to Improve Health Outcomes

With growing evidence on the health effects of too much sitting at work, there is increasing interest in the efficacy and effectiveness of worksite interventions for reducing occupational sitting time. A 2010 review of workplace sitting time interventions found only six studies, but none of these had reducing sitting time as a primary aim. All the studies used self-reported measures of sitting and only one specifically assessed occupational sitting time. There was no evidence of success in reducing sitting time at work (Chau et al. 2010).

Details of additional studies and more in-depth consideration of the challenges of changing sitting time at work are provided in Chapter 24 of this book. If the deleterious effects of sitting in most workplaces are confirmed, there will be a need for more studies to test the effectiveness of interventions to reduce sitting in different workplace settings. Some studies are currently using computers to prompt standing every 30 minutes, but this does not take into account the wide daily variation in individual sitting patterns. The sitting pad has the potential to provide feedback to employees to interrupt their sitting time in real time and to measure and prompt individualized sitting behavior change in office environments (Ryde et al. 2012). More large-scale trials that aim to reduce and interrupt workplace sitting time over long periods of time are now required.

Summary

Occupations have changed remarkably in the last 100 years, and this change has been accompanied by marked increases in sitting time at work. Although research in this area is in its infancy, innovative measures of occupational sitting time are developing, leading to better understanding of patterns of sitting and activity in workplaces. However, because of the difficulties of isolating the effects of occupational sitting from those of sitting in other domains, understanding the health effects of occupational sitting in the 21st century is a relatively new area of research. Although many workers sit for long periods at work, the patterns of interruptions to occupational sitting time are highly variable. Frequent interruptions may mitigate some of the ailments of chair workers. It is also feasible that physical activity in leisure time may offset the detrimental effects of sitting at work, except in situations of extreme sitting where sitting time is both prolonged and uninterrupted.

From the evidence presented in this chapter, it is clear that there is a need for more measurement studies with different occupational groups (not only office workers) in both developing and developed countries. With rapid technological developments, new objective measures are continually emerging that will help to clarify the variety of sitting patterns in different occupational groups. More details about the durations of sitting bouts and frequency and duration of interruptions to sitting time would help us to better understand the relationships between patterns of occupational sitting time and health outcomes. Clarification of the role of physical activity as a potential moderator of any health effects is also required, especially as published evidence shows that an hour of physical activity each day can attenuate, or even eliminate, the long-term ill-effects of prolonged sitting (Ekelund et al. 2016).

KEY CONCEPTS

- **Occupational epidemiology:** The study of the effects of workplace exposures on patterns of diseases and injuries in the population.
- **Occupational sedentary behavior:** This is conceptualized in this chapter as sitting at work.
- **Occupational sitting time:** The amount of time spent sitting while at work.
- **Sitting pad:** A cushion containing a pressure sensor and switch to determine when someone is sitting, with capability of alerting people when it is time to interrupt their sitting (see Ryde et al. 2012).
- **Sitting patterns:** The total time spent sitting, in association with the duration of bouts of sitting and the number of interruptions or breaks in sitting time each day.
- Although occupations have changed greatly over the last 100 years, with marked increases in sitting at work, patterns of sitting vary enormously across occupations. Sitting time at work is higher in men than in women, and increases with seniority.
- Although most research has been conducted with office and call center workers, other occupational groups may be at increased risk, especially if they are more tied to their seats because of the nature of their work (e.g., drivers) or workplace policies (e.g., production workers). Innovative measures are leading to better understanding of patterns of sitting in a range of occupations.
- Growing epidemiological evidence confirms the ill effects of sitting at work, but these may be different from the effects of transport and TV sitting, which may be characterized by different sitting patterns.

STUDY QUESTIONS

1. How has the changing nature of work in the last 50 to 100 years affected sitting and overall energy expenditure? Which occupational groups have experienced the largest change over time? Which ones now sit most in developed and developing countries?

2. In Western developed countries, how much of the day is typically spent at work, and approximately what proportion of this work time is spent sitting? By how much does sitting time vary in people in "sitting all day" and "on their feet all day" jobs?

3. How do patterns of sitting time vary in different occupations? Approximately how many times per day do office workers interrupt their sitting time?

4. If you were to design a study to measure occupational sitting time, which measure would you use and why?

5. What health risk factors have been associated with sitting at work?

6. How do occupational status and sitting time influence weight gain?

7. How strong is the evidence for a prospective association between sitting and diabetes?

8. Why might the health effects of sitting at work be different from those of travel-related and leisure-time sitting?

I am extremely fortunate to have worked with doctoral students Helen Brown, Gemma Ryde, Alessandro Suppini, and Sarah Wane, who contributed to the ideas and work presented in this chapter. My thanks, too, to Nick Gilson and others who have shaped the occupational sitting work we are doing at the Centre for Research on Exercise, Physical Activity and Health at the University of Queensland.

CHAPTER 20

SEDENTARY BEHAVIOR OF OLDER ADULTS

Jorge A. Banda, PhD; Sandra J. Winter, PhD; and Abby C. King, PhD

The reader will gain an overview of the complex relationship between sedentary behavior and older adult health and will encounter novel public health strategies aimed at reducing sedentary behavior in this unique population. By the end of this chapter, the reader should be able to do the following:

▸ Define sedentary behavior in older adults and its potential effects on health, function, and well-being

▸ Describe a conceptual model of sedentary behavior in older adults

▸ Explain the putative drivers of sedentary behavior in older adults

▸ Identify the array of contexts in which older adults are sedentary

▸ Highlight potentially useful interventions aimed at decreasing sedentary activity in older adults

A large body of epidemiological research has identified sedentary behavior (SB) as an important determinant of health independent of physical activity (PA) (Thorp et al. 2011). National surveillance data demonstrate that older adults (defined here as ≥60 years) are disproportionately affected by SB, with the 2003-2004 National Health and Nutrition Examination Survey (NHANES) data showing that older adults engage in greater amounts of accelerometer-measured SB than any other age group (Matthews et al. 2008). Based on 2003-2006 NHANES data, adults aged 60 years and older engaged in 8.5 hours per day of accelerometer-measured SB (Evenson, Buchner, and Morland 2012). Despite being a high-risk group for this health behavior, older adults are underrepresented in the current literature; few studies have examined determinants of SB specific to older adults or tested the efficacy of intervention efforts in this age group.

An ecological model of SB for adults has been proposed that has identified determinants of SB, described contexts in which SB takes place, and proposed interventions for reducing SB in adults (Owen et al. 2011). Although this model provides an important heuristic for the field, it is important to acknowledge that older adults face life transitions (e.g., retirement) and changes in physical and mental health that are typically not observed in other populations. Current research suggests that older adults are driven toward SB in ways that are different and unique from younger adults. The contexts in which older adults are sedentary may also differ. It is therefore worthwhile to consider how models of SB might best be adapted to the circumstances of the older adult population. Thus, we present a conceptual model of SB specific to older adults in order to do the following:

1. Highlight putative factors surrounding older adults' SB

2. Guide research examining determinants of SB and the development of interventions for this population

Our conceptual model of SB for older adults (see figure 20.1) consists of three sections: putative drivers of SB, possible contexts of SB, and potential outcomes of SB. Due to the limited research available in older adults, support for our conceptual model is also derived from the adult SB literature, the adult PA literature, and our extensive experience working with older adults in research and community settings.

Measuring Sedentary Behavior in Older Adults

A continuum of SB through PA that may have particular relevance for older adults is presented in figure 20.2. Although physical inactivity and SB are often used interchangeably, they have been increasingly acknowledged to be, in a number of respects, distinct behaviors. Physical inactivity often is defined as not meeting current national guidelines for PA (U.S. Department of Health and Human Services 2008), and SB is often defined as activity that results in low energy expenditure (≤1.5 METs) (Tremblay et al. 2010). Sedentary behavior can also differ from physical inactivity with regard to measurement and intervention approaches as well as the physiological effects it places on the body (Tremblay et al. 2010).

Sleep presents some complexities related to SB. Tremblay and colleagues (2010) note that sleep should not be considered SB, arguing that it is a separate behavior with different physiological effects on the body. However, they argue that unintentional sleep (e.g., daytime napping) can be considered SB. The latter issue is of particular relevance for older adults, who can engage in significant amounts of napping throughout the day (Foley et al. 2007).

Sedentary behavior can be characterized by the acronym SITT: sedentary behavior frequency (e.g., number of bouts of a certain duration), interruptions (e.g., standing up while viewing television), time (e.g., duration of television viewing), and type (e.g., reading a book, using a computer) (Tremblay et al. 2010). These characteristics play an important role both with respect to more clearly defining the relations between sedentary activity and health outcomes, as well as in fashioning appropriate interventions, and should be incorporated into measures of SB. For example, increased breaks in accelerometer-measured SB have been associated with improvements in cardiometabolic health independent of total sedentary time and moderate- to vigorous-intensity PA in adults (Healy et al. 2008). In addition, different types of sedentary activities can have different cognitive effects in older adults; computer use, for example, has been associated with better cognitive outcomes than television viewing (Kesse-Guyot et al. 2012).

Sedentary behavior occurs throughout the day in a variety of contexts (e.g., work, leisure, and transport) and through a range of activities (e.g.,

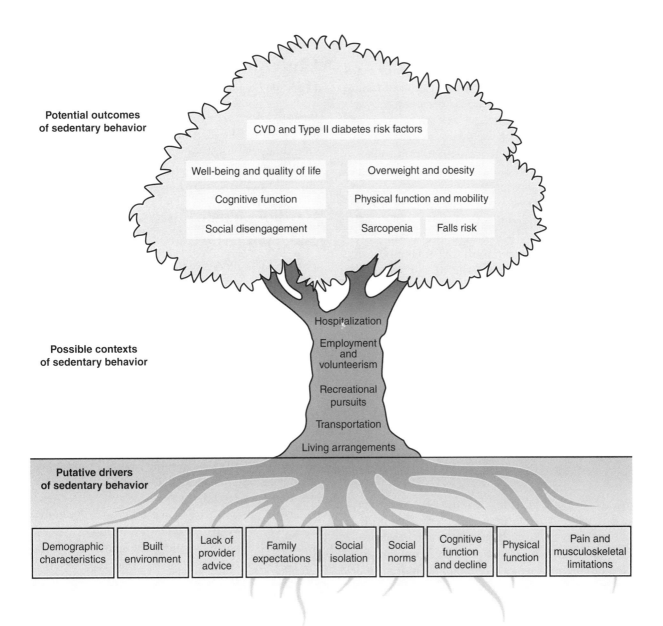

Figure 20.1 Conceptual model of sedentary behavior in older adults.

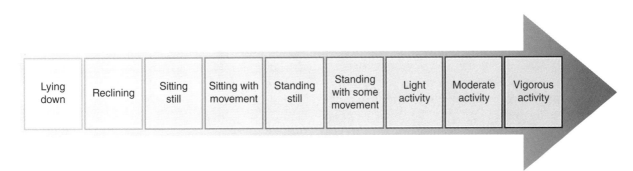

Figure 20.2 Continuum of sedentary behavior and physical activity.

Based on Tremblay et al. 2010.

viewing television, using a computer, driving). As a result, measuring SB in a reliable, valid way is challenging, particularly among older adults who may be affected to a greater degree by recall bias when self-reporting SB due to memory loss or declining cognitive function. Although accelerometers are increasingly being used to objectively measure SB, currently there are limitations related to using accelerometers to characterize SBs in older adults. For example, a majority of the accelerometer cut points used to determine the amount of time spent in different activity intensities were developed on young, healthy populations, offering little generalizability to older adults. This is important because research has shown that as adults age and experience decreases in cardiorespiratory fitness, accelerometer cut points are poorly correlated with effort and perceived exertion (Evenson, Buchner, and Morland 2012). In addition, accelerometers are currently unable to distinguish among lying, reclining, sitting, or standing—behaviors that may be particularly important to differentiate in older populations (Tremblay et al. 2010). Further research validating the use of accelerometer cut points to determine SB in older adults is strongly warranted.

As reflected in figure 20.2, differentiating between various points along the continuum of SBs and their relations with outcomes of interest may be particularly important for older populations, who tend to spend a disproportionate amount of their day at the lower end of this continuum. For example, it is unclear for older adults as well as other age groups whether breaking up extended bouts of sedentary time by simply standing (as opposed to moving to even a small degree) is sufficient to reduce the negative physiological effects of SB. For older adults, it would also be important to differentiate between any accumulated benefits of moving up this continuum—for example, by replacing daytime napping or lying down with reclining or reclining with sitting.

Related to this issue is the importance of considering the relative versus absolute levels of energy expenditure and other physiological processes of particular relevance to older adults relative to other age groups. Given the substantial heterogeneity of the older adult population in relation to fitness, function, and health, definitional and measurement issues in this area become more challenging, and are worthy of specific attention.

Health and Functional Outcomes of Sedentary Behavior

Potential outcomes linked with SB in older adults are presented in figure 20.1. Although this is not an exhaustive list of outcomes, it is representative of different types of key health outcomes in older adults (e.g., physical, cognitive).

Cardiovascular Disease and Type 2 Diabetes Risk Factors

The available literature indicates that objective and self-report measures of SB are associated with risk factors for cardiovascular disease and type 2 diabetes in older adults. A cross-sectional study of older adults (≥65 years) using the 2003-2006 NHANES data found a significant positive association between accelerometer-measured SB and C-reactive protein and plasma glucose (Gennuso et al. 2013). Similar results were observed in a cross-sectional study of older adults (≥60 years) from a population-based sample in England, where accelerometer-measured SB and total self-report leisure-time SB were significantly positively associated with the prevalence of diabetes (Stamatakis et al. 2012). In addition, a cross-sectional study of older adults (≥60 years) from a population-based survey in Australia found a significant positive association in men between overall self-reported sitting time and trigylceride levels, HDL-cholesterol levels, and the presence of metabolic syndrome, and a significant positive association in women between overall self-reported sitting time and trigylceride levels and the presence of metabolic syndrome (Gardiner, Healy, et al. 2011).

Physical Function and Mobility

The available literature indicates that increased SB is associated with reduced physical function in older adults. A cross-sectional study of older adults (≥65 years) using 2003-2006 NHANES data found a significant positive association between accelerometer-measured SB and number of functional limitations (Gennuso et al. 2013). Similarly, a cross-sectional study of older adults (≥65 years) from a population-based sample in Canada found that less self-reported sedentary time was significantly associated with successful physical aging (i.e., physical function) (Dogra and Stathokostas

2012). In addition, a study using data from the Women's Health Initiative found that older women (50-79 years at baseline) who self-reported greater amounts of sedentary time were significantly more likely to report lower physical function at follow-up (mean follow-up length = 12.3 years) (Seguin et al. 2012).

Sarcopenia

The literature has demonstrated that PA is important for the prevention of sarcopenia (i.e., the degenerative loss of skeletal muscle mass, strength, and quality associated with aging) among older adults (Wang and Bai 2012). Although limited, evidence exists that SB may result in sarcopenia in older adults. An experimental study among 11 healthy older adults (mean age = 67 years) found that 10 days of bed rest resulted in significant decreases in leg strength and power (Kortebein et al. 2008). In addition, a recent cross-sectional study among older adults (mean age = 79 years) found that accelerometer-measured SB was significantly negatively associated with leg strength and muscle mechanical quality among men (Chastin et al. 2012).

Falls Risk

The literature examining the effect of SB on falls suggests that there may be an important link between the two that deserves further systematic investigation. For example, a meta-analysis of observational studies found that increased PA was significantly associated with a reduction in falls in older adults, particulary falls with injuries (Thibaud et al. 2012). Since falls are a major public health concern among older adults, examining the effect of SB on the risk of falling is an important research priority.

Overweight and Obesity

The available literature demonstrates that SB is positively associated with body weight and body composition in older adults. A cross-sectional study of older adults (≥65 years) using 2003-2006 NHANES data found significant positive associations between accelerometer-measured SB and body weight, BMI, and waist circumference (Gennuso et al. 2013). Similar significant results have been observed in population-based cross-sectional studies of older adults in England (Stamatakis et al. 2012) and Australia (Gardiner, Healy, et al. 2011).

Cognitive Function

The literature examining the effect of SB on cognitive function is limited. However, results from the 2008 PA Guidelines Committee Report indicate that PA delays the incidence of dementia and the onset of cognitive decline associated with aging (Physical Activity Guidelines Advisory Committee 2008). A prospective study of older women (70-81 years) using Nurses' Health Study data found that higher levels of long-term PA were significantly associated with higher levels of cognitive function and less cognitive decline (Weuve et al. 2004). A cross-sectional study of older adults (50-85 years) in a population-based study in China found a significant dose–response relationship between PA and cognitive function (Xu et al. 2011). Similar results were found in a meta-analysis of prospective studies, where older adults who engaged in low to moderate PA levels (35% reduced risk) and high PA levels (38% reduced risk) were significantly protected against cognitive impairment (PA was categorized as low, moderate, and high from PA volume and intensity) (Sofi et al. 2011).

Thus, it is plausible that decreasing SB may be associated with more favorable cognitive function outcomes as people age. Apropo to this supposition, a cross-sectional study of older adults (mean age = 66 years) in a population-based study in France found that higher television use was significantly associated with lower executive functioning (Kesse-Guyot et al. 2012). However, this study demonstrated the differential effects of specific sedentary activities on cognitive function, showing that increased computer use was significantly associated with better verbal memory and executive functioning (Kesse-Guyot et al. 2012). These results suggest that certain types of sedentary activities, particularly those involving active cognitive engagement (e.g., crossword puzzles, computer use) or social engagement, may benefit cognitive function. Because cognitive function is an important health outcome in older adults, further research is recommended examining the effects of different types and volumes of SB on cognitive function among older adults. It would also be worthwhile to explore the different mechanisms through which SB can affect cognitive function and decline.

Social Disengagement

Similar to cognitive function, it is likely that different types of SB can have different effects on older adults' levels of social disengagement. In a cross-sectional study of older adults (≥65 years) representing a population-based Canadian sample, decreased self-reported sitting time was significantly associated with successful sociological aging (i.e., a strong sense of belonging and low levels of loneliness) (Dogra and Stathokostas 2012). In contrast to this finding, social engagement through primarily sedentary activities (e.g., bingo and other sedentary group activities) may have positive relations with health.

A prospective study of older adults in the United States (baseline mean age = 79 years) found that sedentary leisure activities such as playing board games and playing a musical instrument (which often involve social engagment with others) were significantly associated with a reduced risk of dementia (74% and 69% risk reduction, respectively) at follow-up (median follow-up = 5 years) (Verghese et al. 2003). In addition, a prospective study of older adults in Sweden (baseline mean age = 81 years) found that engaging in social activities (e.g., attending the theatre, concerts, or art exhibits; playing cards or other games; participating in social groups) was significantly associated with a reduced risk of dementia at follow-up (mean follow-up = 6 years) (Wang et al. 2002). Because social disengagement is an important area of study for older adults, we recommend that future research examine the effect of sedentry behavior on social disengagement and whether differential effects exist by type of sedentary behavior (e.g., viewing television, using a computer for social networking purposes, participating in group-based sedentary recreational activities).

Well-Being and Quality of Life

A literature review found that a high level of television viewing was associated with lower psychologocial well-being in adults (Rhodes, Mark, and Temmel 2012). Results from a prospective study of older adults in Spain (baseline mean age = 70 years) found that decreased sitting time was associated with favorable changes in six components of health-related quality of life (i.e., physical functioning, physical role, bodily pain, vitality, social functioning, and mental health) at follow-up (mean follow-up = 6 years) (Balboa-Castillo et al. 2011). Similar results were found in a prospective study of Australian adults, where increased SB was significantly associated with declines in physical and mental health–related quality of life (Buckley et al. 2013).

Putative Drivers of Sedentary Behavior

As shown in figure 20.1, a number of factors can affect prolonged SB in older adults. Given that the ways in which older adults are influenced toward SB may differ from those experienced by younger adults, the following sections highlight several potential drivers of relevance to older populations.

Demographic Characteristics

Prevalence data among adults and older adults indicate that demographic characteristics such as gender, race/ethnicity, and socioeconomic status have the potential to influence SB among older adults (Evenson, Buchner, and Morland 2012; King et al. 2010). Although the mechanisms through

RECOMMENDATIONS FOR FUTURE RESEARCH

In addition to conducting additional research on the effects of SB on these health, functioning, and well-being outcomes in older adults, we recommend that future researchers do the following:

1. Examine whether relations between SB and health outcomes differ for self-reported versus objective measures of SB

2. Examine the dose–response relationship between SB and these outcomes

3. Explore how different types of SB (e.g., viewing television, using a computer) are associated with different outcomes

4. Investigate how demographic characteristics (e.g., age and gender) and other putative drivers of SB affect the relations between SB and these different outcomes

which demographic characteristics influence SB are not fully understood, demographic characteristics may interact with or reflect more basic underlying putative drivers influencing SB. For example, lower-income older adults have been found to have higher levels of functional impairment relative to their more affluent peers, which may drive more types of SB (Chen et al. 2012). Additional research to better understand the mechanisms underlying the associations between demographic characteristics and SB would benefit the field as a whole.

Built Environment

Although the evidence base in older adults is limited, research in younger adults indicates that the built environment may have a strong influence on SB. A cross-sectional study of adults (mean age = 45 years) from the Neighborhood Quality of Life Study found that lower neighborhood walkability was significantly associated with more self-reported television viewing and more driving time (i.e., sitting time) (Kozo et al. 2012). Particularly relevant to older adults as they transition to retirement are results from a longitudinal study in Australia (45% of the sample was 51-70 years of age at baseline), which found a significant interaction between neighborhood walkability and work status on television viewing (Ding et al. 2012). This study found that among adults not working (e.g., retired), living in a highly walkable neighborhood was associated with 23% less television viewing at a 4-year follow-up.

It is important to note that environmental characteristics other than objectively measured neighborhood walkability can influence SB. Results from a nationally representative sample of adults in the United States (mean age = 48.2 years) found that perceived aspects of neighborhood environments were associated with high levels of television viewing, including the presence of heavy traffic and crime, lack of neighborhood lighting, unattractive scenery, and lack of other people walking in the neighborhood (King et al. 2010). These results are important because they suggest that negative perceptions of their neighborhood may keep people in their homes, where sedentary activities are more likely. Similar results were found in a cross-sectional study of African-American adults in Texas, where concerns with litter, walking after dark, and lack of places to shop were associated with more television viewing in women (Strong et al. 2013). Since a majority of the built environment and SB literature has been conducted with younger adults, we recommend further research to examine how characteristics (both objectively measured and perceived) such as neighborhood walkability and pedestrian-friendly elements (e.g., lighting, presence and quality of sidewalks, pedestrian crossing aides) are associated with older adult SB.

Lack of Provider Advice

Health care providers can be an important source of PA advice for older adults (King and Guralnik 2010). As a result, they can play an influential role in public health strategies for promoting PA. Important objectives of Healthy People 2020 (U.S. Department of Health and Human Services 2013) and the American College of Sports Medicine's Exercise is Medicine initiative (American College of Sports Medicine 2013) are to increase the proportion of health care provider visits that include counseling or education related to PA.

Discussing SB can be a natural extension of the health advice and education health provider offices are currently providing; this is particularly true given the frequency of older adult visits to their health providers. Data from the 2010 National Health Interview Survey show that 42% of 65- to 74-year-olds, 33% of 75- to 84-year-olds, and 29% of adults 85 years or older received recommendations related to exercise or PA from a physician or other health care provider (Barnes and Schoenborn 2012). For older adults, targeting SB may be easier than enacting PA regimens, and is therefore well worth exploring.

Physical and Cognitive Function or Decline

Similar to the bidirectional relationships among health, function, and PA (King and Guralnik 2010), we hypothesize that there is a bidirectional relationship between SB and physical and cognitive function or decline in older adults. As discussed in this chapter, SB is associated with functional impairments in older adults. However, due to the bidirectional relationship between SB and function, it is likely that older adults with greater functional limitations are more likely to be sedentary than older adults with fewer such limitations, potentially creating a vicious downward cycle between function and SB. Both aspects of this bidirectional relationship merit further study.

Social Isolation

The literature indicates that social isolation and loneliness are associated with decreased PA in older adults (Hawkley, Thisted, and Cacioppo 2009; Shankar et al. 2011). Building on this research, social isolation may be an important driver of SB. Results from a longitudinal, nationally representative cohort of U.S. older adults (mean age = 71 years) provide support for this hypothesis (Perissinotto, Stijacic Cenzer, and Covinsky 2012). In this study, lonely older adults were significantly more likely to experience a decline in daily living activities, develop difficulties with upper extremity tasks, experience a decline in mobility, and experience difficulty climbing stairs. These decreases in physical function are important because they can lead to increased SB. As a result, preventing social isolation in older adults may be an important method of preventing functional limitations and SB. One approach to doing this is through interventions aimed at increasing social engagement through volunteerism and other generative roles (King and Guralnik 2010).

Pain or Musculoskeletal Limitations

Little doubt exists that increased pain and musculoskeletal limitations in older adults can influence SB. Support for this association comes from research demonstrating that pain is associated with decreased PA and less healthful aging in older adults. Results from a population-based cohort study of adults (25-65 years) in England found that, compared to adults free of chronic widespread pain at baseline, adults with chronic pain engaged in significantly less PA at a 32-month follow-up (McBeth et al. 2010). In addition, results from a population-based cohort study of adults (≥50 years) in the United Kingdom found that the onset of widespread musculoskeletal pain was significantly associated with a decrease in healthy aging (i.e., an index of physical, biomedical, psychosocial, and social factors) at a 6-year follow-up (Wilkie, Tajar, and McBeth 2013). It is a reasonable extension to posit that increased pain and musculoskeletal limitations can likely result in increased SB among older adults.

Family Expectations and Social Norms

A large segment of the older adult population experiences the demands of family roles and expectations related to informal caregiving (often of spouses with infirmities) as well as social norms that may strongly influence SB. Results from a trial in the United States from the National Heart, Lung, and Blood Institute found that family caregivers (mean age = 50 years) of cardiac patients were significantly more likely to be less physically active than noncaregivers (Aggarwal et al. 2009). Similarly, in a prospective cohort study of older adults in the United States (mean age = 81 years) in which poorer self-rated health was significantly associated with a decline in walking speed (i.e., an important predictor of disability) among women, a greater involvement in family caregiving exacerbated the decline in walking speed (Ashburner et al. 2011). Cultural factors are also associated with reduced levels of PA among older adults, including a lack of culturally appropriate programs and role models that promote PA, language barriers, and normative duties related to the home and family (King and King 2010). Whether these factors are associated with SB among older adults is relatively unknown, and should be explored in additional research.

Possible Contexts of Sedentary Behavior

A variety of contexts can set the stage for prolonged SB that can impair health and function. Several such contexts that are particularly germane to older adults are highlighted in the following sections.

Hospitalization

Hospitals can be a pernicious contextual driver of SB among older adults, since hospitalization is a critical event in many older adults' lives. Despite being ambulatory prior to admission and the presence of health care provider orders to engage in out-of-bed activities, older patients typically spend the majority of their hospitalization time being sedentary (e.g., sitting or lying in a bed or chair) (Brown et al. 2009). These results are important because research has shown that hospitalized older adults are typically discharged with worsened levels of physical function, despite the successful treatment of the illness that caused them to be hospitalized (Covinsky et al. 2003; Covinsky, Pierluissi, and Johnston 2011).

As discussed earlier in this chapter, decreased physical function can be a strong influence on SB in older adults. Unfortunately, hospitalization may result not only in immediate sedentariness, but in longer-term SB as well. Based on these observations, it would be worthwhile to examine the effect of hospitalization on subsequent SB among older adults, in concert with intervention efforts to reduce SB in hospitals and on discharge. Because increased PA is associated with a lower probability of a hospital stay as well as a reduced number of days spent in the hospital (Sari 2010), promoting PA in conjunction with less SB may be an effective method.

Living Arrangements

Although the literature exploring associations between senior living arrangements and SB is limited, the available evidence indicates that living arrangements can have a large effect on SB. Data from a longitudinal multilevel study among Australian adults (40-65 years) found that adults who were single and living alone spent more time sitting as part of television viewing, computer use, and general leisure activities than adults who were single and living with others or who were living with a significant other (Burton et al. 2012). Similar results were found in a population-based study of Japanese older adults (65-74 years), where older adults living alone were more likely to engage in prolonged television viewing (>2 hr/day) than older adults living with others (Kikuchi et al. 2013). Future research is needed to determine the mechanism (e.g., social isolation, loneliness, the physical layout of the living space, fewer opportunities to engage in more active pursuits) through which living arrangements influence SB. Further research is also needed to determine how other common living arrangements among older adults (e.g., congregate housing, living in an extended family situation) affect SB.

Employment and Volunteerism

The literature indicates that despite having greater control over their time, retired adults engage in more SB than working adults of similar age. Results from a nationally representative sample of U.S. adults (≥20 years) found that 74.2% of retired adults viewed television for more than 2 hours per day, compared to 69.6% of unemployed, 56.2% of part-time employed, and 51.1% of full-time employed adults (Bowman 2006). Similar results were found in a separate population-based longitudinal study of U.S. adults (45-64 years): Adults who retired were more likely to increase their television viewing time relative to adults who continued to work through a 6-year follow-up (Evenson et al. 2002).

Although research in this area is limited, results from intervention trials indicate that volunteering can be an effective method for increasing PA among older adults (Fried et al. 2004). These results can be extended to SB, suggesting that volunteering could be used as a method for not only increasing PA, but decreasing SB as well. Examining mechanisms through which retirement results in increased SB, developing effective interventions for decreasing SB and promoting PA as older adults transition into retirement, and examining the potential of volunteering to decrease SB among retirees are important areas of future research.

Recreational Pursuits

Current evidence indicates that older adults engage in a number of leisure-time sedentary activities, including viewing television, sitting and socializing, engaging in hobbies, using a computer, listening to music, reading, driving, and talking on the telephone (Clark et al. 2009; Lee and King 2003). This observation notwithstanding, prevalence data indicate that older adults spend a preponderance of their time viewing television. Data from a nationally representative sample of U.S. adults found that 66- to 75-year-olds spent more than 25% of their day viewing television and adults aged 76 years and older spent more than 30% of their day viewing television (Depp et al. 2010).

An interesting finding from the study by Depp and colleagues (2010) is that despite engaging in three times more television viewing than younger adults, older adults (>65 years) enjoyed television less. Missing from much of this research is the anecdotally reported multitasking that can accompany television viewing among older adults and other populations. That is, older adults may be engaging in other types of tasks while the television is on. In addition, little is known about the amount of time older adults spend in different types of sedentary activities in addition to television viewing (e.g., reading, socializing, using a computer), given that, to date, most surveillance systems and research publications focus on children and younger adults.

Transportation

Although limited primarily to younger adults, the literature indicates that urban design characteristics can have a large effect on the amount of time older adults spend traveling in automobiles (i.e., sitting time). A cross-sectional study of adults (mean age = 45 years) from the Neighborhood Quality of Life Study found that lower neighborhood walkability was significantly associated with increased driving time (Kozo et al. 2012). Similar results were found in the pooled analysis of adults (20-65 years) living in the United States, Australia, and Belgium; higher levels of land use mix diversity, walking and cycling facilities, traffic safety, and the absence of cul-de-sacs were significantly associated with less time spent in motorized transport (Van Dyck et al. 2012). Research has also shown that limited transportation options can be associated with increased SB among older adults. Results from a population-based survey of Japanese older adults (65-74 years) found that nondriving status among women was significantly associated with prolonged television viewing (>2 hr/day) (Kikuchi et al. 2013). The authors hypothesized that the lack of convenient transportation options available to these older adults hindered them from leaving their homes, resulting in increased sedentary activities like television viewing. Additional research would be useful in this area.

Interventions Aimed at Reducing Sedentary Behavior

The intervention literature among older adults is limited. We identified seven interventions that targeted decreases in SB or increases in PA, but also examined changes in SB as a secondary outcome. Of these seven interventions, five were pilot studies (De Greef et al. 2010; Fitzsimons et al. 2013; Gardiner, Eakin, et al. 2011; Hawkes et al. 2009; Steeves et al. 2012) and two used a single-arm pretest–posttest design (Gardiner, Eakin, et al. 2011; Hawkes et al. 2009). One intervention tested the effects of stepping in place during television commercials (Steeves et al. 2012), while the other interventions relied on traditional approaches, including in-person and telephone-based behavioral intervention strategies and the use of self-monitoring and feedback (De Greef et al. 2010; De Greef et al. 2011; Fitzsimons et al. 2013; Gardiner, Eakin, et al. 2011; Hawkes et al. 2009; Lee and King 2003). Although these interventions make important contributions to the literature and have had success in reducing SB as a primary or secondary outcome, comprehensive public health approaches are needed to decrease SB among older adults on a population level.

The older adult SB literature has generally followed the prevailing problem-oriented research paradigm (Robinson 2012), focusing primarily on the identification of determinants and health outcomes of SB. Although this research has provided some useful insights into older adult SB, we advocate for a more solution-oriented research approach, which has greater potential to inform policy and practice decisions (Robinson 2012). The following are suggestions for interventions that can be used to stimulate a solution-oriented approach to designing, evaluating, and implementing interventions for older adults at the individual, community, and population levels.

Use Health-Promoting Information Technology

The use of technology is pervasive in our society and is a promising pathway for providing low-cost, convenient, individually tailored, and evidence-based health interventions (Atienza et al. 2007). Older adults are increasingly using technology: 53% of U.S. adults aged 65 years and older use the Internet or e-mail and 69% own a cell phone (Zickuhr and Madden 2012). Previous research targeting PA promotion in older adults has used automated telephone-linked computer (interactive voice response) systems (King et al. 2007), personal digital assistants (King et al. 2008), embodied conversational agents (King et al. 2013), web-based platforms (Irvine et al. 2013), and smartphone applications (King et al. 2012). These technologies can also be used to reduce SB.

Promote Volunteerism

In 2015, approximately 11 million volunteers in the United States were aged 65 years and older (U.S. Department of Labor 2015). Volunteering has been associated with improvement in physical and mental health (U.S. Department of Health and Human Services 2011). Experience Corps is a nonprofit organization that connects older adults with school-aged children for the purposes of improving child academic outcomes. This program has been successful in increasing not only the social and cognitive activities of older adults, but also PA in older adults (Fried et al. 2004). This model could be replicated in other settings (e.g., religious institutions, social service organizations, hospitals, and civic and arts organizations) and focused more directly on reducing SB by getting older adults out of their homes and engaged in more social and physical activities throughout the day.

Enhance Interior Design

Universal design is a concept that simplifies the environment to promote functional independence and safety for everyone regardless of age or disability. Design elements that make it easier for older adults to see include increased visual contrast among floors, walls, doorways, and furniture; more lighting, including natural lighting; and glare-reduction strategies (Bowerman 2006). Design elements that improve walkability include corridors that have continuous and graspable handrails, carpeted floors and seating, the presence of an elevator, conveniently located activity spaces and restrooms, and the presence of aesthetic features such as artwork, plants, and windows with views (Lu et al. 2011).

Develop Transportation Solutions

As discussed earlier in this chapter, older adults with limited transportation options may be more likely to stay home and engage in SB activities. Options to increase transportation for older adults include safe driving programs, volunteer driver programs, paratransit services (e.g., wheelchair accessibility), door-to-door escort services, transportation voucher programs (i.e., fare assistance programs), and travel training (National Center on Senior Transportation, n.d.). An example of travel training is the Mobility Ambassadors program in San Mateo County, California. This program is a peer-driven initiative that shows older adults and people with disabilities how to use public transport through educational presentations, group and one-on-one rider training, and organized group trips. In addition, older adults partner with "mobility ambassadors" to learn how to use route maps and schedules, plan which bus stops to use, where to transfer, and what and how to pay (Senior Mobility Initiative 2013).

Improve Built Environments

Older adults living in low-walkability neighborhoods (including neighborhoods with high traffic and crime, poor neighborhood lighting, unattractive scenery, litter, and few places to shop) are more likely to engage in SB (e.g., watch television). Although organizations such as Smart Growth America (www.smartgrowthamerica.org) and Active Living Research (www.activelivingresearch.org) advocate for environmental changes, older adults can also play a role. Applications of a citizen scientist model have shown that older adults can be important data gatherers about features of their environment that may hinder or facilitate healthful active living. Using such data, older adults can be powerful advocates for change in their communities (Buman et al. 2013).

Reduce Television Viewing

The strategies that are employed in children to reduce television viewing (e.g., parental rules, electronic screen time controllers) cannot readily be translated for older adults. However, many of the public health strategies discussed previously may result in reduced television viewing among older adults. In addition, public awareness campaigns may be an important population-level approach to reducing television viewing in this population segment. Mass media campaigns specifically targeted at an older adult population that provide compelling messages concerning the negative effects of excessive television viewing for seniors may be useful. These campaigns should educate older adults on the potential links between excessive sitting and decrements to health and functioning, provide information about alternatives to television watching, reduce barriers to alternative activities that are more socially and physically engaging, and recommend no more than 2 hours per day of television. Further research is needed to identify feasible and effective strategies for accomplishing this.

Prevent Falls

Prevalence data demonstrate that one-third of adults aged 65 years and older fall each year, and falls are the leading cause of injury and death in older adults (Centers for Disease Control and Prevention 2012). In 2010, more than 2 million older adults were treated in emergency departments for nonfatal fall-related injuries (Centers for Disease Control and Prevention 2012). Fear of falling has been associated with the avoidance of PA in older adults (Kempen et al. 2009). Interventions that can be used to reduce falls include regular PA, review of medication side effects that may increase the likelihood of dizziness, regular eye exams, and improvements in home safety (Centers for Disease Control and Prevention 2012). In addition, people who have fallen should be provided with effective treatment, rehabilitation, and long-term support to reduce the likelihood of future falls, including exercise programs that target balance, strength, and endurance (National Collaborating Centre for Nursing and Supportive Care 2004).

Use Stealth Interventions

Stealth interventions include integrating health promotion efforts with social movements that are highly motivating to different segments of the population (Robinson 2010). In these interventions, people are motivated to change their health behaviors through the objectives of the movement or cause, not for the purposes of improving health per se, with benefits to health being seen as potential side effects (Robinson 2010). Environmental sustainability and climate change may be a powerful stealth intervention for older adults that encourages older adults to engage in active transportation and municipalities to improve mass transit systems and community walkability (Egger 2007; Robinson 2010). Social engagement is another potential stealth intervention for reducing SB in older adults (King and Guralnik 2010), with programs such as Experience Corps (Fried et al. 2004) demonstrating that volunteering can result in significant increases in PA in older adults.

Promote Education and Skills Building

At the individual level, the behavior-change concepts that have been applied to promoting PA, such as goal setting, social support, self-efficacy, active problem solving around barriers, and self-monitoring, can also be used to decrease SB in older adults. At the population level, increased education regarding the substantial detrimental effects of SB in all age groups, but particularly in older adults, is required. A useful framework for such a population-level approach is to adapt the MPOWER concept initially developed by the World Health Organization to reduce smoking for the reduction of SB (Wen and Wu 2012). Strategies for reducing SB on a population level would include improving measurement and surveillance of SB, providing opportunities for older adults to be physically active in safe environments, conducting mass media campaigns that highlight the particular detriments of SB for older adults, and encouraging health care providers to query their patients about SB and make appropriate recommendations for decreasing SB.

Summary

Sedentary behavior in older adults is an important but understudied public health issue. The evidence that does exist suggests that increased time in SB by older adults is associated with a number of health-compromising conditions. This chapter describes how the definition and measurement of SB in older adults may differ from other age groups. In addition, it presents a conceptual model of SB for older adults that describes the putative drivers, possible contexts, and potential outcomes of SB in older adults. Further research is needed in the areas of measuring SB, studying the effects of SB characteristics (i.e., frequency, interruptions, time, and type) on health outcomes, and investigating interactions between SB drivers and health outcomes. A solution-oriented research approach that targets people within neighborhoods and communities is advocated.

KEY CONCEPTS

‣ **Continuum of SB and PA:** A continuum of movement that displays incremental increases in energy expenditure from lying down to vigorous activity.

‣ **Putative drivers of SB:** Factors that can affect prolonged SB in older adults. These include demographic characteristics, built environment, lack of provider advice, family expectations, social isolation, social norms, cognitive function or decline, physical function, and pain or musculoskeletal limitations.

‣ **Sarcopenia:** The degenerative loss of skeletal muscle mass, strength, and quality associated with aging.

‣ **SITT:** An acronym used to characterize SB, including SB frequency, interruptions, time, and type.

‣ Sedentary behavior in older adults differs in important ways from sedentary behavior in other age groups and warrants specific, focused attention.

‣ Older adults engage in more sedentary behavior than other age groups and are at greater risk for poorer cognitive, social, and physical outcomes.

‣ A multifaceted solution-oriented approach to the design and implementation of interventions for reducing sedentary behavior in older adults is needed.

STUDY QUESTIONS

1. Define physical inactivity and sedentary behavior.
2. Describe limitations of using accelerometry to measure activity in older adults.
3. Describe the continuum of sedentary behavior through physical activity.
4. Discuss how the sedentary behavior–physical activity continuum may be different in older adults compared to younger adults.
5. Describe three putative drivers of sedentary behavior in older adults.
6. Describe three possible contexts of sedentary behavior in older adults.
7. Describe three potential outcomes of sedentary behavior in older adults.
8. Discuss why health care provider advice regarding reducing sedentary behavior may be particularly useful in achieving behavior change in older adults.
9. Discuss key life transitions and changes in older age that may result in increased sedentary behavior.
10. Describe stealth interventions that can be used to reduce sedentary behavior in older adults.

This work was supported in part by PHS grant #T32HL007034 (for Banda and Winter) and grant #R01HL109222 (King). We would like to thank Dr. William L. Haskell for his advice and expertise during the writing of this chapter.

CHAPTER 21

SEDENTARY BEHAVIOR IN RACIAL/ETHNIC MINORITY GROUPS

Melicia C. Whitt-Glover, PhD; and Tyrone G. Ceaser, PhD

The reader will gain an overview of definitions of sedentary behavior and physical inactivity and the factors associated with and consequences of these behaviors. By the end of this chapter, the reader should be able to do the following:

▶ Understand how the terms *sedentary* and *physically inactive* are defined in data sets estimating sedentary behavior

▶ Understand the prevalence of sedentary behavior among racial/ethnic minorities in the United States

▶ Identify at least three factors that are correlated with sedentary behavior among racial/ethnic minorities in the United States

▶ Identify health-related consequences of sedentary behavior

▶ Identify strategies that have been used to reduce sedentary behavior in racial/ethnic minority groups

▶ Understand potential future research questions that can lead to successful strategies for decreasing sedentary behavior among racial and ethnic minorities

▶ Consider how previous strategies for influencing sedentary behavior could be improved to be more effective

According to the 2014 American Community Survey, more than 318 million people live in the United States (U.S. Census Bureau 2014). A large proportion of the U.S. population is racial and ethnic minorities (~24%), including ~40 million Blacks and African Americans (13%), ~17 million Asians (5%), ~2.6 million American Indian and Alaska Natives (1%), just over 550,000 Native Hawaiians and other Pacific Islanders (<1%), and ~55 million Hispanics and Latinos (17%).

Although racial and ethnic minorities make up only 24% of the U.S. population, they share a disproportionate burden of chronic disease (National Center for Health Statistics 2016). In 2014, 4 of the 10 leading causes of death among racial and ethnic minorities were chronic diseases directly related to modifiable risk factors associated with lifestyle behaviors (National Center for Health Statistics 2016). These chronic diseases were heart disease, cancer (specifically colon and breast cancer), diabetes, and stroke. For each health outcome and its related risk factors, morbidity and mortality rates were higher among racial and ethnic minorities compared to non-Hispanic whites. The prolonged course of illness and disability from disease and related risk factors, such as obesity and hypertension, result in a decreased quality of life with much pain and suffering as well as enormous health care costs among racial and ethnic minorities (National Center for Health Statistics 2016). Lack of physical activity is a major contributor to the development of many chronic diseases that disproportionately affect racial and ethnic minority populations in the United States, and it has been associated with a variety of social, biological, and environmental factors (U.S. Department of Health and Human Services 1996; 2001). Despite major advances in public health, medicine, economic prosperity, and wealth, health disparities have persisted during the 20th century and have even increased for certain health indicators, such as diabetes. Because physical activity is modifiable and a primary risk factor for many of the diseases that are observed in higher proportions among racial and ethnic minority groups, focusing on physical activity has been viewed as an important step toward reducing or eliminating health disparities for certain health outcomes (U.S. Department of Health and Human Services 1996; 2001).

Recent research has identified sedentary behavior, separate from low levels of physical activity, as an independent risk factor for morbidity and mortality (Katzmarzyk et al. 2009; Thorp et al.

2011). Although they are part of the same health-related continuum, physical activity and sedentary behavior have distinct characteristics and so should be addressed as separate concepts, particularly among underrepresented racial/ethnic minority groups. This chapter provides statistics about the prevalence of sedentary behavior and factors and health outcomes associated with sedentary behavior among racial/ethnic minority groups. The chapter also provides suggestions for future research needs and directions for reducing sedentary behavior in racial/ethnic minority groups.

Statistics

Three major national surveys—the Behavioral Risk Factor Surveillance System (BRFSS), the National Health and Nutrition Examination Survey (NHANES), and the National Health Interview Survey (NHIS)—provide population-level estimates of self-reported (BRFSS, NHANES, NHIS) and objectively monitored (NHANES) physical activity participation among U.S. adults and children. Only NHANES provides information specifically about sedentary behavior. The other national surveys provide the proportion of respondents who report doing no physical activity or exercise (BRFSS) or report on the proportion of respondents meeting physical activity recommendations (NHIS). Data from the Centers for Disease Control and Prevention report that between 1988 and 2008, the percentage of the U.S. population reporting no leisure-time physical activity on the BRFSS dropped from 31% to 25% (CDC 2010a). In 2001, 34.7% of African Americans and 39.8% of Hispanics reported no leisure-time physical activity compared to 22.5% of whites (CDC 2010b). In 2008, 31.9% of African-Americans and 34.6% of Hispanics reported no leisure-time physical activity compared to 22.2% of whites (CDC 2010c).

With regard specifically to sedentary behavior, Matthews and colleagues (2008) used NHANES' objectively monitored physical activity data from 2003-2004 to describe sedentary behavior in U.S. residents 6 years or older. NHANES used accelerometers to assess physical activity, and sedentary behavior was defined as <100 counts per minute. Children aged 6 to 11 years spent 5.9 to 6.1 hours per day in sedentary behavior and those ages 12 to 15 spent 7.4 to 7.6 hours. Young non-Hispanic black girls were significantly less sedentary than non-Hispanic whites and Mexican Americans. No other gender or racial/ethnic differences in sedentary behavior were present in these age groups. Among 16- to 19-year-olds, the average time in sedentary behavior ranged from 7.6 to 8.2 hours per day. Mexican Americans were significantly less sedentary than non-Hispanic whites overall, but these differences did not persist when data were further stratified by gender. Whitt-Glover and colleagues (2009) showed similar findings in a study focused on sedentary behavior among children and adolescents, also using 2003-2004 NHANES data. Another large national data set, the 2003 National Survey of Children's Health, measured physical activity participation and sedentary behavior in immigrants and showed that the prevalence of no sports participation was 42% and the prevalence of television viewing ≥ 3 hours per day was 17% (Singh et al. 2008).

Beginning at age 20, racial/ethnic differences in sedentary behavior become more apparent. Mexican Americans reported less sedentary behavior than other racial/ethnic subgroups across all ages, overall and when stratified by gender. On average, non-Hispanic blacks spent a mean (standard error) of 7.61 (0.05) hours per day in sedentary behavior, compared with 7.18 (0.05) hours per day in Mexican Americans and 7.74 (0.06) hours per day in non-Hispanic whites. Mexican Americans were significantly less sedentary than non-Hispanic whites and blacks. Non-Hispanic black males reported 7.54 (0.06) hours per day in sedentary behavior, compared with 7.74 (0.08) in non-Hispanic whites and 6.89 (0.07) in Mexican Americans. Again, Mexican American men were significantly less sedentary than non-Hispanic black and white men. Trends were similar in women (7.74 [0.04], 7.67 [0.06], and 7.47 [0.05] in non-Hispanic white, non-Hispanic black, and Mexican American women, respectively), and Mexican American women were significantly less sedentary than the other two subgroups. Data from NHANES 2003-2006 also showed that non-Hispanic black adults aged 60 years and older spent an average of 516.7 (95% CI: 504.7–528.6) minutes per day in sedentary behavior, compared with 507.6, 479.4, and 528.7 minutes per day in non-Hispanic whites, Hispanics, and people in the "other" race/ethnicity category, respectively (Evenson, Buchner, and Morland 2012).

Self-reported data from smaller regional samples provide similar estimates. A study of elementary school–aged American Indian children and caregivers indicated 3.0 hours of screen time daily in children and 2.4 hours daily in parents. A South Carolina study found that preschool children spent an average of 32.8 ± 3.9 minutes per hour engaged in sedentary behavior (Byun, Dowda, and Pate 2011). Estimated sedentary behavior among adolescents from regional data sets is ~2 to 3 hours per day of television or video games (Babey, Hastert, and Wolstein 2013; Hanson and Chen 2007; Norman et al. 2005) and ~10 hours per week of computer use for nonschool activities (Babey, Hastert, and Wolstein 2013). Participants in the multiethnic study of atherosclerosis reported spending 2,205 MET-minutes per week (46% of waking time) in sedentary behavior (Allison et al. 2012). The Southern Community Cohort Study, which included 22,948 black and 7,830 white women living in the southeastern United States, found that women engaged in sedentary behavior for 8 to 10 hours per day (Buchowski et al. 2010). Shuval and colleagues (2013) found that African Americans and Hispanics reported ~5 hours per day sitting, 2.3 hours per day on the computer, and 2.5 hours per day in motor vehicles. A study of Hispanic women estimated that women spent a mean (standard deviation) of 97.4 (110.0) minutes per week sitting in a car, 415.4 (252.4) minutes sitting during the week, and 323.0 (228.3) minutes sitting during the weekend, much lower than estimates reported by non-Hispanic blacks and whites (Lee, Mama, and Adamus-Leach 2012). Hispanic women enrolled in the Chicago Breast Health Project reported 1,478 minutes per week (~25 hours) of sitting.

Correlates of Sedentary Behavior

Studies describing the prevalence of sedentary behavior among children, adolescents, and adults in the United States have also identified factors associated with increased or decreased prevalence of sedentary behavior. Primarily, the correlates are associated with demographic characteristics of participants; however, several studies have also identified factors in the built environment that affect sedentary behavior.

Demographics

Although it is commonly accepted that racial/ethnic minority groups report higher rates of sedentary behavior than non-Hispanic whites, the findings vary depending on the method used to assess sedentary behavior (e.g., objective versus self-reported data) and the population of comparison. For example, objectively monitored data from NHANES 2003-2004 indicated that 6- to 11-year-old non-Hispanic black girls engaged in more sedentary behavior than non-Hispanic white girls and 12- to 15-year-old middle income non-Hispanic blacks engaged in more sedentary behavior than non-Hispanic whites with the same income (Whitt-Glover et al. 2009); no other racial/ethnic differences were identified. Matthews and colleagues (2008) found that Mexican American adolescents were less sedentary than whites and that Mexican American men aged 20 to 39 years were the least sedentary of all racial/ethnic subgroups. In the same data set, non-Hispanic white men aged 40 to 59 were more sedentary than non-Hispanic black men in the same age group.

Smaller, regional self-reported data sets consistently report higher sedentary behavior in racial/ethnic minorities compared to whites (Barr-Anderson and Sisson 2012; Hanson and Chen 2007; Sidney et al. 1996). For example, Singh and colleagues compared sedentary behavior, defined as lack of sports participation and television viewing, among U.S.-born non-Hispanic white children and adolescents and U.S.-born parents with non-Hispanic blacks and Hispanics with and without U.S.-born parents (Singh et al. 2008). Children and adolescents with at least one foreign-born parent were more likely to report no sports participation than non-Hispanic whites with U.S.-born parents. However, children and adolescents with two immigrant-born parents were less likely than non-Hispanic whites with U.S.-born parents to watch ≥3 hours of television daily. Foreign-born Hispanics were more likely than other groups to watch ≥3 hours of television daily. A California sample found that American Indian and African American adolescents spent more time in sedentary behavior than white, Latino, and Asian adolescents (Babey, Hastert, and Wolstein 2013).

Most data sets comparing physical activity participation in males and females indicate that females are less active than males (Troiano et al. 2008; National Center for Health Statistics 2013). Associations between gender and sedentary behavior are not as conclusive, however. Some data from local and national surveys indicate that a higher proportion of girls and women compared to boys and men report engaging in sedentary behavior across all age groups (Adegoke and Oyeyemi 2011). Others report higher participation in sedentary behaviors among boys and men compared to girls and women, particularly when sedentary behavior is assessed as computer or video game usage (Barr-Anderson et al. 2011; Babey, Hastert, and Wolstein 2013; Evenson, Buchner, and Morland 2012).

Although not specifically focused on racial/ethnic minorities or sedentary behavior, research on correlates of physical activity suggests that girls are less likely to engage in physical activities like walking to school or participating in after-school activities away from the home because parents do not feel safe letting girls travel alone (McDonald 2008). This increases the likelihood that girls would choose more sedentary activities (e.g., being driven to school; engaging in sedentary behavior at home) if they are not allowed to engage in physically active pursuits. Depending on the types of physical activities in which children are engaging, girls may feel physically incompetent or embarrassed and, thus, may choose to sit out an activity or engage in sedentary behavior rather than participate in physical activity and risk discomfort or embarrassment (Rees et al. 2006). As girls age into adolescence and early adulthood, focus on personal appearance increases, and many young women avoid physical activity to avoid sweating or disturbing their hairstyles (Boyington et al. 2008). A focus group among adolescent African American girls indicated that girls believed that weight gain was a natural part of progression that they should not attempt to control, that African American girls preferred a larger body size, and that when the option is given between physical activity and other choices, African American girls would choose to do something else they enjoy (likely a sedentary behavior) over engaging in physical activity (Boyington et al. 2008).

Among adults, women often report feeling guilty about engaging in physical activity because of demands related to work and caregiving that take precedence over leisure-time pursuits (Henderson and Ainsworth 2000a; 2000b; 2000c; 2001; 2003). The notion of collectivism, which prioritizes the needs of the group over individuals within the group, is ingrained in African, African American, and Latino cultures (Airhihenbuwa et al. 2000; Airhihenbuwa 1995). Collectivism would suggest that until everyone in a group is taken care of, people within the group should not engage in activities that would benefit only the individual (e.g., leisure-time physical activity). Participation in work and caregiving can also leave women feeling exhausted, thus increasing sedentary behavior in the form of rest (Chang et al. 2008; Miller et al. 2012; King et al. 2000). In addition, racial/ethnic minority women often do not perceive that they have leisure time (Sanderson et al. 2003; Ainsworth et al. 2003; Parra-Medina et al. 2011); thus, self-report studies that define sedentary behavior by lack of participation in leisure-time physical activity may overestimate sedentary behavior in racial/ethnic minority women because physical activities related to daily living, transportation, or occupation are not considered. Certain demographic characteristics (e.g., increasing age) or health conditions (e.g., pregnancy, chronic illness, physical disability) may lead family members to demand that people engage in sedentary behavior as a safety precaution (Stathi et al. 2012; Sander et al. 2012; Mathews et al. 2010; Eyler et al. 1998; Evenson et al. 2009).

Age can also play a factor in engaging in sedentary behavior. NHANES provides the most thorough estimates of sedentary behavior participation across a wide range of ages. Data from NHANES 2003-2004 indicate that sedentary behavior increases from ~6 hours per day at 6 to 11 years to ~8 hours per day at 16 to 19 years (Evenson, Buchner, and Morland 2012). Most elementary schools provide some form of recess or physical education; as children age, physical activity during the school day decreases and sedentary behavior during the school day increases, since recess is not offered in middle and high school and physical education requirements vary (Moore et al. 2010). A study of correlates of physical activity among 11- to 16-year-old boys and girls in the UK indicated that as girls aged, they saw physical activity as babyish and not part of becoming a woman, while physical activity confirmed masculinity for young men (Rees et al. 2006). NHANES data on adults ≥20 years showed a positive association between age and sedentary behavior—that is, as age increases, sedentary behavior increases (Matthews et al. 2008). Sedentary behavior continues to increase with age in older adulthood (to ~8 to 10 hours per day), with higher sedentary behavior among those ≥80 years compared to those 60 to 79 years of age (Evenson, Buchner, and Morland 2012).

A few studies have linked education, socioeconomic status, and employment to sedentary behavior. In general, these studies have shown an inverse relationship between each factor and sedentary behavior. Parental factors also affect sedentary behavior among children and adolescents. For example, adolescents whose parents did not work in the previous year reported more television viewing than adolescents with working parents (Babey, Hastert, and Wolstein 2013). However, adolescents with two working parents watched more television than adolescents with at least one parent at home. Adolescents with college-educated parents reported less television viewing than adolescents whose parents had less education. Adolescents residing in low-income neighborhoods reported less computer use than adolescents in high-income neighborhoods. Data from adults in the CARDIA study identified inverse associations between education, income, and working full time and sedentary behavior (Sidney et al. 1996). Further discussion about the influence of education, socioeconomic status, and employment on sedentary behavior is included in the following section on environmental barriers.

Body mass index (BMI), a ratio of weight to height, is positively correlated with engagement in sedentary behavior (Adegoke and Oyeyemi 2011; Buchowski et al. 2010; Shuval et al. 2013). BMI z-score in preschool children was inversely associated with objectively monitored sedentary behavior (Byun et al. 2011). People who have higher BMI levels may choose sedentary behaviors over engaging in physical activity for a variety of reasons, including the additional energy expenditure necessary for them to perform the same activities as normal-weight people, lack of experience with physical activity, potential embarrassment when engaging in physical activity, stigma associated with being overweight, and potential pain (e.g., joints) associated with engaging in physical activity. Parental BMI is also positively correlated with sedentary behavior in children and adolescents, likely because of the direct association between BMI and sedentary behavior among adults. Children and adolescents mimic parental behavior. If parents with high BMI levels engage in more sedentary behavior, it stands to reason that their children will also engage in sedentary behavior, regardless of the child's BMI.

General Physical Activity

As expected, observational research suggests an inverse association between participation in general physical activity and sedentary behavior (Hanson and Chen 2007). Among preschool children, athletic coordination and presence of physical activity equipment in the home were negatively correlated with sedentary behavior (Byun, Dowda, and Pate 2011). Adolescents who reported no participation in physical activity had higher levels of television viewing than those who spent at least 1 hour engaged in physical activity daily (Babey, Hastert, and Wolstein

2013). Fewer days of physical activity were also associated with more computer use among adolescents. Among adults, low levels of physical activity were associated with high levels of television viewing (≥4 hr daily) (Sidney et al. 1996).

Parental participation in sedentary behavior also affects sedentary behavior in children and adolescents. In a study of American Indian children, parental television viewing time was positively associated with children's television viewing time (Barr-Anderson et al. 2011). Interestingly, in the same study, 23% of parents thought children spent too much time watching television, 15% thought children spent too much time playing video games, and 81% thought it would be easy to limit their child's television viewing time. Parental perception that the child spent too much time playing video games was positively associated with screen time; the likely rationale for this association is that parents were more likely to notice children who spent long periods of time playing video games. Conversely, parental perception of how often they limit the child's television time was negatively associated with screen time—meaning parents who had higher perceptions of limiting television time had children who watched less television. Among Hispanics, perceived parental support for an active lifestyle was associated with lower levels of sedentary behavior; girls were less affected by parental support than boys (Cong et al. 2012).

Knowledge, Attitudes, and Beliefs

An additional correlate of sedentary behavior among African Americans could be related to attitudes about the importance of rest and sleep relative to physical activity. A seminal qualitative study by Airhihenbuwa and colleagues (1995) included 10 focus groups with 53 African American participants about the importance of rest, sleep, and exercise. Findings from the study indicated that participants in the sample placed more importance on rest than exercise and felt that rest was necessary before engaging in exercise. This suggests that people who increase physical activity participation might also increase sedentary behavior to compensate for exercise and to prepare for additional physical activity. Participants also indicated that jobs most readily available to African Americans were manual labor jobs that required physical exertion, thus reducing the need for additional leisure-time physical activity outside of work settings (Airhihenbuwa 1995).

Focus group participants also believed that exercise helped young African American men to obtain better physiques and to be tough, which allowed them to survive in low-income areas or attract women; the fact that physical activity was not noted as good or as a necessity in other subgroups suggests more encouragement and acceptance of sedentary behavior in these subgroups (i.e., women, older African American men). In fact, focus group participants argued that older African American men earned the right to engage in sedentary behavior after a lifetime of physical labor and that they had been forced to retire because of physical problems that would promote sedentary behavior.

In general, most people understand the benefits of physical activity, but it is not clear that they truly understand the dangers of sedentary behavior. In addition, because many parents work or are otherwise occupied, they may not be aware of their children's screen time and sedentary behavior. Data on adolescents in California showed that children with both parents working or those whose parents admitted not knowing how their children spent their free time were more likely to report sedentary behavior than children who had at least one parent at home or whose parents were aware of how the children spent their free time (Babey, Hastert, and Wolstein 2013). Among African American girls, caregivers admitted to being more concerned about the *quality* of television viewed by their daughters rather than the quantity; also, they were generally unaware of the amount of television their daughters watched (Gordon-Larsen et al. 2004). Caregivers also noted that television fills an important role as safe and affordable child supervision, which is particularly critical in neighborhoods with high crime and in households with limited disposable income that can be used for childcare.

Built Environment

Environmental factors have been linked with physical activity participation and might also influence sedentary behavior (Whitt-Glover, Bennett, and Sallis 2013; Casagrande et al. 2009). Previous research has highlighted racial and ethnic disparities in access to parks and recreation facilities (Wolch, Wilson, and Fehrenbach 2005; Powell, Slater, and Chaloupka 2004; Gordon-Larsen et al. 2006; Moore et al. 2008). Concerns about poor environmental quality (e.g., crime, poor maintenance, and aesthetics) might serve as barriers to physical activity in low-income racial/ethnic minority communities and may promote sedentary behavior as a safety precaution (Boslaugh et al. 2004). Park and recreational facilities that lack safe or adequate equipment might promote sedentary behavior, even among park users, if there is nothing to do in the park except to sit and relax. Living in a neighborhood with adequate built environment resources may not necessarily equate to less time spent in sedentary behavior, however. A study of Hispanic and Latina women found a positive association between attractiveness of a neighborhood for walking and cycling and time spent in a motor vehicle—time spent in a motor vehicle increased as attractiveness increased (Lee, Mama, and Adamus-Leach 2012). The surprising finding is likely because participants in attractive neighborhoods lived in the suburbs, had longer commute times, and thus spent more time in motor vehicles. The same study showed a negative association between neighborhood attractiveness and time spent sitting on the weekends, suggesting that women in the study engaged in more physical activity and less sitting on weekends, presumably when they did not have to make long daily commutes.

Much of the research linking the environment to sedentary behavior has been focused on general populations, and there is limited evidence about which factors in the environment affect sedentary behavior in racial/ethnic minority groups specifically or whether environmental factors that affect racial/ethnic minority groups are different from environmental factors that influence other population subgroups. Generally, research suggests that people living in older urban neighborhoods and neighborhoods with mixed land use are more active than people living in suburban neighborhoods and neighborhoods without walkable destinations (Trowbridge and McDonald 2008; Ewing et al. 2003; Rosenberg et al. 2009; Grow et al. 2008). This association is likely because people who live in the suburbs or neighborhoods without walkable destinations spend more time in motorized vehicles for transportation. Additional research is needed to understand the effect of the built environment on sedentary behavior in racial/ethnic minority subgroups.

Interventions for Reducing Sedentary Behavior in Racial/Ethnic Minorities

Most interventions related to the continuum between sedentary behavior and physical activity have focused on increasing physical activity levels; however, a few intervention studies have focused solely on decreasing sedentary behavior or on decreasing sedentary behavior while increasing physical activity. The majority of interventions designed to reduce sedentary behavior have primarily focused on children and adolescents. Of those reported, less than half of the studies included samples primarily consisting of African Americans, Latinos, Native Americans, or other minority groups (Gortmaker et al. 1999; Fitzgibbon et al. 2002; Fitzgibbon et al. 2005; 2006; Fitzgibbon et al. 2011; Robinson et al. 2003; Weintraub et al. 2008). On average, interventions lasted as little as 5 days to as long as 2 years. Most studies used subjective measures of media use (e.g., time children spend watching TV or videos, video game use, overall household TV use) reported by the parent or guardian to assess

DISPARITIES IN HEALTH OUTCOMES

In a study of Latino and African American adolescents, people with metabolic syndrome spent more time in sedentary behavior than those without metabolic syndrome (Hsu et al. 2011). The multiethnic study of atherosclerosis showed that every 1 standard deviation unit increase in sedentary behavior was associated with an increase in leptin and tumor necrosis factor, which are both markers of adiposity-associated inflammation (Allison et al. 2012). A study of 95 Hispanic women in the Chicago Breast Health Project showed no association between sedentary time and insulin, HOMA, or percentage of breast density (Wolin et al. 2007). Other studies on the effect of sedentary behavior on health outcomes have not been specific to racial/ethnic minority populations. Stratified analyses are important for clearly delineating the association and assisting with planning for effective interventions that can be used to reduce screen time and, consequently, reduce disparities in health outcomes.

sedentary behaviors. Few studies included objective measures of sedentary behavior such as electronic TV monitors. Most interventions, full or pilot, used randomized control trials, included parental involvement, and attempted to intervene on multiple behaviors (e.g., diet modification, social support, and physical activity). Additionally, these trials primarily occurred in school settings (mostly preschool and middle school), either during the school day or immediately following the school day. Of those trials occurring in school settings, teachers often served as the primary deliverer of the intervention, especially in those interventions simultaneously targeting multiple schools. The second most utilized intervention setting was the home.

Although several studies reported positive changes in reducing sedentary time (e.g., screen time, DVD use, TV viewing) among children and adolescents, these changes appear to be minimal at best. Most studies, on average, showed significant reductions in screen time ranging from 30 minutes to 150 minutes per day. However, no study was able to reduce video game time in children or adolescents. Since the average child accumulates approximately 7 to 8 hours of screen time per day, 30 minutes to 150 minutes per day would represent approximately a 6.5% to 32% reduction in daily screen time. Whether this is a clinically meaningful reduction in screen time is yet to be determined. Furthermore, it is unknown how people use time previously allocated for screen time. Is the time replaced with other sedentary pursuits, or do children use the time to engage in physical activity?

Limited evidence exists regarding the design, implementation, and effectiveness of interventions to reduce sedentary behavior in adults. To date, most studies of adult sedentary behavior are cross-sectional in nature. Even fewer have either focused on or included a representative sample of minorities. Given the positive association between increasing age and sedentary behavior, additional research on effective strategies for reducing sedentary behavior in adults is warranted.

Summary

Sedentary behavior is associated with myriad poor health outcomes, many of which appear in higher rates in racial/ethnic minority subgroups. Interestingly, objectively monitored physical activity data show lower levels of sedentary behavior among racial/ethnic minority youth and adolescents compared with non-Hispanic white youth and adolescents. Among adults, Mexican Americans report the lowest and non-Hispanic whites report the highest levels of sedentary behavior. Factors that are associated with higher levels of sedentary behavior include being female, caregiving responsibilities, increasing age, having two working parents (adolescents), higher BMI, little or no physical activity participation, parental participation in sedentary behavior (children), attitudes about the importance of rest and sleep relative to physical activity, and limited access to recreational facilities or safe places to exercise. Factors associated with lower levels of sedentary behavior include higher socioeconomic status, employment, having at least one parent at home (adolescents), having college-educated parents (adolescents), athletic coordination, and the presence of physical activity equipment in the home. Little is known about the most effective strategies for reducing sedentary behavior in racial/ethnic minority children and adults. Strategies that incorporate physical activity into typically sedentary behaviors (e.g., walking meetings) show promise; however, additional research using randomized, controlled trial designs is needed.

KEY CONCEPTS

▸ **Correlates of sedentary behavior:** Factors or variables that can make a person more or less likely to engage in a sedentary behavior.

▸ **Low physical activity:** Refers to levels of physical activity that are *below* the national guidelines for physical activity for healthy children and adults.

▸ **Racial/ethnic minority:** In the United States, racial/ethnic minority groups include Black or African American, American Indian or Alaska Native, Hispanic or Latino, Native Hawaiian and other Pacific Islander, Asian, and multiracial.

STUDY QUESTIONS

1. Why is it important to pay attention to sedentary behavior among racial/ethnic minority sub-groups?

2. What do national data tell us about physical activity levels in racial/ethnic minority groups compared to non-Hispanic whites? Do the data look the same when comparing sedentary behavior in racial/ethnic minority groups compared to whites?

3. How does sedentary behavior affect health outcomes among racial/ethnic minority subgroups?

4. Describe at least three correlates of sedentary behaviors and how each correlate might work to increase or decrease sedentary behavior.

5. Describe at least one strategy that could be used to reduce sedentary behavior for each of the correlates described previously.

The authors gratefully acknowledge the support of Stepheria Hodge Sallah, MPH, Shanice L. Borden, BS, and Mrs. Bobbi Wright in preparing this chapter.

PART V

CHANGING SEDENTARY BEHAVIOR

For sedentary behavior and health, fundamental questions relate to the extent to which sedentary behavior realistically can be changed and the options that may exist for doing so. Thus, part V has six chapters covering conventional intervention methods based on behavioral theories and psychological models, plus environmental, social, community, worksite, and technology-based interventions.

In chapter 22, Kevin O. Moran and John P. Elder provide insightful perspectives on psychological and behavior-based interventions. They describe the mainstream social cognitive theories that have been used to develop behavioral-change interventions and emphasize the importance of environment–behavior relationships, proposing an ecological perspective to guide thinking about sedentary behavior change. The central theme and emphasis of chapter 22 are further elaborated throughout chapter 23, where Jordan A. Carlson and James F. Sallis deal specifically with environment and policy interventions for changing sedentary behavior. This chapter emphasizes the importance of setting-specific approaches and the creation of opportunities for sitting less through environmental innovations, regulations, and policy. The initial chapters in part V remain strongly thematic in regard to context and

environmental influences on sedentary behavior. In chapter 24, Nicolaas P. Pronk addresses worksite interventions for changing sedentary behavior. He shows how relatively simple innovations such as the availability of low-cost sit-to-stand workstations can significantly reduce sedentary time at work.

The latter three chapters of part V deal with interrelated but distinct aspects of sedentary behavior change. In chapter 25, Adrian Bauman and Josephine Y. Chau consider community-based interventions for influencing sedentary behavior. This chapter provides a thorough and informative perspective on what has been learned through community-wide approaches to reducing sedentary behavior, including the role of physical activity. In Chapter 26, John B. Shea and Kelly J. Baute present an ergonomic view of issues around redesigning sitting. They provide an excellent reminder for the many of us who have found a way into the workplace sitting field through an interest in physical activity, sedentary behavior, and health. Dealing with sitting has been a traditional concern of the field of the ergonomics, particularly occupational ergonomics. This is an excellent tutorial chapter, engaging the reader with ergonomic issues of particular relevance to fine-tuning approaches to sedentary behavior change and drawing on lessons from a highly-relevant and well-established field of research and practice.

Echoing some of the themes that emerged in part III related to applications of new information-technology capacities, chapter 27 deals with emerging communication systems for influencing physical inactivity. Dolores Albarracin and colleagues not only describe the evidence and potential of new communication capacities (particularly as delivered through the Internet, smartphones, tablets, and other devices), but also provide a strong, theoretically informed perspective about how such technologies may be used for the purposes of behavioral change.

This final section of the book contains novel and compelling material. That said, these are yet early days for the field of sedentary behavior interventions. Much remains to be developed and tested before strong evidence-based claims can be made about the potential options for pursuing sedentary behavior change.

CHAPTER 22

PSYCHOLOGICAL AND BEHAVIOR-BASED INTERVENTIONS

Kevin O. Moran, MPH; and John P. Elder, PhD, MPH

The reader will gain an overview of the psychological, behavioral, and socioecological theoretical frameworks that are relevant to understanding and influencing sedentary behavior. By the end of this chapter, the reader should be able to do the following:

▶ Develop a broad perspective on ways to understand sedentary behavior from behavioristic and ecological model perspectives

▶ Understand the main characteristics of psychosocial models of behavior and behavioral change and their limitations in guiding public health approaches

▶ Identify the key constructs of the transtheoretical model of behavior change and their potential applications for understanding and influencing sedentary behavior

▶ Understand the underlying philosophical perspective of operant conditioning, contingency management, and positivistic models of behavioral change

▶ Identify key applications of operant conditioning and contingency management constructs for practical sedentary-behavior change initiatives

▶ Identify the ways in which ecological models can provide integrative perspectives on sedentary behavior change in different contexts

In the decades since health behavior change has replaced health education as the dominant thrust in the behavioral science approach to public health, a variety of psychosocial models have come to dominate the theoretical constructs in health behavior. More recently the implied individual focus of psychosocial models has been deemed inadequate to inform the development of wide-scale behavior change. Over the years, models and theories have increasingly emphasized the need to intervene beyond the individual level, with applications to group, organizational, community, and even national levels and programs.

Ecological and socioecological models of health behavior change extend beyond direct change of knowledge, attitudes, and behavior to indirect strategies through policy, technology, and other interventions. Multilevel models have long been widely accepted in areas such as tobacco control and the prevention and control of infectious diseases, both in developing and developed countries. The development of these models and theories may be largely grouped as socioecological models, lending themselves to better understanding, measurement, and change strategies for behavior. However, any psychological model still implicitly emphasizes human cognitive and behavioral functions, at least at the individual level. Behavior change researchers and program developers have yet to agree on a common theoretical structure for addressing a wide range of health behaviors and targeting populations in various public health programs.

Sitting is pervasive in so many aspects of daily life that it is easily ignored. By contrast, smoking and tobacco use are relatively very easy to measure. People remember whether they had a cigarette yesterday and can easily ascertain how many they smoke on a typical day. Bioassays can confirm the validity of this self-report. With respect to broader socioecological levels, clean indoor air, sales to minors, and regional and national levels of tobacco sales are relatively easy to measure. The measurement of sedentary behavior, however, is still at an early stage of its development. Although there are no healthy levels of cigarette smoking, the cutoff points for the amount of sedentary time that is deleterious to health remain to be established. Because much of sedentary behavior is such an integral part of daily life in multiple settings, it is largely invisible.

Sedentary behavior presents a specific challenge to the development and application of psychosocial and socioecological models. It is often viewed as the converse of physical activity. Research has identified sedentary behavior as a distinct risk for various diseases and illness conditions. Thus, it is important to understand sedentary behavior from both measurement and intervention perspectives.

However, from a simple postural perspective, sedentary behavior is not really a behavior. The criterion for operationalization in years past that would apply to sedentary behavior was "Can a dead person do it?" In other words, if a person or object without life can be said to do the same things that someone who is alive can (e.g., be sedentary), this is not good operationalization. Therefore, when specifying sedentary behavior, we must identify a positivistic definition of the cluster of the construct of sedentary behavior or the cluster of behaviors that contribute to being sedentary. Moreover, a certain level of sedentariness is healthy. The body needs rest, for example. One must distinguish healthy levels of resting and recovery from unhealthy levels of sitting while watching TV in terms of targeting sedentary behaviors. This has important implications not only for measurement and intervention but also for the theories and models that frame them.

Theories of Reasoned Action and Planned Behavior

The theory of reasoned action (TRA) aims to explain the roles of attitudes and intentions in predicting behaviors. Whereas attitude theorists prior to the TRA focused on attitudes toward an object of interest (say, being overweight), the TRA's foundational research explored attitudes with respect to the object (say, prevention of overweight through physical activity). Fishbein (1967) showed that attitudes about a preventive health behavior were more predictive of that behavior than attitudes about the condition itself. These attitudes are driven by expectations or beliefs about the behavior, whether positive or negative, high or low cost. The theory of planned behavior (TPB) was later proposed to account for situations in which a person is not in complete control of a behavior's occurrence, proposing the notion of *control* as a separate predictive variable (Fishbein and Ajzen 1975).

The TRA proposes the following constructs:

▸ *Attitude.* This consists of a person's beliefs about the consequences that will follow from a behavior (*behavioral beliefs*), along with subjective valuations of those consequences. As mentioned previously, *attitudes* here are specific to the behavior, rather than to the condition or disease the behavior is intended to mitigate.

▸ *Subjective norms.* Considered an ancillary predictor of behavior, subjective norms consist of two constructs: normative beliefs and motivation to comply. The TRA posits that a person will consider the opinions of peers and other esteemed people with regard to whether they approve or disapprove of a behavior. Termed *normative beliefs*, this notion is theorized to affect behavior only if a person has a strong *motivation to comply* with the expectations of these referent individuals.

▸ *Intention.* One of the TRA's primary assumptions is that intention to perform a behavior is the primary determinant of its occurrence. According to the TRA, attitude and subjective norms both influence the intention to perform a behavior.

The TPB considers another construct predictive of behavioral intention:

▸ *Perceived control.* TRA is largely dependent on a behavior being under conscious individual control, but begins to fail when the degree of people's control over their behavior diminishes. Perceived control is determined by the presence of hindering or enabling factors (*control beliefs*) and the *perceived power* those factors maintain. Factors that maintain little perceived power will not largely influence perceived control.

The TRA and TPB are well supported in the literature; however, researchers comparing TRA and TPB in physical activity interventions have noted that TPB better predicts behavioral intention (Hagger, Chatzisarantis, and Biddle 2002). Physical activity studies intervening on the attitudes of preventive behaviors as well as subjective norms have been found to positively influence behavioral intent (Hagger, Chatzisarantis, and Biddle 2002); the challenge, however, is to link such intent prospectively to actions.

Social Cognitive Theory

Social cognitive theory (SCT; called social learning theory in its earlier incarnations) explains human behavior as the interplay among individual, social, and environmental variables, while recognizing the individual's ability to create environments that are conducive to productive behaviors. Initially closely aligned with operant psychology (Bandura 1969), SCT gained popularity among health behavior researchers as it pivoted toward a more cognitive basis. Central to this theory is the concept of *self-efficacy*, which refers to the confidence a person has in being able to carry out a skill or behavior (Bandura 1977; 1986). SCT posits that, regardless of skill level, increasing levels of self-efficacy lead to a greater likelihood of engaging in a specific behavior. Self-efficacy also extends to people's beliefs about their ability to alter their behavior and influence the events that affect their lives. People with an efficacious attitude, for example, are more likely to incorporate more leisure-time physical activity than to have a high level of fitness. Self-efficacy is the most widely cited construct of SCT, and has been incorporated into several other models of health behavior (discussed in the following sections).

SCT proposes *outcome expectations* as another critical psychological determinant of behavior. Defined as the belief about the likelihood of positive reinforcement as a consequence of action, outcome expectations are founded on the idea that people desire to maximize benefits and minimize costs. An extension of this is the concept of *social outcome expectations*, which are beliefs about how others will evaluate our behavior. This social consideration is analogous to *social norms*, as posited by the theories of reasoned action and planned behavior.

SCT theorizes that both individual and social outcomes govern behavior, but that self-evaluative outcomes can be more powerful. This might explain how people can act differently from the sedentary behavior of their friends or family to meet their own standards of action.

SCT also suggests that people learn vicariously through observation and reinforcement of peer, family, or media models. Evidence consistently shows that peer models that are similar to the observer are likely to affect behavior (Schunk 1987). This is seen most fundamentally with children learning from their siblings and parents or through popular role models. In an effort to alter the individual and social outcome expectations of behavior change, physical activity interventions have championed the peer-leader model to promote active lifestyles.

SCT has been widely used in health behavior change efforts, especially with regard to peer-led interventions and health promotion campaigns through electronic, print, and social media. SCT-derived variables have also been used to help explain physical activity in youth (Sallis, Prochaska, and Taylor 2000).

Health Belief Model

Traditionally, health education was aligned with the health belief model (HBM), which still has important parallels in popular theories in the field (such as the notion of outcome expectations in social cognitive theory). Thus, health education largely embodied an approach of knowledge, attitudes, and behavior (KAB) to improving public health. The KAB assumption is that either on an individual level or through mass communication, changing knowledge (and in many cases, corresponding attitudes), if done properly, would result in risk factor reduction and other forms of behavior change. By accessing the correct facts and feelings through introspection, the logical person would arrive at a healthy choice.

The HBM seeks to explain why people take action in preventing, screening, or controlling illness (Hochbaum 1958). It theorizes that people perceive a level of threat regarding a particular disease. In order to take action to mitigate this threat, however, people must believe that these actions will have an advantageous outcome and will come at an acceptable cost (Hochbaum 1958). The HBM core constructs are as follows:

▸ *Perceived threat.* This construct represents a person's feelings regarding how hazardous a condition or disease is. It is comprised of two factors: perceived susceptibility and perceived severity. Perceived susceptibility represents a person's ideation regarding the likelihood of getting a condition, while perceived severity represents the seriousness (medically, such as risk of death, and socially, such as stigmatization) associated with that disease.

▸ *Perceived benefits.* These are the attitudes about how much there is to gain by engaging in a particular preventive action. Included here may be health-related benefits like better physical functioning, as well as non-health-related gains such as a decrease in medical bills.

▸ *Perceived barriers.* These represent feelings associated with the potential negative aspects of a particular health behavior. These deterrents to action are weighed against perceived benefits, in effect conducting a cost–benefit analysis of the targeted preventive health action.

The HBM posits several other concepts considered integral in the process of preventive action. The first is the notion of *cues to action*, which are thought to be prompts that trigger action such as environmental factors or biological events (Hochbaum 1958). A lack of empirical evidence exists for this construct, however, since cues are difficult to define and measure. Second, the notion of self-efficacy (Bandura 1997) was later added to the HBM to account for whether people feel they have sufficient competence to overcome the perceived barriers of an action (Rosenstock, Strecher, and Becker 1988).

Core to the assumptions underlying the HBM is people's logical and reasonable thinking with regard to their health behaviors and susceptibility to disease. In contrast to the behavioral explanations posited by Watson and Skinner (Watson 1925; Skinner 1938), the HBM grew from the cognitive theory perspective that subjective valuations of behavioral outcomes drive action (Tolman 1932; Lewin 1939). Critical to this model are the roles of reasoning, hypothesizing, and anticipating behavioral outcomes. More specifically, it is assumed that people (*a*) value illness avoidance or being healthy and (*b*) expect certain actions to prevent or remedy illnesses.

The HBM has been largely tied with health behavior studies that emphasize health education. The KAB approach stems from the same cognitive theory as HBM. KAB is founded on the principle that changing someone's knowledge will change their corresponding attitudes as well, which will be reflected in their behavior. Take, for example, sedentary behavior intervention in a workplace. The aims may be raising awareness about the risks of prolonged sedentary time (threat) as well as the benefits of mitigating actions (benefits). Simultaneously, practitioners may seek to enable action by encouraging and promoting frequent standing or walking breaks (perceived barriers).

Transtheoretical Model

The transtheoretical model (TTM) is an integration of behavior modification processes across stages of change. The fundamental concept here is the notion that behavior change occurs in stages. The foundation of this concept arose from studying smokers' intention (or lack thereof) to quit. DiClemente and colleagues (1982) identified 10 processes of change that were tied to smoking cessation. More telling, though, was that smokers employed various processes at different times throughout their struggle to quit. This reflected a vital shift in the conceptual framework of behavior change—one that now considered change as a chronological, rather than discrete, process.

TTM outlines six stages of change:

1. *Precontemplation* is the earliest stage, in which people do not intend to change within the next 6 months.

2. *Contemplation* identifies people who intend to change within the next 6 months.

3. *Preparation* is achieved when a person is planning to change soon, likely within the next month.

4. *Action* is reserved for people who have made a change in their lifestyle within the last 6 months.

5. *Maintenance* is reached when a person has made a significant modification in lifestyle longer than 6 months and is working to avoid relapse.

6. *Termination* is the stage that represents complete transition to a new behavior, where the risk of relapse is operationally zero.

The processes of change outlined by TTM are understood to be the method by which people move through the stages of change. These processes include concepts from various psychological approaches (hence, *transtheoretical*). Most notable are the notions of contingency management, stimulus control, and counterconditioning from the Skinnerian tradition of operant psychology (Skinner 1972). Other processes include helping relationships, as outlined by Carl Rogers (1951), as well as raising consciousness from the Freudian tradition (Freud 1969).

Also of note regarding the TTM is the application of three supplemental constructs of health behavior theory. The first is the notion of *decisional balance*, by which people weigh the pros and cons of a particular change. The second is Bandura's self-efficacy theory (1982). Although not strictly a method for change, this construct is the valuation by which the ability to begin or maintain a change is measured. Finally, *temptation* is generally referred to as the

reverse of self-efficacy, or the urge to relapse in a difficult situation.

The TTM has gained considerable popularity in physical activity behavior interventions as well as interventions targeting multiple risk factors (Prochaska et al. 2008). The strength of the model is its ability to guide a tailored intervention approach. People can be placed into stages with a simple questionnaire, which helps researchers target processes of change most commonly associated with a given stage. TTM-tailored communication interventions have been shown to be effective in worksite settings (Prochaska et al. 2008), which is encouraging for sedentary behavior research because sedentary behavior is highly prevalent in the workplace (Matthews et al. 2012). TTM interventions guiding people from contemplation to action (even modest action) have relevance for substantial health effects. In fact, evidence has shown that interrupting sedentary behavior with light-activity breaks as short as 2 minutes will reduce glucose levels (Dunstan et al. 2012).

Although it is widely applied across behaviors and settings, the TTM does have limitations. Most notable of these is its application to primary prevention of detrimental health behaviors. TTM-guided interventions aimed at prevention of substance abuse have had limited success (Hollis et al. 2005). Although prevention trials have proven difficult regardless of theoretical framework, the tenets of the TTM do suggest that its application is best suited to those who already engage unhealthy behaviors and therefore can be placed in either precontemplation or contemplation. Additionally, health behavior change studies using the TTM have at times shown no stage change in spite of behavior change, perhaps because the people involved in the interventions were already in contemplation or action as a function of being in the program in the first place.

Positivistic Models

The branch of the philosophy of science known as *positivism* (associated with the thinking of philosophers Mach, Wittgenstein, and Russell) asserts that only phenomena that can be directly and reliably assessed through observation (i.e., seeing and hearing; for sedentary behavior research, behaviors and their effects) are of interest to scientific inquiry (Russell 1950; Wittgenstein 1922). Positivists do not deny the existence of cognitive processes, but question the extent to which they are relevant, given that they are unique experiences to the person who is thinking or feeling them. Thus, positivists challenge the validity of measuring constructs such as decisional balance, self-efficacy, and outcome expectations.

Among health behavior theories, those most aligned with positivism generally fall under the rubric of learning theories, specifically, operant psychology. The terms *operant psychology, instrumental* or *operant conditioning, behavior modification, behaviorism, contingency management*, and other expressions have been used interchangeably by some while taking on different connotations by others. In this chapter, we are referring to the collective expression of these concepts with its modern heritage in the work of B.F. Skinner's operant conditioning. Over the past 125 years, a theory of learning emerged that emphasized the relationship between behavior and environment. One of the early pioneers of this learning theory was E.L. Thorndike (1911) who established the law of effect, emphasizing that behavior was most likely to recur if it was followed by a reward and less likely to do so if followed by some sort of aversive consequence. Soon after, John Watson (1913) became one of the first to use the term *behaviorism*. Watson's behaviorism deviated from the field of psychology in general in that it was fully based in positivism. Behaviorism has different roots than do other cognitively oriented psychosocial theories. Watson held that with respect to environment–behavior relationships, both humans and lower animals were governed by similar response–consequence relationships.

In 1938, B.F. Skinner expanded on Watson's behaviorism to develop a refined form of learning theory that he labeled operant conditioning. Specifically, Skinner invoked the Darwinian tradition in defining distinctions between primary and secondary reinforcers. Primary reinforcers are those thought to contribute to natural selection and survival, such as sex, food, and, naturally, rest. Secondary reinforcers are other objects that might be considered neutral in and of themselves (e.g., paper money or coinage, which have no inherent or intrinsic survival value). However, since they are paired with primary reinforcers, secondary reinforcers take on their own reinforcing value.

Thus, of all socioecological models, operant theory is simultaneously most closely connected to true ecological models that derive from biology and relevant to physical activity and sedentary behavior. Behavior–consequence relationships are easily demonstrated across animal species. For example, a male bird will select a habitat and define its boundaries based on three interrelated parameters: the amount of energy needed to define the habitat (e.g., the amount of flight needed to monitor its borders), the opportunity costs associated with selection or expansion (e.g., potential loss of a mate or nest), and the potential for injury (or death) from exposure to competition, predators, and the elements (e.g., Stamps, Krishnan, and Reid 2005). Thus, the bird's decision to become less active may be every bit as logical as the converse.

Skinner described contingencies that govern behavior, specifically behavior–consequence relationships. He emphasized that reasons for behavior change could not be inferred by making guesses about a person's cognitive processes but instead must be observed through contingent behavior–environment relationships. Among his many contributions to the theory of behavior was his notion of *negative reinforcement*, which is often misused in health behavior circles. Specifically, negative reinforcement is the strengthening of behavior through the offset of an aversive condition contingent on the behavior. It should not be confused with punishment, which involves a decline in response rate as a function of a specific type of consequence.

The application of operant conditioning for understanding various types of sedentary behavior presents a special but very important challenge. Specifically, a person may engage in screen time, television watching, and other forms of sedentary activity to escape an unpleasant situation. This is distinct from punishment; for example, the person may have found a form of physical activity to be unpleasant and thus uses sedentary behavior as a fallback response pattern. Clearly, far more needs to be known about the antecedent behavior–consequence relationships that govern sedentary behavior.

Within the operant framework, what behavior-environment contingencies apply to sedentary behavior? The following are examples:

▸ *Positive reinforcement.* Sedentary behaviors may be reinforcing in their own right. Popular culture expressed through cinematic arts, books, and magazines requires that users to be sedentary to enjoy it. The use of the Internet, cell phones, and other communication devices provides social and professional rewards. Sitting or lying down may result in rested muscles and a sense of relaxation. Sedentary behavior may require minimal skills, making it easy to engage in relative to certain physical activities such as skilled sports.

▸ **Extinction.** As noted previously, sedentary behavior is not necessarily just the absence of physical activity. However, the two behavioral categories (MVPA and sedentary behavior) are indeed incompatible, that is, they cannot occur at the same time in the same person. Thus, when MVPA is no longer positively reinforced, it may diminish over time and be replaced by sedentary behavior. Thus, we can say that the MVPA was extinguished. For example, a young adult may have enjoyed playing soccer over many years, but can no longer find a group of peers to play with. Thus, this healthy behavior is extinguished because it no longer provides social reinforcement. (At the same time, a more mature peer group may get together to watch soccer on TV, providing additional positive reinforcement for this decidedly sedentary substitute.)

▸ *Negative reinforcement.* Not to be confused with punishment, negative reinforcement is the escape from or avoidance of aversive conditions. The "no pain, no gain" concept of becoming physically fit arguably does not have a broad appeal. Sore feet, injuries, or the social embarrassment of an unskilled performance on a public athletic field may contribute to people reducing their level of MVPA and becoming more sedentary.

Operant theory provides an objective basis for examining behavior–environment relationships without resorting to hypothetical cognitive constructs. However, it cannot account for all of human behavior with simple reference to the immediate environment, given complex and long-preexisting histories of reinforcement. Fisher articulates this point very well: "A common misconception about behaviorism is that it views the actions of the individual as responses only to current stimuli. This fails to recognize the fundamental point that behavior is learned, that past experience guides present behavior" (2008, page 4).

Socioecological Models

Psychosocial models have been dominant in guiding the design of health behavior change programs. Interventions based on such models have shown promise (Glanz, Rimer, and Viswanath 2008), at least within the limits of small-number experimental contexts (Fisher 2008). However, psychosocial models alone cannot inform the development of intervention strategies that target changes beyond the individual level. Indeed, Craig and his colleagues note:

> The science of how to change individual behaviours has overshadowed efforts to understand true population change. Because of this unbalanced focus, the structural and systemic changes necessary to promote physical activity in populations across various sectors have not yet been addressed. (2012, page 72)

METACONTINGENCIES: ECONOMICS, POLICY, AND SOCIETY

Ultimately, neither operant theory nor mentalistic formulations can prove that it accounts for all sedentary activities. An operant framework, however, is arguably better able to accommodate the broad social and economic forces that may contribute either to sedentariness or active lifestyles, since this framework makes no reference to the existence (or nonexistence) of complex and subjective cognitive pathways. Public transportation, bike paths, and clean and safe parks and playgrounds reduce barriers to physical activity, while higher gasoline taxes and parking prices may make sedentary transportation less reinforcing. Parents who change the home environment to remove televisions from bedrooms and restrict the number of hours children engage in any screen time may directly reduce sedentary activities and increase physical activity, as would worksites that provide regular activity breaks and even standing desk options for workers. These broader changes in physical and social environments that in turn lead to behavior changes in many or most of the people who encounter these environments are sometimes referred to as *metacontingencies*, or contingencies of reinforcement that are applied not at individual but instead at group or even population levels (Hovell, Wahlgren, and Gehrman 2002). Parallel constructs derived from other social sciences are implicit in systems change theory (Kohl, Rief, and Glombiewski 2012), behavioral economics (Bickel and Vuchinich 2000), and other relatively recent schools of thought.

At least from this perspective, individual models of behavior change grounded in health education and traditional psychology and other behavioral sciences may have even impeded public health progress in the physical activity field. They may similarly impede progress in the new public-health initiatives for reducing sedentary behavior.

From the beginning years of the health promotion field, guiding frameworks have emphasized the need to intervene in domains beyond psychological and social variables, such as supportive environments, policies, and a reorientation of health services (WHO 1986; Green and Kreuter 1991). Analogous to behavioral economics or behaviorism's metacontingencies, socioecological models of health behavior characterized by multiple and interacting layers of influence on behavior and an emphasis on environmental and policy influences have become common (McLeroy et al. 1988; Stokols 1992; Cohen, Scribner, and Farley 2000). Multilevel ecological models have been widely accepted and guide the public health and science policy agendas of Healthy People (U.S. Department of Health and Human Services 2000) and the Institute of Medicine (Smedley and Syme 2001). Despite the use of these models to explain health behavior and set broad policy agendas, many health behavior change programs continue to be targeted to the individual level only (Richard et al. 1996).

The development of ecological models for intervention purposes presents challenges distinct from the use of psychosocial models. Ecological frameworks typically comprise a broad range of variables to be considered and do not give guidance on which specific variables might be applicable to sedentary activity or other target behaviors. However, other models and theories need to be integrated into ecological frameworks to provide specificity for selected domains. Thus, ecological models need to be tailored for each behavior or health condition and population because, for example, adolescents will perform different physical activities in different settings using different equipment than older adults. Therefore, implementation strategies could differ for each population, but components of the model could be used across various populations. Given the political and logistical limits of the scientific method, psychosocial and metacontingency models are often developed with reference to correlational rather than experimental studies (Sallis, Owen, and

Fisher 2008). Thus, such models must often be based on the consensus of practitioners and participants rather than on direct scientific proof.

In any case, interest in ecological models is particularly strong in the physical activity field, possibly because physical activity must be done in specific settings and early studies showed consistent associations with a wide range of environmental variables (Humpel, Owen, and Leslie 2002). Several multilevel models specific to physical activity have been proposed that include variables at the individual, social, environmental, and policy levels (Sallis and Owen 1999; Booth et al. 2001; Saelens, Sallis, and Frank 2003). The socioecological framework has provided the structure for successful interventions combining environmental and individual approaches in school- and community-based programs (Sallis et al. 2003; Stevens et al. 2005). However, researchers do not yet understand the degree to which the narrower individual and broader ecological layers respectively contributed to the successful results of these efforts or the degree to which these layers interact (Fisher 2008).

Summary

To a great extent, psychosocial theories have failed to produce solutions to what Kohl, Rief, and Glombiewski (2012) labeled a global pandemic of physical inactivity. As they note, "a systems approach to physical activity beyond a reliance on behavioural science needs coordinated changes at the individual, social and cultural, environmental and policy levels" (page 67). These authors assert that progress in addressing this pandemic compares unfavorably to previous efforts in the control of noncommunicable risks such as cigarette smoking. Within these concerns, there are important lessons for understanding and influencing sedentary behavior.

This criticism from the physical activity field is well taken, but perhaps itself does not take into account the pervasive nature of sedentary behaviors that compete so strongly with physical activity and the context in which theories and models based in individualistic perspectives on the determinants of behavior have come to predominate.

A focus on change that is directed at the level of the individual is also pervasive. Scientific norms (and research funding) requiring statistical power at the individual level lead to small-number randomized studies with overly intensive cognitive-behavioral assessment and limited follow-up (Fisher 2008). Operant and socioecological models lend themselves to more objective and comprehensive measurement, but may fail to account for complex learning histories and interactions among levels of influence. Also, no solid evidence exists that systems-level interventions perform any better than individual-level programs. Advances in actigraphy and ecological momentary assessment (Marshall et al. 2003) at the individual level combined with observational assessment (McKenzie and Cohen 2011) at the environmental level offer at least the hope of advances in the science of sedentary behavior interventions and population-wide promotion of healthy levels of physical activity. Should time-series designs emphasizing behavioral settings with many participants rather than a single person's actions become more broadly accepted, positivistic theories of behavior change may yet prove valuable to this endeavor.

KEY CONCEPTS

▶ **Health belief model:** *Perceived threat* represents a person's feelings regarding how hazardous a condition or disease is. This construct involves two factors: perceived susceptibility and perceived severity. *Perceived benefits* are attitudes about the how much there is to gain by engaging in a particular preventive action. *Perceived barriers* represent feelings associated with the potential negative aspects of a particular health behavior.

▶ **Social cognitive theory:** *Self-efficacy* and *outcome expectations* are cognitive processes that may make behaviors more likely to occur. Self-efficacy refers to the confidence a person has in being able to perform a specific behavior. Outcome expectations are the anticipated consequences of engaging in the behavior. Social cognitive theory also emphasizes the notion of *reciprocal determinism* among three entities: behavior, the environment, and the person (i.e., an individual's cognitive processes). The addition of the latter element represents its departure from operant theory.

▶ **Theories of reasoned action and planned behavior:** An *attitude* consists of a person's beliefs about the consequences that will follow from a behavior (*behavioral beliefs*), along with subjective valuations of those consequences. *Subjective norms* consist of two constructs: normative beliefs and motivation to comply. *Normative beliefs* affect behavior only if a person has a strong *motivation to comply* with the expectations of their family, peers, or other important people within in their community. Attitudes and subjective norms both influence the *intention* to perform a behavior. *Perceived control* is determined by the presence of hindering or enabling factors (*control beliefs*) and the *perceived power* those factors maintain. Factors that maintain little perceived *power* will not largely influence perceived control.

▶ **Transtheoretical model's stages of change:** *Precontemplation* is the earliest stage, in which people do not intend to change within the next 6 months. *Contemplation* identifies people who intend to change within the next 6 months. *Preparation* is achieved when a person is planning to change soon, likely within the next month. *Action* is reserved for people who have made a change in their lifestyle within the last 6 months. *Maintenance* is reached when a person has made a significant modification in lifestyle longer than 6 months and is working to avoid relapse. *Termination* is the stage that represents complete transition to a new behavior, where the risk of relapse is operationally zero.

STUDY QUESTIONS

1. Identify and explain the three most important ways in which psychosocial models of behavior change might act to hinder public health approaches to reducing excessive sitting time.

2. Taking into account the transtheoretical model's precontemplation and contemplation stages of change, identify how an older adult who sits for 11 hours each day might be persuaded to reduce and break up sitting time.

3. Describe three examples of how the positive reinforcement, extinction, and negative reinforcement constructs could be used to reduce the daytime television viewing of an unemployed teenager.

4. What do you consider to be the three most useful attributes of ecological models for understanding and influencing the determinants of health behaviors? Explain why you have chosen these attributes.

5. Using an ecological model, identify the individual, social, and environmental factors that would be most important in determining prolonged, unbroken sitting among computer-based office workers.

6. What are the metacontingencies that would be of most relevance for reducing prolonged sitting among office-based workers?

The authors would especially like to thank Kathleen A. Butler, department of geography at San Diego State University, for her assistance in conducting the background research for the writing of this chapter.

CHAPTER 23

ENVIRONMENT AND POLICY INTERVENTIONS

Jordan A. Carlson, PhD; and James F. Sallis, PhD

The reader will gain an overview of environment and policy interventions for reducing sedentary behavior in varied settings. By the end of this chapter, the reader should be able to do the following:

- ▸ List promising environment or policy approaches for reducing sedentary time for home, school, and community settings
- ▸ Describe barriers to implementing environment and policy interventions
- ▸ List advantages and disadvantages of implementing environment or policy interventions for reducing sedentary time
- ▸ List opportunities for research on environment and policy approaches for reducing sedentary time

---

What if every school classroom and office had height-adjustable desks? What if insurance companies gave discounts to workers with treadmill desks? What if every restaurant and bar had standing tables? What if half of the conference rooms at worksites had no chairs? What if employers had policies to encourage standing meetings and walking meetings? What if furniture makers made tall coffee tables without chairs for home entertainment rooms where people would stand to watch TV? What if theaters had labeled standing sections with premium views? What if padded comfortable chairs were taxed more than hard, less-comfortable chairs? Would any of these changes in our society make a difference in sitting time or risk for chronic diseases?

The preceding questions raise possibilities about how we could create environments and policies that might lead to less sitting. These environments and policies would make it easier for people to choose to stand or be active. Such interventions would likely need to be combined with educational and motivational programs to encourage people to take advantage of these standing-friendly environments. The interventions would not take away anyone's freedom but would make it easier to choose standing over sitting. If evidence keeps mounting about the negative health effects of the extraordinary amount of sitting done by most people, interventions could be justified that *require* less sitting and more standing. Standing desks, standing meetings, standing sections in theaters, standing tables at restaurants, and standing by retail workers could be required. Interventions to prohibit sitting or require standing in certain situations would no doubt be controversial, but they might be effective in reducing sitting by a substantial amount.

The focus of this chapter is on built or physical environment interventions for replacing sitting time with standing or physical activity. We consider several types of policies, both formal (legislative, regulatory) and informal (not legally binding). Policies that can affect sitting could be adopted by companies and school districts, health care organizations, community organizations, parents, and local, state, or federal governments. They would focus on where people spend the most time: home, the workplace, and school. Many options exist for environment and policy interventions, but relatively few have been evaluated for their effectiveness in controlled studies or even for their feasibility in free-living situations. So, we both review the available studies and suggest more intervention approaches that could be attempted.

Many opportunities exist for environment and policy interventions because so many environment attributes and policies in our current world have been created to facilitate, encourage, or require sitting. Sitting is virtually, though not legally, required by informal policies throughout most of the school day, in most occupations, and in entertainment settings like restaurants and movie theaters. Sitting is legally required at times while flying on airplanes. The design of items we use every day makes it essentially impossible to stand while driving, working at a normal desk, or eating at a sit-down restaurant. How are we going to reduce unhealthful levels of sitting unless substantial changes in environments and policies are made? Our contention is that environment and policy changes will be required to reduce sitting time by a large amount in most people.

Interventions to reduce sitting can replace it with standing, which appears to have beneficial physiological effects (Owen et al. 2010; see also chapter 3), or with physical activity, which would seem to have the double benefits of reducing sitting and increasing physical activity. To maximize health benefits of interventions, replacing sitting with physical activity is preferable when possible.

There are unavoidable overlaps to be found with other chapters in this book, such as those on workplace (chapter 24), community (chapter 25), ergonomics (chapter 26), and technology interventions (chapter 27). We briefly discuss environment and policy interventions related to each of these topics, so the present chapter is relatively comprehensive, but we try to avoid redundancy. Other overlaps occur because it is difficult to clearly distinguish environment and policy changes from other types of interventions. For example, replacing sedentary video games with active ones is an environment intervention that is also a technological intervention. Another example of overlap is policies that provide incentives to use software that reminds people to stand or to attend group sessions on reducing sedentary time.

Comprehensive Multilevel Approaches

Will environment and policy interventions be sufficient by themselves to dramatically reduce the health risks of prolonged sitting? Probably not, for two reasons. The first is that many people are likely to resist environment and policy changes that reduce the convenience of sitting. We do not have sitting-friendly environments by accident. Humans conserve energy for evolutionary reasons, such as surviving famines. Sitting conserves more energy than standing or moving, so it is logical that people who were well adapted for prolonged sitting would survive famines and pass on their tendencies or preferences for sitting to their progeny. The biological mechanisms for sitting preference have not been documented, but there are biological mechanisms that lead animals and likely people to prefer less physical activity as they age (Ingram 2000). From this perspective, it would seem politically difficult to make big enough environment and policy changes that have large effects on sitting.

A second reason that environment and policy interventions may not be enough is the growing evidence that interventions are most effective when they operate on multiple levels. A principle of ecological models of behavior is that behavior is affected by individual (e.g., psychological, biological), social and cultural, organizational, built environmental, and policy levels of influence (Sallis, Owen, and Fisher 2008). Interventions carried out on multiple levels can build on the strengths of each component. Environment and policy changes can make it easier to reduce sitting time by removing barriers and providing incentives. Organizational and social changes can create supportive norms throughout the community and through media channels. Educational and motivational programs targeted at individuals can encourage people to use supportive environments and build a favorable political climate for policy change. An ecological model of sedentary behavior has been developed that suggests interventions at all levels that can be applied to reduce sitting in work, school, transport, recreation, and home settings (Owen et al. 2011).

Connections exist between environments and policies that are helpful to keep in mind. Policies can influence behaviors through several mechanisms. Policies can provide incentives to engage in a behavior or not. Policies to encourage standing could include health insurance discounts for having a standing or treadmill desk or making employees buy their chairs for work. Budgeting can change behavior by encouraging consumers to buy less comfortable chairs or funding educational programs to discourage prolonged sitting. Envi-

ronment changes like those suggested in the first paragraph of this chapter are usually the result of formal or informal policies. The effect on behavior should be greater when environments and policies are complementary. For example, if a company has a policy to have standing meetings but its conference rooms are full of chairs, the company sends an inconsistent message.

Evaluating Environment and Policy Interventions

Environment and policy interventions can be difficult to implement and evaluate, particularly when they affect large geographic areas and numbers of people. Using randomized controlled experimental trials is typically not feasible when evaluating macro-level environment interventions. Because large-scale environment modifications are so expensive, they are typically initiated by governments or companies rather than researchers. Thus, investigators do not control decisions about the intervention, and finding appropriate comparison groups can be difficult when a state or large city adopts a policy. Another barrier to documenting effects of environment and policy interventions is that governments or companies usually do not evaluate the effects of environment modifications. Thus, multisector collaborations among governments, researchers, and health departments are needed to build evidence on the influence of environment and policy interventions on sedentary time. Other barriers to conducting experimental studies of environment and policy interventions have been identified (Sallis, Story, and Lou 2009).

Environment and policy interventions in settings such as homes, schools, and worksites are more feasible to conduct and evaluate within grant periods. Settings can be randomized to experimental conditions and direct observations can be conducted relatively easily within a specific setting. One evaluation challenge of special relevance is that interventions may not be implemented as intended. For example, policies may be adopted but not enforced or environment changes may be planned and announced, but funding may be delayed or lost. In other situations, control schools or companies may decide to implement the intervention. Another evaluation challenge is the lack of validated measures of sitting-related environment attributes and policies.

Interventions in the Home Setting

Evaluated interventions for reducing sedentary time at home have primarily focused on reducing the amount of time youth spend watching television, playing video games, and using computers (i.e., screen time). A majority of these interventions have used educational sessions to increase participants' motivation and skills for reducing television viewing time in combination with environment modification. The types of environment modification that have been used fall within three categories: restricted screen time, contingent screen time, and active screen time (i.e., replacing sedentary behaviors with more active behaviors during screen time).

Restricted Screen Time

Environment interventions for restricting screen time have used devices such as the TV Allowance, which plugs into the television or other screen-based device and monitors and regulates the amount of time the device can be used. In forced restriction studies, the TV Allowance was programmed by the interventionist to shut off the TV after a specified amount of viewing time (e.g., 2 hr/day) (Epstein et al. 2008). In open restriction studies, the TV Allowance monitored viewing time and participants were encouraged but not forced to follow an upper limit of viewing time (Ni Mhurchu et al. 2009; Robinson

1999). Parents were often encouraged to enforce a specified amount of viewing time.

Target TV times in these interventions ranged from a reduction of 1 hour per day (Ni Mhurchu et al. 2009) to a 50% reduction (Epstein et al. 2008; see figure 23.1). The interventions led to reductions in TV time of 5 hours per week in two studies (Ni Mhurchu et al. 2009; Robinson 1999) and more than 10 hours per week in another study (Epstein et al. 2008). Epstein and colleagues also found reductions in children's BMI z-score and energy intake over a 2-year period.

Evidence of efficacy in reducing TV time is promising because large reductions were documented. One limitation is that few studies assessed total sedentary time for the day. Little evidence exists to support the acceptability of restricting screen time on a large scale and in diverse populations. Sustainability is an important question because the majority of youth screen-time interventions did not include a long-term follow-up assessment.

Contingent Screen Time

Contingent screen-time interventions have required participants to engage in physical activity to earn time for viewing screen-based devices. One study tested an intervention where children earned 1 hour of TV viewing for every 400 steps they walked, assessed by pedometer (Goldfield et al. 2006). Parents monitored their child's pedometer and

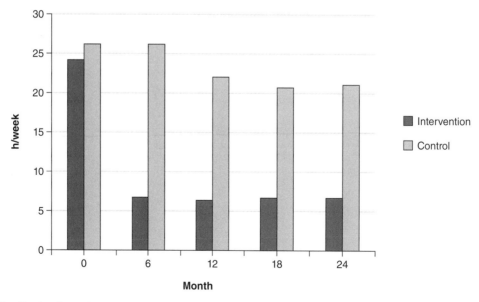

Figure 23.1 Reductions in sedentary behavior for TV restriction with TV allowance.
Data from Epstein et al. 2008.

presented the child with tokens to be used in a TV Allowance device. The intervention led to reductions in TV viewing by almost 2 hours per day as well as increases in moderate- to vigorous-intensity physical activity (MVPA).

Active Screen Time

Some interventions have required children to ride a stationary bicycle (Faith et al. 2001) or walk on a treadmill (Lanningham-Foster et al. 2006) while watching TV. These interventions can be considered both contingency interventions and active screen-time interventions because they required children to engage in physical activity to earn screen time and they replaced sedentary time with physical activity during screen time. In one study, pedaling on a stationary bicycle while watching TV reduced TV viewing to less than 2 hours per day (Faith et al. 2001). In another study, walking on a treadmill while watching TV led to significant increases in energy expenditure, although the authors did not assess changes in TV viewing time (Lanningham-Foster et al. 2006).

Active video games such as Dance Revolution, XBox Kinect, and Nintendo Wii have been substituted for sedentary video games to increase energy expenditure. Intervention studies have generally found that active video games lead to increased energy expenditure and moderate-intensity physical activity over sedentary video games (Barnett, Cerin, and Baranowski 2011; Lanningham-Foster et al. 2006; Maloney et al. 2008). However, effect on reducing sedentary time was usually not assessed. Studies on active video games have found that game play decreases rapidly within a few weeks (Barnett, Cerin, and Baranowski 2011), so lack of sustainability is of particular concern.

Interventions in the Work Setting

Many occupations involve prolonged sitting for office and retail work. Most worksite interventions to date have been conducted with participants who spend a majority of their day working at a desk, typically on a computer. Interventions are believed to be particularly promising in this population because they have high baseline rates of sitting and thus have substantial room for reducing sedentary time.

Standing Desks

Replacing standard desks with standing or sit-to-stand desks is the most common strategy used in workplace sedentary interventions. Several studies have reported good feasibility and acceptability for using standing desks, suggesting this is a promising environment modification strategy (e.g., Beers et al. 2008; Gilson et al. 2012; Healy et al. 2013). The largest study to date used sit-to-stand workstations and behavioral coaching in office work-

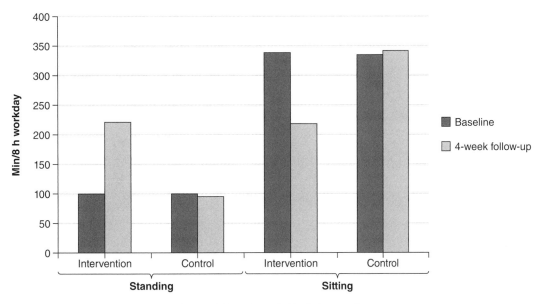

Figure 23.2 Sedentary reductions for multilevel worksite interventions.

Data from Healy et al. 2013.

ers and achieved a reduction in sitting of 125 minutes per 8-hour workday (Healy et al. 2013; see figure 23.2).

A major barrier to implementing environment interventions in worksites is that sit-to-stand desks are often cost prohibitive on a large scale, but as more evidence on the health consequences of prolonged sedentary time accumulates, buy-ins from business owners may increase. Increasing demand for sit-to-stand desks or computer risers can be expected to lead to better designs and cost reductions. Studies that document the effect of sitting interventions on work performance and productivity could accelerate adoption of such workplace interventions.

Computer Prompts

Computer software has been used to send prompts to users at given intervals. The software is typically programmed to open a window on the computer screen that displays a message for the user to take a standing break. One study investigating computer prompts found some evidence of reductions in sitting time and sitting episodes when using prompts every 30 minutes (Evans et al. 2012). Prompts could be incorporated with other strategies, such as linking a sensor to the prompt system so prompts are displayed only when the user has been sitting for a given amount of time. The software could be modified so the computer is locked for a certain amount of time when a prompt appears, thus restricting computer use during that interval and potentially increasing user compliance.

Providing Activity Breaks

Workplace policies have been evaluated that interrupt sedentary jobs several times per day with brief physical activity breaks. This is an intervention with a potential double benefit of reducing sitting and increasing physical activity. This strategy has been feasible in several worksites and has led to outcomes of interest to employers such as reductions in sick days and ergonomic injuries (Lazarovici 2012).

Interventions in the School Setting

Traditionally, classroom learning involves large amounts of sitting. However, evidence exists that children's learning improves when they are more physically active and potentially when they are less sedentary (Singh et al. 2012). Few interventions have targeted reducing or interrupting sedentary time during school. The environment

and policy strategies that have been investigated include incorporating movement into academic lessons and modifying classroom desks to allow students to stand. Interventions for reducing sedentary time at school are particularly promising because they could reach large numbers of youth and thus have great potential for affecting public health.

Active Lessons

The goal of an active lesson is to incorporate physical activity into an existing academic lesson or teach through activity (e.g., Kibbe et al. 2011). Active lessons could involve subjects such as mathematics, science, or language arts. Although the primary goal of active lessons is to get children to be physically active, the lessons also serve to interrupt and reduce sedentary time. However, the effect of active lessons on classroom sedentary time has not been evaluated. Some evidence exists that these interventions led to improved academic performance and classroom concentration (Kibbe et al. 2011). A barrier to modifying academic curricula to include active lessons is that it would require significant resources and teacher training. Also, current norms are for teachers to encourage young children to be still during class because moving around too much is often perceived as disruptive (De Decker et al. 2012).

Standing Desks

Standing desk interventions have recently emerged as a promising strategy for decreasing sedentary time at school, but most studies have included only a small number of classrooms (Blake, Benden, and Wendel 2012; Cardon et al. 2004; Clemes et al. 2015; Hinckson et al. 2013). One study aimed to create a moving school, where classroom furniture is organized to provide students with an open area for walking around and some standing desks are provided. Results showed that 31% of children's sitting time was replaced by standing and 10% was replaced by walking (Cardon et al. 2004). There were no negative effects on children's reading and writing productivity. A study in primary schools in the UK and Australia replaced standard desks with sit-to-stand desks and observed that sitting time was reduced from 70% to 60% of the school day (Clemes et al. 2015).

Evidence about the efficacy and feasibility of standing desks in the classroom is promising, but substantial barriers likely exist to modifying school environments on a large scale, including that modifying classrooms to include sit-to-stand desks for all students would have significant financial costs. However, few studies have investigated these barriers.

Interventions in Community Settings

Many places within communities involve prolonged sedentary time. Examples include restaurants, movie theaters, airports, sporting events, and conferences. To date, environment and policy intervention studies have not targeted these settings, but some modifications are occurring that should be evaluated for their influence on sedentary behavior. Some restaurants and pubs are incorporating standing tables, and many have taller tables with stools that are the appropriate height for standing. Standing workstations that could affect users' sedentary behavior have recently begun to appear in airports. Incorporating a standing section or standing prompts in movie theaters would likely need to be supported by educational interventions, but this may be a viable strategy for reducing sedentary behavior.

Conferences, large meetings, and sporting events may affect each attendee infrequently, but such events often require prolonged sitting for hundreds and thousands of people. Active Living Research incorporates active applause into its 3-day annual conference, which involves standing ovations for all conference presenters. This practice has been adopted at several other conferences. In many public health conferences, it is becoming more common to observe participants standing in the side and back of meeting rooms than sitting in chairs. Prompts and standing sections could be used during events of many types to promote standing breaks.

Many community settings could be targeted to reduce sedentary behavior. Environment and policy strategies in these settings are promising, but will likely require community support and buy-in. Evaluations of naturalistic experiments are needed because many environment modifications that affect sedentary behavior are currently occurring.

Interventions in Transportation, Land Use, and Parks

Transportation and land use policies affect travel patterns by supporting pedestrian and bicycle

INTERVENTIONS IN UNIQUE COMMUNITY INSTITUTIONS

Environment and policy interventions in institutions such as retirement communities, senior centers, day care centers, and churches and places of worship would likely use similar strategies as home, school, and worksite interventions. Targeting retirement communities and day care centers could reach a substantial portion of older adults and preschool-aged children on a daily basis, so these settings are promising for intervention. Time spent at places of worship is typically low, so strategies in this setting have lower reach. A benefit of intervening in institutions is the potential for making the changes permanent. However, no published evaluations of sedentary interventions in these settings could be located.

- **Retirement communities.** Given the potentially major effect of reductions in sedentary time on healthy aging, targeting older adults appears a promising public health strategy. Adapting home and worksite strategies, such as restricting TV time and using standing break prompts, could be especially effective in these settings.

One study targeted policy interventions by training older adults at senior centers and retirement communities to advocate for standing breaks during meetings and events that involved prolonged sitting (Kerr et al. 2012).

- **Day care centers.** Children watch substantial amounts of TV at some day care centers (McWilliams et al. 2009), so strategies for reducing sedentary time might include policies that require standing breaks or limit TV viewing to educational purposes only.

- **Places of worship.** Though it appears that most worship services have substantial amounts of sedentary time, the amount of standing in places of worship varies during prayer or other aspects of worship. Potential environment and policy strategies could include distributing (rather than front-loading) standing breaks throughout a service or incorporating a standing section in the worship area.

infrastructure as well as smart growth land use (Handy 2005). Built environment attributes have good evidence of association with physical activity (Bauman et al. 2012), but they likely also play a role in influencing sedentary behavior.

Transportation

Driving and riding in motor vehicles is a major source of sitting. Transportation policies can offset other sedentary behavior by providing bicycle and pedestrian infrastructure that allows users to choose active over automobile transportation. Though many cities have shown that long-term, multicomponent, multilevel interventions can be effective at increasing bicycling (Pucher, Dill, and Handy 2010), it is unclear whether increases in active transportation lead to decreases in sedentary behavior.

Transportation policies also affect public transportation, which is relevant to reducing sedentary behavior because buses and trains usually include standing areas. Environment and policy interventions for reducing sedentary behavior in public transportation could increase standing room on vehicles and include prompts to promote standing. Targeting these strategies on long-distance train and airplane rides may be effective for reducing sedentary behavior.

Land Use and Smart Growth

Smart growth and urban development land use policies aim to reduce automobile dependency and facilitate active travel, primarily through increased residential density and land use mix, where homes, retail sites, schools, and worksites are in close proximity. Smart growth usually incorporates pedestrian-oriented transportation infrastructure, and is closely tied to transportation policies (Handy 2005). Good evidence exists that people of all ages living in mixed-use walkable communities do more walking for transportation and total physical activity (Bauman et al. 2012; Sallis et al. 2012).

Walkable neighborhood designs have also been related to spending less time in specific sitting behaviors in a few studies. Though no studies to date have shown a significant relationship between living in a walkable neighborhood and total sedentary time, lower levels of TV time (Kozo et al. 2012; Sugiyama et al. 2007) and driving in a motor vehicle (Kozo et al. 2012) have been documented in walkable neighborhoods. However, a study in Belgium using objective measures did not show the expected

association of less sedentary time in residents of walkable neighborhoods (Van Dyck et al. 2010).

Controlled intervention studies to evaluate smart growth are nearly impossible to conduct because neighborhood development or redevelopment is a slow process and people self-select into neighborhoods, which prohibits randomized controlled trials. Though quasiexperimental prospective studies are finding that moving to different built environments is related to changes in physical activity (Giles-Corti et al. 2013), sedentary behavior outcomes have not been reported. Similar to transportation policies, the mechanism by which land use policies may reduce sedentary behavior likely increases MVPA and also potentially increases light activity.

Parks

Parks are a specific land use in the public domain, and good evidence exists that proximity and design of parks are related to physical activity (Bauman et al. 2012; Sallis et al. 2012). Parks serve many purposes, including providing space for quiet relaxation, contemplation of nature, and respite from hectic urban living. Opportunities may exist for designing parks so they reduce sedentary behavior without interfering with more contemplative activities. For example, spectator areas for amateur sports facilities could have designated standing areas close to the action or, better yet, walking areas and outdoor exercise equipment to give attractive alternatives to sitting. Why couldn't children's playgrounds also have adult exercise equipment so parents could be active instead of sitting and watching while children are playing?

Ensuring that virtually every park has linear features like sidewalks and trails that facilitate movement could balance the allure of plentiful benches. It is worthwhile to explore standing tables in picnic areas. It may not be wise to remove most park benches. Places to rest are important for older adults in particular, so removing benches may result in fewer trips to parks by older adults. Even if people mostly sit while in the park, they can get some activity by walking to the park and walking to the bench.

Well-placed and well-designed parks may contribute to reducing sedentary travel to parks. Developing more parks that are smaller or linear within walking or biking distance to a greater number of people would be more effective than emphasizing larger regional parks. The roads leading to parks should be optimized for safe pedestrian and bicycle access to reduce driving.

Integrating Environment and Policy Interventions With Other Approaches

Many of the sedentary behavior interventions suggested in the preceding sections are likely to seem unfamiliar, even radical. Seeing a restaurant or living room without chairs or a movie theater with a standing section would be jarring for many people. Thus, public acceptance or support for many of the suggested interventions should not be expected in the short term. Consistent with ecological models, educational interventions to inform people about the health effects of too much sitting and media campaigns to change social norms and build support for environmental and policy interventions will almost certainly be needed before most of these interventions can be applied in practice. Even after environmental and policy interventions are implemented, complementary interventions at the individual, social, and organizational levels will likely be required to achieve desired effects.

A further impediment to implementing many of the suggested environmental and policy interventions is the near certainty of opposition. Much opposition can be expected from industries whose products and services rely on or require sitting. Policies that would take chairs out of offices or schools would not be popular among many furniture makers. However, increasing demand for standing desks and tables already is giving rise to new product lines and design innovations. The costs of ret-rofitting existing schools and offices with standing furniture and making time for activity breaks may lead to resistance to new health-promoting interventions. Parents may be unwilling to pay for TV allowance devices and uncomfortable enforcing screen-time limits that are unpopular with their children. Interventions that provide options, prompts, and incentives for reducing sitting time are probably going to be more acceptable than interventions that remove options to sit or require standing. Overcoming resistance to sedentary behavior interventions will require continued strengthening of evidence on the negative health consequences of sitting and the effectiveness of recommended interventions. Barriers and opposition to environment and policy interventions are a useful area for research.

Practical Guidelines

Evidence of serious negative health effects of sitting is new and interventions for reducing sedentary behavior are even newer. Though environment and policy interventions have the potential advantages of wide reach and long-term effects, few such interventions have been evaluated to date. Only worksite interventions with adults and television reduction approaches for youth have been evaluated in multiple studies, so it is premature to develop many evidence-based recommendations. It may be useful to offer some tentative guidelines based on the existing evidence along with encouragement to expand the research in all directions, both further testing existing approaches and evaluating novel interventions. Table 23.1 presents a summary of the settings and strategies for reducing sedentary behavior that are presented in this chapter.

Table 23.1 Settings and Strategies for Environment and Policy Interventions for Reducing Sedentary Behavior

Setting	Evaluated strategies	Examples of unevaluated strategies
Homes	Restricted screen time, contingent screen time, active screen time	Redesigning furniture and room layout
Worksites	Standing desks, computer prompts, physical activity breaks	Redesigning occupational vehicles, conference rooms with no chairs
Schools	Active lessons, standing desks	Regular breaks from sitting
Other institutions	Same as home and worksite strategies	Standing breaks during meetings
Community settings	None	Standing applause, standing sections at events, standing tables
Transportation and land use	Walkable neighborhoods	Redesigning or increasing availability of public transit and parks

One of the most promising studies evaluated a multilevel approach that included education and skills building to reduce sedentary behavior in addition to environment modification (e.g., adding standing desks) (Healy et al. 2013). Some interventions with evidence of efficacy may have limited reach, sustainability, and external validity, such as those aimed at reducing children's screen time (e.g., Epstein et al. 2008). Thus, future interventions should be designed to maximize sustainability, and studies should include long-term assessments of sustainability. Perhaps mass media campaigns could help build support for environment and policy changes that seem far from current cultural norms. Since sedentary interventions are a relatively new topic in public health, there are many avenues to explore, making this area a particularly rich research opportunity.

Next Steps for Research

Next steps for developing interventions to reduce home-based sedentary time are to evaluate low-cost, high-reach, and sustainable strategies. Interventions are needed in adults, and novel ideas need to be investigated. For example, family rooms could be redesigned to remove the TV as the centerpiece of the room or move the sofa away from the TV. Designers could be challenged to create appealing furniture, such as standing coffee tables, to facilitate standing during electronic entertainment. These could be effective strategies for reducing TV time, although they are likely to be viewed as drastic changes from current cultural norms.

Although most sedentary worksite environment interventions to date have been conducted with office workers, interventions could have a great influence in other sedentary occupations. Sedentary interventions for other occupations may include strategies such as promoting standing breaks in vehicle operators (e.g., bus drivers, taxi drivers) or standing meetings in occupations that involve substantial time in meetings. Large vehicles like buses and trucks could have seats that fold up, giving the driver the opportunity to alternate sitting and standing.

For the school setting, next steps should include investigating other school-based strategies, including those aiming to interrupt sitting time. Low-cost environment modifications, such as environmental prompts or simply standing beside desks, could be effective at interrupting students' sedentary time.

In the community setting, more evidence is needed to determine whether transportation, land use, and parks policies can reduce sedentary behavior. These policies and environments are difficult to change because they involve political decisions and large investments, but built environments are constantly changing. The potential effects of transportation and land use improvements are great, due to high reach and sustained effects. Transportation and land use strategies may be particularly effective in people who spend large amounts of time in sedentary travel. Parks designed to reduce sedentary leisure behavior and encourage users to travel to reach them could affect all segments of the population.

Summary

Environment and policy interventions for reducing sedentary behavior could include standing desks and tables at workplaces and schools, policies to encourage standing meetings and activity breaks, and standing sections in commonly used settings such as restaurants, movie theaters, and meeting rooms. Small numbers of studies conducted in homes, schools, and workplaces demonstrated that environment changes can be effective and provide proof of concept, but questions remain. Transportation and land use policies can reduce driving, which is a common sedentary behavior. Numerous potential environment and policy interventions are suggested in this chapter that could be evaluated in a wide range of settings. Changing environments and policies are promising in terms of reducing sedentary behaviors because such changes could reach many people and have long-term effects, in contrast to most interventions at the individual and social levels that tend to have limited reach and short-term effects.

The major challenges to environment and policy changes are likely to be political feasibility and population acceptance, because many of the interventions would be considered unfamiliar or even radical. Thus, efforts to build political will and individual motivation need to precede and accompany environment and policy changes in a coordinated multilevel approach. Constraints exist to evaluating environment and policy interventions because they are seldom controlled by investigators, so opportunistic evaluations of natural experiments are recommended. The emphasis in the next few years should be on prioritizing research questions and building an evidence base about environment and policy interventions that can guide later efforts to create change on a scale sufficient to affect population levels of sedentary behavior.

KEY CONCEPTS

▶ **Environment and policy interventions:** Time spent sitting is a pervasive aspect of the everyday lives of adults and children. Individual motivational approaches to reducing sedentary time are unlikely to result in substantial or sustainable changes. Wide-reaching influences are needed so that the environments in which people spend their time and the relevant social norms, regulations, or sometimes laws are such that opportunities are more widely available for activities other than sitting for the majority of time.

▶ **Multilevel influences on sedentary behavior:** Ecological models suggest that individual, interpersonal, and environmental factors interact to influence behavior. Although motivation for reducing sedentary behavior varies among people, even highly motivated people engage in prolonged sedentary time because numerous aspects of the environment make sitting the normative and default behavior. Thus, to maximize effectiveness, interventions should target environmental modifications, awareness, cultural shifts, and individual skills and motivation.

▶ **Settings-based approaches to sedentary behavior:** Much of the sitting in people's daily lives takes place in the workplace, in schools, in automobiles, and in front of screens in the domestic environment. Interventions in these different contexts will need to differ in important ways. For example, the provision of sit-to-stand workstations for office employees might be the most powerful approach in the workplace setting. For time spent sitting in cars, more widespread availability of public transport options and other aspects of urban design might be most relevant. For time in front of screens in the domestic environment, changes to public awareness and social norms might be most effective.

STUDY QUESTIONS

1. Compare environmental versus individual-level approaches for reducing sedentary time. Give two examples of each.

2. Describe three features of the environment that promote sedentary time and explain how you would overcome these environmental barriers when designing a sedentary intervention.

3. Identify which settings are most promising for targeting reductions in sedentary behavior and why.

4. Choose either a school or worksite setting and describe your ideal vision of a multilevel sedentary intervention in this setting.

5. Provide two examples of collaborations you could form to facilitate development of a new environment or policy intervention for reducing sedentary time.

6. Describe two major societal barriers to modifying environments to support reductions in sitting time.

CHAPTER 24

SEDENTARY BEHAVIOR AND WORKSITE INTERVENTIONS

Nicolaas P. Pronk, PhD, MA

The reader will gain an overview of the potential that exists to address the risks associated with sedentary behavior in the workplace setting and will consider critical design elements needed for programs to achieve such potential. By the end of this chapter, the reader should be able to do the following:

▸ Better understand the workplace as a context for programs that reduce sedentary behavior
▸ Identify and consider implications of approaches used to reduce sedentary behavior and prolong standing time at work
▸ Identify recommendations for future research and practice

Within the context of the worksite setting, this chapter provides an overview of approaches and interventions designed to reduce sedentary behavior among workers and outlines recommendations for future developments and research in this emerging field of study.

Sedentary behavior is being rediscovered as a health hazard, and recommendations for avoiding prolonged exposures to sedentary tasks and behaviors are increasingly being heeded. Particular relevance to this concern relates to the worksite setting. Historically speaking, messages related to the ill-health effects of sedentary work tasks were highlighted as early as the 1700s by Italian physician Bernardino Ramazzini (1713/1940). Ramazzini, widely recognized as the father of industrial medicine, published his book *Diseases of Workmen* (*De Morbis Artificum Diatriba*) in 1700, a publication that became the foundation of the occupational medicine discipline. He observed that cobblers, tailors, and women who did needlework suffered ill-health effects due to the sedentary nature of their work tasks. On the other hand, compared to sedentary workers, messengers (whose work involved running to deliver messages) avoided many health problems suffered by the cobblers and tailors. As a result, Ramazzini advised that sedentary workers "take to physical exercise, at any rate on holidays" to counteract the harm done by many days of sedentary life (1713/1940, 285).

Another landmark study in the field of physical activity epidemiology is the London bus study conducted in 1953 by Dr. Jeremy Morris and colleagues. These researchers carefully documented the effect of sedentary work on coronary heart disease (CHD) by comparing the rates of CHD between the active bus conductors, who spent most of their working time on their feet and climbing the stairs of double-deck buses, and those of the bus drivers, who spent almost 90% of their work time seated. The increase in CHD rates among the more sedentary bus drivers was basically doubled compared to the more active conductors.

More recently, Owen and colleagues (2010) reviewed the available evidence on sedentary behavior and health outcomes and concluded that sedentary behavior should be considered separate and distinct from a lack of moderate- to vigorous-intensity physical activity (MVPA) and that prolonged sitting is an independent predictor of disease. Defined as activities characterized by minimal movement and a very low level of energy expenditure (<1.5 METs), sedentary behavior was associated with obesity, diabetes, impaired glucose uptake, and insulin resistance. These associations remained important even after statistically adjusting for MVPA and waist circumference. Furthermore, these researchers observed that adults, on average, spent approximately 60% of their waking hours being sedentary. The effect of this much daily sedentary time is compromised health, even among people who meet the recommended levels of 150 minutes or more of MVPA per week (Owen et al. 2010; Physical Activity Guidelines Advisory Committee 2008). These observations extend to the workplace as indicated by the work of Mummery and colleagues (2005), who showed that Australian workers who sit more than 6 hours per day are twice as likely to be obese compared to those who sit less than 45 minutes per day.

The health-related concerns around sedentary behavior in general and prolonged sitting time in particular in the workplace setting are exacerbated by the observation that occupation-related physical activity is becoming increasingly sedentary. Church and colleagues (2011) noted that during the five decades between 1960 and 2010, occupations classified as sedentary activity have increased from 15% to 23% and light-activity jobs have increased from 37% to 57%. On the other hand, moderate-activity jobs decreased from 48% to 20%. The net result constitutes a shift away from occupations that require moderate-intensity physical activity to jobs that are mostly sedentary. The estimated effect is a decrease of more than 100 calories in daily occupational energy expenditure, which in turn accounts for a large portion of the increase in average body weight among U.S. men and women during this time period (Church et al. 2011).

Attempts to deal with the increasingly sedentary nature of work in the contemporary workplace may be considered a strategic priority for business and industry (Pronk and Kottke 2009; Pronk 2009a). The challenges associated with sedentary behavior at the workplace are not limited to health alone. Research has shown the influence of physical activity–related variables on health care costs (Pronk et al. 1999; Goetzel et al. 2012; Pronk, Tan, and O'Connor 1999) and productivity-related concerns such as absenteeism (Proper et al. 2002), presenteeism (Cancelliere et al. 2011; Brown et al. 2011), or the effect of musculoskeletal disorders on worker performance (Straker 1998). However, in general, the literature lacks strong evidence on the relationship between sedentary behavior and productivity outcomes as well as the effect of interventions for reducing sedentary behavior and the associated changes in cost, productivity, and worker performance outcomes. Additional important research findings include the notion that employment in itself is important for maintaining physical activity levels. Van Domelen and colleagues (2011) showed that based on cross-sectional data from the National Health and Nutrition Examination Survey, full-time employment, even in sedentary occupations, is associated with higher levels of physical activity compared to unemployment, among both men and women. Furthermore, based on longitudinal surveys and economic modeling of the data, regular exercise has been associated with a 6% to 9% wage increase (Kosteas 2013). Reducing sedentary behavior represents an important objective from a variety of perspectives. It may be considered a shared objective among employers and employees, as well as from the perspective of public health.

Characteristics of Worksite Interventions

Cross-sectional studies have documented the problems associated with sedentary behavior and linked those to the worksite setting. However, *changing* the sedentary behavior of the workforce may be considered a different task altogether. Attempts to reduce sedentary behavior depend on a wide variety of factors, characteristics, and contexts related to the worksite setting. As noted previously, the workplace has become increasingly sedentary over the past five decades (Church et al. 2011). Furthermore, estimates indicate that those in sedentary occupations are engaged in sedentary behavior for approximately 11 hours per day (Tudor-Locke et al. 2011). Hence, although ample evidence indicates the need to reduce sedentary time, there does not appear to be much time left during the remainder of the waking hours to increase physical activity.

Yet, the workplace provides many opportunities and great potential for health improvement. As a complex social environment, the workplace allows many strategies to be deployed for the purpose of reducing sedentary time. Employees may be reached for extended periods of time with a high frequency of health-related interventions; multiple tools, resources, and vehicles may be mobilized to increase awareness, change behaviors, modify environments, and influence organizational policy;

and companies may collaborate with each other to influence broader social policy at a local, statewide, provincial, or national level (Pronk 2009a; Pronk et al. 1999). Yet workplace health programs designed to change behavior are not limited to those focused on physical activity or sedentary behavior. In fact, systematic reviews have repeatedly shown that the most effective programs tend to be multicomponent comprehensive programs that engage as many employees as possible over extended periods of time (Pronk 2009a; Pronk et al. 1999; Goetzel and Pronk 2010; Pronk and Goetzel 2010; Soler, Leeks, Razi, et al. 2010; Soler, Leeks, Buchanan, et al. 2010). Several benchmark studies and summary documents have derived a list of key characteristics of health programs that are associated with effective workplace programs and policies (O'Donnell 2002; Chapman 2004; Goetzel et al. 2007; Pronk 2009b; NIOSH 2008; Sparling 2010; Berry, Mirabito, and Baun 2011). Specific to the promotion of physical activity at the worksite, Pronk and Kottke (2009) applied various domains of the socioecological model against the list of "Essential Elements of Effective Workplace Programs and Policies for Improving Worker Health and Wellbeing" from the National Institute for Occupational Safety and Health (NIOSH 2008) and presented examples from the literature for each of the elements. As a result, this particular paper outlines evidence-based support related to physical activity interventions for each of the essential elements.

Whereas all these benchmark projects propose various lists of characteristics, there is substantial overlap among them. In an attempt to consolidate, I (2009b) compiled all original benchmark studies (O'Donnell 2002; Chapman 2004; Goetzel et al. 2007, NIOSH 2008) and organized them into a list of best-practice characteristics for employee health management. The list recognized four major dimensions: leadership and strategy, operations, evaluation, and integration and data practices. Under each dimension, key components are outlined that, taken together, present a comprehensive, multicomponent list of characteristics related to design features of successful worksite health programs. Specifically, these features include the following:

▸ Leadership and strategy
- Organizational commitment
- Shared program ownership (leadership at all levels of the company)

- Identification of wellness champions
- Program connected to business objectives
- Supportive policy, physical, and cultural environment
  ▸ Operations
    - Clearly defined plan of operations
    - Effective communication
    - Scalable, sustainable, and accessible programs
    - Scalable and effective assessment, screening, and triage
    - Effective interventions
    - Meaningful participation incentives
  ▸ Evaluation
    - Program measurement and evaluation
  ▸ Integration and data practices
    - Integration of program components at the point of implementation
    - Integration across multiple organizational functions and departments
    - Integrated data systems
    - Efficient and effective data practices
    - Relentless focus on safeguarding privacy and confidentiality of personal health information

Therefore, a key consideration in the application of workplace interventions designed to reduce sedentary behavior is the way in which such interventions fit into the larger health improvement strategy for the company. It is important for any organization to consider this context and place intervention activities into a framework for action. One such framework was proposed as part of the recommendations for a national physical activity plan for business and industry and is organized according to relevance of the program to stakeholders and across multiple levels of influence that align with the socioecological model (Pronk 2009a). Figure 24.1 presents this framework as applied to reducing sedentary behavior instead of promoting physical activity. In this framework, each cell may hold specific interventions or implementation processes that, taken together, add up to the total set of interventions. All these activities generate a certain set of experiences for the audiences of those interventions or programs. Regardless of the type of program or intervention, the experience of the

user or consumer of that activity should be exceptional. If not, those users may not readily return or continue to participate, and such poor experiential outcomes may put the entire program in jeopardy or, at a minimum, suboptimize outcomes. All experiences add up to participation and consumption of the interventions and drive outcomes in multiple domains, including reduced sedentary behavior, cost reduction, and productivity improvement.

Applications of Worksite Interventions

Programs designed to reduce sedentary behavior at the workplace come in various forms. By definition, sedentary behavior is characterized by minimal movement and an energy expenditure level of less than 1.5 METs—primarily sitting behaviors that manifest themselves in the context of work, such as sitting while commuting, doing computer work, or conducting meetings. The minimum necessary requirement of such programs would be to increase energy expenditure from less than 1.5 METs by introducing situations in which workers expend more than 1.5 METs. Using this criterion, interventions that move workers from a sitting into a standing, walking, or running position would meet the standard of successful programs. Additionally, as outlined by Owen and colleagues (2010), Healy and colleagues (2008), and Thorp and colleagues (2012), the major culprit to be addressed is *prolonged* sitting time. The goal is therefore to reduce sedentary behavior by breaking up prolonged sitting time with periods of standing, walking, or running. As Ramazzini already noted in the 1700s, standing too long is associated with its own set of health concerns.

A systematic review of workplace interventions for reducing sitting by Chau and colleagues (2010) included studies up to April 2009 that specifically measured sitting as a primary or secondary outcome and found only six studies that met criteria for inclusion. All six studies had increasing physical activity as the primary aim and reducing sitting time as the secondary outcome. No studies showed reductions in sitting time compared to a control or comparison group. Barr-Anderson and colleagues (2011) conducted a systematic review of short bouts of physical activity integrated into the organizational routine and included 12 studies in their search related to the worksite setting. This review indicated that short bouts of physical activity

Make reducing sedentary behaviors...	Level of influence			
	Individual	Team or group-based	Organizational	Environmental
Possible				
Simple				
Socially rewarding				
Financially rewarding				
Personally relevant				
Organizationally relevant				
Community connected				

Figure 24.1 A framework for action for reducing sedentary behavior in the workplace.

Adapted, by permission, from N.P. Pronk, 2009, "Physical activity promotion in business and industry: Evidence, context, and recommendations for a national plan," *Journal of Physical Activity and Health* 6 (Suppl. 2): S220-S235.

tended to be around 10 to 15 minutes in duration. These programs were structurally integrated into the workflow of the organizations and manifested themselves as activity breaks during the workday or the promotion of stair use through changes in building design. The studies considered the effects of these changes for an average of approximately 10 months. Positive outcomes were noted across a variety of outcomes, including employees feeling supported in their efforts to be more active and to eat more healthfully, improved mood states, and improved psychosocial factors. Outcomes related to employee performance were mixed. Work ability showed improvement (e.g., data entry speed and accuracy), yet other studies showed no significant effects on worker productivity.

However, despite the fact that limited evidence exists of effectiveness of workplace interventions designed to reduce (prolonged) sitting time (Chau et al. 2010), pilot and small-scale studies have shown promising results. Feasibility studies among working and nonworking populations (Gardiner et al. 2011; Kozey-Keadle et al. 2012; Thompson et al. 2008), exploratory research on policy development related to commuting to and from work (Panter, Desousa, and Ogilvie 2013), and pre–post stud-

ies without comparison groups (e.g., Yancey et al. 2006) have emerged that indicate potential to create intervention programs with reasonable likelihood for success or policies that may stimulate changes in worker behaviors. In addition, studies have also been noted that test interventions that not only focus on reducing prolonged sitting time, but include programmatic efforts to increase the number of physical activity breaks in order to break up the prolonged sedentary situation (Galinsky et al. 2000). Not all such studies are explicit in their attempt to reduce sedentary behavior; instead, they position their intervention so as to increase or stimulate more physical activity. However, in so doing, they pursue a goal that breaks up sedentary time or reduces prolonged sitting time. Table 24.1 provides a summary of studies that have emerged in the literature that have ideas consistent with the intent of this chapter and are appropriate to consider for further study and application. Although this summary is not intended to be an exhaustive review of the literature, it does provide a useful insight into the state of the field in terms of research and promising practices.

Results of this summary of studies indicated that short breaks in the sedentary work routine that last about 10 to 15 minutes each can bring about

Table 24.1 Description of Interventions for Reducing Sedentary Behavior in the Workplace

Group	Intervention	Study design	Results
Alkhajah et al. 2012	Sit-to-stand workstation	Quasiexperimental design with comparison group	The intervention group reduced sitting time and increased HDL cholesterol.
Balci and Aghazadeh 2003	PA breaks	RCT with 3 intervention groups; no control (60 min work/10 min rest, 30 min work/5 min rest, and 15 min work/ micro breaks)	The 15 min work/micro break schedule resulted in significantly lower discomfort in the neck, lower back, and chest than the other schedules.
Dishman et al. 2009	PA breaks, pedometer, organizational support	Cluster RCT; a group-randomized 12-week intervention consisting of organizational action and personal and team goal-setting	The proportion of participants who met recommendations for physical activity increased to 51% at intervention sites compared to no change at control sites.
Evans et al. 2012	Prompting software	RCT; education group compared to education plus prompting software to take breaks from prolonged sitting	Prompted group reduced (improved) number and duration of sitting events that were greater than 30 min.
Galinsky et al. 2000	PA breaks	Experimental design; comparing two rest break schedules—2 × 15 min/day and same plus supplementary short 5 min breaks for every hour without a break	Increased use of breaks for the supplementary breaks group reduced discomfort in forearm, wrist, and hand and reduced eyestrain. No differences were noted in productivity and accuracy.
Galinsky et al. 2007	PA breaks	RCT; one stretching group and a no stretching (control) group	Discomfort, eyestrain, and data-entry speed were significantly improved with supplementary breaks.
Gilson et al. 2012	Standing desk	Single group, repeated measures	Desk use did not alter overall sedentary work time in this sample.
John et al. 2011	Treadmill work-stations	Single-group, repeated measures trial	Significant increases were seen in the median standing and stepping time and total steps/ day.
John et al. 2009	Treadmill work-stations	Counterbalanced, within subjects' design; seated and walking conditions on 2 separate days	Compared with the seated condition, treadmill walking caused a 6–11% decrease in measures of fine motor skills and math problem solving, but did not affect selective attention and processing speed or reading comprehension.
McLean et al. 2001	PA breaks with software prompt	Experimental study; 3 randomly assigned groups: microbreaks at own discretion, every 20 min, or every 40 min	All conditions showed positive effect on reducing discomfort; the condition with microbreaks every 20 min showed best results.
Nicoll and Zimring 2009	Stairwell walking and skip-stop elevators	Controlled trial; use of and attitude toward stairs in an office building where the main elevators stop only at every third floor ("skip-stop" elevators)	The skip-stop elevator was used 33 times more than the enclosed stair of the traditional elevator core, with 72% of survey participants reporting daily stair use.
Pronk et al. 1995	PA breaks, exercises, organizational support	Pre–post with comparison pilot groups and all-population main study	Flexibility and mood showed modest improvements following the implementation of a plant-wide 10 min daily flexibility and strength program.
Pronk et al. 2012	Sit-to-stand workstation	2-group pre–post comparison interrupted time series study	Reduced time spent sitting, reduced upper back and neck pain, and improved mood states. Removal of the device largely negated all observed improvements within 2 weeks.
Robertson, Ciriello, and Garabet 2013	Sit-to-stand workstations	RCT; 8 hr per day over 15 days, assigned to ergonomics trained or comparison group	The ability to mitigate symptoms, change behaviors, and enhance performance through training combined with a sit-to-stand workstation had implications for preventing discomforts in office workers.
Roelofs and Straker 2002	Sit-to-stand vs. just sit and just stand worksta-tions	Field study among bank tellers; sit-to-stand condition required alternating between sitting and standing every 30 min. All participants worked in each of the three conditions for 1 day.	Musculoskeletal discomfort outcomes were measured. The sit-to-stand alternating condition reported the least discomfort and was favored by 70% of participants.

HDL = high-density lipoprotein cholesterol, PA = physical activity, RCT = randomized controlled trial.

significant short- and longer-term improvements in a variety of outcomes that reflect how employees feel, how they view their employer regarding the support they receive to be healthy, and several indicators of physical fitness (e.g., hand strength, flexibility, eyestrain). Sit-to-stand workstations are a promising practice solution to breaking up prolonged sitting time, since several studies have reported decreased sitting time, improved work performance, improved mood states, and slight improvements in blood lipid profiles. On average, it appears that sit-to-stand desks can reduce sitting time by 1 to 3 hours per day. Standing desks, facilitating a standing workstation by use of a motorized option to raise or lower the desk when desired, did not see an overall reduction in sitting time. Treadmill workstations represent another promising practice because they appear to be effective in increasing overall energy expenditure and therefore reducing sedentary behavior, although decreases in fine motor skills while on the treadmill were noted as well. Prompting software installed on work computers to remind workers to stand up periodically appears to be effective as well.

However, little is known about long-term health and worker performance effects of continued use of the various options to reduce prolonged sitting time. In addition, most studies tend to have small sample sizes. More rigorous methods are warranted in order to generate more robust conclusions.

Practical Approaches

In a typical day, after a good night's rest, many workers get up only to sit back down for breakfast, sit in their car to drive to work, sit at the computer at work in the morning, sit for lunch, sit at the computer for work in the afternoon, sit in their car to drive home, sit at the table for dinner, and sit on the couch to watch television in the evening. Even after including a 30- to 45-minute exercise session to ensure they meet guidelines for physical activity (Physical Activity Guidelines Advisory Committee 2008), it may be impossible to offset the negative influence of so much sitting time throughout the course of the day (Owen et al. 2010). Given that much of people's daily time is spent at work, designing interventions to counteract the negative effect on health of too much sitting at the workplace makes good sense (Pronk and Kottke 2009; Pronk 2009a; Pronk 2010).

The workplace is a complex social system. Prolonged sitting time is a result of not only the specific job task an employee is engaged in, but also the net effect of the multiple interactive relationships among the working conditions at the workplace, the design of the workstations, organizational policies, operational systems, individual employee's beliefs and behaviors, and leadership engagement, as well as the social norms and corporate culture that shape the way of doing things at the workplace. As a result, interventions designed to reduce sedentary behavior in general and prolonged sitting time in particular need to fit the local, site-specific situation and be supported with company-wide policies and organizational culture.

In order to implement a successful effort to reduce sedentary behavior at the workplace, it behooves any company to treat the program as a strategic business priority (Pronk and Kottke 2009). As such, the business case for implementation of programs to reduce sedentary behavior needs to go beyond health alone and include operational efficiency, quality, worker productivity and performance, human resource management, safety, cost reduction, cultural fit, and other factors that are valued by any given company (Pronk 2009a; 2009b). To support efforts such as these, the framework presented in figure 24.1 is intended to help organize tactics according to the level at which they influence outcomes and the relevance they have to the key stakeholders involved, principally the employer and the employee. In addition to the framework, other practical guidelines are included in the highlighted box.

Additional useful guidance is presented by other organizations as well. For example, the Centers for Disease Control and Prevention (CDC), NIOSH, the World Health Organization (WHO), and the International Association for Worksite Health Promotion (IAWHP) represent organizations and associations that provide ongoing support for practitioners and employers related to these issues. The CDC and NIOSH provide guidance through the Total Worker Health program (see www.cdc.gov/niosh/twh) and their essential elements list, described previously (Pronk and Kottke 2009; NIOSH 2008). The WHO has introduced a healthy workplace model that integrates health improvement and safety activities in an improvement model (see www.who.int/occupational_health/en) and provides robust guidance to support it. Finally, the IAWHP (see www.iawhp.org) has endorsed the WHO healthy workplace model and provides worldwide support for worksite health promotion practitioners (Pronk 2011).

EMPLOYER GUIDANCE TO REDUCE SEDENTARY BEHAVIOR

- *Comprehensive programming.* Include the specific strategies for reducing sedentary behavior as part of the overall approach to worksite health at the company (Pronk 2009b).

- *Collaborative approach.* Using a participatory collaborative approach that includes employees in the process may enhance acceptability of the program (e.g., microbreaks, sit-to-stand work-stations) and provide individual workers with a sense of control over the choices they have available to them.

- *Integration.* Connect and integrate the program into organizational structures and product-specific processes and explicitly link to the mission of the company (Pronk 2009b; Carnethon et al. 2009).

- *Intervention strategies.* Use a variety of strategies and tactics to achieve the objectives:
  - Ongoing communication to ensure awareness
  - Behavior modification strategies
  - Meaningful incentives
  - Behavioral economics
  - Prompting and reminder systems
  - Self-monitoring
  - Health coaching
  - Web portal and access to online resources
  - Social support
  - Supportive organizational policy
  - Supportive physical, social, and economic environments
  - Education and skill development
  - Training

- *Multimodal delivery.* Provide a variety of ways in which the intervention may be delivered. In many cases, the optimal delivery represents multiple options provided simultaneously:
  - Organizational policy
  - Modifications in the physical (built) and social environment
  - Group based, onsite
  - Telephonic
  - Internet based

- *Evaluation.* Use a practical evaluation model that will allow for data to be reported to management and improvement of the program based on experience (Langley et al. 2009):
  - Plan-Do-Check-Act (PDCA) cycles
  - Continuous quality improvement (CQI)
  - Rapid cycle improvement models
  - Action research spirals

Summary

This chapter presents an overview of the opportunity the workplace provides for reducing overall sedentary behavior and outlines several strategies that have emerged from the literature related to this potential. It is clear from cross-sectional studies that sedentary behavior has detrimental effects on health and that prolonged sitting time at work is a major determinant of overall sedentary time. Intervention studies specifically designed to reduce sitting time at work have only recently begun to emerge from the literature. Interventions, such as physical activity microbreaks, stair walking, sit-to-stand devices, treadmill workstations, and software that prompts workers to stand up every so often, may be promising practices. This emerging field of study is in need of additional high-quality research and appears to be poised for growth in the coming years.

KEY CONCEPTS

▸ **Complex social system:** Future research and practice initiatives need to recognize the workplace as a complex social system and recognize the importance of operating at multiple levels of influence and with efforts that are relevant to the stakeholders involved.

▸ **Employee health management best-practice characteristics:** Elements and factors related to highly successful programs that may be highlighted for use in programs designed to not only effectively reduce sedentary time but also fit well in the workplace setting.

▸ **Microbreaks:** Short breaks from sitting that occur throughout the day and effectively break up prolonged periods of sitting.

▸ **Promising practices:** Programs designed to reduce sedentary behavior and prolonged sitting time at work show promise but are in need of additional research.

▸ **Workplace setting:** The workplace represents an important venue for interventions designed to reduce sedentary behavior.

STUDY QUESTIONS

1. Name two historical sources that noted the effect of sedentary work tasks on worker health.

2. By how much has the average energy expenditure of occupational physical activity reduced over the past 50 years?

3. By how much have sit-to-stand desks been shown to reduce daily sitting time?

4. Name four practical considerations for the successful implementation of programs designed to reduce sedentary behavior in the workplace.

5. Name three organizations that provide ongoing support for workplace health promotion services and practitioners.

CHAPTER 25

COMMUNITY-BASED INTERVENTIONS

Adrian Bauman, MD, MPH, PhD; and Josephine Y. Chau, PhD, MPH

The reader will gain an overview of the characteristics and approaches to community-based interventions targeting sedentary behavior. By the end of this chapter, the reader should be able to do the following:

- Identify the characteristics of community-based interventions that are effective for reducing sedentary behavior
- Understand the settings and approaches for community interventions for reducing sedentary time
- Provide a framework for sedentary behavior interventions in community settings
- Identify the characteristics of and evidence for community-based interventions for reducing sedentary behavior
- Understand the strengths and limitations of current community-based sedentary behavior interventions
- Provide future research directions

The concept of community settings for healthy lifestyle interventions arose in the 1980s in response to the mostly clinical settings in which preventive programs were delivered. The need for extending preventive programs into community settings was based on the need to increase population reach beyond that achieved through clinical settings alone. The concept of community interventions was sometimes divided into community-wide settings that targeted a whole population and community-based settings that focused on a particular population group or specific setting, such as a single school or a workplace. In this chapter, we combine these uses into the term *community-level intervention* and propose a definition that includes any settings outside of the workplace or clinical context.

Many sedentary behavior (SB) interventions target the workplace (see chapter 24), but this chapter considers preventive settings outside the workplace, such as schools, community centers, and whole communities, as well as interventions that target specific population subgroups. In this chapter we include primary care or other community locations as *nonworkplace settings*. Community interventions are further divided into those for adults and those targeting children and adolescents. This is because the determinants and settings for SB are different for children and adolescents than adults, particularly screen time during leisure and passive commuting time.

An approach to behavioral interventions can be adapted from the CDC community guide to physical activity interventions (Kahn 2002) and applied to SB interventions. In this chapter we used this guide to classify interventions, three of which are relevant to community SB interventions:

▸ **Informational approaches** to change individual or community knowledge and attitudes about the potential health consequences of sedentary behavior. Informational approaches provide education to children, parents, and clinicians about the potential benefits of reducing sedentary behavior (typically time spent watching TV, videos, or DVDS and using the computer or playing video games). Typically, these are in the context of interventions that encourage spending less time in SB and more time on physical activity.

▸ **Behavioral and social approaches** to teach the skills needed for adopting and managing behavior change (i.e., reducing SB). These the-

ory-based programs include self-regulation and social cognitive theory approaches to restricting SB time as well as peer-led interventions and modeling to encourage behavior change.

▸ **Environmental and policy approaches** to change physical and organizational environments to reduce sedentary behavior or decrease barriers to being sedentary (see chapter 23).

Interventions may use single strategies or include multiple intervention components in efforts to reduce sedentary behavior. Further, many SB interventions are not specific to sedentary behavior. Rather, they are primarily physical activity or obesity interventions with intervention elements and outcome measures specific to SBs. To date, community interventions have rarely focused exclusively on SB reduction.

Framework for Assessing Sedentary Behavior–Reducing Interventions

A logical, linear framework for interventions is often proposed using a socioecological model. A linear framework for developing interventions for reducing SB includes evidence generation, descriptive studies, efficacy studies, and policy responses. Figure 25.1 shows this linear model, which has particular relevance to community interventions (but also applies to workplace interventions). A public health framework suggests that assembling the evidence for health effects of a behavior should be the first step, followed by understanding the magnitude of the problem in populations (steps 1 and 2) and then conducting intervention testing (done by researchers). Because of the nature of funded research, these are usually efficacy or effectiveness studies that focus on the achievement of reductions in sitting behaviors (step 3). Most interventions assess either physical activity or obesity rather than SB. Among children, SB reduction is often secondary to obesity prevention interventions. In the published research to date among adults, sedentary behavior is often explored as a secondary outcome within physical activity interventions. This means that limited data exist on primary SB interventions, making it difficult to discern true efficacy.

A major concern is that evidence from efficacy studies (step 3) is often considered to be directly relevant to policy makers, who review the intervention evidence to date and build policy responses in terms

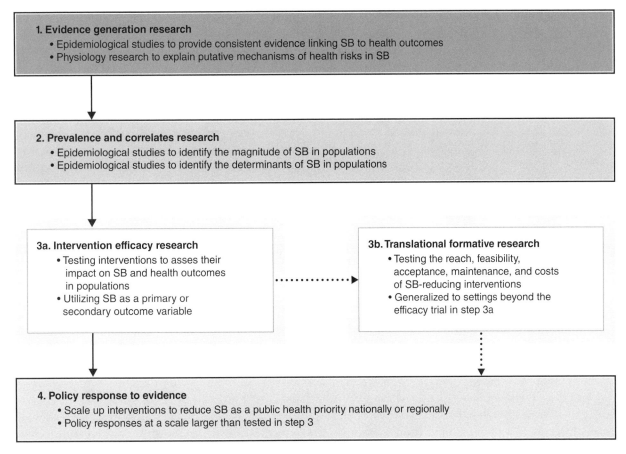

Figure 25.1 A conceptual framework for interventions for reducing SB.

of considering adapting interventions for reducing sitting time at a much larger scale than tested in the evidence-generating efficacy interventions and trials (step 4). An additional stage, translational formative research (step 3b), is seldom funded or conducted (O'Hara 2014), although it should follow efficacy studies (step 3a). This kind of research is essential for research translation and would assess the feasibility of SB interventions to be scaled up and to achieve high population reach if generalized to settings beyond the efficacy trial. In addition, elements of any diffusion process are relevant to scaling up SB interventions into wider community settings, including affordable costs, acceptability, trialability (Rogers 2002), and long-term maintenance of SB by incorporating nonsitting behaviors into healthy lifestyles.

The relevance of this conceptual framework is to guide understanding of current research and guide future research into reducing SB in communities. Most of the published literature available for review is of efficacy testing in nature (step 3a), namely studies to assess the effects of interventions on SBs. A mini-

mal amount of formative research exists (step 3b) to inform scaled-up public health practice in this area. There is also the assumption of temporal sequence in public health actions (linearity), with intervention studies presumed to follow from epidemiologic evidence sufficient for characterizing risk and prevalence research sufficient for characterizing the population of the behavior in question. In practice, this seldom occurs, since intervention studies are developed concurrently with the evidence. In the absence of public health scaling-up exemplars, the literature reviewed in this chapter is mostly of the typology expressed in step 3a.

Evaluating Community-Based Interventions

Several reviews have been published on the effects of interventions for reducing SBs, especially for children. The number of reviews is almost as great as the number of primary studies. Review papers identified some of the same intervention studies, but curiously, even accounting for literature searches carried out on the same time period, around a quarter of studies differed from review to review.

Only two reviews of adult SB interventions were located, one specifically for worksite studies (Chau et al. 2010) and one for more generic interventions (Owen 2011). The latter review located two intervention studies, one in the community that was targeted at reducing television time (Otten et al. 2009) and the other in workplaces. The community-based intervention for reducing television time was a small randomized control trial (RCT) that sampled only 36 overweight and obese adults and used an electronic lockout to restrict television time as one of the intervention outcomes (Otten et al. 2009).

Several reviews have assessed programs for reducing television time among children and adolescents. These interventions were carried out in domestic settings or as community-based or school interventions. Many reported weight or obesity prevention as the primary outcome measure and assessed the outcomes of reduced SB only as secondary variables in the context of an obesity prevention program.

One of the earlier reviews, done by Kamath and colleagues (2008), provided quantitative estimates of the effect size and concluded from 10 reports that the mean effect size (ES) was -0.29 ($p < 0.01$), indicating that interventions showed small to moderate effects in reducing SB. In a narrative review, DeMattia, Lemont, and Meurer (2007) reported that 6 of 7 studies had reduced SB and that all reduced weight or body mass index (BMI). A contrary conclusion was reported by Salmon and colleagues (2011), who assessed the potential for interventions to reduce SB among young people. This narrative review concluded that "few recent studies aiming to reduce TV viewing or sedentary time among young people have been successful" (page 197),with very limited evidence for the success of interventions in reducing total sedentary time. Salmon and colleagues identified that four previous reviews had been carried out, nearly as many as primary studies.

Biddle and colleagues (2011) reported on a meta-analysis of 17 trials for reducing SB among children or adolescents. They reported a different effect size metric, Hedges g coefficient, as -0.192 ($p < 0.01$), indicating that on average, reduction in SBs was one-fifth of a standard deviation greater in intervention compared to control groups. Although this overall ES was small, only 2 of the 17 studies did not show any effect at all. There was a greater

ES for community-based interventions (-0.61) and for short-term SB outcomes, but effects did not differ on whether the interventions were theory based. The small but consistent overall ES suggests program efficacy, but the review further noted that sedentary behavior might be resistant to change and that types of SB are maintained due to their strong cues and behavioral reinforcers (Biddle et al. 2011). The review also noted the lack of process evaluation measures in that studies did not assess program delivery fidelity or behavioral maintenance of nonsedentary behavioral choices.

Campbell and Hesketh (2007) assessed interventions focusing on children aged 0 to 5 years and found nine studies in community and primary care settings. These studies mostly addressed obesity prevention, but most showed some level of effectiveness in obesity prevention behavior (change), including reducing sedentary behaviors.

Wahi and colleagues (2011) examined interventions for reducing screen time in children as part of obesity prevention trials. The mean sample size in these studies was 90 participants. Outcomes were BMI and screen time, and studies were reported up to 2011 and among children younger than 18 years. Thirteen studies were located from school and community settings, but only six were suitable for meta-analysis. The mean BMI reduction was 0.1 (not significant) greater in intervention than control children. From nine studies that assessed SB, half the studies showed some decline but half did not. Overall, no significant difference in SB reduction was noted between intervention and controls; a small effect was seen when the analysis was confined to preschool age children (a reduction of 3.7 hr/week more in the intervention children, $p = 0.04$). The review concluded that despite enthusiasm in the literature, no clear evidence existed to demonstrate effective interventions for decreasing SB in studies targeting SB reduction as a strategy for preventing childhood obesity.

Leung and colleagues (2012) carried out a narrative review of interventions for reducing SB and childhood obesity among school-aged children. They located 12 studies with a primary outcome of reducing SB and identified methodological issues including design and measurement limitations. The chosen studies largely overlapped with those in the review by Wahi and colleagues (2011). Their qualitative conclusion was that interventions focusing on SBs tended to show decreases in SB time, but they did not provide quantitative estimates.

The variation in studies chosen and in conclusions reached is interesting, since although these literature reviews were usually systematic, they reached somewhat different conclusions. Different summary metrics were reported, so that effects are not directly comparable. The broader conclusions also differed among review papers, with some citing clear evidence of small to moderate effects and others deeming the evidence to be inconclusive.

In order to review primary community intervention studies in this field, the next section describes individual studies. This will add to an understanding of the strengths and limitations of the field of community interventions for reducing SBs. We identified specific community-based intervention studies in the past decade that reported a clear SB intervention component and a measured SB outcome. Our approach to study identification was systematic, but we did not explore all possible databases. The aim was to provide a range of illustrative examples of informational, behavioral, and environmental interventions that attempted to reduce SB time among adults and children.

Community Interventions Among Adults

The studies in the first section of table 25.1 illustrate interventions with SB outcomes assessed in adults. Six studies with outcomes for adults were noted, although some were family interventions that reported outcomes for their children as well. An example of this was the study by Sepulveda and colleagues (2010), which showed small but significant decreases in daily screen time for both parents and children. The intervention illustrates the principles of behavioral economics and was a financial reinforcement trial based around healthy lifestyle changes at the family level. Generalizability is partly addressed in this study, since half of those eligible from the large workforce participated in the study. A similar family study was reported by French and colleagues (2011) in Minnesota, who saw household TV time decreasing in intervention compared to control families. Reported television reductions were apparent for parents but not for adolescent children. Of these six interventions, three were focused on individual behavior change and one on environment or policy changes, and two used multicomponent strategies. The two multicomponent approaches were comprehensive community interventions. A Belgian study called 10,000 Steps

Ghent primarily targeted physical activity behavior and had SB as a secondary outcome (de Cocker et al. 2008). This multistrategy intervention included a SB component and showed small decreases in total sitting time in the intervention community and no change in the control town. This difference was significant for weekday and weekend total sitting time. Another community intervention in Scotland that primarily targeted walking (Fitzsimons et al. 2012) showed that reported sitting declined substantially more among intervention group participants.

A church-based peer-education program for obese adults was reported by Goldfinger and colleagues (2008). This small single-group study showed significant and maintained reductions in screen time following the program. The project was theory based around social cognitive principles and individual behavior change. By contrast, an intervention among Canadian Aboriginal families targeted diet and physical activity with a behavior change program and showed no difference in screen time among intervention families (Anand et al. 2007).

Community Interventions Among Children and Adolescents

The interventions for children covered all three areas of intervention: behavior change, organizational change, and environment change strategies. Only one study used information alone, 11 focused on individual behavior change strategies, and 5 reported multicomponent interventions. Environmental approaches are beyond the scope of this section but are described elsewhere (chapter 23).

Two studies focused on community-based interventions (see table 25.2). Cong and colleagues (2012) carried out a large study of Hispanic families in Texas and developed a multicomponent intervention addressing active living. Children in the intervention families showed a significant decline in screen time compared to controls, especially among girls, but the intervention effect waned after the 4-month follow-up. Another family study described by Ford and colleagues (2002) was delivered through an urban community clinic and provided brief counseling about SB. Children's and household TV time were not significantly changed by the intervention.

Some studies primarily targeted childhood obesity (see table 25.3), but used SB as part of the program delivery and measured it as a secondary outcome. Shrewsbury and colleagues (2011) examined adolescents attending a community obesity

Table 25.1 Adult-Focused Community-Based Interventions

Sepúlveda et al. 2010: IBM's Children's Health Rebate program, United States (pre–post study)

SB outcome	Intervention	Results
Daily screen time (exposure to electronic entertainment modes)	Cash incentive ($150) given to parents to complete 12-week Internet-delivered program targeting self-selected activities in family food planning and meals, family PA, and screen time (electronic entertainment).	Significant increase in proportion of children and adults reaching target of <1 hr/day screen time. **Children**: 22.4% at baseline, 30.7% at follow-up, $p < 0.001$. **Adults**: 18.1% at baseline, 24.2% at follow-up, $p < 0.001$.

Goldfinger et al. 2008: Project HEAL: Healthy Eating, Active Lifestyles, United States (pre–post study)

SB outcome	Intervention	Results
Time spent watching TV, videos, and DVDs (sedentary time)	Modified version of Stanford University chronic disease self-management program for use with local community; included weekly action plans, group feedback, support for change, and modeling of self-management and problem solving.	Baseline mean sedentary time: 5.4 hr/day. At **10 weeks**, mean sedentary time 4.1 hr/day (Δ: $p = 0.034$). At **22 weeks**, mean sedentary time 4.5 hr/day (Δ: $p = 0.246$). At **1 year**, mean sedentary time 2.5 hr/day (Δ: $p < 0.001$).

De Cocker et al. 2008: 10,000 Steps Ghent, Belgium (quasiexperimental, pre–post study)

SB outcome	Intervention	Results
Total sitting time (IPAQ), sitting for transport (IPAQ)	Campaign promoting pedometer use and 10,000 steps per day, incidental activity, and MVPA; used local media campaign, website, workplace projects, projects for older adults, and environmental (street signs with number of steps, walking in parks).	**Daily sitting time**: Ix group showed nonsignificant decrease in sitting time (396 min baseline) to follow-up (384 min) (Δ: –12 min; 95% CI: –24, 0); Cx nonsignificant increase from baseline (378 min) to follow-up (396 min) (Δ: +18 min; 95% CI: 0, 24); overall significant intervention effect (F = 9.5, $p = 0.002$). **Weekday sitting time**: Ix showed nonsignificant decrease (baseline 378 to follow-up 366 min/day (Δ: –12 min; 95% CI: –24, 0), while Cx no change from baseline (354 to follow-up 360 min); overall significant intervention effect (F = 4.1, $p = 0.044$). **Weekend sitting time**: Ix community showed no change in sitting time baseline 294 to follow-up 288 min); Cx showed a significant increase baseline 276 to follow-up 312 min; overall significant intervention effect (F = 17.7, $p < 0.001$). **Sitting for transport**: No significant intervention effect (F = 1.2, $p = 0.265$).

French et al. 2011: Take Action, United States (RCT)

SB outcome	Intervention	Results
TV-viewing time (hr of TV viewing and computer use)	6 monthly face-to-face group sessions related to weight control; placement of time-limiting devices on all home TVs; behavioral strategies (goal setting, self-monitoring); 12 home-based activities to reinforce behavioral messages (incentive provided for each activity completed, e.g., gift cards). Delivered face to face and via telephone and monthly newsletters.	TV-viewing time significantly declined among Ix households (from 2.82 to 1.70 hr/day) compared to Cx (from 2.67 to 2.04 hr/day) (Ix effect: $p = 0.03$) Significant reductions in "TV being on most of the time" among Ix households (both adults and adolescents) compared to Cx (both $p < 0.0001$). Proportion of participants indicating that "TV is usually on during meals" decreased for adults but not adolescents in Ix compared to Cx. Ix adults: from 52.1% to 29.2%; Cx adults: from 43.7% to 42.8% ($p = 0.02$); Ix adolescents: from 59.8% to 36.8%; Cx adolescents: from 45.2% to 46.0% ($p = 0.23$).

Anand et al. 2007: SHARE-AP ACTION, Canada (RCT)

SB outcome	Intervention	Results
Screen time (TV, video games, computer use)	SHARE-ACTION program; regular home visits by Aboriginal health counselors to assess and set diet and PA goals for each household member; individual and household targets.	No significant difference in the change in screen time for Ix compared with Cx ($p = 0.69$). Ix group (from 3.7 to 3.1 hr/day; change: –0.6) versus Cx group (from 3.5 to 3.4 hr/day; change –0.1).

(continued)

Table 25.1 *(continued)*

Fitzsimons et al. 2012: Walking for Wellbeing in the West, Scotland (RCT)		
SB outcome	Intervention	Results
Total sitting time (IPAQ)	Pedometer-based walking program plus PA consultations.	Overall significant interaction effect for weekday sitting time ($F = 4.16$; $p < 0.05$). Post hoc significant differences between groups across time points. **Preintervention to week 12** ($p = 0.035$, $d = 0.48$): Ix (mean change: −325.00 min) and Cx group (mean change: −36.25 min). **Week 24 to week 48** ($p = 0.042$, $d = 0.47$): Ix (Δ 44.6 min) and Cx (Δ 27.0 min). Overall significant main effect for time for weekday sitting ($p < 0.05$). Significant decrease between baseline (mean = 615.70) and 12 weeks (mean = 505.8 min, $p = 0.030$, $d = 0.35$) and between baseline and 24 weeks ($p = 0.030$, $d = 0.19$). Overall significant interaction effect found for total sitting time ($p < 0.05$). **Preintervention to week 12** ($p = 0.046$, $d = 0.46$): Ix (Δ: −451.1 min); Cx (Δ: −130.2 min).

Ix = intervention, Cx = control, PA = physical activity, RCT = randomized control trial

Table 25.2 Youth-Focused Community-Based Interventions

Cong et al. 2012: Transformacion Para Salud, United States (quasiexperimental pre–post study)		
SB outcome	Intervention	Results
Parent-reported screen time (TV, DVD, computer, Internet, and video games)	Modified school curriculum (martial arts, gardening); resources (worksheets, newsletters) provided to children, parents, schools, and community (family fun nights, home visits for overweight and obese children from trained health services staff who provided individualized education and social support).	Children in Ix showed significantly reduced hours of screen time per day ($p < 0.05$). Children in Cx showed no change over study period ($p > 0.05$). Children with parental support had lower screen time ($p < 0.05$). Girls were less sedentary than boys at baseline but their screen time was less influenced by parental support than boys' were ($p < 0.05$). Intervention effects diminished over time; screen time decreased from 4th to 12th month, increased from 12th to 22nd month.
Ford et al. 2002: United States (RCT)		
SB outcome	Intervention	Results
Time spent watching TV and videos and playing games Days eating breakfast and dinner with the TV on	BC provided (5-10 min) about potential problems associated with excessive media use, discussion on how to set TV budgets, plus electronic TV time manager.	No difference found between groups in weekly TV, video, and video game use pre to post. B: −13.7 ± 26.1 hr/week; BC: −14.1 ± 16.8 hr/week, $p = 0.71$. No difference found between groups in overall household TV use, B: −3.4 ± 6.8 hr/week, BC: −2.0 ± 7.5 hr/week, $p = 0.57$. No difference found between groups in number of days of breakfast with TV on. B: −1.7 ± 2.6 days, BC: −1.1 ± 1.9 days, $p = 0.52$. No difference found between groups in number of days of dinner with TV on. B: −1.4 ± 2.7 days, BC: −0.4 ± 1.6 days, $p = 0.29$.

B = behavioral, BC = brief counseling, Ix = intervention, Cx = control, RCT = randomized control trial

Table 25.3 Youth-Focused Interventions Targeting Obesity

Shrewsbury et al. 2011: The Loozit Study (2-month outcomes), Australia (pre–post study)		
SB outcome	Intervention	Results
Screen and non-screen SB (Children's Leisure Activities Study Survey)	Low- to moderate-intensity (1 contact per week) community-based lifestyle program given to both arms of RCT; delivered separately for adolescents and their parents or carers.	No change in % adolescents with ≥2 hr/day of screen-based leisure time (i.e., exceed guidelines): $n = 82$, 28% at baseline, 32% at 2 months, $p = 0.664$. Total SB time significantly decreased: $n = 82$, from baseline mean 39.7 min to 2 months 34 min; $p = 0.004$. Screen-based leisure time significantly decreased: from baseline 22.4 min to 2 months 19.9 min; $p = 0.04$: TV, video, and DVD time significantly decreased: from baseline 14.0 min to 2 month mean 11.9 min; $p = 0.02$. No change found in time spent using computer or time spent playing electronic games. Non-screen-based SB significantly decreased: from baseline 17.3 min to 2 months mean 14.1; $p = 0.009$:

Nguyen et al. 2012: The Loozit Study (12-month outcomes), Australia (RCT)		
SB outcome	Intervention	Results
Screen time	Lifestyle modification, behavior change focusing on self-efficacy, motivation, perseverance, and self-regulation related to diet and PA. **RCT group 1**: booster group session every 3 months from 2 months to 24 months. **RCT group 2**: booster group sessions plus additional telephone coaching, mobile phone text messages, and e-mail messages.	Significant reductions in screen time at 12 months: geometric mean −0.8 hr; $p = 0.045$. Significant reductions in TV viewing: geometric mean −0.8 hr, $p = 0.02$. No significant group × time interactions. Additional telephone and electronic contact provided no extra benefit at 12 months.

Sacher et al. 2010: Mind, Exercise, Nutrition, Do it (MEND) Program, UK (RCT)		
SB outcome	Intervention	Results
Time in SB (TV, computer)	Parents and children attended 18 group educational (nutrition, PA, inactivity) and PA sessions 2× week in sports centers and schools, given 12-week free family swimming pass.	At 6 months, SB time significantly decreased: Ix mean 15.9 hr/week versus Cx mean 21.7 hr/week; Δ: −5.1 hr/week, $p = 0.01$ Analyses Ix children only: no change from 0-12 months in sedentary time; Δ: −2.0 hr/week, $p = 0.10$

Stahl et al. 2011: 5-4-3-2-1 Go!, United States (quasiexperimental pre–post study)		
SB outcome	Intervention	Results
Screen time	Brief training for pediatric residents to deliver behavioral intervention during clinical care for childhood obesity prevention. Residents completed brief online training program (<60 min) and their patients received intervention. SB-related component: decrease TV-viewing time.	Residents' knowledge of screen time guideline (<2 hr/day) improved significantly pre to post training (38% at pre vs. 96% at post, $p < 0.0001$). TV viewing decreased significantly in Ix group patients vs. Cx (36% vs. 24%, $p < 0.01$).

Faith et al. 2001: United States (randomized pre–post study)		
SB outcome	Intervention	Results
TV-viewing time	Ix participants given TV powered by pedaling stationary cycle ergometer. Cx participants given stationary cycle, but TV power not contingent on pedaling.	Over 10-week intervention phase, TV viewing in Ix group was significantly lower than in Cx group (1.6 hr/week vs. 2.1 hr/week; $p = 0.006$).

Foster et al. 2008: School Nutrition Policy Initiative, United States (RCT)		
SB outcome	Intervention	Results
Time spent watching TV, videos	Schools implemented the School Nutrition Policy Initiative; components include school self-assessment, staff training, nutrition education, nutrition policy, social marketing, and parent outreach. SB-related aspect included education and family outreach on being less sedentary (≤2 hr/day of TV, video games).	At follow-up, TV hr/day significantly lower in Ix (2.92 hr/weekday at baseline, 2.89 hr/weekday at 2 years) compared to Cx (2.81 hr/weekday at baseline, 3.02 hr/weekday at 2 years); adjusted odds ratio showed Ix group had 5% less likelihood of TV watching on weekdays, but no significant differences found on TV viewing on weekend.

Ix = intervention, Cx = control, PA = physical activity, RCT = randomized control trial clinic and delivered a theory-based behavior change program; this resulted in a decline in the absolute number of SB minutes but no change in the proportion who achieved the guideline, less than 2 hours of leisure-based screen time daily. In a subsequent report from the same study, Nguyen and colleagues (2012) examined 12-month outcomes and noted a reduction in screen time of 0.8 hours per day. Faith and colleagues (2001) reported on a small study of obese children that used cycle-powered television watching; this behaviorally reinforcing intervention lowered TV time and increased physical activity. Sacher and colleagues (2010) reported on the MEND trial with obese children and showed a sizeable reduction of around 50 fewer minutes of SB time per day among intervention participants compared to controls. Foster and colleagues (2008) also reported an obesity prevention trial with a small effect on screen time.

In the 5-4-3-2-1 Go! intervention, pediatric residents received brief training to deliver a childhood obesity prevention intervention to patients they saw in routine care (Stahl et al. 2011). This was an information-only intervention that targeted health professionals. Awareness of the guidelines of 2 hours per day for SB in children increased among doctors who were trained. At a 6-month follow-up, a significantly greater proportion of patients in the intervention group reported TV viewing of less than 2 hours per day compared to patients of control doctors (36% versus 24%, $p < 0.01$).

School-based studies formed the largest group of interventions (see table 25.4). Robinson (1999) described an elementary school intervention in California that used behavior change approaches of self-regulation and showed a marked decline in TV time compared to controls. Salmon and colleagues (2008) described an Australian trial among elementary school children involving curriculum-based skills development that showed that the behavioral modification intervention group *increased* their reported TV time, a counterintuitive finding. Gortmaker and colleagues (1999) reported a school curriculum intervention with small but significant decreases in TV time. Another school program (Platcha-Danielzik et al. 2007) described a large trial in Germany with relatively small effect on TV watching (0.3 hr/day) among intervention group children, and only at short-term follow-up. Cui and colleagues (2012) reported on a trial of junior high school students in Beijing that used a peer-led approach and showed only small effects on total

SB time. Simon and colleagues (2004) presented data from junior high school students in France with a multicomponent intervention compared to controls. SB declined only among adolescents with high baseline SB time. Jones and colleagues (2008) reported on a trial of 6th and 7th grade girls aimed at improving physical activity and bone health. TV time was lower among intervention group girls at follow-up (around 15 min/day less total SB).

Several studies addressed infants and preschool-aged children (see table 25.5). Wen and colleagues (2012) reported a healthy beginnings trial in Australia and showed that by 2 years of age, intervention children were less likely to have meals in front of the television. However, the authors found no decline in the mother's TV time. Dennison and colleagues (2004) also described an educational program targeting preschool children and demonstrated a difference of 5 hours per week between intervention and control children in weekly screen time. De Silva-Sanigorski and colleagues (2011) also described a program for preschool children that showed significant intervention effects on TV time and other types of SB.

Practical Guidelines

For policy makers and practitioners interested in implementing evidence-based programs, the different conclusions reached in the research thus far may prove to be barriers to implementation and policy action. More primary studies with a central focus on SB reduction would be useful for this field and further systematic reviews will be less important in the near future.

The field of SB reduction among adults is mostly confined to interventions for reducing workplace sitting, with less focus on community SB. Future research could consider alternate community settings as well as other types of SB beyond television time, which is used as a proxy for SB in nonworking time among adults. Interventions could consider prolonged commuting time as part of inactive travel, as well as other non-screen-time forms of domestic SB, in developing new intervention questions and populations. Further, the determinants of domestic forms of SB in adults may be deeply culturally ingrained. Rather than just correlate studies (step 2 in figure 25.1), determinant studies with observations of SB over time may provide more causal evidence. In addition, other contexts for community sitting and SB may be amenable to change,

Table 25.4 Youth School-Based Interventions

Robinson 1999: United States (RCT)		
SB outcome	Intervention	Results
Time spent watching TV, watching videos, playing video games Other SB time (using computer, doing homework, reading, listening to music, doing art or crafts, talking with parents, attending classes or clubs)	Children in 1 school received 18-lesson curriculum focused on reducing TV, video, and video game use over 6 months (approx. 18 hr class time in total); parents received newsletters to help children stay within time budgets, strategies for the family to reduce screen time, and a TV-locking device.	**Child self-report** TV-viewing time. Ix: 15.35 hr/week to 8.8 hr/week; Cx: 15.46 to 14.46 hr/week; adjusted Δ: −5.53 (95% CI: −8.61, −2.42), $p < 0.001$. Ix group had significant reduction in video game time compared to Cx: 2.57 to 1.32 hr/week in Ix vs. 2.85 to 4.24 hr/week in Cx; Δ: −2.54 (95% CI: −4.48, −0.60) $p = 0.01$. No difference found between groups in time spent watching videos ($p = 0.11$) or other SB ($p = 0.44$). **Parent report on child's SB** Ix: significant reduction in TV-viewing time compared to Cx (12.43 hr/week to 8.86 hr/week Ix, and 14.90 to 14.75 hr/week in Cx, $p < 0.001$). No difference found between groups in time spent watching videos ($p = 0.60$) or playing video games ($p = 0.13$) or in time in other SB ($p = 0.16$).

Salmon et al. 2008: Switch-Play, Australia (RCT)		
SB outcome	Intervention	Results
Screen behaviors (TV viewing, computer use, electronic games)	**Intervention A**: Behavioral modification only (BM); self-monitoring, decision-making skills, goal setting for screen-based entertainment, parent newsletters to match children's goals and help children maintain switch-off behaviors. **Intervention B**: Fundamental movement skills only (FMS); games and activities focused on mastery of six FMS. **Intervention C**: BM + FMS Each Ix condition had 19 lessons (40-50 min) from qualified PE teacher.	BM children reported significantly more TV viewing on average than Cx time (at 6 months: 229 min/week, $p < 0.05$; at 12 months: 239 min/week, $p < 0.05$). This effect is in the *opposite direction* from expected. No significant intervention effects observed on other screen behaviors (electronic games, computer use) for BM. No intervention effects on SB found in other study arms.

Gortmaker et al. 1999: Planet Health, United States (RCT)		
SB outcome	Intervention	Results
Time spent watching TV, videos	Planet Health curriculum (teacher training workshops, classroom lessons, PE materials, wellness sessions and fitness funds). SB-related component: Students were encouraged to make space for more activity in their lives by reducing TV time.	Boys and girls significantly reduced TV and video hours from baseline to follow-up: Ix vs Cx. Boys: Ix decreased TV time 2.98 hr/day to 2.28 hr/day at follow-up, (Cx 3.10 hr/day to 2.99 hr/day at follow-up), Δ: −0.58, $p = 0.001$. Girls: Ix decreased TV time 3.73 hr/day to 3.03 hr/day at follow-up vs. Cx 3.78 hr/day to 3.43 hr/day, Δ: −0.40, $p = 0.0003$.

Plachta-Danielzik et al. 2007: Kiel Obesity Prevention Study (KOPS 4-year follow-up), Germany (RCT)		
SB outcome	Intervention	Results
Time spent watching TV, playing video games (high: ≥1 hr/week; low: <1 hr/week)	Behavioral education intervention targeted health diet and PA in students, plus provided teacher training and parental support. SB-related component: Reduce TV time to <1 hr/day.	Sedentary behavior outcomes were analyzed using only a subsample, $n = 775$ (Ix: $n = 164$; Cx: $n = 611$). At 3 months post intervention, significant decrease found in TV viewing in Ix (from 1.9 to 1.6 hr/day, $p < 0.05$) (Muller et al. 2001). At 4-year follow-up, there was no significant improvement in TV viewing in the Ix vs. Cx groups.

(continued)

Table 25.4 *(continued)*

Plachta-Danielzik et al. 2011: Kiel Obesity Prevention Study (KOPS 8-year follow-up), Germany (RCT)		
SB outcome	Intervention	Results
Time spent watching TV, playing video games In 6-year-olds at baseline, high: >1 hr/week In 14-year-olds, high: >3 hr/week	Behavioral education intervention targeted health diet and PA in students, plus provided teacher training and parental support. SB-related component: Reduce TV time to <1 hr/day.	At 8-year follow-up, no significant differences were found in TV time between Ix and Cx groups.

Cui et al. 2012, China (RCT)		
SB outcome	Intervention	Results
7-day PA questionnaire; 8-item SB score, including TV, DVD, games, and other types of SB	Peer-led theory-based intervention (social cognitive theory, empowerment education, goal setting) with 4 components: food, carbonated drinks, PA, and SB. Older peers delivered multiple intervention elements, including games, discussions, and presentations.	Total SB trend, but NS ($p = 0.06$) for total sedentary time at baseline, 3 months, and 7 months; Ix: 248, 237, and 229 min; Cx: 256, 256, and 258 min. Weekday SB decreased significantly in Ix (by 20 min/day) and computer use reduced by 14 min/day (both $p < 0.02$). Nonsignificant differences were noted for other types of SB.

Simon et al. 2004: Intervention on physical activity and sedentary behavior (ICAPS), France (RCT)		
SB outcome	Intervention	Results
Time spent watching TV, playing video games	Multilevel intervention focusing on adolescent PA involving educational, environmental, and family components. SB-related component: time spent watching TV and playing video games each day.	Significant decrease found in % girls with high SB (>3 hr/day TV and video games) in Ix vs. Cx groups (OR: 0.54, 95% CI: 0.38–0.77, $p < 0.01$). Significant decrease found in % boys with high SB (>3 hr/day TV and video games) in Ix vs. Cx groups (OR: 0.52, 95% CI: 0.35–0.76, $p < 0.01$).

Jones et al. 2008: Incorporating More Physical Activity and Calcium in Teens (IMPACT) study, United States (RCT)		
SB outcome	Intervention	Results
TV and video viewing time Time spent using computer or playing video games Total daily sedentary time	Physical activity intervention to improve bone health based on social cognitive theory and transtheoretical model, delivered via school curriculum.	At follow-up: Ix students had significantly lower daily TV or video viewing time than Cx students (94.7 min/day vs. 106.8 min/day; mean difference = –12.1, 95% CI: 11.7–12.5; $p = 0.05$). No difference found between Ix and Cx students for daily time spent using computer or playing video games (38.0 min/day vs. 44.4 min/day; $p = 0.16$). Ix groups had significantly lower total daily sedentary time than Cx group (134.9 min/day vs. 151.9 min/day; mean difference = –16.99, $p = 0.04$).

Ix = intervention, Cx = control, NS = not significant, PA = physical activity, RCT = randomized control trial, OR = odds ratio

including exploration of the potential to reduce SB in diverse social situations, restaurants, and community centers. Similarly, reported intervention effects are typically short term. The maintenance of nonsitting behavior change over time is essential to policy makers, but the current research base is very limited.

Among children and adolescents, interventions targeted obesity and inactivity as the usual primary outcomes, with SB often reported as a secondary outcome. The main form of SB assessed was television or screen time, and this may make up a major proportion of home-based SB among young people. For children and older adolescents, other forms of SB need to be included as more specific behavioral outcomes, including (mostly sedentary) online gaming, smartphone use, and time spent on social networking behaviors such as Facebook.

Table 25.5 Studies With Infants and Preschool-Aged-Children

Wen et al. 2012: Healthy Beginnings Trial, Australia (RCT)		
SB outcome	Intervention	Results
TV-viewing time when child aged 2 years old	8 home visits by trained community nurse over first 2 years of life (promote health feeding, PA, enhanced parent–child interaction) with proactive telephone support between visits, visits based on child developmental milestones.	Proportion of children eating dinner in front of the TV was significantly lower in Ix vs. Cx groups: 56% vs. 68%, $p = 0.01$. Proportion of children watching TV for >60 min/day was significantly lower in Ix vs. Cx groups: 14% vs. 22%, $p = 0.02$. No difference found by group in proportion of mothers watching TV $\geq$120 min/day: 65% vs. 64%, $p = 0.84$.
Dennison et al. 2004, United States (RCT)		
SB outcome	Intervention	Results
Time spent watching TV or videos, playing computer games	Trained early childhood teachers and music teachers visited each day care or preschool once per week to provide a 1-hr session on musical activities or education on promoting healthy eating (22 sessions) and less TV viewing (7 sessions) for total of 39 weeks.	Parent-reported child screen time: Mean weekly TV and video viewing decreased 3.1 hr/week among children in Ix compared with an increase of 1.6 hr/week among Cx (Δ: –4.7 hr/week; $p = 0.02$). Proportion of children watching TV and videos $\geq$ 2 hr/day significantly decreased in Ix (33% to 18%) and increased in Cx (41% to 47%); Δ: –21.5% ($p = 0.046$).
De Silva-Sanigorski et al. 2011: Romp and Chomp, Australia (post only)		
SB outcome	Intervention	Results
Screen-based SB (TV viewing, using computer, playing electronic games)	Multicomponent intervention involving capacity building for staff (day care providers), awareness raising in media, integration of policies in early childhood information guides, advocacy, and partnership building.	Children in Ix sites spent significantly less time watching TV compared to those in Cx group ($p = 0.03$). Children in Ix group spent significantly less time using computer or playing electronic games compared to those in Cx group ($p = 0.03$).

Ix = intervention, Cx = control, PA = physical activity, RCT = randomized control trial

This suggests further methodological refinement in the assessment of SB and in interventions to reduce sitting and SB in different contexts among young people, rather than the blanket categorization of these behaviors as screen or television time. As with adults, specific interventions report short-term effects; whether reducing SBs can be maintained is not known.

More studies are needed with a primary outcome of specifically reducing SB rather than embedding SB in more complex lifestyle or activity programs. This will allow for research testing of interventions addressing the primary target of SB and for best-case effect sizes to be determined. In addition, policy-relevant intervention research needs to be conducted to ensure the scalability of SB interventions (Milat et al. 2013). In other words, the longer-term effects of interventions, their generalizability to broader populations and communities, and the intervention sustainability remain to be explored (step 3b in figure 25.1). These areas are required before public health authorities and decision-makers are likely to implement SB interventions on a larger scale.

USING MEDIA CAMPAIGNS

As community awareness of SB increases, SB components may be more seriously regarded by the community. Some large-scale social marketing and mass media campaign efforts have begun to target sedentary behavior and inform the population about the risks of prolonged SB. These may eventually have community-wide effects through influencing the cultural and social norms that underpin high levels of maintained SB, which may contribute to future community-wide strategies. Currently, national social marketing campaigns in England and in Australia have used the reduction of SB as one of the communication components when targeting middle-aged adults (e.g., Public Health England's Change for Life, Commonwealth Department of Health and Ageing, Canberra Australia's Swap It). Although these campaigns primarily focused on increasing physical activity, they both included sitting-specific mass media messages.

Summary

This chapter focuses on sedentary behavior interventions conducted in community settings such as schools and community centers, as well as whole-community interventions targeting adults, children, and adolescents. SB interventions may be developed following a linear conceptual framework consisting of (1) evidence on epidemiological associations between SB and health outcomes and sitting physiology research about underlying mechanisms, (2) prevalence and correlates of SB, (3) efficacy studies of SB reduction strategies, (4) formative research to assess reach, feasibility, and generalizability, and (4) policy response and use of evidence to upscale efficacious SB interventions at the population level.

Conclusions from systematic reviews suggest that the effectiveness of community interventions for reducing SB is inconsistent and more policy-informing studies are needed. To date, intervention evidence has been based largely on trials that have assessed SB as secondary to other primary outcomes like physical activity or BMI. Much of the literature in community settings is around SB (TV viewing and screen time in particular) in children and adolescents; only recently has attention been paid to adult SB. Examination of specific SB interventions in community settings highlights a gap in the literature for intervention studies that focus on SB as the primary outcome and for studies that examine SB in a wider range of contexts than TV viewing and screen time. Furthermore, research is needed to investigate approaches to reducing SB in adults outside of the workplace. Finally, there is a need for more formative research to increase understanding of the feasibility, generalizability, and particularly the maintenance and sustainability of specific community SB-reduction strategies and, in turn, to inform the translation and expansion of these strategies to a community-wide level.

KEY CONCEPTS

▸ **Applying a public health framework:** This approach starts by collecting evidence about the health associations of sedentary behavior and the extent to which sedentary behavior is prevalent in the general population and population subgroups. Next, researchers conduct efficacy trials to test the effectiveness of interventions for reducing sedentary behavior (e.g., Did the intervention reduce sitting time? If so, by how much, and is this meaningful to health?). In addition to efficacy testing, researchers also carry out studies to determine the generalizability of the intervention for application at a population level. The final step involves a policy response and scaling up of effective and feasible interventions into wider community settings. When we apply this public health framework as an overarching guide for examining community-based sedentary behavior interventions, it is apparent that the bulk of the published literature is about testing the effects of interventions on sedentary behavior (i.e., efficacy).

▶ **Community-based intervention:** A community-based intervention targets a setting outside of the clinical or workplace context (e.g., schools, community centers) and a specific population group or subgroup. Community-based interventions may take informational, behavioral, or environmental approaches to reducing sedentary behavior and focus on one sedentary behavior or more, such as daily sitting time, watching television, computer use, and passive commuting. However, to date, few interventions have focused exclusively on reducing sedentary behavior; instead, sedentary behavior outcomes tend to be secondary to outcomes related to physical activity and obesity.

STUDY QUESTIONS

1. What is a community-based intervention for reducing sedentary time?
2. What evidence is needed to develop a sedentary behavior intervention in community settings?
3. What are the strengths of current community-based sedentary behavior interventions?
4. What are the limitations of current community-based sedentary behavior interventions?
5. What future steps are needed to build on the current evidence base about community-based sedentary behavior interventions

The initial research paper search through PubMed and Ovid Medline was carried out by Karla Fedel, MPH, whose work is gratefully acknowledged.

CHAPTER 26

ERGONOMICS OF REDESIGNING SITTING

John B. Shea, PhD; and Kelly J. Baute, PhD

The reader will gain an overview of the evolution of chair sitting as a workplace positional behavior and the circumstances in which ergonomic modification of this behavior may reduce the risk of health-related issues. By the end of this chapter, the reader should be able to do the following:

▸ Review the evolution of human working positional behaviors and postures

▸ Discuss early human positional behaviors

▸ Consider the importance of modern human's selective pressures that led to our highly evolved existence

▸ Describe the history of the chair (how the chair emerged and what the chair's initial purpose was)

▸ Describe how the traditional chair contributes to musculoskeletal disorders

▸ Understand the conditions and circumstances in which revising sedentary behavior may reduce the risk of health-related issues and categorize this information in order to apply it to common professional scenarios

▸ Identify future directions for assessing sedentary behavior and apply this content in professional settings to enhance client or patient knowledge of sedentary behavior

The study of ergonomics has progressed from its early emphasis on increasing worker productivity to an emphasis on health promotion in the places of daily living. This perspective encourages consideration of our evolutionary adaptations and the ecological contexts that provided the framework that perpetuated the development of our highly evolved and unique biological systems. This perspective must be included in any discussion regarding sedentary behavior and health. The ecological contexts in which we evolved provided the substrates in which the strategies and activity patterns for procuring resources advanced our unique combination of physiological, anatomical, and morphological characteristics, which in return provided affordances for our success. Åstrand suggests, "Insight into our biological heritage may help us to modify our current lifestyle in a positive way" (1992, page 1235S). The significant changes in the ecological contexts and the associated activity patterns in which we currently subsist are the culprits of today's current health crisis.

Procuring resources to ensure survival is a biological necessity of all organisms, and *Homo sapiens* are no different. Strategies to secure those resources have changed dramatically in the past 10,000 years. Ninety-nine percent of (anatomically) modern human's existence was spent with procurement strategies and activity patterns that involved both gross and fine motor movements representative as what would today be classified as physical activity (Malina and Little 2008). The rapid change in our ecological contexts altered these activity patterns and the associated positional behaviors of the past to the sedentary, constrained positional behaviors of today, which have exacted a dramatic and negative effect on our physiology and represented as an increase in mortality resulting from all causes and cardiovascular disease (Katzmarzyk et al. 2009). These behaviors have also exacted a dramatic and negative effect on the musculoskeletal system, represented as musculoskeletal disorders and experienced as (but not limited to) lower back, neck (Kumar 2001; Magnusson and Pope 1996), and shoulder pain (Lundberg 2002). "Movement is the substrate of activity" (Malina and Little 2008, page 373), and our biological systems have evolved based on a life cycle that includes regular physical activity and its associated movements. Our current activity patterns and subsequent sedentary subsistence strategies are methods of resource procurement that are generating a great cost to our health. This

provokes the question, Is our survival still based on successful fitness?

Modern human's biological phylogeny stems from a movement-based lifestyle. Hunter-gatherers' existence and success depended on movement of a variety of patterns (walking, carrying, some running, climbing, chopping, play, and rest) (Hill et al. 1985) and a variety of complexities (agility, accuracy, and speed of gross and fine motor movements) (Malina and Little 2008). For instance, early *Homo* would have needed to walk and occasionally run to track or stalk prey. In looking at today's extant hunter-gatherer groups, rarely is it seen that long distance running at high speeds is common (Hill et al. 1985). Conversely, Malina and Little noted that modern hunter-gatherers move in intermittent activity patterns. They wrote that in the past, we were required to have high-level, cardiovascular demands, but only as a small percentage of our activity budget. Additionally, our hunter-gatherer predecessors did not place themselves in behaviors that were isolated or confined in movement. These behaviors placed demands on the system of early *Homo*; however, these demands were more along the lines of intermittent activities as well as occasional periods of continuous activity. As Malina and Little pointed out, it is not in our biological lineage to work in the static, confined postures of the present.

Subsistence strategies of an agricultural lifestyle maintained intermittent activity patterns similar to those of hunter-gatherers and persisted until the industrial revolution at the dawn of the 20th century. This was immediately followed by the technological revolution beginning in the 1950s, as the first wave of sedentary occupations, ranging from office and clerical work to long-haul driver-operators, appeared. This dramatic change to our biological system contributed to disease and degeneration of the physical systems. The 1950s also saw the first signs of what would become a major health epidemic, cardiovascular disease (CVD).

By the 1970s, CVD was reaching an epidemic proportion. Fitness-based interventions were introduced in the form of cardiovascular exercise guidelines (ACSM 1978) as well as fitness programs, including running (Morgan 2013) and aerobics (Cooper 2013). The first ACSM guidelines were developed by health and exercise science researchers to provide a framework for improving the cardiovascular health of the U.S. population; thus, the guidelines' sole focus was on cardiorespiratory fitness and health. Not until 1990 did the ACSM recognize the importance of muscle conditioning by including it in a revision. And not until 1998 was flexibility added, with a neuromuscular focus appearing in 2009.

Whereas the ACSM, Cooper, and others were instrumental in the development of fitness-based programs to improve cardiovascular health, these interventions have not been successful in fostering healthy activity patterns of the U.S. population. When combined with the sedentary behaviors of most work-related tasks, the result on our biology is profound and has identified a need for a new field of study: inactivity physiology (Ekblom-Bak, Hellenius, and Ekblom 2010). Katzmarzyk and colleagues (2009) describes inactivity physiology as more than just not moving enough and using physiological and biomechanical systems. Rather, it is a mechanism leading to the onset of multiple degenerative diseases that are deteriorating the quality of life of those affected, even in the presence of planned exercise. Inactivity physiology studies have demonstrated a link between sitting time and nonexercise activity as contributors to rates of metabolic syndrome, type 2 diabetes, obesity, and cardiovascular disease (Hamilton, Hamilton, and Zderic 2007). These findings highlight the need to redesign or consider alternatives to traditional seat design and sitting behaviors.

Characteristics and Influence of Chair Designs and Positional Behaviors

Historically, sitting positional behaviors have been used to provide the best affordances for completing specific tasks: squatting to gather, chop, mash, and clean (Hill et al. 1985). The sitting positional behaviors or modes from which our preindustrialized ancestors could select include crouching, kneeling, and squatting (Hill et al. 1985; Kroemer and Grandjean 2005). But where did the chair originate? Anthropological evidence suggests that the chair or seats were first used for status within a group such that higher-ranking individuals were seated above individuals of lower rank (Kroemer and Grandjean 2005).

Kroemer, Kroemer, and Kroemer-Elbert (2001) provide an account of how chairs came to be used in China. Cultural relics from the Shang through the Han dynasties (1600 BC to 220 AD) show people sitting on mats in either kneeling or sitting

positions. The opening of the Silk Road allowed travel to western Asia, where Chinese visitors were introduced to chairs. Folding stools appeared in the Chinese imperial court around the 3rd century AD. By the 4th century, stools in China were about the same height as those used in the Western hemisphere. During the 7th to 10th centuries, the use of mats gradually disappeared and the use of stools for sitting became popular. Around the year 1200, complete sets of raised furniture existed in China.

Thus began the development of chairs, which are still considered a status symbol; generally, as salary goes up, so, too, does the sophistication of the chair (Kroemer and Grandjean 2005). So how did seats or chairs become associated with occupational tasks? In short, physiology. As reviewed in Kroemer and Grandjean (2005), well-being of workers was best achieved if they were allowed to sit, which reduced the muscular effort required by the lower body during prolonged standing. Four primary factors are associated with sedentary work:

1. Taking the weight off the legs
2. Stability of upper body posture
3. Reduced energy consumption
4. Fewer demands on the circulatory system

Unfortunately, prolonged sitting has the same negative effect on the musculature of the torso that prolonged standing has on the musculature of the lower body, contributing to the development of musculoskeletal disorders (MSDs). Research has associated prolonged sitting with lower back pain and discomfort (Kroemer and Grandjean 2005; Magnusson and Pope 1998; Vieira and Kumar 2004). In addition to the effects prolonged sitting has on the musculature of the back, the associated compression of the intervertebral discs decreases nutrient flow into those tissues. It is suggested that frequent changes in posture allow for changes in both musculature demands and intervertebral pressures (Kroemer and Grandjean 2005; Magnusson and Pope 1998). Other investigations suggest that work-related musculoskeletal disorders (WMSDs) can be reduced by managing the biomechanical factors associated with sitting and evaluating the task to be performed and the seat design (Magnusson and Pope 1998; Vieira and Kumar 2004). For example, tasks such as line assembly or benchwork allow the worker to use a semisitting (Magnusson and Pope 1998) positional behavior, thus allowing the worker to change between sitting and standing and consequently changing the musculature recruitment and intervertebral pressures. The design of the seat, such as height and inclination, and position of the armrest and backrest are of primary importance because these factors affect the posture seated workers assume to complete their task, essentially creating positional or postural affordance. Grandjean, Hünting, and Pidermann's (1983) investigation of computer workstations concluded that workstation operators' postural adjustments were limited by the constraints of the workstation's design.

In addition to the negative effects sedentary behavior exacts on our physiological systems, sedentary, static, and constrained positional behaviors constitute the vast majority of occupational tasks. Complaints triggered by prolonged, constrained positional behaviors thus contribute to the majority of worker compensation claims. Compensation is paid to 1 in 10,000 workers for a minimum of 3 days' paid leave due to back pain associated with working conditions. This leads to a 2% to 4% loss of net profits. Malina and Little (2008) describe working conditions of today to be grossly different from work-associated tasks of the past. The majority of today's occupational task systems are designed to meet production demands and are not concerned as to whether the biological systems of the workers have the capacity or capability to meet those demands (Vieira and Kumar 2004; Westgaard and Winkel 2011). If a production line is required to produce a specified number of units, then the production line will move at a speed to meet that quota. The workers must then maintain that pace and speed of movement or risk job loss. Thus, workers are forced into working behaviors that most likely are or will become beyond their biological systems' capacity.

Magnusson and Pope (1998) found that confined or constrained static postures are a risk factor for WMSDs. Specifically, when workers are confined to the same static posture for prolonged periods of time, their soft tissues are subjected to poor physiological conditions. For instance, when a muscle is not allowed or able to move through appropriate ranges of motion, the reduction of blood flow into that tissue is diminished. This reduces oxygen to the tissues and cells and increases the buildup of metabolic waste. This places the soft tissues in a poor physiological state and increases the risk of injury. The authors suggest that workers need to have the freedom to move into different postures. People who are able to move from a sitting to a standing position are less likely to sustain WMSDs. Magnusson and Pope (1998) further state that our bodies are accustomed to movement. Even during sleep, our bodies move in order to provide changes of postures and redirect stresses and forces on joints and soft tissue.

Lungberg (2002) studied the psychophysiological stresses associated with office workers. He found that the trapezius muscle was activated and remained activated even though work tasks were not requiring its contribution. He associated these higher levels to be associated with the physical and psychological stress of the job demands. Lundberg concluded that the higher and prolonged activation of the trapezius muscles is associated with upper body WMSDs in office (desk) workers.

Many investigations have been conducted on lower back pain associated with constrained static postures (Hodges and Richardson 1997; Hodges 2001; Hodges et al. 2003; Kumar 1990; 1999; 2001; Urquhart et al. 2005). These investigations have deduced that poor posture, repetitive forces, and awkward movements produced from positional or postural constraints are the primary contributors to conditions. Interventions have been proposed suggesting that lower back pain is an artifact of weak spinal stabilizers. Thus, improving the strength of the spinal stabilizers will prevent lower back pain. Companies have promoted the use of a stability ball at workstations as an intervention for improving strength of the core musculature. Researchers have thus investigated the efficacy of the stability ball in improving core strength. McGill, Kavcic, and Harvey (2006) found no difference between sitting on a stability ball and sitting on a stool without a backrest. Callaghan and McGill (2001) found similar results. Urquhart and colleagues (2005) investigated the musculature involvement in spinal stability and were unable to conclude if any specific muscle contributed more in producing spinal stability. They concluded that interventions designed to improve spinal stability should not focus on conditioning one muscle or a muscle in isolation; rather, the system should be conditioned with a systems approach.

Applications of Sitting Redesign

Sitting in the workplace has continued to be equated with the use of a chair with legs, seat pan, backrest, and armrests. Discussion on chair designs that promote healthier sitting behaviors has centered on the appropriate configuration of these components. Thus, research findings related to the biomechanics and physiology of sitting posture have been interpreted within the constraints imposed by traditional chair design. This has limited innovation in sitting design, and it is possible to find defined lists for what constitutes good office chair design. Kroemer and Grandjean (2005, page 81-82) cite the following golden rules for office chairs:

- ▸ Office chairs must be adapted to both the traditional office job and the modern equipment of information technology, especially to jobs at computer workstations.

- ▸ Office chairs must be conceived for forward and reclined sitting postures.

- ▸ The backrest should have an adjustable inclination.

- ▸ The backrest height must be at least 500 mm vertically above the seat surface.

- ▸ The backrest must have a well-formed lumbar pad, which should offer good support to the lumbar spine between the third vertebra and the sacrum.

The primary health problem motivating research on office chair design has been back problems related to the strain on muscles and vertebral discs from assuming static postures for extended periods of time. Andersson and Ortengren (1974) showed that increasing the seat angle reduces both disc pressure and muscle strain. Krämer (1973) studied the nutritional needs of intervertebral discs. The interior of a disc has no blood supply and must be fed by diffusion through the fibrous outer ring. Krämer showed that pressure on the disc creates a diffusion gradient from the interior to the exterior so that tissue fluid leaks out. When the pressure is taken off, this gradient is reversed and tissue fluid diffuses back, taking nutrients with it. Thus, the discs need to be subjected to positional change to keep them well nourished. From a medical point of view, therefore, an occasional change of posture is beneficial. However, modern workstation design has constrained the movement of operators in rather subtle ways defined by the keyboard–monitor relationship (Grandjean, Hünting, and Pidermann 1983). In addition, many orthopedists still recommend an upright sitting posture because it holds the spine in a shape of an elongated S with a lordosis of the lumbar spine. They believe that disc pressure is lower in such a posture than when the body is

curved forward with kyphoses in the lumbar and thoracic sections. This orthopedic advice is at odds with the fact that a slightly forward or reclined sitting posture relieves strain on the back muscles and makes sitting more comfortable (Andersson and Ortengren 1974; Lundervold 1951; 1958). Andersson and Ortengren found that workstation operators instinctively do the right thing when they prefer a reclined sitting posture and ignore the recommended upright trunk position. According to Kroemer, Kroemer, and Kroemer-Elbert (2001), there is no one healthy posture. Research does not support the idea of a single sitting posture that is healthy, comfortable, and efficient. They go on to point out that furniture should allow body movement and various postures. There have been numerous innovations to achieve this goal.

One innovation in chair design that has challenged the existing paradigm and gained popularity is the use of a stability ball in place of a chair for sitting. There has been increasing interest in the use of a stability ball in place of an office chair in order to improve core muscle strength and to create a dynamic sitting opportunity (McGill, Kavcic, and Harvey 2006). Numerous stability ball manufacturers claim that sitting on a stability ball improves the strength of the core muscles and decreases the risk of back pain. However, research has not demonstrated this to be true. McGill, Kavcic, and Harvey (2006) determined that prolonged sitting on an exercise ball relative to a stool has "little effect on spine loads, muscle activity and the resulting spine stability" (page 359). Additional research found little alteration in the way people sit while using a stability ball during prolonged sitting and that the use of a stability ball may not provide the comfort that a traditional office chair provides (Gregory, Dunk, and Callaghan 2006). Gregory and colleagues found that people performing office tasks were less comfortable while sitting on a stability ball than while sitting on a chair. Interestingly, Merritt and Merritt (2007) presented two case studies in which patients had incorporated stability ball sitting, one using the ball at work in place of an office chair and the other using the ball for exercise. Both patients found a reduction in pain severity and frequency of pain. These authors further suggested that stability ball sitting is advantageous by activating "proprioception, balance and equilibrium control" (page 50).

Additional considerations for workstations are the movements associated with job tasks. For instance, reaching to grasp an object, press a button, or operate a lever are common actions that alter balance and muscle mechanics. The increased demand placed on both the upper and lower body in response to reaching tasks includes the musculature recruitment to maintain posture as well as to balance the upper body on the base of support, the lower body. Dean, Shepherd, and Adams (1999) found that lower limbs contributed significantly to the distance of the reach and the effect reaching distance has on leg muscle activation. They also noted, "the varying times of onset of muscle activity suggest that individual muscles play different roles during reaching" (page 142). This is further evidence for the need to investigate the varying range of seated workstation postures and tasks. Kingma and van Dieën (2009) showed that enhanced spine motion did not differ whether sitting on a stability ball or sitting on a chair while performing a typing task. To date, research has been conducted on seated postures that use chairs and stools. A few investigations have also been done on torso muscle activity and spine loads during static sitting on a stability ball.

No research had been conducted to investigate the lower limb contributions during sitting on a stability ball at a workstation while the upper body is performing a job-related task until 2008. Baute investigated the contribution of lower-extremity musculature to a reaching task while sitting on a stability ball. Specifically, subjects were seated on a stability ball at a desk. EMG readings were recorded for the quadriceps, hamstrings, tibialis anterior, and the gastrocnemius muscles of the dominant and nondominant legs while the participants reached to move a cup of water from one position (either target A or B) to another (either target A or B) with either their dominant or nondominant hands. The subjects were instructed to begin the task with their reaching hand on their lap and return their hand back to their lap when not moving the cup. Each movement was comprised of seven phases: (1) move hand from lap to pick up a cup at target position A, (2) move cup from target position A to target position B, (3) return hand to lap, (4) pause or rest, (5) move hand from lap to pick up cup at target position B, (6) move cup from target position B to target position A, and (7) return hand to lap. While reaching with the dominant side, EMG recordings were collected from the dominant lower limb; conversely, while reaching with the nondominant hand, EMG recordings were collected from the nondominant lower limb. Muscle onset, duration,

and intensity data were measured for all trials for each movement phase.

Figure 26.1 shows duration of muscle contraction measures for all muscles and movement phases. Analyses conducted on these measures showed that the duration of the hamstring contraction and the onset of the tibialis anterior had the highest effect size. The duration of hamstring activity quite possibly reflects the stabilizing mechanism the hamstring provides while moving forward and back on a stability ball. Consider that hamstring duration is lowest in phase 4, where the hand is resting in the lap and no forward or backward movement is made. The onset of the tibialis anterior could reflect the lifting of the front of the foot in response to movement being initiated, specifically forward movement to reach out, since the tibialis anterior was the only muscle active in reaching forward. Additionally, it is likely that the stability ball allows for easier forward movements by rolling. The transfer of weight into the forefoot is controlled by activation of the tibialis anterior.

Figure 26.2 shows the intensity of muscle contraction measures for all muscles and movement phases. Analysis of intensity of muscle contraction between dominant and nondominant sides across all four muscle groups determined that the anterior muscles of the dominant side have greater firing intensity than those of the nondominant side. Conversely, the posterior muscles of the nondominant side have greater firing intensity than those of the dominant side. This comparison of sides between reaching forward and moving back suggests that the anterior dominant side muscles anticipate movement more so than the anterior nondominant side. This finding is likely related to practice or experience of the dominant or preferred side. The quadriceps on the dominant side activate quickly and briefly while the onset of the hamstrings of the dominant side is significantly delayed. This may indicate that handedness is a factor that affects reciprocal inhibition. Muscle firing intensity was highest during the reaching or moving back movement phases. Additionally, only the tibialis anterior was active during the reaching or moving forward phases. The stability ball creates an environment to allow for easier forward movement by rolling in which the tibialis anterior responds to control movement, such as braking; however, when rolling back, there are no contributors to controlling the movement. This heightens the person's awareness; thus, this is a factor in why we

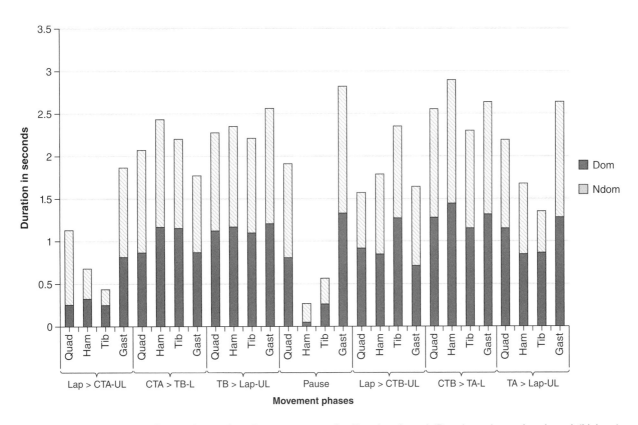

Figure 26.1 Duration of muscle contraction measures for the dominant (Dom) and nondominant (Ndom) leg muscles (quadriceps, hamstrings, tibialis anterior, and gastrocnemius) and movement phases: (1) (Lap > CTA-UL) Move hand from lap to pick up a cup at target position A, (2) (CTA > TB-L) move cup from target position A to target position B, (3) (TB > Lap-UL) return hand to lap, (4) (Pause) pause or rest, (5) (Lap > CTB-UL) move hand from lap to pick up cup at target position B, (6) (CTB > TA-L) move cup from target position B to target position A, and (7) (TA > Lap-UL) return hand to lap.

CTA = cup at target A, CTB = cup at target B, L = hand loaded with weight of cup, UL = hand not loaded with the weight of the cup, TA = target A, TB = target B

see highest intensity elicited during reaching back in all muscles.

Practical Guidelines

In order to limit risk for WMSDs, we must consider the traditional chair and talk about design. But first, a discussion of anthropological factors and design of the sitting substrate should be viewed from a bottom-up rather than a top-down perspective. That is, consider what are the fundamental physiological, anatomical, and morphological requirements of sitting rather than what the task requires: The take-home message is that the constraints of the traditional chair are unrealistic. Seating design is for *context*, not the *interaction*. The traditional chair was designed without knowledge of physiological, anatomical, or morphological factors. Additionally,

the traditional chair constrains our perception of what chairs are, and solutions are viewed from the top-down perspective. Looking from the bottom up, the stability ball provides the affordances chairs do not. By turning a stability ball into a traditional chair or by using roller bases, you limit the affordances of the stability ball. Considering all these data, the most efficient chair is the stability ball.

Whereas the energy expenditure of stability ball sitting is not significantly higher than sitting on a chair, when factoring in all relative components of the affordances generated by sitting on a stability ball, it is obvious to suggest the stability ball as an ideal alternative to traditional chairs. Additionally, evidence supports the use of a stability ball in the intervention of various disabilities. Previous investigations of stability ball sitting have identified the muscle synergies.

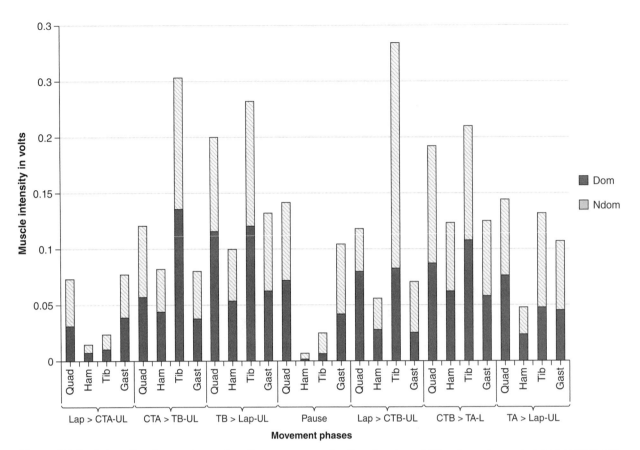

Figure 26.2 Intensity of muscle contraction measures for the dominant (Dom) and nondominant (Ndom) leg muscles (quadriceps, hamstrings, tibialis anterior, and gastrocnemius) and movement phases: (1) (Lap > CTA-UL) Move hand from lap to pick up a cup at target position A, (2) (CTA > TB-L) move cup from target position A to target position B, (3) (TB > Lap-UL) return hand to lap, (4) (Pause) pause or rest, (5) (Lap > CTB-UL) move hand from lap to pick up cup at target position B, (6) (CTB > TA-L) move cup from target position B to target position A, and (7) (TA > Lap-UL) return hand to lap.

CTA = cup at target A, CTB = cup at target B, L = hand loaded with weight of cup, UL = hand not loaded with the weight of the cup, TA = target A, TB = target B

Physical Activity Benefits

Inactivity physiology studies have demonstrated a link between sitting time and nonexercise activity as contributors to rates of metabolic syndrome, type 2 diabetes, obesity, and cardiovascular disease (Hamilton, Hamilton, and Zderic 2007). These findings highlight the need to redesign or consider alternatives to traditional seat design and sitting behaviors. One emerging alternative has been the use of the stability ball in place of the chair. Few studies have reported the effect of the stability ball on electromyography (EMG) during sedentary sitting (Gregory, Dunk, and Callaghan 2006; McGill, Kavcic, and Harvey 2006; O'Sullivan et al. 2006). A recent study on EMG during submaximal arm ergometry while sitting on a chair or stability ball was reported by Markes, Hylland, and Terreall (2012). Sitting on a stability ball resulted in greater EMG values for rest and for three levels (15%, 30%, and 45%) of age-predicted maximum heart rate (HR) for the rectus femoris muscle. With the exception of the external oblique muscles at 45% predicted maximum HR, trunk EMG differences were not different between ball and chair sitting. Sitting on the stability ball also resulted in 10% to 16% greater oxygen consumption ($\dot{V}O_2$) than chair sitting, but HR was unaffected. This finding suggests that exercise during ball sitting may be a useful exercise intervention for cardiac rehabilitation programs.

Classroom Performance Benefits

Stability balls have been increasingly adapted as a replacement for classroom chairs. Although research concerning the benefits of stability balls in comparison to chairs is relatively recent, evidence is accumulating that ball sitting enhances classroom performance of children (Illi 1994; Witt and Talbot 1998; Schilling et al. 2003). Sensory modulation deficits that reflect an adjustment in ongoing physiological processes to ensure internal adaptation to new or changing sensory information (Miller and Lane 2000; Miller et al. 2007) have been suggested as a factor contributing to attention deficits, and stability ball sitting has been suggested as an intervention for improving attention and school performance. This possibility was investigated by Schilling and colleagues (2003), who showed that stability ball sitting improved classroom performance in students with attention deficit hyperactivity disorder (ADHD). This finding was explained as reflecting self-modulation of personal sensory needs by each student in order to maintain an optimal state of arousal. Additional support for the use of stability balls in place of chairs for students with ADHD was provided by Fedewa and Erwin (2011), who used a larger population of students than Schilling and colleagues (2003). In addition to being beneficial to children with ADHD, Schilling and Schwartz (2004) provided evidence that stability ball sitting can benefit classroom behavior in children with autism spectrum disorders (ASD). This research was extended by Bagatell and colleagues (2010), who demonstrated that research on the use of the stability ball should consider differences between children. The authors suggested that the stability ball may be more useful for children who seek out vestibular-proprioceptive input than for children with other sensory processing characteristics.

Summary

Over the past 10,000 years, physical activity patterns have changed from those involving gross and fine movements necessary for procurement of resources for survival to the sedentary and constrained positional behaviors of today. Åstrand (1992) and Malina and Little (2008) as well as others have identified sedentary behavior as in opposition to our biology. Research on inactivity physiology has demonstrated a link between

DUAL-TASK TRAINING AND COGNITIVE BENEFITS

The speculation that the stability ball provides important vestibular-proprioceptive input that facilitates cognitive performance in children, and especially those with ADHD and ASD, is a plausible one. In addition, increasing evidence on dual-task training suggests that the stability ball may provide a learning context that facilitates executive function by aiding the capability to flexibly allocate attention across different tasks. We offer the speculation that this capability may be general in nature and not tethered to motor performance as exemplified by stability ball sitting. This view challenges the interpretation offered by movement theorists that dual-task training benefits represent a unique combination of exercise and cognitive function (e.g., Pesce 2012). Early evidence that dual-task training may promote the coordination of multiple processes, tasks, and skills, especially in old adults, was provided by Kramer, Larish, and Strayer (1995). This finding was later extended to the case of two motor tasks that required similar motor responses (Bherer et al. 2005). Erickson and colleagues (2007) later demonstrated neural correlates for learning-induced plasticity as the basis for dual-task performance gains. They suggested that these gains reflect enhanced reliance on central executive operations. Pellecchia (2005) provided evidence that dual-task training can reduce postural sway in comparison to no training or single-task training for dual-task performance. This finding was extended to improvements in gait performance by Silsupadol and colleagues (2009), who used a double-blind design. The relationship of dual-task training on gait and executive function was discussed by Yogev-Selingmann, Hausdorff, and Giladi (2008) in relation to clinical populations. The view that motor control in aging is influenced by executive control was advanced by Li and colleagues (2010). This important study demonstrated improvements on measures of dual-task standing balance and mobility as a result of nonmotor cognitive dual-task training.

sitting time and nonexercise activity to rising rates of metabolic syndrome, type 2 diabetes, obesity, and cardiovascular disease. These findings suggest the need to redesign the seat to promote active sitting behaviors. This is a unique event in the evolution of seat design. Throughout history, seat design has been solely focused on the accomplishment of the task being performed. It therefore focused on only one goal—increasing job performance—and this was accomplished by eliminating any other potentially competing secondary tasks. For the first time in history, we are faced with the possible need for seat design to consider the goals of promoting task performance as well as health through an increase in physical activity. The challenge is that seat design should provide as many opportunities for movement as possible, yet still maintain support of the lower body to stabilize the upper body for task performance (Baute 2008; McGill, Kavcic, and Harvey 2006).

It is further suggested that frequent changes in posture are beneficial. The evidence reviewed in this chapter suggests the stability ball is the ideal option for redesigning sitting. The stability ball provides a context for sitting that the traditional chair does not, allowing the freedom to move and alter postures. It also creates a coordinative structure or functional synergy between the stability ball and the worker (Baute 2008). This functional synergy does not increase cognitive demands while working; the same cannot be said for other chair alternatives like the treadmill-type desk, which ultimately limits task performance. Instead, it appears that using a stability ball in place of a traditional chair affords for dual-tasking yet still provides freedom for movement. Stability balls have been increasingly adapted as a replacement for classroom chairs. Evidence is accumulating that ball sitting enhances the classroom performance of children (Illi 1994; Witt and Talbot 1998), including children with ADHD (Shilling et al. 2003).

KEY CONCEPTS

▸ **Activity patterns:** The activities of daily life and behaviors used within a person's life span.

▸ **Biological phylogeny:** The evolutionary or genealogical relationships among a group of organisms.

▸ **Ecological contexts:** Refers to those factors external to the individual that work to influence behavior; the person and environment are viewed as interdependent (Dunn, Brown, and McGuigan 1994).

▸ **Ergonomics:** In the context of this chapter, refers to the design of the environment to fit the job as opposed to fitting the worker to the job with the purpose of alleviating physical and environmental stresses.

▸ **Functional synergies:** In the context of this chapter, refers to the coordination of physical and environmental components to execute a task (e.g., coordinating an arm reach afforded by the movement of a stability ball).

▸ **Human positional behaviors:** Postures assumed during activities of daily life, such as sitting, standing, and any task-related postures. These include but are not limited to operating heavy machinery or performing assembly-line work.

▸ **Positional or postural affordance:** Positional behavior used to facilitate the successful performance of a task.

▸ **Sensory modulation deficits:** These reflect a change in physiological processes in response to changing sensory information and have been suggested as contributing to attention deficits.

▸ **Subsistence strategies:** The methods, plans, and actions people rely on to procure resources for survival and consider the positional behaviors used to execute tasks.

▸ **Substate:** Within a bioanthropological context (field dependent), refers to the structures acted on that promote a specific locomotive or positional behavior. Extended into a kinanthropological context, refers to the equipment or furniture used in activities of daily living. Specifically, within the context of this chapter, refers to the stability ball.

STUDY QUESTIONS

1. What evolutionary factors should be considered during discussions of sedentary behavior?

2. What is the history of the chair?

3. What alternative sitting behaviors provide intervention effects for musculoskeletal disorders (MSDs)?

4. Does using the stability ball provide additional benefits outside of preventing WMSDs?

5. What are the future possibilities for assessing sedentary behavior?

6. Do prolonged sitting or other positional behaviors detract attention from cognitive tasks?

7. Can the stability ball be useful in dual-task learning?

8. Does the stability ball provide an alternative to classroom chairs for schools?

CHAPTER 27

EMERGING COMMUNICATION SYSTEMS TO CURB PHYSICAL INACTIVITY

Dolores Albarracin, PhD; Q. Vera Liao, PhD; Jessica Yi, BS; and ChengXiang Zhai, PhD

The reader will gain an overview of how emerging systems can contribute to curbing physical inactivity and how critical psychological processes can shape the design of systems in this domain. By the end of this chapter, the reader should be able to do the following:

▸ Understand how exposure, attention, and behavior change can be influenced by information systems

▸ Identify how online information technologies and data transfer systems may be facilitated by the Internet or telecommunications, including Twitter, Facebook, and the use of simpler forms such as text messaging

▸ Identify key attributes of stand-alone electronic delivery systems (e.g., counseling websites), social networks, monitoring and tracking systems, search engines, recommender systems, and gamification systems

▸ Understand information processing stages from a psychological perspective

▸ Understand ways of characterizing information systems that are relevant to influencing physical inactivity

Physical inactivity and sedentary behavior now constitute troubling health care issues of the 21st century, and lack of physical activity has been shown to be among the top 10 leading causes of death and disability in moderate- to high-income countries (Davis et al. 2014; O'Reilly et al. 2011). Physical activity comprises movements resulting in increased energy expenditure and improved physical fitness (Pettee et al. 2012). Its absence, physical inactivity, is a significant public health risk that must be reduced to decrease coronary heart disease, breast and colon cancer, and diabetes, among many other conditions directly or indirectly linked to this risk factor (Lee et al. 2012).

Increasing physical activity can confer important benefits on 39 diseases and health conditions (Hillsdon et al. 2005). A systematic review of 29 randomized controlled trials to promote physical activity or combat inactivity showed that the interventions have a positive moderate effect in increasing physical activity (Hillsdon et al. 2005). These programs entail counseling, activity prescriptions, social support, provision of written information, and self-monitoring—all techniques that continue to be important in the current generation of behavioral interventions using emerging media and electronic systems with the same objectives.

Exposure and attention to the information are prerequisites for the influence of any intervention, including online programs and new electronic systems for curbing sedentary behavior. *Exposure* implies reading, viewing, or listening to the information, whereas *attention* involves focusing on the presented content to ensure understanding and subsequent recall. Both exposure and attention must occur for the information to be received by the audience. Exposure and attention are thus prerequisites of the behavior change sought by researchers and practitioners trying to elicit physical activity. Emerging electronic systems (e.g., websites, search engines, expert recommendation systems) have been designed to ensure that materials reach their relevant audiences, potential viewers can search for the information in a systematic fashion, and materials are presented in an interactive, engaging fashion.

The effects of emerging electronic interventions on increasing activity can be measured in terms of changes in behavioral, clinical, or biological outcomes in direct and indirect recipients of the program. *Behavior change* is the modification of the intensity and duration of a behavior performed at an earlier (arbitrary) time. Biological outcomes of import in this domain include weight loss, blood pressure, and blood glucose measures, as well as the prevention of physical conditions (e.g., cancer, diabetes). Interventions for promoting physical activity are often concerned with increasing the frequency of the behavior and moving people from inactivity to initiation. Interventions for increasing sport performance have the objective of increasing movement duration and precision.

In this chapter, we provide a perspective on emerging communication systems for addressing physical inactivity, which have important potential implications for the sedentary behavior field in terms of how exposure, attention, and behavior change can be influenced by information systems. Online information technologies are characterized by using data transfer systems facilitated by the Internet or telecommunications, including Twitter, Facebook, and the use of simpler forms such as text messaging. These technologies include, but are not limited to, stand-alone electronic delivery systems (e.g., counseling websites), social networks, monitoring and tracking systems, search engines, recommender systems, and gamification systems. We first describe the information processing stages from a psychological perspective and then characterize the information systems that are relevant to influencing physical inactivity. We discuss established contributions and, when available, system efficacy and consider future opportunities for this exciting area.

Determinants of Exposure and Attitude

The classic assumption in attitude research is that people are motivated to defend their attitudes from challenges (e.g., Festinger 1957; Hart et al. 2009; Olson and Stone 2005) and that this defense leads them to seek out and disseminate attitude-consistent information. In attitude theory (e.g., Albarracín et al. 2005; Eagly and Chaiken 1993; Zanna and Rempel 1988), the term *attitude* represents an evaluation of an entity (an issue, person, event, object, or behavior; e.g., jogging, President Obama). Selective exposure and selective dissemination both enable people to defend their attitudes, beliefs, or behaviors by restricting challenging information and ensuring the availability of consistent information. Selectivity of this type results in what is known as a *congeniality bias*, traditionally referring to exposure but here used to encompass information dissemination as well (see Hart et al. 2009).

Festinger was probably the first to formalize the notion of attitudinal selectivity (1957; 1964). His work states that people avoid information inconsistent with their attitudes and decisions to prevent the unpleasant state of arousal known as *cognitive dissonance*. The potential for learning that one is mistaken can cause dissonance and trigger a search for consistent information to reestablish the more pleasant state of cognitive consonance. In this chapter (see also Cappella et al. 2015), we also propose that cognitive dissonance can trigger *dissemination* of consistent information to avoid the presence of dissonant, threatening information in a social network.

The *congeniality principle* has often been examined with a laboratory paradigm in which participants select information from alternatives. Prior to this selection, participants make a decision (e.g., about the guilt of a defendant in a mock trial), form an attitude (e.g., toward works of art), report an existing attitude (e.g., on abortion), or report a prior behavior (e.g., whether they have smoked in the past). Afterward, participants can select information about the same issue (e.g., abortion, smoking) from a list of options usually presented as titles or abstracts of available articles. Typically, half of these options support the participant's attitude and the other half contradict it. Selection of more articles that agree and fewer that disagree with prior attitudes or behavior indicates a congeniality bias, whereas selection of fewer agreeable articles and more disagreeable ones indicates an *uncongeniality bias*.

In one of the first studies ever investigating selective exposure (Adams 1961), mothers reported their belief that child development was predominantly influenced by genetic or environmental factors. They could choose to hear a speech supporting either point of view. Consistent with the congeniality bias, mothers overwhelmingly chose the speech that favored their view on the issue. Despite periodic challenges to the existence of attitudinal selectivity (e.g., Freedman and Sears 1965), findings from research synthesis indicate a bias favoring congenial information, even though there are important moderators of the phenomenon. Hart and colleagues' (2009) meta-analysis synthesized 67 eligible reports of selective exposure that contained 91 studies incorporating 300 statistically independent groups with around 8,000 participants. The average effect indicating a congeniality bias was estimated at $d = 0.36$ (95% CI = 0.34, 0.39) according to fixed-effects analysis and $d = 0.38$ (95% CI = 0.32, 0.44) according to the random-effects analysis, both indicating a moderate congeniality bias.

Hart and his colleagues (2009) proposed a model of selective exposure determinants. This model can be expanded to also incorporate attitudinal selectivity in *dissemination* of information (see also Cappella et al. 2015). In this model, information choices are meant to fulfill goals to defend attitudes, beliefs, and behaviors and to accurately appraise and represent reality (Chaiken et al. 1989). Defense and accuracy motives have been popular in analyses of how people process attitude-relevant information (Chaiken et al. 1996; Eagly et al. 1999; Johnson and Eagly 1989; Prislin and Wood 2005; Wyer and Albarracín 2005). *Defense motivation* can be defined as the desire to defend one's existing attitudes, beliefs, and behaviors; *accuracy motivation* is the desire to form accurate appraisals of stimuli (Hart et al. 2009). Although previous theorists also proposed a third motive (e.g., see Lundgren and Prislin 1998), which here we term *social motivation*, the desire to form and maintain positive interpersonal relations, Hart and colleagues did not include this motive because it was not well represented in their synthesized research. This motive, however, is included in this chapter due to its role in the inherently social character of information transmission through emerging electronic systems.

Defense motivation is stronger when people who just engaged in a behavior or reported an attitude or belief receive challenging (versus supporting) information before selecting new information (Frey 1986; Hart et al. 2009). If people encounter a challenge to recently expressed attitudes, beliefs, or behaviors, their effort to diminish the cognitive conflict may increase the selection rate of congenial information (Beauvois and Joule 1996; Festinger 1964). Defense motivation is also enhanced when attitudes are linked to enduring values (e.g., on controversial issues such as euthanasia or abortion) and when people commit to the relevant attitude, belief, or past behavior (Brehm and Cohen 1962; Kiesler 1971). Researchers have operationalized commitment by directly assessing participants' loyalty (e.g., Jonas and Frey 2003) or by asking them to dedicate more or less time or effort to attitude-relevant behavior (e.g., Betsch et al. 2001) or publicly affirm or withhold their opinions (e.g., Sears and Freedman 1965). In addition, individual personality differences may affect the extent to which people are motivated to defend their views and behaviors. Closed-minded people may view challenging information as a threat, whereas open-minded people may view it with curiosity (Adorno et al. 1950; Altemeyer 1981; 1998). Furthermore, people who view themselves as incapable of resisting or counterarguing challenging information may be more motivated to proactively guard against such threats (e.g., Albarracín and Mitchell 2004). If so, the congeniality bias should be stronger for people with less confidence in their attitude, belief, or behavior (e.g., Berkowitz 1965; Brechan 2002; Brodbeck 1956; Feather 1962; Micucci 1972; Thayer 1969).

Accuracy motivation increases attention to and elaboration of attitude-relevant information and preference for valid information, regardless of its consistency with prior views (Chaiken et al. 1989; 1996; Kunda 1990). For example, people who are held accountable for their judgments about a target individual consider and integrate more of the person's characteristics and hence can predict that person's future behavior more accurately (Tetlock and Kim 1987). Also, when accuracy motivation is higher, people who lack sufficient diagnostic evidence are less likely to form an impression of another person (Kassin and Hochreich 1977). Generally, any issue that could have foreseeable effects on future personal outcomes (i.e., high outcome relevance) is likely to increase accuracy motivation (Albarracín 2002; Eagly et al. 1999; Johnson and Eagly 1989; Kruglanski and Freund 1983; Petty and Cacioppo 1986; Tetlock and Kim 1987; but see Darke and Chaiken 2005) and thus engender unbiased exposure to both congenial and uncongenial information.

Any increase in the utility of uncongenial information also diminishes the congeniality bias by enhancing accuracy motivation. Researchers have manipulated utility by assigning participants to either debate an issue or write an essay in support of their attitudes, beliefs, or behaviors (e.g., Canon 1964; Freedman 1965). Expecting to participate in a debate enhances participants' selection of uncongenial information that may be more useful for the debate (Canon 1964). Correspondingly, the expectation of supporting one's view in an essay enhances the selection of congenial information that may facilitate constructing stronger supporting arguments (Canon 1964). In addition, people may select novel information, regardless of its position, because new information is typically of greater value than familiar information (Frey and Rosch 1984). Finally, any increase in information quality can potentially increase the probability that it will

be selected. Contrary to defense motivation, accuracy motivation should direct people to the highest quality information despite the potential negative consequences for cognitive conflict. Hence, congeniality biases in selective exposure may diminish when the uncongenial information is high in quality but be accentuated when the congenial information is low in quality.

Hart and colleagues' (2009) meta-analysis thoroughly examined defense motivation as a source of the congeniality bias. In this synthesis, the congeniality bias was weaker when there was support for the attitude (rather than no challenge or no support) prior to information selection, even though the two latter conditions did not differ from each other. Also, the congeniality bias was larger when the uncongenial or congenial information available for selection was high or moderate in quality than when it was low; it was also larger for samples with high rather than moderate commitment to an attitude, belief, or earlier behavior. Last, the congeniality bias was larger when the value relevance of the issue was high rather than low, samples were high (versus moderate) in closed-mindedness, and participants were low or moderate (versus high) in confidence in the attitude, belief, or behavior.

Hart and team's meta-analysis also found support for the role of accuracy motivation in attitudinal selectivity. First, the congeniality bias was larger when the congenial information was highly useful than when there was no experimental goal, and an uncongeniality bias appeared when the congenial information was not useful. Second, the congeniality bias was weaker when the uncongenial information was high in utility than when the congenial information was low in utility or when there was no goal. Contrary to the moderating role of accuracy motivation, the congeniality bias was larger when the uncongenial information was high or moderate in quality rather than low in quality. This finding suggests that high-quality uncongenial information is threatening because defense motivation dominates decisions.

Various past perspectives have emphasized that attitudes and decisions are used to manage social relationships (Johnson and Eagly 1989; Prislin and Wood 2005; Schlenker 1980; Tetlock and Manstead 1985). Selecting information in public settings can facilitate or hinder social goals (Katz 1960; Tetlock and Manstead 1985). For example, the desire to communicate an attitude to a social group may lead to publicly selecting congenial information (e.g., Katz

1960). In contrast, the desire to appear as motivated by accuracy or openness may lead to the public selection of uncongenial information.

Defense, accuracy, and social motives are also important in information transmission or dissemination, another critical contributor to exposure. An investigation of exposure decisions made for others (Earl et al. 2009) was based on the notion that selective exposure *for others* may follow the same mechanisms as selective exposure for one's self. To the extent that selective exposure for others operates under similar principles, people may choose information guided by their own defense and accuracy motivations. For example, merely choosing congenial information to be presented to others may reduce the selector's cognitive dissonance and generate pleasant affective states. Likewise, people making the choice may feel they are disseminating accurate information, thus satisfying their own need for accuracy. More so than with decisions for the self, selective transmission is likely to be in the service of social motives like relationship maintenance, generating tendencies to meet the goals of the target person in making the selection.

Suppose people disseminate information that is expected to meet the defense motivation of the receivers of the information. This bias may be larger for people we like rather than dislike, since people are more likely to intuit the motives someone they like rather than a neutral or disliked other (Heider 1958). Examples of the probability of experiencing the motives and emotions of liked others include vicarious experiences of pain for liked others (Krebs 1975) and vicarious embarrassment and dissonance for in-group members (Miller 1987; Norton et al. 2003). Consistent with this possibility, Earl and her colleagues (2009) found that people are aware that others prefer to receive congenial to uncongenial information. Furthermore, in making dissemination decisions, selectors honor the assumed or known preferences of others both spontaneously and on command. Interestingly, this selective dissemination occurs even when no interaction with the target is expected, suggesting that the same biases may occur for anonymous Internet audiences.

The research by Earl and colleagues (2009) suggests that the motivation to maintain or enhance social relationships underlies information transmission, producing dissemination of information expected to be congenial to the recipients. However, the defense motivation for the selector and the recipient can suggest very different decisions. For example, if the recipient's attitude is opposite to the selector's attitude, the selector may choose information that meets the defense motivation of the selector or the recipient. Future research needs to establish which of these motivational forces carries the day. Perhaps the recipient's motivation drives decisions when the social motivation is higher than the selector's defense motivation, but this possibility needs to be empirically tested in the future.

Like with many other health behaviors, preaching to the choir can be a significant problem in the area of physical activity as well. As shown by Steel and colleagues (2007a), however, online tools can present significant advantages when it comes to exposure. In their study of adults randomized to different types of programs, the Internet-mediated and Internet-only groups were more likely to have been exposed to at least 75% of the program compared to the face-to-face group. Thus, little doubt exists that emerging information technologies can ensure better exposure and relatively cost-effective capturing and retention of audiences in need of physical activity promotion.

Finally, exposure to emerging media also depends on message factors that have been reviewed elsewhere (Cappella et al. 2015), including utility, novelty, and the type and intensity of emotions evoked by the information. For instance, Thorson (2008) examined news articles providing advice on such issues as medical problems, real estate, finance, personal relationships, and jobs. Findings indicated that articles that remained on the *New York Times*' most e-mailed list were longer, supposedly containing more information (see also Berger and Milkman 2012). Novel content is also more likely to be transmitted than well-known content. Likewise, studies of *New York Times* news articles have shown that surprising articles are more frequently shared than unsurprising ones (Berger and Milkman 2012; Thorson 2008), and individual retransmission of information has been shown to correlate with evaluation of the information as novel (Kim et al. 2013). Further, positive emotionality and emotional intensity both seem to correlate with virality (Berger and Milkman 2012; Carter et al. 2011; Eckler and Bolls 2011).

Determinants of Attitude and Behavior Change

Whether online information and emerging systems influence physical activity depends on the persuasiveness of the information and the degree to which that information is tightly linked to the behaviors being targeted. Like exposure, the persuasiveness of the information depends on defense, accuracy, and social motives, such that information that agrees with the recipients' values is perceived as strong, factually accurate information and data are perceived as strong, and information aligned with social norms is perceived as compelling (see e.g., Hart et al. 2009). However, the ultimate behavioral influence of the information depends on the linkage of the information with the recommended behavior. For example, one may change the perception that exercise helps people to relax, but this belief will be inconsequential for those who do not care about relaxing. Or a message may state that exercise is enjoyable, but such a belief will have no effect in people who fail to exercise because it is difficult or they lack structural opportunities to do so. Therefore, efficacious information connects with the determinants of the behavior.

Considerable past research and theorizing support the point that the ultimate effect of the information depends on its potential to influence immediate determinants of behavior. Several theoretical models have identified motivational and cognitive antecedents of health behaviors (lettered a through e), including physical activity (see Albarracin et al. 2005). For example, the theory of reasoned action (Fishbein and Ajzen 1975) and the theory of planned behavior (Ajzen and Madden 1986; for a meta-analysis, see Albarracín et al. 2001) state that health behaviors stem from (a) the perceived desirability of the behavior (i.e., positive attitudes and expectancies about physical activity) and (b) the normative pressure to engage in the behavior (i.e., social norms). The theory of planned behavior also includes (c) perceptions that physical activity is easy and up to the individual (i.e., perceived behavioral control). Social cognitive theory (Bandura 1986; 1989; 1994) assumes that feeling capable of performing a behavior is central to implementing that behavior, implying that feeling efficacious in the area of physical activity should increase compliance with exercise recommendations. Furthermore, social cognitive theory (Bandura 1989) and the information-motivation-behavioral skills model (Fisher and Fisher 1992) both state that people are more likely to perform a behavior once they acquire relevant (d) knowledge and (e) behavioral skills.

Although other determinants of health behavior have been proposed (see e.g., Janz and Becker 1984; Floyd et al. 2000; Rogers 1975; Rosenstock 1974;

Rosenstock et al. 1994; for a review, see Albarracin et al. 2005), attitudes, norms, self-efficacy, and behavioral skills appear to be the strongest, most consistent pathways leading to intentions and actual behavior. Evidence also exists that interventions containing components for inducing change in these determinants are more efficacious than programs lacking these elements. For example, a health-promotion intervention may attempt to motivate recipients by increasing favorable attitudes and norms. Further, a persuasive communication may not only tout the benefits of the advocated behavior (i.e., attitudinal arguments) or mention groups that support it (i.e., normative arguments), but also describe how success in meeting health goals depends on preparatory actions (i.e., behavioral skills arguments), such as scheduling physical activity in advance. As another example, a widely accepted strategy is to have people role-play skills, including resistance to the behavior by people close to them (i.e., behavioral skills training). Presumably, behavioral practice and instructional feedback facilitate the acquisition of key behavioral skills.

The effect of different intervention strategies has been most intensely investigated in a meta-analysis of the effects of HIV-prevention interventions. As part of this project (Albarracín et al. 2005), more than 350 interventions and around 100 control groups were selected comprising a large number of countries, U.S. states, and years. For each of these groups or conditions, the researchers calculated amount of change in behavior (e.g., increases in condom use frequency) as well as change in various psychological variables as a function of intervention strategies consistent with the theories outlined previously. Messages that mentioned outcomes of the target behavior were coded as including attitudinal messages. Messages that mentioned who in the recipient's network might support the behavior were coded as including normative arguments. Messages that mentioned how recipients may feel more in control of the behavior were classified as including control arguments. Programs with active behavioral skills training were coded as such.

One important conclusion from the meta-analysis by Albarracin and colleagues (2005) was that the inclusion of attitudinal, normative, and control arguments was beneficial, but interventions that included behavioral-skills training had the greatest effect. Furthermore, the benefits of each type of strategy also depended on the degree of control people had over the behavior. Consistent with the possibility that women had less control over condom use than did men, the effect of self-management skills training was stronger for women than for men. Similarly, populations with lower education, ethnic minorities, and younger populations benefitted more from behavioral skills training than did their more educated, older counterparts. Presumably, the lack of resources associated with lower education, ethnic minority status, and younger age created a greater need for behavioral skills to offset obstacles and facilitate compliance with the behavioral recommendation.

Systematic reviews of the efficacy of face-to-face interventions for increasing physical activity suggest that information provision and social support can be effective, but many interventions are dismal failures (Kahn et al. 2002; O'Reilly et al. 2011). A meta-analysis reported a positive effect of online interventions (Davies et al. 2014), which suggests the need to continue to invest in the use of technology for reducing physical inactivity. Several online programs have been designed to influence physical activity using the same theoretical constructs that have proved advantageous in other health-promotion domains. For example, a study by Marshall and colleagues (2003) revealed that a stage-based physical activity website significantly decreased sitting time and increased motivational readiness for physical activity. Steele and colleagues (2007b), however, conducted a randomized trial comparing intervention delivery modes for a 12-week physical activity intervention based on social cognitive theory (Health-eSteps). Results indicated no differences between intervention groups and no increases in activity over time for any group. However, a later study by the same authors (2007a) showed that ensuring exposure led to significant increases in physical activity. Overall, though, there is sufficient interest in making emerging technologies successful in this domain and a need to systematically review the characteristics and efficacy of emerging systems, as we do presently.

Information Systems

The Internet era arrived with the intent to use websites to deliver informational and counseling interventions in all domains, including the promotion of physical activity. Various platforms associated with social networks (e.g., Twitter, Facebook, blogs) allow for delivery of information and social normative influences that can affect physical activity and other

health behaviors. Many monitoring and tracking systems have been designed to provide accurate feedback and reinforcement of physical activity and often involve social networks to strengthen social monitoring and normative pressures. Gamification can be used with social networking and monitoring purposes and search engines enable active, deliberate information seeking. Finally, both search engines and expert recommendation systems influence information exposure through two modes: *push* and *pull*. In the push mode, the information is pushed to a user by a system (e.g., the advertisement displayed by a search engine, or recommendation of movies), whereas in the pull mode, the user takes initiative to seek the relevant information (e.g., seeking relevant information types in a query in a search engine or browsing a collection of items). In general, in the pull mode, a user has a clear information need and thus can be assumed to pay more attention to the information than in the push mode, in which the user can easily choose to ignore the recommended information. Sometimes, however, the boundaries between push and pull are not that clear. For example, a search engine can manipulate the search results to embed recommended information directly in the search results. Such an *implicit* recommendation in response to an information need likely enables effective influences on the user, perhaps even stronger influences than those obtained through direct push-type recommendations. Internet users tend to be unaware of the inevitable bias in the results returned by a search engine, which suggests the possibility to leverage search engines to intentionally tailor content to correct people's sedentary behavior. Table 27.1 describes how each system relates to the stages of exposure, attention, and behavior change. We review details of the systems and available efficacy data in the upcoming sections.

Websites as Information Delivery Systems

Since the advent of the Internet, there has been exponential growth in the use of websites to deliver interventions previously delivered in person or on the phone. The main rational is that online information is accessible irrespective of location and offers the possibility of greater engagement and tailoring relative to a print presentation (see table 27.1). A large number of empirical studies have tested the efficacy of these programs in the domain of

Table 27.1 Electronic Information Systems and Likelihood of Influence at the Stages of Exposure, Attention, and Behavior Change

Psychological stage	Exposure to information and messages and materials	Attention to information and messages and materials	Behavior change
Information delivery systems	Can make information accessible, particularly if presented in ways that high-light congeniality with prior attitudes and behaviors.	Can increase attention if the material is novel and emotionally interesting.	The evidence is mixed. Can occur but depends entirely on the design of the materials.
Social networks	Can make information accessible, particularly if presented in ways that highlight congeniality with prior attitudes and behaviors. Can leverage the social network to ensure information relevance.	Can increase attention if the material is novel and emotionally interesting.	Has not been tested for all platforms. Available evidence for Facebook is mixed.
Monitoring and tracking tools	Not applicable.	Not applicable.	Evidence is mixed. Depends entirely on the design of the materials.
Search engines	Excellent tool for making information available. Biases are prioritizing positive responses to questions, clicks from other users, and negative health outcomes.	Can increase attention if the material is novel and emotionally interesting.	Can probably occur but depends entirely on the design of the materials.
Recommender systems: *implicit or embedded*	Excellent tool for tailoring information exposure to user.	Can increase attention if the material is novel and emotionally interesting.	Can probably occur but depends on the materials.
Recommender systems: *explicit, stand-alone*	Excellent tool for tailoring information exposure to user.	Can increase attention if the material is novel and emotionally interesting. Depends on user's trust in the system. It can increase reactance because it is obvious.	Can probably occur but depends on the materials and trust in the system. System can increase reactance because it is obvious.
Gamification systems	Can make information accessible, particularly if presented in ways that high-light congeniality with prior attitudes and behaviors.	Can increase attention if the material is novel and emotionally interesting.	Depends on the materials. Systems often present simple information but could evolve to include more complex programs. Ideal for training skills if designed with a strong behavioral science basis.

physical activity, and the resulting evidence shows that many programs are effective but many are not. Our literature review identified 16 studies showing at least some improvements in physical activity as a result of an Internet-delivered intervention. Spittaels and colleagues (2007) examined the efficacy of an Internet-delivered physical activity intervention that provides computer-tailored feedback to a general population sample. The researchers compared recipients of Internet-based interventions with or without repeated feedback (two intervention groups) with a no-intervention control group. Results revealed significant increases favoring the intervention group for active transportation and leisure-time physical activity and a decrease for minutes sitting on weekdays, with no significant differences resulting from feedback provision. Irvine and colleagues (2013) evaluated the efficacy of a 12-week Internet intervention for helping sedentary older adults over 55 years of age adopt and maintain an exercise regimen. At post test, intervention participants showed significant improvements in 13 of 14 outcome measures compared to the control group. Glasgow and colleagues (2010) conducted a randomized trial to evaluate minimal and moderate contact versions of an Internet-based diabetes self-management program compared to an enhanced-usual-care condition. The Internet-based intervention produced significantly greater physical activity improvements than the enhanced usual care condition, but the improvements were independent of intervention dosage. Gow and colleagues (2010) evaluated an Internet intervention with first-year college students randomly assigned to one of four treatment conditions: no treatment, 6-week online intervention, 60-week weight and caloric feedback only (through e-mail), and 6-week combined feedback and online intervention. Following the intervention administration, the combined intervention group had lower BMI at posttesting than the other three groups. Carr, both individually (2009) and with colleagues (2008), sought to determine whether the Active Living Every Day Internet-delivered physical activity program was effective (intervention versus delayed intervention control) and found that the intervention increased physical activity. Similarly, promising results were reported in other studies (De Bourdeaudhuij et al. 2010; Carr el al. 2013; Dunton et al. 2008; Huang et al. 2009; Lau et al. 2012; Liebreich et al. 2009; Mailey et al. 2010; Napolitano et al. 2003; Winett et al. 2007; Schwinn et al. 2014; Van Wier et al. 2011), suggesting that online interventions can be efficacious at inducing physical activity.

In addition to the successful studies suggesting the efficacy of Internet-delivered programs, we also identified 12 showing null effects and 3 reversals for which the intervention decreased physical activity. For example, Cullen and colleagues (2013) tested the influence of a website promoting nutrition and physical activity for adolescents. Over 8 weeks, participants were asked to weekly log on to either an intervention or a control condition website to review web content and set goals to improve dietary and physical activity behaviors. At a post test occurring after 8 weeks, a greater proportion of intervention-group participants reported eating three or more daily vegetable servings in the past week compared to the control group. Although both groups reported significant increases in physical activity and significant decreases in TV watching, there were no differences across conditions (for similar results, see Bosak 2007; Cooperberg 2014; Kosma et al. 2005; Leung 2011; Morgan et al. 2009; Maher et al. 2010; Pekmezi et al. 2010; Skår et al. 2011; Van Genugten et al. 2012; Webber et al. 2008; Whittemore et al. 2013). Studies showing boomerang effects of online physical activity interventions are rarer but not inexistent. For example, Marks and colleagues (2006) compared the effectiveness of a web-based physical activity intervention with identical content delivered in a printed workbook among a sample of adolescent girls. Both groups had significant changes in physical activity self-efficacy and intentions, but the print group demonstrated greater increases in intentions and self-reported activity than the Internet group. Thus, online programs offer promise but must be carefully pretested; they are as good as the materials they present (see table 27.1).

Social Networks as Information Delivery Systems

Because social networks have great capacity to diffuse innovations, it is not surprising that online communities have been touted as a sort of magic bullet for the promotion of all kinds of health behaviors, including physical activity. Networks can effectively disseminate information by tapping interpersonal connections; they are also a repository of information (see table 27.1). In this section, we review these platforms and their potential, which is clearly vast if the associated programs can ensure attention and behavior change efficacy.

Twitter

Twitter is a platform that allows for rapid dissemination of information in a network. Born in 2006, Twitter now has more than 200 million active users who post more than 300 million tweets per day. Not surprisingly, as with any emerging media that acquires popularity, people use it to find and spread information and to network with others. The delivery of short and frequent messages and the easy and casual access to information that does not require approval or ad hoc mutual connections have made Twitter an effective and powerful platform for delivering health information and promoting public health awareness and positive behavior change. By following existing social networks (e.g., friends, colocated users), health providers (Chretien, Azar, and Kind 2011), and government users such as state health departments (e.g., CDC) (Neiger et al. 2012), Twitter users may receive a wide range of health-related information on various topics such as promoting dental health (Heavilin et al. 2011), improving sleeping habits (Jamison-Powell et al. 2012), smoking cessation (Prochaska et al. 2012), managing diabetes and cancer (De la Torre-Díez et al. 2012), and treating concussions (Sullivan et al. 2012). Twitter has also been shown to be useful for patients with chronic diseases, who seek advice, discuss treatment options, and find support and role models that would otherwise be unavailable (Jamison-Powell et al. 2012; Sullivan et al. 2012). For instance, researchers have examined the discussion of antibiotics on Twitter and found that the relevant conversations cover a wide range of topics related to the treatment such as general use and advice, as well as side effects and misuse (Scanfeld et al. 2010). Moreover, Twitter-based interventions (e.g., from the CDC) directly target behavior change by delivering information or reminders through Twitter updates. Twitter can thus increase exposure to very brief messages or links to more complex programs through websites. The ultimate attention and exposure depend on the content of the disseminated materials (see table 27.1).

Facebook

Facebook is currently the most popular form of online social media. It allows users, groups, and organizations to create their own web pages, publish various content (e.g., texts, external links, images, video), and connect with each other by either adding someone as a friend (mutual connection) or following another user (one-sided connection). Facebook was founded in 2004 and currently has more than 1 billion active users.

Unlike Twitter, Facebook is based on users' existing ties, such as family members and friends. As a result, social motivations play a prominent role in users' information sharing and seeking. For example, research has shown that Facebook is often used to update others about one's health goals and progress toward goals, increasing personal accountability, as well as seeking and providing emotional support. These characteristics make Facebook ideal for maintaining behavior change and inducing self- and social monitoring, although the public nature of information sharing may lead to greater reporting of successes than failures (see e.g., Newman et al. 2011). Facebook, however, is less frequently used to seek information advice compared to presently discussed social media surrounding specific

health issues (e.g., a health forum; Skeels et al. 2010; Newman et al. 2011).

Up to now, however, the effects of Facebook-based programs are mixed at best. On the one hand, there is a comparison between a 12-week Facebook-based intervention aimed at increasing moderate- to vigorous-intensity physical activity (MVPA) and a Facebook-based self-help comparison condition. Over 12 weeks, both groups increased self-reported weekly minutes of MVPA, but there was no significant difference between groups. However, increases in light physical activity were greater relative to the control group, and the experimental group reported significant weight loss over time (Valle et al. 2012). On the other hand, a test of the efficacy and feasibility of a social support intervention primarily delivered through Facebook revealed no differences in physical activity outcomes across groups (Cavallo 2013).

Specialized Online Health Communities

Online health communities are made up of groups formed around common health interests or concerns. They offer the benefits of asynchronous communication and thus wide temporal access to the information, anonymity, and ample accessibility regardless of isolation and mobility (White and Dorman 2001; Farnham et al. 2002; Hwang et al. 2010). For example, PatientsLikeMe is an online social platform that can automatically identify and suggest connections with others sharing similar concerns or background information (for its effects, see Wicks et al. 2010).

Content analysis of online health communities has shown them to be important sources of informational support and emotional support (Fogel et al. 2002; Rodgers and Chen 2005; Mo and Coulson 2008; Ziebland and Wyke 2012). Users can exchange information about the course of diseases, treatments, side effects, communication with physicians, financial and other burdens, and treatment outcomes (Rodgers and Chen 2005; Coulson 2005). Users can also obtain emotional support, including encouragement and compassion from other members, a greater sense of community, reduced feelings of isolation, as well as improved self-confidence (Salem et al. 1997; Preece 1998; White and Dorman 2001; Klemm et al. 2003). A longitudinal content analysis on a breast cancer online community revealed a positive shift in patients' affect toward the disease and treatments, as well as improved psychosocial outcomes (Blanchard et al. 1995; Rodgers and Chen 2005).

Online health communities also provide first-person accounts from people with similar experiences or with more experience dealing with particular health issues. The communities can satisfy patients' information needs, especially for people with low health literacy and the desire to learn from others who have actual experience in an area (Hibbard and Peters 2003). From an informational perspective, peer patients' accounts of disease and treatment may make the information more relevant (Sillence et al. 2007), facilitate comprehension (Hibbard and Peters 2003), and provide contexts to support reasoning about disease causes and outcomes (Rothman and Kiviniemi 1999). Sharing and learning about personal experience in online health communities can also contribute to behavior change (Ziebland and Wyke 2012). Online social groups that aim at facilitating behavior change, such as those focusing on weight loss, smoking cessation, and chronic disease management, can increase confidence and self-efficacy (Anderson-Bill et al. 2011), provide social support for making changes, increase social pressure and competition to promote adherence (Hwang et al. 2010), and enhance attention to and comprehension of information (Ziebland and Wyke 2012).

The effects of a specialized online community were examined in a study of an Internet-mediated program to promote physical activity (Richardson et al. 2010). The study compared an Internet-mediated walking program (participants could post and read messages from other participants) with no online community. Both arms significantly increased their average daily steps between the baseline and the post test, but there were no significant differences in increase in step counts between the two arms. Online health community interventions, however, are in their infancy, and their contents and methods must be refined before solid efficacy conclusions can be reached (see table 27.1).

Blogs and Vlogs

Blogs and vlogs (video blogs) are sites typically created and maintained by an individual, or a group of people, who posts original entries presented in reverse chronological order. These posts are read by users who can make online comments. These days, many patients, health professionals, health issue activists, and organizations use blogs to record experiences, express views, and promote public health awareness. Compared to online health communities, blogs provide more author control over the information and are easy to set up, but they often require a high level of commitment to regular posting and response monitoring. Blogs and vlogs also help to disseminate information by sharing external links to website repositories, linking to and citing from other blogs, and encouraging communication between authors and audiences (e.g., by commenting on the posts).

Blogs provide many informational and social benefits for health promotion and management. For example, by surveying bloggers who write about chronic pain and illness, Ressler and colleagues (2012) found that by providing opportunities to articulate illness narratives, blogs increased connection with others, decreased isolation, promoted social accountability, and created opportunities to help others and gain new insights. For example, cancer patients (Chung and Kim 2008) use blogs for emotion management, information sharing, and problem-solving on issues such as seeking alternative care options. More recently, video blogging has become popular. Patients with chronic illnesses, such as HIV, diabetes, and cancer, vlog to create rich and strong connections with viewers, engage in a form of self-therapy, and seek and provide social support (Liu et al. 2013; see also Hoff et al. 2008).

Computer-Mediated Communication Tools

The wide adoption and frequent, often daily, use of computer-mediated communication tools, such as e-mail, texting, and instant messaging, make them convenient and useful for delivering health-related information. For instance, by sending regular messages to consented or subscribed users, e-mail-based interventions have been shown to be effective in promoting physical activities and healthy diets (Franklin et al. 2006). Patients widely use computer-mediated communication to communicate with providers, family members, friends, and other patients. By offering fewer communication barriers and greater flexibility, computer-mediated communication can lead to higher satisfaction with communication, more sharing of psychosocial content, and better health outcomes than traditional communication channels such as the telephone (Lin et al. 2005). Disease-specific mailing lists are an important tool for patients with chronic diseases such as cancer or rare diseases such as primary biliary cirrhosis (Lasker et al. 2005). Patients can seek advice on treatment-related issues, receive validation and support from peers, learn about the experiences of others, receive suggestions on how to communicate with health care providers, obtain information for problem management, and learn to cope with disease recurrence. All computer-mediated communication is helpful for patients with limited mobility, communication difficulties, chronic diseases, and mental health problems (see e.g., Burke et al. 2010).

However, evidence is mixed about the efficacy of using computer-mediated technologies such as e-mail for the promotion of physical activity. For example, Wadsworth (2006) evaluated the efficacy of an e-mail intervention based on social cognitive theory to increase physical activity in college women. In this study, the intervention group received e-mails every week for 6 weeks and then every other week until 22 weeks. They also received access to an e-counselor and a Blackboard account. Meanwhile, the control group received paper information on starting an exercise program and information from their baseline physical activity measurements. Results indicated that the intervention increased behavioral skills and days of self-reported moderate physical activity at 6 weeks, but no difference for vigorous physical activity and no effects were found at 22 weeks. Similarly, a web-based physical activity intervention showed some effects at 6 weeks but no effects at 13 months (Wanner et al. 2009). Other programs have had similarly disappointing results (Kelders et al. 2011; Spittaels et al. 2007).

Other studies, however, show greater promise. Oenema and colleagues (2008) evaluated the short-term efficacy of an Internet-delivered, computer-tailored lifestyle intervention targeting saturated fat intake, physical activity, and smoking cessation, compared with a wait-list control. This intervention resulted in significantly lower self-reported saturated fat intake and a higher likelihood of meeting the physical activity guidelines among the respondents who were insufficiently active at baseline. Likewise, an evaluation of a 12-week intervention for sedentary patients recovering from breast cancer performed by Hatchett (2009) showed that receiving e-mails and being e-counseled increased days of self-reported moderate physical activity at 12 weeks and days of self-reported vigorous physical activity at 6 and 12 weeks. This intervention was based on social cognitive theory, suggesting that the content

of the associated materials is key to behavior change (see table 27.1).

Electronic Monitoring and Tracking Systems

Many technologies have been developed to measure and track physical activity, weight loss (Purpura et al. 2011), sleep (Kim et al. 2008), biometric data, disease management, and mental health (Bardram et al. 2012; Matthews et al. 2008). Computer-based monitoring and tracking tools often focus on improving self-management and adherence by providing timely feedback through enhanced records presentation and summarization. For example, visualization technology is often used to make the results easy to comprehend but sometimes also serves to motivate users through nudges such as progress made, goals, and social comparison. For example, *UbiFit Garden* (Consolvo et al. 2006) used a garden metaphor to help users visualize activity and complete goals. *Breakaway* (Jafarinaimi et al. 2005) used an ambient display on a computer screen—a sculpture slumping over time—responsive to deficits in physical activity.

Social sharing, typically in the form of light-hearted comments, accompanies many of the tracking and monitoring applications in the market. In many monitoring applications, users can choose to broadcast to their social network by reporting progress, initiating discussion, and seeking social support. For example, *BuddyClock* (Kim et al. 2008) tracked users' sleeping status and enabled users to share data with others with the objective of increasing health awareness and motivate healthy behavior. MAHI (Mobile Access to Health Information) was a mobile monitoring application that tracked food intake and also served as a social platform for users to share and discuss information with peers (Mamykina et al. 2008). Research has found that sharing such information promotes awareness and can increase motivation, adherence to plans, and reflection about health behavior (Maitland et al. 2006). Social sharing of tracked results may also provide incentives in the form of social support, feedback, positive reinforcement, and social pressure.

The degree to which monitoring systems have demonstrated effects on the promotion of physical activity seems less clear, however. On the positive side, Lubans and colleagues (2009) evaluated the effect of a school-based intervention incorporating pedometers and e-mail support on physical activity in adolescents and found that the intervention group increased step counts more than the control group. In contrast to this success, however, failures abound. For instance, Slootmaker and colleagues (2009) evaluated the feasibility and efficacy of a 3-month intervention in which Dutch office workers were provided with a personal activity monitor coupled to simple and concise web-based advice on physical activity. After 3 months, there were no significant effects on sedentary behavior or any physical activity outcome. Likewise, Cavallo (2013) tested the efficacy of a physical activity intervention that combined education, physical activity monitoring, and online social networking (Facebook) to increase social support for physical activity compared to an education-only control. Although participants experienced increases in social support and reported increased physical activity over time, no differences were noted across monitoring and control conditions. In a third illustrative failure, Robroek and colleagues (2012) evaluated the cost-effectiveness of a long-term workplace program promoting physical activity. The intervention included online action-oriented feedback, self-monitoring, a forum to ask questions, and monthly e-mail messages but did not differ from the standard program (physical health check with face-to-face advice and personal feedback on a website). Overall though, a meta-analysis of pedometer interventions (Kang et al. 2009) showed moderate increases in activity as a result of electronic monitoring. Therefore, more sophisticated tracking systems that can be built in with other components offer promise.

Search Engines

The most influential information systems are various search engines, notably web search engines like Google and Bing, which are used routinely by many people in the world every day. A major Internet search engine like Google processes more than 1 million queries daily and delivers content that can have significant influences on users and their health. According to a recent survey by the Pew Internet and American Life Project (Fox and Duggan 2013), 59% of U.S. adults have looked for health information online in the past year, primarily using search engines such as Google, Bing, and Yahoo. Moreover, a survey of health-information-seeking practices (Sillence et al. 2006) found that more than 73% of respondents used the World Wide Web for

health advice, support, or preparation for a medical appointment. Moreover, online contents influence people's decisions regarding whether to visit their general practitioner or a medical specialist (Baker et al. 2003; White and Horvitz 2009a; 2013).

A recent study involving a combination of web search log analysis and user studies showed that web searchers exhibit their own biases and are also subject to biases introduced by the search engine (White 2013). White studied search-related biases through multiple probes in the health domain, including an exploratory retrospective survey, human labeling of the captions results returned by a web search engine, and a large-scale log analysis of search behavior on that engine. Results revealed that users of web search engines tend to seek evidence to confirm a belief that they already held before searching, a clear form of congeniality bias (see Cappella et al. 2015; Hart et al. 2009; see table 27.1). Furthermore, most seekers of health information are searching for answers to questions, but search engines strongly favor a particular, usually affirmative, response irrespective of the truth. This bias is introduced when searchers click through on links that confirm information when they ask a question, a practice that induces propagation of both the positional bias (i.e., users tend to click on highly ranked results regardless of whether they are really relevant; Joachims et al. 2005; Pan et al. 2007) and the tendency to seek information that agrees with the initial belief that guided the question (another form of the congeniality bias).

Recommender Systems

Recommender systems (Ricci et al. 2011) can take different forms, including stand-alone platforms that e-mail recommendations to users and embedded systems (e.g., the advertising components in a web search engine) that push information through a search engine (i.e., contextual advertising; Broder et al. 2007). Regardless of its specific form, a recommender system generally attempts to infer a user's interests or information needs, matches users' interests with a set of recommendations, and chooses and delivers well-matched items. Relevant to the theme of this book is the recommendation of such products as exercise equipment or health information to promote physical activity. Recommender systems can also be used to suggest interventions and online materials that have the potential to change the user's physical activity patterns (see table 27.1).

CYBERCHONDRIA

Another bias introduced by search engines favors emotionally negative, anxiety-provoking information. Specifically, people are often overly concerned with serious diseases and thus click on fear-inducing items, leading to that information being featured more prominently online than in traditional media (White and Horvitz 2009b). The bias in search engine results in the medical domain leads to a phenomenon referred to as *cyberchondria*, the unfounded escalation of concerns about common symptomatology based on the review of search results and literature online. This bias further shows the great potential of a web search engine to influence users and, in particular, to influence people's sedentary behavior in a positive way. Search engines outside the Web operate in a similar way and also hold the potential to be leveraged to promote physical activity. The degree to which they can ignite behavior change, however, ultimately depends on the information and programs users find (see table 27.1).

In contrast to a search engine that responds to a user's request, a recommender system simply imposes the information on a user. As a result, in general terms, exposure to the recommended information may not be as effective as exposure when the user has taken the initiative to seek relevant information. However, if relevant and interesting to a user, a recommended item might be particularly influential because the information may not be what the user expected to find or even knew existed. A key technology barrier for recommender systems is ensuring that the recommended information is sufficiently interesting and novel to capture users' attention (see table 27.1). Many computational techniques can be leveraged to achieve this goal, notably information retrieval (Shen et al. 2005; Zhai 2008) and machine learning technologies (Liu 2009; Wang et al. 2013).

Although little research exists on how users respond to recommended online information, information recommended by a trusted friend may have more influence on a person than information directly recommended by a system. For example, Berger and Milkman (2010) have shown why some online content is more viral than others. Using a news data set, they examined how emotion shapes virality and found that positive content tends to be more viral than negative content and that information of both positive and negative valence (items evoking either awe or anger and anxiety) more frequently becomes viral than depressing information. These findings suggest that online social networks can be potentially leveraged to recommend selected positive content to users who need to change their sedentary behavior.

To facilitate behavior change, recommender systems can also work as a persuasive technology by pushing forward healthier and more beneficial information or choices to users (Felfernig et al. 2013). For instance, a substantial amount of research exists on the development of recommender systems that encourage healthier food choices (Mankoff et al. 2002; Lee et al. 2011; Wagner et al. 2011). Research has also started to explore activity recommender systems that can facilitate physical activity and lifestyle changes. For example, Hammer and colleagues (2010) proposed a recommender system to support diabetes patients' self-management by providing recommendations on food intake and exercise. In particular, Bielik and colleagues (2012) developed *Move2Play*, a system designed to make activity recommendations that also has tracking, evaluation, and gamification elements. Although most of these studies so far have focused on developing relevant recommendation algorithms, preliminary user evaluation has revealed positive user reception. Recommender systems can be hoped to ultimately increase exposure to physical activity programs, although the ultimate effects on attention and behavior change will be driven by the nature of the materials users access (see table 27.1).

Gamification Systems

Besides its use for entertainment, a game may deliver various benefits that depend on how the game is designed. This has led to the emergence of a new field called *gamification* (Deterding et al. 2011), which refers to the use of game thinking and game mechanics in nongame contexts with the objective of engaging users in problem-solving. The reported benefit of gamification systems for business corporations spans a wide spectrum, including improving employee training, attracting talent, and enhancing motivation, productivity, and innovation (Object Frontier 2013). Quite a few games have been created to promote well-being and physical fitness, such as *SuperBetter* (www.superbetter.com) and *Zombies, Run!* (www.zombiesrungame.com).

With the increasing adoption of smartphones, such games can become easily available in mobile contexts and ubiquitous. Moreover, compared with search engines and recommender systems, gamification systems have the significant advantage of going beyond exposing users to the desired content to further enable longer-term engagement of users. Many games use stories, fantasy, and visual and audio experience, to attract and maintain attention, create an immersive experience and engage users through interactivity, emotions, and persuasion (e.g., tailored messages, goal setting; Baranowski et al. 2008).

In terms of their content, gamification systems that focus on health behavior change include games promoting physical activity, diet intervention games, and educational games on health and disease management. Among games that promote physical activity, exergames are best received. These are typically video games that use players' energy expenditure from physical activity as input to drive the games, achieved by mapping the physical input into points or rewards in the virtual games (Orji et al. 2013). Many of these games use sensors to track users' movement, but some use biometric data such as heart rate (De Oliveira and Oliver 2008). Popular exergames include *Dance Dance Revolution* (DDR) and various video games played on *Nintendo Wii* and Xbox *Kinect*. Previous research has found that exergames contribute to fitness and weight loss (Biddiss and Irwin 2010; Staiano and Calvert 2011; Unnithan et al. 2006). In a meta-analysis, Peng and colleagues (2011) concluded that playing exergames leads to increases in heart rate, oxygen consumption, and energy expenditure comparable to light- to moderate-intensity physical activity. Exergames have also been reported to have psychosocial and cognitive benefits such as increased self-esteem, social interaction, motivation, attention, and visual-spatial skills (Gao and Mandryk 2012; Staiano and Calvert 2011). Encouraging sustained use is likely the challenge for these systems, so integrating them into daily life tasks may be the next item of the agenda.

Another category of virtual games focuses on promoting users' daily life activity. These rely on pedometer or mobile devices to track users' steps or movements and integrate gamification elements such as goal setting, rewarding, and reinforcement. Moreover, an emerging trend in these applications is to use social gameplay to elicit social facilitation, social comparison, normative influence, and social learning (Maitland and Chalmers 2011). For instance, *Fish 'n' Steps* (Lin et al. 2006) tracked users' physical activities and mapped them onto the activity of a virtual fish in a virtual tank. In a 14-week evaluation study, the game was found to act as a catalyst for promoting exercise beyond the trial period and improving game players' attitudes toward physical activity. *American Horsepower Challenge* is a web-based game that follows users' daily activity and translates activity amounts into points in a virtual race (Poole et al. 2011). A large-scale field trial with 61 schools found that the game significantly increased the number of steps in youth.

Diet-intervention games attempt to promote healthy eating behavior for weight control and improved health. Some focus on tracking and monitoring food intake, some provide just-in-time information or messages to remind users to make appropriate food decisions at the time of eating, and others educate users about healthy eating habits (Consolvo et al. 2006; Grimes et al. 2010; Orji et al. 2013). For instance, *OrderUP!* is a goal-based role-playing game in which the player (assuming the role of a waiter) recommends healthy food to customers (Grimes et al. 2010). *LunchTime* was a role-playing multiplayer game in which a group of users with specific health goals collaboratively chooses food from a restaurant menu (Orji et al. 2013). Past evaluations of these games has shown positive effects on learning, reflection, and attitude and behavior change (Consolvo et al. 2006; Grimes et al. 2010; Orji et al. 2013).

Video games may provide several advantages over didactic education and disease management, including vicariously practicing behavioral skills, facilitating complex problem-solving and contingency-based learning, and acquiring procedural knowledge in an interactive manner (Thomas et al. 1997). Previous studies have examined the effects of video games for stroke rehabilitation (Brown et al. 2009), physical therapy (Herndon et al. 2001), mental-health care (Wilkinson et al. 2008), pain management (Hoffman et al. 2001), and management for such conditions as diabetes, cystic fibrosis, cancer, and asthma (Bartholomew et al. 2006; Brown et al. 1997; Davis et al. 2004; Kato et al. 2008; Lin et al. 2005; Mamykina et al. 2008). The scientific evidence so far promises to link game use to effective disease management, medication adherence, self-efficacy, disease-related knowledge, and health service use. The ultimate efficacy, however, will be driven by efficacious contents informed on the science of behavior change (see table 27.1).

Summary

In this chapter, we use a psychological framework to systematically examine the potential effects of various technological systems, namely delivery systems such as websites, social networks, monitoring and tracking tools, search engines, recommender systems, and gamification systems. Our general conclusion is that all these forms offer opportunities to potentially influence people's beliefs, attitudes, and behaviors, but each requires different strategies (see table 27.1). Several important recommendations follow from the information reviewed in this chapter.

1. Social networks can potentially be leveraged to create a viral effect and ensure high exposure and attention, but the ultimate effect on exposure, attention, and behavior change depends on the degree to which the content influences those stages. More novel information will attract more attention and materials that successfully improve behavioral skills will likely reduce inactivity.

2. Search engines can be modified to encourage physical activity by promoting specific content at the top of search results, thus increasing exposure to efficacious content and demoting unhealthy messages. These innovations can decrease the negative effects and potentially increase the positive effects of the congeniality bias. For example, search items may be described as confirming the question of a user who seeks information that negates the need for physical activity even though the contents ultimately refute the user's belief.

3. Recommender system technologies can be exploited to automatically infer a user's need and adapt the recommended content or products to those needs. Such technologies, however, are likely to be most effective in combination with search engine results or embedded in a social network that increases the trustworthiness of the content relative to delivery from an explicit, stand-alone recommender system.

4. Gamification systems are among the most effective ways to influence people through online games or interactions or with a combination of online games and physical activities. Nevertheless, how to motivate people to play a game may be a challenge that requires creativity and ongoing updates to a constantly evolving game.

5. It is also desirable to combine multiple strategies whenever possible. For example, games recommended through a social network or through a search engine in the right search context are more likely to be adopted.

In closing, the efficacy of emerging communication systems depends on the availability of intelligent information processing technologies developed in the computer science field, particularly in relation to information retrieval, data mining, human–computer interaction, and machine learning. Fortunately, all these areas have made significant progress in the last two decades, and many useful technologies are available for intelligently modeling and inferring a user's interests and preferences, analyzing and understanding online contents, and recommending information in a context-sensitive and personalized way. These technologies are now available to maximize the efficacy of behavioral interventions for curbing physical inactivity and its associated health risks.

KEY CONCEPTS

▸ **Accuracy motivation:** The desire or goal to hold accurate information and reach factually correct conclusions.

▸ **Behavior change**: Modification of the intensity and duration of a behavior performed at an earlier (arbitrary) time.

▸ **Defense motivation:** The desire to approach and disseminate information that is consistent with prior beliefs and thus feels personally validating or reassuring.

▸ **Electronic intervention delivery:** Websites to deliver interventions previously delivered in person or on the phone.

▸ **Electronic monitoring and tracking systems:** Technologies to measure and track physical activity, weight loss (Purpura et al. 2011), sleep (Kim et al. 2008), biometric data, disease management, and mental health (Bardram et al. 2012; Matthews et al. 2008).

▸ **Gamification systems:** In this context, a game designed to deliver health and fitness benefits.

▸ **Recommender systems:** Include stand-alone platforms that e-mail recommendations to users and embedded systems that push information through a search engine. These systems attempt to infer a user's interests or information needs, match users' interests with a set of recommendations, and choose and deliver well-matched items.

▸ **Search engines:** Web search engines like Google and Bing are used routinely by many people in the world every day.

▸ **Selective exposure and dissemination:** These terms refer to biases in attention, selection, and dissemination of information on the basis of defense, accuracy, and social motives.

▸ **Social motivation:** The desire to create and maintain positive relationships with other people.

▸ **Social network information delivery systems:** Systems to develop information to networks, including Twitter, Facebook, specialized online communities, blogs and vlogs, and computer-mediated communication such as e-mail or text messaging.

STUDY QUESTIONS

1. How do the defense, accuracy, and social motives influence exposure to information in emerging systems?
2. Is the influence of each motive likely to be different across different platforms?
3. How are characteristics of a population likely to determine which system would you use to reduce physical inactivity?

Epilogue: Where to Go From Here?

The fast-growing body of evidence on sedentary behavior and health is a rapidly emerging element of the chronic disease prevention agenda. There are also many potential implications for well-being, workplace practice and policy, and other social, community, and environmental concerns. The fact that humans now spend so much of their time sitting is a consequence of technological, economic, and social changes. Now sedentary behavior must be part of the broader debate about the determinants of human health, quality of urban life and work, and the design of the broader environment.

Here in the Epilogue, the editors provide selected overall conclusions about the state of this new field and identify some of the most promising research strategies and future directions. In doing so, we borrow from several of our key chapters, further emphasizing specific perspectives of broad relevance. This material provides excellent pointers for guiding the development of research, as well as practical and policy implications for the field of sedentary behavior and health.

A Broadly Informed Perspective

Addressing sedentary behavior and dealing with the implications of new research evidence in the broader public, political, and policy domains will require nuanced and informed perspectives. Considering, for example, the historical role and social functions of the chair (as we are invited to do so engagingly by Galen Cranz in chapter 4), identifying the roles of screen-based behaviors in the lives of children (chapter 5), and having an informed sense of the fundamental role of gravity and historical roots in space science (chapter 2) provide contextual sophistication and a depth and breadth of perspective to guide future research on sedentary behavior and health, research translation, and practical and policy applications.

The first three chapters in part I place a strong emphasis on the causal logic of experimental research. Observational studies, both cross-sec-

tional and prospective, have opened up the field of sedentary behavior and health research, generated influential hypotheses, and provided strong guidance to subsequent experimental investigations. Hopefully, the sedentary behavior and health research field will further develop through strong and explicit cross talk between observational and experimental evidence. Both of these types of evidence are important. Observational study evidence greatly assists in understanding the relevance and potential applicability of experimental evidence. Experimental evidence provides rigorous investigative tools through which the hypotheses generated by observational studies may be tested.

In Chapters 4 and 5, the main environmental drivers of sedentary behavior—the chair and the screen—are addressed. Chapter 6 deals with regulation. The thoughtful reader will identify our biases in how we have selected contributors and developed the overall shape of the book. These final three chapters of part I reflect, each to a greater or lesser extent, a theme that runs through much of the material covered in the chapters that make up part V: What can be done to change sedentary behavior? In that section, the balance of emphasis is on behavioral settings: how can the environmental contexts of sedentary behavior be reshaped in order to reduce sitting time and increase physical activity? Those chapters, nevertheless, acknowledge the importance of individual choice, volitional initiative, and motivation. Environmental change is the central concern, but environments include, and are shaped by, people—individually and collectively.

Complementary Relationships of Experimental and Observational Studies

As the chapters in parts I and II of the book make clear, there is the particular need to better understand the biological and behavioral mechanisms by which sedentary behavior affects health outcomes and to identify dose–response relationships for sedentary behavior and health. For example:

▶ How much sitting is too much?

▶ How often should sitting time be broken up to reduce adverse health effects?

▶ If someone sits for the majority of the day, how much exercise or physical activity might be needed to provide protective benefit?

These and other questions can be addressed through carefully controlled laboratory research (as illustrated in chapter 3) and through epidemiologic observational studies (as illustrated particularly in chapters 7, 8, 9, and 10). Both types of investigative logic are crucial for the development of the field. Here, there is the need to better understand the relationship of sedentary behavior and physical activity as they exert their distinct and interrelated influences to determine health outcomes.

As Archer and colleagues explain in chapter 9, strong evidence on health outcomes needs to be followed through with real-world initiatives. If, for example, further reductions in CVD mortality and morbidity are to be realized, then increasing the proportion of the population that is active and reducing sedentary behaviors must be a primary goal. Although there is compelling evidence of the efficacy and effectiveness of behavioral interventions for reducing the burden of CVD in both primary and secondary prevention contexts, the translation of empirically supported interventions into practice has been limited and only a small fraction of clinically effective interventions has been adopted. Archer and colleagues make a strong case that, although research is still needed before empirically based guidelines can be widely promulgated, basic recommendations of limiting time spent in sedentary behavior are well justified in relation to both children and adults.

Other areas of sedentary behavior research that are less well developed can provide useful lessons. As Boscolo and Zhu make clear in chapter 11, there is still a need to clarify the existence of the causal relationship between lower back pain and sedentary behavior. They make the case that, for lower back pain, the current epidemiological evidence is insufficiently strong to support that a causal relationship is likely to exist. For the field of lower back pain research and indeed for other fields where sedentary behavior may be important but not yet well understood, the need exists for developing relevant problem-specific research tools. As is the case for lower back pain research, the research strategies and measurement techniques need to be developed and their methodological quality needs to be refined.

Future studies on the range of potential health problems that may be influenced by sedentary behavior will be particularly informative over the next several years. In conducting epidemiological analyses on differential health risks and the potential independent influences of sedentary behavior on health outcomes, highly informative bodies of evidence are likely to emerge:

▶ How will the consequences of sedentary behavior for particular health outcomes be influenced by different levels of moderate- to vigorous-intensity physical activity?

▶ How might sedentary behavior exert its effects on different health problems for different age groups in the context of ubiquitous dietary exposures, including widely available sugary drinks?

▶ What will future estimates of the overall burden of disease attributable to sedentary behavior tell us about its importance relative to other health risk exposures?

High-Quality Research Designs, Measurements, and Analysis

Part III of the book highlights matters of particular importance for a new field like sedentary behavior research. High-quality measures, strong evidence, and good evaluations of practical initiatives are needed if the field is to progress in science and in practice. Chapters 14, 15, and 16 highlight the enormous potential of new measurement technologies, while chapters 13 and 17 provide some solid and sober reminders of the importance of well-established measurement methodologies and established and newly emerging analytic capacities. Measures of sedentary behavior of relevance to the overall evidence spectrum are needed for clinical studies, intervention trials, large-scale observational studies, and systematic evaluations of practical programs and of the regulatory and policy initiatives that we are likely to see emerging in workplaces over the next several years. It is particularly important to employ high-quality measurement approaches in population-based studies, as is illustrated by chapters 13 and 14. In this context, there is the need for variations in sedentary behavior within and between populations to be identified and for trends over time to be characterized accurately.

Chapter 10 nicely illustrates how applications of advanced statistical theory and methods have greatly improved the capacity for causal inference from observational data in cancer research. In chapter 10, Lynch and Friedenreich identify opportunities for future research using complex modeling strategies such as marginal structural models or structural nested models to estimate causal effects. These approaches will help to account for variation in sedentary behavior over time as well as time-varying confounding and mediation.

Methodological Research Issues That Arise Across the Life Span

The issues raised by Welk and Kim in chapter 18 not only highlight research priorities in understanding and influencing sedentary behavior in children and youth; They also raise several key issues that are of broader importance for all age groups and life stages:

▶ *Improve measures of sedentary behavior.* Self-report instruments specific for assessment of those at different life stages need to be developed and validated. More-refined measurement error modeling should be developed to correct for measurement errors inherent in various types of self-report instruments. Accelerometer-derived measures may preclude comparing estimates of sedentary time across studies due to the application of different cut-point values.

▶ *Conduct detailed time-use studies.* Studies capitalizing on time-use surveys are needed for better understanding how adults and youth allocate and accumulate sedentary time over a day (e.g., discretionary vs. nondiscretionary, active gaming vs. inactive gaming, single-tasking vs. multitasking at work).

▶ *Emphasize a wide range of types of sedentary behavior.* Previous studies on youth and adult sedentary behavior have focused primarily on screen-based activities or have used a single behavioral indicator. Broader approaches with multiple sedentary behavior indicators are needed.

▶ *Run longitudinal studies of the tracking of sedentary behavior from childhood to adulthood.* Many sedentary behavior studies have been cross-sectional or longitudinal studies conducted only during childhood or adult life. Therefore, longitudinal studies are needed that investigate how patterns, correlates, and health effects observed during childhood would carry over into future adult life stages.

▶ *Examine effects of sedentary behavior on cognition.* A number of studies have linked physical activity and fitness with indicators of academic achievement and several aspects of cognitive function, but fewer studies have examined the potential negative effects of sedentary behavior. It is possible that sustained sedentary behavior may negatively affect cognition in children and adults.

Focus on Racial/Ethnic Minority Subgroups

In chapter 21, Whitt-Glover and Ceaser point out that physical activity research has primarily focused on getting people up and moving; however, over time, efforts to increase leisure-time physical activity have produced only small changes at the population level but almost no change in racial/ethnic minority groups. This suggests that efforts to increase the proportion of people who choose deliberately to engage in physical activity during their leisure time may be ineffective, particularly among segments of the community with low internal motivation to engage in physical activity.

As an alternative strategy with broader potential for inclusiveness, there has been a call for active-by-default strategies to decrease sedentary behavior and increase physical activity. Such strategies make the healthy choice the easy choice by incorporating physical activity into organizational practices through such efforts as group calisthenics, walking meetings, restricting close parking to people who need it, and physical activity breaks during meetings, throughout the workday, or in the classroom. Most active-by-default strategies have been incorporated with children in school settings; however, a few examples such as Instant Recess have been used in adults in workplace settings and have been successful at breaking up long bouts of sitting.

Viable Behavioral Change

Changing sedentary behavior, as the chapters in part V make clear, presents many new challenges. In order to change behavior, it is important to change the determinants of behavior. Much remains to be understood about the personal, social, and environmental determinants of sedentary behavior, particularly since these different levels of determinate factors may be used in behavioral-change programs and other initiatives. Interventions for influencing sedentary behavior on a large scale will require initiatives at multiple levels. Translational formative research and policy-relevant studies are needed for examining the feasibility of scaling-up sedentary behavior interventions in multiple contexts.

In chapter 23, Carlson and Sallis describe research on environment and policy interventions for reducing sedentary behaviors and give specific recommendations, including the following:

▶ A systematic process for identifying the most promising environment and policy interventions could include expert consensus meetings, qualitative and quantitative assessment of perceptions of people from high-risk groups, and polling about feasibility and barriers to interventions. We suggest engaging political scientists and market researchers in these studies.

▶ Suggested criteria for selecting environment and policy interventions for further development should target the most prevalent sedentary behaviors, reach populations at high risk for chronic diseases, have promising political and popular feasibility, likely have favorable cost-effectiveness ratios, and provide dual benefits of reducing sitting time and increasing physical activity.

▶ Multilevel, cost-effective interventions that combine environment and policy changes with individual or social interventions.

Pronk outlines several practice-based recommendations for the workplace context in chapter 24, including the use of multilevel frameworks, the guidance of behavior-change interventions by available evidence of effectiveness, the integration into a comprehensive programmatic solution (ensuring that the initiative is being measured and evaluated), the connection to community resources, and the testing of policy-level approaches while safeguarding personal data and information. In addition, Pronk emphasizes including diverse populations to address health equity and disparities (as is highlighted by Whitt-Glover and Ceaser in chapter 21) and evaluating the economic and financial effects of workplace initiatives. He identifies challenges that remain where additional research will be an important factor in the successful application of practice-based solutions, including the following:

▶ Real-world practice-based trials to identify effective interventions using (experimental) study designs with high external validity

▶ Studies that test creative solutions and innovations designed to effectively and efficiently reduce sedentary behavior in the workplace

▶ Practice-based trials that optimize the workplace context and recognize this setting as a complex adaptive system

▶ Single- and multilevel studies that allow the identification of best choices for intervention

▶ Studies that inform us about the relative influence of reducing sedentary behavior on cost reduction, productivity improvement, and financial return on investment

We hope that you, the reader, have enjoyed and gained new insights from the 27 chapters of *Sedentary Behavior and Health*, each written by experts in their fields, and that you will now feel well informed and well prepared to engage with too much sitting as a significant agenda for research, practical action, and public policy debate into the future.

REFERENCES

Chapter 1

Alkhajah, T., M. Reeves, E. Eakin, E. Winkler, N. Owen, and G. Healy. 2012. Reducing sitting time in office workers: Efficacy and acceptability of sit-stand workstations. *American Journal of Preventive Medicine* 43:298-303.

Anuradha, S., D.W. Dunstan, G.N. Healy, J.E. Shaw, P.Z. Zimmet, T.Y. Wong, and N. Owen. 2011. Physical activity, television viewing time, and retinal vascular caliber. *Medicine & Science in Sports & Exercise* 43:280-286.

Barker, R.G., ed. 1968. *Ecological psychology*. Stanford, CA: Stanford University Press.

Bauman, A., B.E. Ainsworth, J.F. Sallis, M. Hagstromer, C.L. Craig, F.C. Bull, M. Pratt, et al. 2011. The descriptive epidemiology of sitting. A 20-country comparison using the International Physical Activity Questionnaire (IPAQ). *American Journal of Preventive Medicine* 41:228-235.

Bauman, A., J. Sallis, D. Dzewaltowski, and N. Owen. 2002. Toward a better understanding of the influences on physical activity: The role of determinants, correlates, causal variables, mediators, moderators, and confounders. *American Journal of Preventive Medicine* 23:5-14.

Brown, W.J., A.E. Bauman, and N. Owen. 2009. Stand up, sit down, keep moving: Turning circles in physical activity research? *British Journal of Sports Medicine* 43:86-88.

Centers for Disease Control and Prevention (CDC), National Center for Health Statistics (NCHS). 2011. *National Health and Nutrition Examination Survey Data*. Hyattsville, MD: Authors.

Chau, J.Y., H.P. Van Der Ploeg, S. Dunn, J. Kurko, and A.E. Bauman. 2011. A tool for measuring workers' sitting time by domain: The Workforce Sitting Questionnaire. *British Journal of Sports Medicine* 45:1216-1222.

———. 2012. Validity of the occupational sitting and physical activity questionnaire. *Medicine & Science in Sports & Exercise* 44:118-125.

Clark, B.K., G.N. Healy, E.A. Winkler, P.A. Gardiner, T. Sugiyama, D.W. Dunstan, C.E. Matthews, and N. Owen. 2011. Relationship of television time with accelerometer-derived sedentary time: NHANES. *Medicine & Science in Sports & Exercise* 43:822-888.

Clark, B.K., T. Sugiyama, G.N. Healy, J. Salmon, D.W. Dunstan, and N. Owen. 2009. Validity and reliability of measures of television viewing time and other non-occupational sedentary behaviour of adults: A review. *Obesity Reviews* 10:7-16.

Clark, B.K., A. Thorp, E. Winkler, P.A. Gardiner, G.N. Healy, N. Owen, and D.W. Dunstan. 2011. Validity of self-report measures of workplace sitting time and breaks in sitting time. *Medicine & Science in Sports & Exercise* 43:1907-1912.

Davies, S., H. Burns, T. Jewell, and M. Mcbride. 2011. *Start active, stay active: A report on physical activity from the four home countries*. London: UK Department of Health Chief Medical Officers.

Ding, D., T. Sugiyama, and N. Owen. 2012. Habitual active transport, TV viewing and weight gain: A four year follow-up study. *Preventive Medicine* 54:201-204.

Ding, D., T. Sugiyama, E. Winkler, E. Cerin, K. Wijndaele, and N. Owen. 2012. Correlates of change in adults' television viewing time: A four-year follow-up study. *Medicine & Science in Sports & Exercise* 44:1287-1292.

Dunstan, D.W., E.L. Barr, G.N. Healy, J. Salmon, J.E. Shaw, B. Balkau, D.J. Magliano, A.J. Cameron, P.Z. Zimmet, and N. Owen. 2010. Television viewing time and mortality: The Australian Diabetes, Obesity and Lifestyle Study (AusDiab). *Circulation* 121:384-391.

Dunstan, D.W., B. Howard, G.N. Healy, and N. Owen. 2012. Too much sitting—A health hazard. *Diabetes Research & Clinical Practice* 97:368-376.

Dunstan, D.W., B.A. Kingwell, R. Larsen, G.N. Healy, E. Cerin, M.T. Hamilton, J.E. Shaw, et al. 2012. Breaking up prolonged sitting reduces postprandial glucose and insulin responses. *Diabetes Care* 35:976-983.

Dunstan, D.W., J. Salmon, G.N. Healy, J.E. Shaw, D. Jolley, P.Z. Zimmet, and N. Owen. 2007. Association of television viewing with fasting and 2-h postchallenge plasma glucose levels in adults without diagnosed diabetes. *Diabetes Care* 30:516-522.

Dunstan, D.W., J. Salmon, N. Owen, T. Armstrong, P.Z. Zimmet, T.A. Welborn, A.J. Cameron, T. Dwyer, D. Jolley, and J.E. Shaw. 2004. Physical activity and television viewing in relation to risk of undiagnosed abnormal glucose metabolism in adults. *Diabetes Care* 27:2603-2609.

———. 2005. Associations of TV viewing and physical activity with the metabolic syndrome in Australian adults. *Diabetologia* 48:2254-2261.

Epstein, L.H. 1998. Integrating theoretical approaches to promote physical activity. *American Journal of Preventive Medicine* 15:257-265.

Epstein, L.H., J.A. Smith, L.S. Vara, and J.S. Rodefer. 1991. Behavioral economic analysis of activity choice in obese children. *Health Psychology* 10:311-316.

Garber, C.E., B. Blissmer, M.R. Deschenes, B.A. Franklin, M.J. Lamonte, I.M. Lee, D.C. Nieman, and D.P. Swain. 2011. American College of Sports Medicine position stand. Quantity and quality of exercise for developing and maintaining cardiorespiratory, musculoskeletal, and neuromotor fitness in apparently healthy adults: Guidance for prescribing exercise. *Medicine & Science in Sports & Exercise* 43:1334-1359.

Gardiner, P.A., B.K. Clark, G.N. Healy, E.G. Eakin, E.A. Winkler, and N. Owen. 2011. Measuring older adults' sedentary time: Reliability, validity, and responsiveness. *Medicine & Science in Sports & Exercise* 43:2127-2133.

Gardiner, P.A., E.G. Eakin, G.N. Healy, and N. Owen. 2011. Feasibility of reducing older adults' sedentary time. *American Journal of Preventive Medicine* 41: 174-177.

Hamilton, M.T., G.N. Healy, D.W. Dunstan, T.W. Zderic, and N. Owen. 2008. Too little exercise and too much sitting: Inactivity physiology and the need for new recommendations on sedentary behaviour. *Current Cardiovascular Risk Reports* 2:292-298.

Hamilton, M.T., and N. Owen. 2012. Sedentary behavior and inactivity physiology. In *Physical activity and health* (2nd ed.), edited by C. Bouchard, S.N. Blair, and W.L. Haskell, 53-70. Champaign, IL: Human Kinetics.

Healy, G.N., B.K. Clark, E.A. Winkler, P.A. Gardiner, W.J. Brown, and C.E. Matthews. 2011. Measurement of adults' sedentary time in population-based studies. *American Journal of Preventive Medicine* 41:216-227.

Healy, G.N., D.W. Dunstan, J. Salmon, E. Cerin, J.E. Shaw, P.Z. Zimmet, and N. Owen. 2008. Breaks in sedentary time: Beneficial associations with metabolic risk. *Diabetes Care* 31:661-666.

Healy, G.N., E.G. Eakin, A.D. Lamontagne, N. Owen, E.A. Winkler, G. Wiesner, L. Gunning, et al. 2013. Reducing sitting time in office workers: Short-term efficacy of a multicomponent intervention. *Preventive Medicine* 57:43-48.

Healy, G.N., C.E. Matthews, D.W. Dunstan, E.A. Winkler, and N. Owen. 2011. Sedentary time and cardio-metabolic biomarkers in US adults: NHANES 2003-06. *European Heart Journal* 32:590-597.

Healy, G.N., K. Wijndaele, D.W. Dunstan, J.E. Shaw, J. Salmon, P.Z. Zimmet, and N. Owen. 2008. Objectively measured sedentary time, physical activity, and metabolic risk: The Australian Diabetes, Obesity and Lifestyle Study (AusDiab). *Diabetes Care* 31:369-371.

Howard, B.J., S.F. Fraser, P. Sethi, E. Cerin, M.T. Hamilton, N. Owen, D.W. Dunstan, and B.A. Kingwell. 2013. Impact on hemostatic parameters of interrupting sitting with intermittent activity. *Medicine & Science in Sports & Exercise* 45:1285-1291.

Koohsari, M.J., T. Sugiyama, S. Sahlqvist, S. Mavoa., N. Hadgraft, and N. Owen. 2015. Neighborhood environmental attributes and adults' sedentary behaviors: Review and research agenda. *Preventive Medicine* 77:141-149.

Kozo, J., J. Sallis, T. Conway, J. Kerr, K. Cain, B. Saelens, L. Frank, and N. Owen. 2012. Sedentary behaviors of adults in relation to neighborhood walkability and income. *Health Psychology* 31:704-713.

Lakerveld, J., D. Dunstan, S. Bot, J. Salmon, J. Dekker, G. Nijpels, and N. Owen. 2011. Abdominal obesity, TV-viewing time and prospective declines in physical activity. *Preventive Medicine* 53:299-302.

Lappalainen, R., and L.H. Epstein. 1990. A behavioral economics analysis of food choice in humans. *Appetite* 14:81-93.

Latouche, C., J.B. Jowett, A.L. Carey, D.A. Bertovic, N. Owen, D.W. Dunstan, and B.A. Kingwell. 2013. Effects of breaking up prolonged sitting on skeletal muscle gene expression. *Journal of Applied Physiology* 114:453-460.

Lynch, B.M., D.W. Dunstan, G.N. Healy, E. Winkler, E. Eakin, and N. Owen. 2010. Objectively measured physical activity and sedentary time of breast cancer survivors, and associations with adiposity: Findings from NHANES (2003-2006). *Cancer Causes and Control* 21:283-288.

Lynch, B.M., D.W. Dunstan, E. Winkler, G.N. Healy, E. Eakin, and N. Owen. 2011. Objectively assessed physical activity, sedentary time and waist circumference among prostate cancer survivors: Findings from the National Health and Nutrition Examination Survey (2003-2006). *European Journal of Cancer Care* 20:514-519.

Lynch, B.M., C.M. Friedenreich, E.A. Winkler, G.N. Healy, J.K. Vallance, E.G. Eakin, and N. Owen. 2011. Associations of objectively assessed physical activity and sedentary time with biomarkers of breast cancer risk in postmenopausal women: Findings from NHANES (2003-2006). *Breast Cancer Research & Treatment* 130:183-194.

Marshall, A.L., Y.D. Miller, N.W. Burton, and W.J. Brown. 2010. Measuring total and domain-specific sitting: A study of reliability and validity. *Medicine & Science in Sports & Exercise* 42:1094-1102.

Matthews, C.E., S.M. George, S.C. Moore, H.R. Bowles, A. Blair, Y. Park, R.P. Troiano, A. Hollenbeck, and A. Schatzkin. 2012. Amount of time spent in sedentary behaviors and cause-specific mortality in US adults. *American Journal of Clinical Nutrition* 95:437-445.

Morris, J.N., J.A. Heady, P.A. Raffle, C.G. Roberts, and J.W. Parks. 1953. Coronary heart-disease and physical activity of work. *Lancet* 265:1111-1120.

Neuhaus, M., G. Healy, D. Dunstan, N. Owen, and E. Eakin. 2014. Workplace sitting and height-adjustable workstations: A randomized controlled trial. *American Journal of Preventive Medicine* 46(1):30-40.

Oliver, M., G.M. Schofield, H.M. Badland, and J. Shepherd. 2010. Utility of accelerometer thresholds for classifying sitting in office workers. *Preventive Medicine* 51:357-360.

Owen, N. 2012. Ambulatory monitoring and sedentary behaviour: A population-health perspective. *Physiological Measurement* 33:1801-1810.

Owen, N., and A. Bauman. 1992. The descriptive epidemiology of a sedentary lifestyle in adult Australians. *International Journal of Epidemiology* 21:305-310.

Owen, N., G.N. Healy, C.E. Matthews, and D.W. Dunstan. 2010. Too much sitting: The population health science of sedentary behavior. *Exercise & Sport Science Reviews* 38:105-113.

Owen, N., E. Leslie, J. Salmon, and M.J. Fotheringham. 2000. Environmental determinants of physical activity and sedentary behavior. *Exercise & Sport Science Reviews* 28:153-158.

Owen, N., P.B. Sparling, G.N. Healy, D.W. Dunstan, and C.E. Matthews. 2010. Sedentary behavior: Emerging evidence for a new health risk. *Mayo Clinic Proceedings* 85:1138-1141.

Owen, N., T. Sugiyama, E.G. Eakin, P.A. Gardiner, M.S. Tremblay, and J.F. Sallis. 2011. Adults' sedentary behavior determinants and interventions. *American Journal of Preventive Medicine* 41:189-196.

Paffenbarger, R.S., Jr., I.M. Lee, and J.B. Kampert. 1997. Physical activity in the prevention of non-insulin-dependent diabetes mellitus. *World Review of Nutrition and Dietetics* 82:210-218.

Pate, R.R., J.R. O'Neill, and F. Lobelo. 2008. The evolving definition of "sedentary". *Exercise & Sport Science Reviews* 36:173-178.

Rachlin, H., J.H. Kagel, and R.C. Battalio. 1980. Substitutability in time allocation. *Pyschological Review* 87: 355-374.

Reeves, M., G. Healy, N. Owen, J. Shaw, P.Z. Zimmet, and D.W. Dunstan. 2013. Joint associations of poor diet quality and prolonged television viewing time with abnormal glucose metabolism in Australian men and women. *Preventive Medicine* 57(5):471-476.

Sallis, J., and N. Owen. eds. 1999. *Physical activity and behavioral medicine.* Thousand Oaks, CA: Sage.

———. 2015. Ecological models of health behavior. In *Health behavior theory research and practice* (5th ed.), edited by K. Glanz, B.K. Rimer, and K. Viswanath, 43-64. San Francisco: Jossey-Bass.

Sallis, J.F., N. Owen, and E.B. Fisher. 2008. Ecological models of health behavior. In *Health behavior and health education: Theory, research, and practice* (4th ed.), edited by K. Glanz, B. Rimer, and K. Viswanath, 465-486. San Francisco: John Wiley & Sons.

Sallis, J.F., N. Owen, and M.J. Fotheringham. 2000. Behavioral epidemiology: A systematic framework to classify phases of research on health promotion and disease prevention. *Annals of Behavioral Medicine* 22:294-298.

Salmon, J., N. Owen, D. Crawford, A. Bauman, and J.F. Sallis. 2003. Physical activity and sedentary behavior: A population-based study of barriers, enjoyment, and preference. *Health Psychology* 22:178-188.

Salmon, J., M.S. Tremblay, S.J. Marshall, and C. Hume. 2011. Health risks, correlates, and interventions to reduce sedentary behavior in young people. *American Journal of Preventive Medicine* 41:197-206.

Sedentary Behaviour Research Network. 2012. Letter to the editor: Standardized use of the terms "sedentary" and "sedentary behaviours". *Applied Physiology Nutrition and Metabolism* 37:540-542.

Sugiyama, T., G.N. Healy, D.W. Dunstan, J. Salmon, and N. Owen. 2008. Is television viewing time a marker of a broader pattern of sedentary behavior? *Annals of Behavioral Medicine* 35:245-250.

Thorp, A.A., G.N. Healy, N. Owen, J. Salmon, K. Ball, J.E. Shaw, P.Z. Zimmet, and D.W. Dunstan. 2010. Deleterious associations of sitting time and television viewing time with cardiometabolic risk biomarkers: Australian Diabetes, Obesity and Lifestyle (AusDiab) study 2004-2005. *Diabetes Care* 33:327-334.

Thorp, A.A., S.A. McNaughton, N. Owen, and D.W. Dunstan. 2013. Independent and joint associations of TV viewing time and snack food consumption with the metabolic syndrome and its components; a cross-sectional study in Australian adults. *International Journal of Behavioral Nutrition and Physical Activity* 10:96.

Thorp, A.A., N. Owen, M. Neuhaus, and D.W. Dunstan. 2011. Sedentary behaviors and subsequent health outcomes in adults: A systematic review of longitudinal studies, 1996-2011. *American Journal of Preventive Medicine* 41:207-215.

Troiano, R.P., K. Pettee Gabriel, G. Welk, N. Owen, and B. Sternfeld. 2012. Reported physical activity and sedentary behavior: Why do you ask? *Journal of Physical Activity and Health* 9(Suppl. 1): S68-S75.

Trost, S.G., N. Owen, A.E. Bauman, J.F. Sallis, and W. Brown. 2002. Correlates of adults' participation in physical activity: Review and update. *Medicine & Science in Sports & Exercise* 34:1996-2001.

Vallance, J.K., E.A.Winkler, P.A. Gardiner, G.N. Healy, B.M. Lynch, and N. Owen. 2011. Associations of objectively-assessed physical activity and sedentary time with depression: NHANES (2005-2006). *Preventive Medicine* 53:284-288.

Van Der Ploeg, H.P., T. Chey, R.J. Korda, E. Banks, and A. Bauman. 2012. Sitting time and all-cause mortality risk in 222 497 Australian adults. *Archives of Internal Medicine* 172:494-500.

Van Dyck, D., G. Cardon, B. Deforche, N. Owen, K. De Cocker, K. Wijndaele, and I. De Bourdeaudhuij. 2011. Socio-demographic, psychosocial and home-environmental attributes associated with adults' domestic screen time. *BMC Public Health* 11:668.

Van Dyck, D., G. Cardon, B. Deforche, N. Owen, J.F. Sallis, and I. De Bourdeaudhuij. 2010. Neighborhood walkability and sedentary time in Belgian adults. *American Journal of Preventive Medicine* 39:25-32.

Veerman, J.L., G.N. Healy, L.J. Cobiac, T. Vos, E.A. Winkler, N. Owen, and D.W. Dunstan. 2012. Television viewing time and reduced life expectancy: A life table analysis. *British Journal of Sports Medicine* 46:927-930.

Vernikos, J. 2004. *The G-connection: Harness gravity and reverse aging.* Lincoln, NE: iUniverse.

———. 2011. *Sitting kills, moving heals: How simple everyday movement will prevent pain illness and early death—and exercise alone won't.* Fresno, CA: Quill Driver Books.

Wicker, A.W., ed. 1979. *An introduction to ecological psychology.* Monterey, CA: Brooks/Cole.

Wijndaele, K., G.N. Healy, D.W. Dunstan, A.G. Barnett, J. Salmon, J.E. Shaw, P.Z. Zimmet, and N. Owen. 2010. Increased cardiometabolic risk is associated with increased TV viewing time. *Medicine & Science in Sports & Exercise* 42:1511-1518.

Winkler, E.A., P.A. Gardiner, B.K. Clark, C.E. Matthews, N. Owen, and G.N. Healy. 2011. Identifying sedentary time using automated estimates of accelerometer wear time. *British Journal of Sports Medicine* 46:436-442.

Chapter 2

Alkner, B.A., and P.A. Tesch. 2004a. Efficacy of a gravity independent resistance exercise device as a countermeasure to muscle atrophy during 29-day bed rest. *Acta Physiologica Scandinavica* 181:345-357.

———. 2004b. Knee extensor and plantar flexor muscle size and function following 90 days of head down bed rest with or without resistance exercise. *European Journal of Applied Physiology* 93:294-305.

Asher, R.A. 1947. The dangers of going to bed. *British Medical Journal* 2:967-968.

Bacabac, R.G., T.H. Smit, J.J. Van Loon, B.Z. Doulabi, M. Helder, and J. Klein-Nulend. 2006. Bone cell responses to high frequency vibration stress: Does the nucleus oscillate within the cytoplasm? *The FASEB Journal* 20(7):858-864.

Bacabac, R.G., T.H. Smit, M.G. Mulender, S.J. Dicks, J.J. Van Loon, and J. Klein-Nulend. 2004. Nitric oxide production by bone cells is fluid shear stress rate dependent. *Biochemical Biophysical Research Communications* 315(4):825-829.

Bergouignan, A., F. Rudwill, C. Simon, and S. Blanc. 2011. Physical inactivity as the culprit of metabolic inflexibility: Evidence from bed-rest studies. *Journal of Applied Physiology* 111:1201-1210.

Bey, L., and M.T. Hamilton. 2003. Suppression of skeletal muscle lipoprotein lipase activity during physical inactivity: A molecular reason to maintain daily low intensity activity. *Journal of Physiology* 551(2):673-682.

Biolo, G., B. Clocchi, M. Lebenstedt, R. Barazzoni, M. Zanetti, P. Platen, M. Heer, and G. Guarnieri. 2004. Short-term bed rest impairs amino-acid-induced protein anabolism in humans. *Journal of Physiology* 558:381-388.

Browse, N.L. 1965. *The physiology and pathology of bed rest.* Springfield, IL: Charles C. Thomas.

Convertino, V.A., D.F. Doerr, D.I. Eckberg, J.M. Fritsch, and J. Vernikos-Danellis. 1990. Head-down bedrest impairs vagal baroreflex responses and provokes orthostatic hypotension. *Journal of Applied Physiology* 68:1458-1464.

Convertino, V.A., W.C. Adams, J.D. Shea, C.A. Thompson, and G.W. Hoffler. 1991. Impairment of the carotid-cardiac vagal baroreflex in wheelchair-dependent quadriplegics. *American Journal of Physiology Regulatory Integrated Comparative Physiology* 260:R576-R580.

Cooke W.H., and V.A. Convertino. 2002. Association between vasovagal hypotension and low sympathetic neural activity during presyncope. *Clinical Autonomic Research* 12:483-486.

Dallman, M.F., L.C. Keil, V.A. Convertino, D. O'Hara, and J. Vernikos. 1984. Hormonal, fluid and electrolyte responses to 6° antiorthostatic bedrest in healthy male subjects. In *Stress: Role of catecholamines,* edited by E. Usdin and R. Kvetnansky, 1057-1078. New York: Gordon Breach.

Delp, M.D. 2007. Arterial adaptations in microgravity contributing to orthostatic tolerance. *Journal of Applied Physiology* 102:836.

Dietrick, J.E., G.D. Whedon, E. Shorr, V. Toscani, and V.B. Davis. 1948. Effect of immobilization on metabolic and physiologic functions of normal men. *American Journal of Medicine* 4:3-35.

Dunlop, D., J. Song, E. Arnston, P. Semanik, J. Lee, R. Chang, and J.M. Hootman. 2015. Sedentary time in US older adults associated with disability in activities of daily living independent of physical activity. *Journal of Physical Activity & Health* 12(1):93-101.

Dunstan, D.W., A. Kingwell, R. Larsen, G.N. Healy, E. Cerin, M.T. Hamilton, J.E. Shaw, et al. 2012. Breaking up prolonged sitting reduces post-prandial glucose and insulin responses. *Diabetes Care* 35(5):976-983.

Duvivier, B.M., N.C. Schaper, M.A. Bremers, G. van Crombrugge, P.P. Menheere, M. Kars, and H.H. Savelberg. 2013. Minimal intensity physical activity (standing and walking) of longer duration improves insulin action and plasma lipids more than shorter periods of moderate to vigorous exercise (cycling) in sedentary subjects when energy expenditure is comparable. *PLoS One* 8(2):e55542.

Dyckman D.J., C.L. Sauder, and C.A. Ray. 2012. Effects of short-term and prolonged bed rest on the vestibule-sympathetic reflex. *American Journal of Physiology. Heart Circulation Physiology.* 302(1):H368-H374.

Ekblom-Bak, E., E. Ekblom, M. Vikstrom, U. de Faire, and M.L. Hellenius. 2014. The importance of non-exercise physical activity for cardiovascular health and longevity. *British Journal of Sports Medicine* 48:233-238.

Engelke, K.A., D.F. Doerr, and V.A. Convertino. 1995. A single bout of exhaustive exercise affects integrated baroreflex function after 16 days of head-down tilt. *American Journal of Physiology* 269: R614-R620.

Gratas-Delamarche, A., F. Debre, S. Vincent, and J. Cillard. 2014. Physical inactivity, insulin resistance and the oxidative-inflammatory loop. *Free Radio Research* 48(1): 93-108.

Hilton, J. 1863. *Rest and pain,* edited by E.W. Walls and E.E. Phillips (1950). London: G. Bell & Sons.

Ingber, D.E. 2008. Tensegrity-based mechanosensing from macro to micro. *Progress in Biophysical and Molecular Biology* 97:163-179.

Keyak, J.H., A.K. Koyama, A. LeBlanc, Y. Lu, and T.F. Lang. 2009. Reduction in proximal femoral strength due to long-duration spaceflight. *Bone* 44:449-453.

Klein-Nulend, J., R.F. van Oers, A.D. Bakker, and R.G. Bacabac. 2014. Nitric oxide signaling in mechanical adaptation of bone. *Osteoporosis International* 25(5):1427-1437.

Kolegard, R., I.D. Mekjavic, and O. Eiken. 2013. Effects of physical fitness on relaxed G-tolerance and the exercise pressor response. *European Journal of Applied Physiology* 113:21-29.

Krebs, J.M., V.S. Schneider, H. Evans, M.C. Kuo, and A.D. LeBlanc. 1990. Energy absorption, lean body mass, and total body fat changes during 5 weeks of continuous bed rest. *Aviation Space and Environmental Medicine* 61:314-318.

Lang, T., A. LeBlanc, H. Evans, Y. Lu, H. Genant, and A. Yu. 2004. Cortical and trabecular bone mineral loss from the spine and hip in long duration spaceflight. *Journal Bone of Mineral Research* 19:1006-1012.

Leblanc, A.D., C. Lin, L. Shackelford, V. Sinitsyn, H. Evans, O. Belichenko, B. Schenkman, et al. 2000. Muscle volume, MRI relaxation times (T2) and body composition after spaceflight. *Journal of Applied Physiology* 89:2158-2169.

LeBlanc, A.D., V.S. Schneider, H.J. Evans, C. Pientok, R. Rowe, and E. Spector. 1992. Regional changes in muscle mass following 17 weeks of bedrest. *Journal of Applied Physiology* 73:2172-2178.

LeBlanc, A.D., V.S. Schneider, H.J. Evans, D.A. Engelbretson, and J.M. Krebs. 1990. Bone mineral loss and recovery after 17 weeks of bed rest. *Journal of Bone Mineral Research* 5:843-850.

Levine, B.D., J.H. Zuckerman, and J.A. Pawelczyk. 1997. Cardiac atrophy after bed-rest deconditioning: A non-neural mechanism for orthostatic intolerance. *Circulation* 96: 517-525.

Lutwak, L., G.D. Whedon, P.A. Lachance, M. Reid, and H. Lipscomb. 1969. Mineral electrolyte and nitrogen balance studies of the Gemini VII fourteen-day orbital space flight. *Journal of Clinical Endocrinology and Metabolism* 29:1140-1156.

Luxa, N., M. Salanova, G. Schiff, M. Gutsmann, S. Besnard, P. Denise, A. Clarke, and D. Blottner. 2013. Increased myofiber remodeling and NFATc1-myonuclear translocation in rat postural skeletal muscle after experimental vestibular deafferentation. *Journal of Vestibular Research* 23(4):187-193.

McGavock, J.M., M. Hastings, P.G. Snell, D.K. McGuire, E.L. Pacini, B.D. Levine, and J.H. Mitchell. 2009. A forty-year follow-up of the Dallas bed-rest and training study: The effect of age on the cardiovascular response to exercise in men. *Journal of Gerontology & Biological Science Medicine* 64:293-299.

Mikines, K.J., E.A. Richter, F. Dela, and H. Galbo. 1991. Seven days of bed rest decrease insulin action on glucose uptake in leg and whole body. *Journal of Applied Physiology* 70:1245-1254.

Monk, T.H., S.K. Kennedy, L.R. Rose, and J.M. Linenger. 2001. Decreased human circadian pacemaker influence after 100 days in space: A case study. *Psychosomatic Medicine* 63(6):881-885.

Muller-Delp, J.M., S.A. Spiers, M.W. Ramsey, and M.D. Delp. 2002. Aging impairs endothelium-dependent vasodilation in rat skeletal muscle arterioles. *American Journal of Physiology: Heart Circulation Physiology* 283:1662-1672.

Narici M.V., B. Kayser, P. Barattini, and P. Ceretelli. 2003. Effects of 17-day spaceflight on electrically evoked torque and cross-sectional area of the human triceps surae. *European Journal of Applied Physiology* 90:275-282.

Paloski, W.H., F.O. Black, and E.J. Metter. 2004. Postflight balance control recovery in an elderly astronaut: A case report. *Otological Neurotology* 25:53-56.

Paloski, W.H., F.O. Black, M.F. Reschke, D.S. Calkins, and C. Shupert. 1993. Vestibular ataxia following shuttle flights: Effects of microgravity on otolith-mediated sensorimotor control of posture. *American Journal of Otology* 14:9-17.

Pavy-LeTraon, A., M. Heer, M.V. Narici, J. Rittweger, and J. Vernikos. 2007. From space to Earth: Advances in human physiology from 20 years of bed rest studies (1986-2006). *European Journal of Applied Physiology* 101:143-194.

Payne, M.W., H.K. Uhthoff, and G. Trudel. 2007. Anemia of immobility: Caused by adipocyte accumulation in bone marrow. *Medical Hypotheses* 69(4):778-786.

Peddie, M.C., J.I. Bone, N.J. Rehrer, M.C. Skeaff, A.R. Gray, and T.L. Perry. 2013. Breaking prolonged sitting reduces postprandial glycemia in healthy normal weight adults: A randomized crossover trial. *American Journal of Clinical Nutrition* 98(2):358-365.

Peper, E., and I.M. Lin. 2012. Increase or decrease depression—How body postures influence your energy level. *Biofeedback* 40(3):126-130.

Pietramaggiori, G., P. Liu, S.S. Scherer, A. Kaipanen, M.J. Prsa, H. Mayer, J. Newalder, et al. 2007. Tensile forces stimulate vascular remodeling and epidermal cell proliferation in living skin. *Annals of Surgery* 246:896-902.

Prisby, R.D., A.G. Nelson, and E. Latsch. 2004. Eccentric exercise prior to hindlimb unloading attenuated reloading muscle damage in rats. *Aviation Space and Environmental Medicine* 75:941-946.

Rittweger, J., and D. Felsenberg. 2009. Recovery of muscle and bone loss from 90 days bed rest: Results from a one year follow up. *Bone* 44:214-221.

Robieson, L.E., E.K. Webster, S.W. Logan, W.A. Lucas, and L.T. Barber. 2012. Teaching practices that promote motor skills in early childhood settings. *Early Childhood Education Journal* 40:79-86.

Rubin, C.T., A.S. Turner, R.S. Muller, E. Mittra, K. McLeod, W. Lin, and Y.X. Qin. 2002. Quantity and quality of trabecular bone in the femur are enhanced by a strongly anabolic, non-invasive mechanical intervention. *Journal of Bone Mineral Research* 17:349-357.

Rubin, C.T., E. Capilla, Y.K. Luu, B. Busa, H. Crawford, Y.D.J. Nolan, V. Mittal, C.I. Rosen, J.E. Pessin, and S. Judex. 2007. Adipogenesis is inhibited by brief, daily exposure to high frequency extremely low magnitude mechanical signals. *Proceedings of the National Academy of Sciences* 104:17879-17884.

Sandler, H., and J. Vernikos, eds. 1986. *Inactivity: Physiological effects.* New York: Academic Press.

Schild, H.H., and M. Heller, eds. 1982. *Osteoporose.* Stuttgart, Germany: Georg Thieme.

Sibonga, J.D., H.J. Evans, H.G. Sung, E.P. Spector, T.F. Lang, V.S. Oganov, A.V. Bakulin, L.C. Shackelford, and A.D. LeBlanc. 2007. Recovery of spaceflight-induced bone loss: Bone mineral density after long-duration missions as fitted with an exponential function. *Bone* 41:97973-97978.

Silver, F.H., D. DeVore, and L.M. Siperko. 2003. Role of mechanophysiology in aging of ECM: effects of changes in mechanochemical transduction. *Journal of Applied Physiology* 95:2134-2141.

Smorawinski, J., H. Kaciuba-Uscilko, K. Nazar, P. Kubata, E. Kaminska, A.W. Ziemba, J. Adrian, and J.E. Greenleaf. 2000. Effects of three-day bed-rest on metabolic hormonal and circulatory responses to an oral glucose load in endurance or strength trained athletes and untrained subjects. *Journal of Physiology and Pharmacology* 51:279-289.

Sun, X., Y.J. Yao, C.B. Yang, S.Z. Jiang, C.L. Jiang, and W.B. Liong. 2005. Effect of lower-body negative pressure on cerebral blood flow velocity during 21 days head-down tilt bed rest. *Medical Science Monitor* 11:1-5.

Trappe, S., D. Costill, P.M. Gallagher, A. Creer, J.R. Peters, H. Evans, D.A. Riley, and R.H. Fitts. 2009. Exercise in space: Human skeletal muscle after 6 months aboard the international Space Station. *Journal of Applied Physiology* 106:1159-1168.

Vernikos, J. 1996. Human physiology in space. *Bioessays* 18:1029-1037.

———. 2004. *The G-connection: Harness gravity and reverse aging.* Lincoln, NE: iUniverse.

———. 2011. *Sitting kills, moving heals.* Fresno, CA: Quill Driver Books.

Vernikos, J., D.A. Ludwig, A.C. Ertl, C.E. Wade, L.C. Keil, and D. O'Hara. 1996. Effect of standing or walking on physiological changes induced by head down bed rest: Implications for spaceflight. *Aviation Space and Environmental Medicine* 67(11):1069-1079.

Vernikos, J., M.F. Dallman, G. Van Loon, L.C. Keil, D. O'Hara, and V.A. Convertino. 1993. Gender differences in endocrine responses to posture and 7 days of –6 degrees head-down bed rest. *American Journal of Physiology* 265:E153-E161.

Vernikos, J., and V.S. Schneider. 2010. Space, gravity and the physiology of aging: Parallel or convergent disciplines? A mini-review. *Gerontology* 56:157-166.

Vico, J., D. Chappard, C. Alexandre, S. Palle, P. Minaire, G. Rittat, B. Morukov, and S. Rakhmanov. 1987. Effects of a 120 day period of bed rest on bone mass and bone cell activities in man: Attempts at countermeasures. *Bone Mineral* 2:383-394.

Vigneaux, G., S. Besnard, J. Ndong, B. Philoxene, P. Denise, and F. Eleftheriou. 2013. Bone remodeling is regulated by inner ear vestibular signals. *Journal of Bone and Mineral Research* 28:2136-2144.

Weinert, B.T., and P. Timiras. 2003. Theories of aging. *Journal of Applied Physiology* 95:1706-1716.

Wilkerson, M.K., L.A. Lesniewski, E.M. Golding, R.M. Bryan, Jr., A. Amin, E. Wilson, and M.D. Delp. 2005. Simulated microgravity enhances cerebral artery vasoconstriction and vascular resistance through endothelial nitric oxide mechanism. *American Journal of Physiology: Heart Circulation Physiology* 288:1652-1661.

Winget, C.M., J. Vernikos-Danellis, S. Cronin, C.S. Leach, P.C. Rambaut, and P.B. Mack. 1972. Circadian rhythm asynchrony in humans during hypokinesis. *Journal of Applied Physiology* 33:640-645.

Yanagibori, R., Y. Suzuki, K. Kawakubo, Y. Makita, and A. Gunji. 1994. Carbohydrate and lipid metabolism after 20 days of bed rest. *Acta Physiologica Scandinavica* 616(Suppl.):51-57.

Yates B.J., M.J. Holmes, and B.J. Jian. 2000. Adaptive plasticity in vestibular influences on cardiovascular control. *Brain Research Bulletin* 53(1):3-9.

Chapter 3

American Diabetes Association. 2001. Postprandial blood glucose. American Diabetes Association. *Diabetes Care* 24:775-778.

Australian Government. 2014. Australia's physical activity and sedentary behaviour guidelines. Canberra: Department of Health.

Bailey, D.P., and C.D. Locke. 2014. Breaking up prolonged sitting with light-intensity walking improves postprandial glycemia, but breaking up sitting with standing does not. Journal of Science and Medicine in Sport. 2015. May 18(3):294-8.

Bergouignan, A., F. Rudwill, C. Simon, and S. Blanc. 2011. Physical inactivity as the culprit of metabolic inflexibility: Evidence from bed-rest studies. Journal of Applied Physiology 111:1201-1210.

Blankenship, J., K. Granados, and B. Braun. 2014. Effects of subtracting sitting versus adding exercise on glycemic control and variability in sedentary office workers. Applied Phsyiology, Nutrition, and Metabolism 39:1286-1293.

Buckley, J.P., D.D. Mellor, M. Morris, and F. Joseph. 2013. Standing-based office work shows encouraging signs of attenuating post-prandial glycaemic excursion. Occupational and Environmental Medicine 71:109-111.

Davies, S., H. Burns, T. Jewell, and M. Mcbride. 2011. Start active, stay active: A report on physical activity from the four home countries' Chief Medical Officers. London:

Department of Health, Physical Activity, Health Improvement and Protection.

Dunstan, D.W., B.A. Kingwell, R. Larsen, G.N. Healy, E. Cerin, M.T. Hamilton, J.E. Shaw, et al. 2012. Breaking up prolonged sitting reduces postprandial glucose and insulin responses. Diabetes Care 35:976-983.

Dunstan, D.W., B.J. Howard, G.N. Healy, and N. Owen. 2012. Too much sitting—A health hazard. Diabetes Research and Clinical Practice 97:368-376.

Duvivier, B.M., N.C. Schaper, M.A. Bremers, G. Van Crombrugge, P.P. Menheere, M. Kars, and H.H. Savelberg. 2013. Minimal intensity physical activity (standing and walking) of longer duration improves insulin action and plasma lipids more than shorter periods of moderate to vigorous exercise (cycling) in sedentary subjects when energy expenditure is comparable. PLoS One 8:e55542.

Garber, C.E., B. Blissmer, M.R. Deschenes, B.A. Franklin, M.J. Lamonte, I.M. Lee, D.C. Nieman, and D.P. Swain. 2011. American College of Sports Medicine position stand. Quantity and quality of exercise for developing and maintaining cardiorespiratory, musculoskeletal, and neuromotor fitness in apparently healthy adults: Guidance for prescribing exercise. Medicine and Science in Sports and Exercise 43:1334-1359.

Hamilton, M.T., D.G. Hamilton, and T.W. Zderic. 2004. Exercise physiology versus inactivity physiology: An essential concept for understanding lipoprotein lipase regulation. Exercise and Sports Science Reviews 32:161-166.

———. 2007. Role of low energy expenditure and sitting in obesity, metabolic syndrome, type 2 diabetes, and cardiovascular disease. Diabetes 56:2655-2667.

Healy, G.N., K. Wijndaele, D.W. Dunstan, J.E. Shaw, J. Salmon, P.Z. Zimmet, and N. Owen. 2008. Objectively measured sedentary time, physical activity, and metabolic risk: The Australian Diabetes, Obesity and Lifestyle Study (AusDiab). Diabetes Care 31:369-371.

Holmstrup, M., T. Fairchild, S. Keslacy, R. Weinstock, and J. Kanaley. 2014. Multiple short bouts of exercise over 12-h period reduce glucose excursions more than an energy-matched single bout of exercise. Metabolism 63: 510-519.

Howard, B.J., S.F. Fraser, P. Sethi, E. Cerin, M.T. Hamilton, N. Owen, D.W. Dunstan, and B.A. Kingwell. 2013. Impact on hemostatic parameters of interrupting sitting with intermittent activity. Medicine and Science in Sports and Exercise 45:1285-1291.

Larsen, R.N., B.A. Kingwell, P. Sethi, E. Cerin, N. Owen, and D.W. Dunstan. 2014. Breaking up prolonged sitting reduces resting blood pressure in overweight/obese adults. Nutrition, Metabolism and Cardiovascular Diseases 24:976-982.

Lunde, M.S., V.T. Hjellset, and A.T. Hostmark. 2012. Slow post meal walking reduces the blood glucose response: An exploratory study in female Pakistani immigrants. Journal of Immigrant and Minority Health 14:816-822.

Mills, E.J., A.W. Chan, P. Wu, A. Vail, G.H. Guyatt, and D.G. Altman. 2009. Design, analysis, and presentation of crossover trials. Trials 10:27.

Miyashita, M., J.H. Park, M. Takahashi, K. Suzuki, D. Stensel, and Y. Nakamura. 2013. Postprandial lipaemia: Effects of sitting, standing and walking in healthy normolipidaemic humans. International Journal of Sports Medicine 34:21-27.

Nygaard, H., S.E. Tomten, and A.T. Hostmark. 2009. Slow postmeal walking reduces postprandial glycemia in middle-aged women. Applied Phsyiology, Nutrition, and Metabolism 34:1087-1092.

Owen, N., G.N. Healy, C.E. Matthews, and D.W. Dunstan. 2010. Too much sitting: The population health science of sedentary behavior. Exercise and Sports Science Reviews 38:105-113.

Owen, N., A. Bauman, and W.J. Brown. 2009. Too much sitting: A novel and important predictor of chronic disease risk? British Journal of Sports Medicine 43:81-83.

Peddie, M.C., J.L. Bone, N.J. Rehrer, C.M. Skeaff, A.R. Gray, and T.L. Perry. 2013. Breaking prolonged sitting reduces postprandial glycemia in healthy, normal-weight adults: A randomized crossover trial. American Journal of Clinical Nutrition 98:358-366.

Stephens, B.R., K. Granados, T.W. Zderic, M.T. Hamilton, and B. Braun. 2011. Effects of 1 day of inactivity on insulin action in healthy men and women: Interaction with energy intake. Metabolism 60:941-949.

Thorp, A.A., B.A. Kingwell, P. Sethi, L. Hammond, N. Owen, and D.W. Dunstan. 2014. Alternating bouts of sitting and standing attenuates postprandial glucose responses. Medicine and Science in Sports and Exercise 46:2053-2061.

Thorp, A.A., N. Owen, M. Neuhaus, and D.W. Dunstan. 2011. Sedentary behaviors and subsequent health outcomes in adults: A systematic review of longitudinal studies, 1996-2011. American Journal of Preventive Medicine 41:207-215.

Thyfault, J.P., and R. Krogh-Madsen. 2011. Metabolic disruptions induced by reduced ambulatory activity in free-living humans. Journal of Applied Physiology 111:1218-1224.

Van Dijk, J.W., M. Venema, W. Van Mechelen, C.D. Stehouwer, F. Hartgens, and L.J. Van Loon. 2013. Effect of moderate-intensity exercise versus activities of daily living on 24-hour blood glucose homeostasis in male patients with type 2 diabetes. Diabetes Care 36:3448-3453.

World Health Organization. 2010. Global recommendations on physical activity for health. Geneva: WHO Press.

Chapter 4

Alexander, F.M. 1918. *Man's supreme inheritance.* London: Dutton.

———. 1985. First printing 1923. *Constructive conscious control of the individual*. Downey, California: Centerline Press: 148-149.

Andersson, G.B. 1980. The load on the lumbar spine in sitting postures. Department of Orthopaedic Surgery, Sahlgren Hospital, Goteborg, Sweden: 231-39.

———. 1981. Epidemiologic aspects of low back pain in industry. *Spine* 6:53-60.

———. 1985. Posture and compressive spine loading: Intradiscal pressures, trunk myoelectric activities, intra-abdominal pressures, and biochemical analyses. *Ergonomics* 28(1):91-93.

Andersson, G.B., R. Ortengren, and A. Nachemson. 1982. Disc pressure measurements when rising and sitting down on a chair. *Engineering in Medicine* 11(4):189-190.

Andersson, G.B., R. Ortengren, A. Nachemson, and G. Elfstrom. 1974. Lumbar disc pressure and myoelectric back muscle activity during sitting. *Scandinavian Journal of Rehabilitative Medicine* 6:104-114.

Cranz, G. 1998. *The chair: Rethinking culture, body and design*. New York: WW Norton.

Donkin, S.W. 1986. *Sitting on the job*. Boston: Houghton Mifflin.

Giedion, S. 1948. *Mechanization takes command*. London: Oxford University Press.

Grandjean, E. 1980. *Fitting the task to the man*. London: Taylor & Francis.

Gross, G.A. 1990. Preventing low back pain. In *Preventing Disease*, edited by R.B. Goldbloom and R.S. Lawrence, New York: Springer-Verlag: 204-211.

Hettinger, T. 1985. Occupational hazards associated with diseases of the skeletal system. *Ergonomics* 28(1):69-75.

Hunting, W., T. Laubli, and E. Grandjean. 1981. Postural and visual load at VDT workplaces: Constrained postures. *Ergonomics* 24:917-931.

Levine, J.A. 2007. The effect of sitting postures on the hemodynamics of the popliteal and femoral veins. Thesis for Master of Consumer and Applied Sciences. University of Otago, Dunedin, New Zealand.

Lucie-Smith, E. 1990. *Furniture: A concise history*. New York: Thames and Hudson.

Opsvik, Peter. 1997. Interview. Olso, Norway. May.Opsvik, Peter. 2009. *Rethinking sitting*. New York: WW Norton.

Ravn, K. 2013. Don't just sit there. Really. *Los Angeles Times*. May 25. http://articles.latimes.com/2013/may/25/health/la-he-dont-sit-20130525

Saunders, T. 2011. Can too much sitting kill you? *Scientific American* (guest blog). January 6. http://blogs.scientificamerican.com/guest-blog/2011/01/06/can-sitting-too-much-kill-you

Sitting down on the job: Not as easy as it sounds. *Occupational Health and Safety* 5(10):24-26.

Zacharkow, D. 1988. *Posture: Sitting, standing, chair design, and exercise*. Springfield, IL: Charles C. Thomas.

Chapter 5

Aggio, D., A.A. Ogunleye, C. Voss, and G.R. Sandercock. 2012. Temporal relationships between screen-time and physical activity with cardiorespiratory fitness in English schoolchildren: A 2-year longitudinal study. Preventive Medicine 55(1):37-39.

Altenburg, T.M., G.H. Hofsteenge, P.J. Weijs, H.A. Delemarre-van de Waal, and M.J. Chinapaw. 2012. Self-reported screen time and cardiometabolic risk in obese Dutch adolescents. PLoS One 7(12):e53333.

Blades, M., C. Oates, and S. Li. 2013. Children's recognition of advertisements on television and on web pages. Appetite 62:190-193.

Borzekowski, D.L., and T.N. Robinson. 1999. Viewing the viewers: Ten video cases of children's television viewing behaviors. Journal of Broadcasting and Electronic Media 43(4):506-528.

———. 2001. The 30-second effect: An experiment revealing the impact of television commercials on food preferences of preschoolers. Journal of the American Dietetic Association 101(1):42-46.

Carlson, S.A., J.E. Fulton, S.M. Lee, J.T. Foley, C. Heitzler, and M. Huhman. 2010. Influence of limit-setting and participation in physical activity on youth screen time. Pediatrics 126(1):e89-e96.

Carson, V., and I. Janssen. 2011. Volume, patterns, and types of sedentary behavior and cardio-metabolic health in children and adolescents: A cross-sectional study. BMC Public Health 11:274.

Chaput, J.P., L. Klingenberg, A. Astrup, and A.M. Sjodin. 2011. Modern sedentary activities promote overconsumption of food in our current obesogenic environment. Obesity Reviews 12(5):e12-e20.

Chaput, J.P., T. Visby, S. Nyby, L. Klingenberg, N.T. Gregersen, A. Tremblay, A. Astrup, and A. Sjodin. 2011. Video game playing increases food intake in adolescents: A randomized crossover study. American Journal of Clinical Nutrition 93(6):1196-1203.

Council on Communications and Media. 2011. Children, adolescents, obesity, and the media. Pediatrics 128(1):201-208.

———. 2013. Children, adolescents, and the media. Pediatrics 132(5):958-961.

de Jong, E., T.L. Visscher, R.A. HiraSing, M.W. Heymans, J.C. Seidell, and C.M. Renders. 2013. Association between TV viewing, computer use and overweight, determinants and competing activities of screen time in 4- to 13-year-old children. International Journal of Obesity 37(1):47-53.

Dembek, C., J.L. Harris, and M.B. Schwartz. 2014. Trends in television food advertising to young people: 2013 update. New Haven, CT: Yale Rudd Center for Food Policy and Obesity.

Epstein, L.H., Roemmich, R.A. Paluch, and H.A. Raynor. 2005a. Influence of changes in sedentary behavior on energy and macronutrient intake in youth. American Journal of Clinical Nutrition 81(2):361-366.

Epstein, L.H. 2005b. Physical activity as a substitute for sedentary behavior in youth. Annals of Behavioral Medicine 29(3):200-209.

Epstein, L.H., J.N. Roemmich, J.L. Robinson, R.A. Paluch, D.D. Winiewicz, J.H. Fuerch, and T.N. Robinson. 2008. A randomized trial of the effects of reducing television viewing and computer use on body mass index in young children. Archives of Pediatrics and Adolescent Medicine 162(3):239-245.

Epstein, L.H., R.A. Paluch, A. Consalvi, K. Riordan, and T. Scholl. 2002. Effects of manipulating sedentary behavior on physical activity and food intake. Journal of Pediatrics 140(3):334-339.

Epstein, L.H., R. Paluch, J.D. Smith, and M. Sayette. 1997. Allocation of attentional resources during habituation to food cues. Psychophysiology 34(1):59-64.

Gebremariam, M.K., I.H. Bergh, L.F. Andersen, Y. Ommundsen, T.H. Totland, M. Bjelland, M. Grydeland, and N. Lien. 2013. Are screen-based sedentary behaviors longitudinally associated with dietary behaviorrs and leisure-time physical activity in the transition into adolescence? International Journal of Behavioral Nutrition and Physical Activity 10:9.

Goldfield, G.S., G.P. Kenny, S. Hadjiyannakis, P. Phillips, A.S. Alberga, T.J. Saunders, M.S. Tremblay, et al. 2011. Video game playing is independently associated with blood pressure and lipids in overweight and obese adolescents. PLoS One 6(11):e26643.

Goldfield, G.S., T.J. Saunders, G.P. Kenny, S. Hadjiyannakis, P. Phillips, A.S. Alberga, M.S. Tremblay, and R.J. Sigal. 2013. Screen viewing and diabetes risk factors in overweight and obese adolescents. American Journal of Preventive Medicine 44(Suppl. 4):S364-S370.

Gortmaker, S.L., A. Must, A.M. Sobol, K. Peterson, G.A. Colditz, and W.H. Dietz. 1996. Television viewing as a cause of increasing obesity among children in the United States, 1986-1990. Archives of Pediatrics and Adolescent Medicine 150(4):356-362.

Gortmaker, S.L., K. Peterson, J. Wiecha, A.M. Sobol, S. Dixit, M.K. Fox, and N. Laird. 1999. Reducing obesity via a school-based interdisciplinary intervention among youth: Planet Health. Archives of Pediatrics and Adolescent Medicine 153(4):409-418.

Hancox, R.J., B.J. Milne, and R. Poulton. 2004. Association between child and adolescent television viewing and adult health: A longitudinal birth cohort study. Lancet 364(9430):257-262.

Harris, J.L., J.A. Bargh, and K.D. Brownell. 2009. Priming effects of television food advertising on eating behavior. Health Psychology 28(4):404-413.

Lapierre, M.A., J.T. Piotrowski, and D.L. Linebarger. 2012. Background television in the homes of US children. Pediatrics 130(5):839-846.

Leibowitz, J., J.T. Rosch, E. Ramirez, J. Brill, and M. Ohlhausen. 2012. A review of food marketing to children and adolescents: Follow-up report. Washington, DC: Federal Trade Commission.

Lipsky, L.M., and R.J. Iannotti. 2012. Associations of television viewing with eating behaviors in the 2009 Health Behaviour in School-Aged Children Study. Archives of Pediatrics and Adolescent Medicine 166(5):465-472.

Madden, M., A. Lenhart, M. Duggan, S. Cortesi, and U. Gasser. 2013. Teens and technology 2013. Washington, DC: Pew Research Center.

Matheson, D.M., J.D. Killen, Y. Wang, A. Varady, and T.N. Robinson. 2004. Children's food consumption during television viewing. American Journal of Clinical Nutrition 79(6):1088-1094.

Matheson, D.M., Y. Wang, L.M. Klesges, B.M. Beech, H.C. Kraemer, and T.N. Robinson. 2004. African-American girls' dietary intake while watching television. Obesity Research 12(Suppl.):32S-37S.

Mitchell, J.A., R.R. Pate, and S.N. Blair. 2012. Screen-based sedentary behavior and cardiorespiratory fitness from age 11 to 13. Medicine and Science in Sports and Exercise 44(7):1302-1309.Nunneley, S. 2013. Minecraft sales hit 20 million mark for all platforms. Accessed April 15, 2013. www.vg247.com/2013/01/22/minecraft-sales-hit-20-million-mark-for-all-platforms

Pearson, N., and S.J. Biddle. 2011. Sedentary behavior and dietary intake in children, adolescents, and adults. A systematic review. American Journal of Preventive Medicine 41(2):178-188.

Plachta-Danielzik, S., B. Kehden, B. Landsberg, A. Schaffrath Rosario, B.M. Kurth, C. Arnold, C. Graf, S. Hense, W. Ahrens, and M.J. Muller. 2012. Attributable risks for childhood overweight: Evidence for limited effectiveness of prevention. Pediatrics 130(4):e865-e871.

Rideout, V. 2013. Zero to eight: Children's media use in America 2013. New York: Common Sense Media.

———. 2015. The common sense census: Media use by tweens and teens. San Francisco: Common Sense Media.

Rideout, V.J., U.G. Foehr, and D.F. Roberts. 2010. Generation M2. Media in the lives of 8-to 18-year-olds. Menlo Park, CA: Kaiser Family Foundation.

Roberts, D.F., U.G. Foehr, and V.J. Rideout. 2005. Generation M. Media in the lives of 8-to 18-year-olds. Menlo Park, CA: Kaiser Family Foundation.

Robinson, T.N. 1999. Reducing children's television viewing to prevent obesity: A randomized controlled trial. Journal of the American Medical Association 282(16):1561-1567.

———. 2001. Television viewing and childhood obesity. Pediatric Clinics of North America 48(4):1017-1025.

Robinson, T.N., D.L. Borzekowski, D.M. Matheson, and H.C. Kraemer. 2007. Effects of fast food branding on young children's taste preferences. Archives of Pediatrics and Adolescent Medicine 161(8):792-797.

Robinson, T.N., M.L. Wilde, L.C. Navracruz, K.F. Haydel, and A. Varady. 2001. Effects of reducing children's television and video game use on aggressive behavior: A randomized controlled trial. Archives of Pediatrics and Adolescent Medicine 155(1):17-23.

Robinson, T.N., M.N. Saphir, H.C. Kraemer, A. Varady, and K.F. Haydel. 2001. Effects of reducing television viewing on children's requests for toys: A randomized controlled trial. Journal of Developmental and Behavioral Pediatrics 22(3):179-184.

Rodin, J. 1974. Effects of distraction on the performance of obese and normal subjects. In Obese Humans and Rats, edited by S. Schachter and J. Rodin, 97-110. Potomac, MD: Erlbaum.

Russ, S.A., K. Larson, T.M. Franke, and N. Halfon. 2009. Associations between media use and health in US children. Academic Pediatrics 9(5):300-306.

Sandercock, G.R., and A.A. Ogunleye. 2013. Independence of physical activity and screen time as predictors of cardiorespiratory fitness in youth. Pediatric Research 73(5):692-697.

Sisson, S.B., C.M. Shay, S.T. Broyles, and M. Leyva. 2012. Television-viewing time and dietary quality among U.S. children and adults. American Journal of Preventive Medicine 43(2):196-200.

Sisson, S.B., and S.T. Broyles. 2012. Social-ecological correlates of excessive TV viewing: Difference by race and sex. Journal of Physical Activity and Health 9(3):449-455.

Sisson, S.B., T.S. Church, C.K. Martin, C. Tudor-Locke, S.R. Smith, C. Bouchard, C.P. Earnest, T. Rankinen, R.L. Newton, and P.T. Katzmarzyk. 2009. Profiles of sedentary behavior in children and adolescents: The US National Health and Nutrition Examination Survey, 2001-2006. International Journal of Pediatric Obesity 4(4):353-359.

Sonneville, K.R., and S.L. Gortmaker. 2008. Total energy intake, adolescent discretionary behaviors and the energy gap. International Journal of Obesity 32(Suppl. 6):S19-S27.

Stamatakis, E., N. Coombs, R. Jago, A. Gama, I. Mourao, H. Nogueira, V. Rosado, and C. Padez. 2013. Type-specific screen time associations with cardiovascular risk markers in children. American Journal of Preventive Medicine 44(5):481-488.

Strasburger, V.C., A.B. Jordan, and E. Donnerstein. 2010. Health effects of media on children and adolescents. Pediatrics 125(4):756-767.

Tandon, P.S., C. Zhou, J.F. Sallis, K.L. Cain, L.D. Frank, and B.E. Saelens. 2012. Home environment relationships with children's physical activity, sedentary time, and screen time by socioeconomic status. International Journal of Behavioral Nutrition and Physical Activity 9:88.

Temple, J.L., A.M. Giacomelli, K.M. Kent, J.N. Roemmich, and L.H. Epstein. 2007. Television watching increases motivated responding for food and energy intake in children. American Journal of Clinical Nutrition 85(2):355-361.

U.S. Department of Health and Human Services. n.d. 2020 Topics and Objectives: Physical Activity. Accessed April 13, 2013. www.healthypeople.gov/2020/topicsobjectives2020/objectiveslist.aspx?topicid=33

Viner, R.M., and T.J. Cole. 2005. Television viewing in early childhood predicts adult body mass index. Journal of Pediatrics 147(4):429-435.

Wansink, B. 2004. Environmental factors that increase the food intake and consumption volume of unknowing consumers. Annual Review of Nutrition 24:455-479.

Zimmerman, F.J., and J.F. Bell. 2010. Associations of television content type and obesity in children. American Journal of Public Health 100(2):334-340.

Chapter 6

Ambec, S., M.A. Cohen, S. Elgie, and P. Lanoie. 2013. The porter hypothesis at 20: Can environmental regulation enhance innovation and competitiveness? Review of Environmental Economics and Policy 7(1):2-22.

Baicker, K., D. Cutler, and Z. Song. 2010. Workplace wellness programs can generate savings. Health Affairs 29(2):1-8.

Bell, D. 1973. The coming of post-industrial society. New York: Basic Books.

Blakely, E.J., and P. Shapira. 1984. Industrial restructuring: Public policies for investment in advanced industrial society. Annals of the American Academy of Political and Social Sciences 475:96-109.

Bleich, S.N., and R. Sturm. 2009. Developing policy solutions for a more active nation: Integrating economic and public health perspectives. Journal of Preventive Medicine 49(4):306-308.

Bluestone, B. 2013. Detroit and deindustrialization. Dollars & Sense 308:18-24.

Bluestone, B., and B. Harrison. 1982. The deindustrialization of America: Plant closings, community abandonment, and the dismantling of basic industry. New York: Basic Books.

Bodenheimer, T. 2005. High and rising health care costs. Part 1: Seeking an explanation. Annals of International Medicine 142(10):847-854.

Boles, M., B. Pelletier, and W. Lynch. 2004. The relationship between health risk and work productivity. Journal of Occupational and Environmental Medicine 46(7):737-745.

Brady, D., and R. Denniston. 2006. Economic globalization, industrialization and deindustrialization in affluent democracies. Social Forces 85(1):297-329.

Brownson, R.C., C.M. Hoehner, K. Day, A. Forsyth, and J.F. Sallis. 2009. Measuring the built environment for physical activity: State of the science. American Journal of Preventive Medicine 36(4):S99-S123.

Brownson, R.C., T.K. Boehmer, and D.A. Luke. 2005. Declining rates of physical activity in the United States: What are the contributors? Annual Review of Public Health 26(1):421-443.

Carey, M.P. 2013. Counting regulations: An overview of rulemaking, types of federal regulations, and pages in the Federal Register. Washington, D.C.: Congressional Research Service.

Cawley, J., and C. Meyerhoefer. 2012. The medical care costs of obesity: An instrumental variables approach. *Journal of Health Economics* 31(1):219-230.

Cerina, F., and F. Mureddu. 2013. Structural change and growth in a NEG Model. *Review of Development Economics* 17(2):182-200.

Church, T.S., D.M. Thomas, C. Tudor-Locke, P.T. Katzmarzyk, C.P. Earnest, R.Q. Rodartel, C.K. Martin, S.N. Blair, and C. Bouchard. 2011. Trends over 5 decades in U.S. occupation-related physical activity and their associations with obesity. *PLoS ONE* 6(5): e19657.

Clark, C. 1957. *The conditions of economic progress*, 3rd ed. London: Macmillan.

Claxton, G., M. Rae, N. Panchal, A. Damico, H. Whitmore, N. Bostick, and K. Kenward. 2013. Health benefits in 2013: Moderate premium increases in employer-sponsored plans. *Health Affairs* 32(9):1667-1676.

Clemes, S.A., S.E. O'Connell, and C.L. Edwardson. 2014. Office workers' objectively measured sedentary behavior and physical activity during and outside working hours. *Journal of Occupational and Environmental Medicine* 56(3):298-303.

Council of Economic Advisers (U.S.). 2012. *Smarter regulations through retrospective review*. Washington, D.C.: Executive Office of the President, Council of Economic Advisors.

Daltroy, L.H., M.D. Iversen, M.G. Larson, R. Lew, E. Wright, J. Ryan, C. Zwerling, A.H. Fossel, and M.H. Liang. 1997. A controlled trial of an educational program to prevent low back injuries. *New England Journal of Medicine* 337:322-328.

Dimitri, C., A. Effland, and N. Conklin. 2005. *The 20th century transformation of U.S. agriculture and farm policy.* U.S. Department of Agriculture, Economic Research Service 59390.

Driessen, M.T., K.I. Proper, M.W. van Tulder, J.R. Anema, P.M. Bongers, and A.J. van der Beek. 2010. The effectiveness of physical and organisational ergonomic interventions on low back pain and neck pain: A systematic review. *Occupational and Environmental Medicine* 67(4):277-285.

Drucker, P.F. 1968. *The age of discontinuity: Guidelines to our changing society.* New York, NY: Harper & Row.

———. 2001. *The essential Drucker.* New York, NY: Harper Collins.

Duncan, M.J., C. Short, M. Rashid, N. Cutumisu, C. Vandelanotte, and R.C. Plotnikoff. 2015. Identifying correlates of breaks in occupational sitting: a cross-sectional study. Building Research and Information 43(5): 646-658. DOI: http://dx.doi.org/10.1080/09613218.2015.1045712.

Ermolaeva, E., and J. Ross. 2010. *Unintended consequences of human actions.* Lanham, MD: University Press of America.

Executive Order 13563. 3 C.F.R. 2011. *Improving Regulation and Regulatory Review.* 76(14):3821-3823.

Federal Regulatory Directory. 2009. *Federal regulatory directory: The essential guide to the history, organization, and impact of U.S. federal regulation*, 14th ed. Washington, D.C.: CQ Press.

Finkelstein, E.A., C.J. Ruhm, and K.M. Kosa. 2005. Economic causes and consequences of obesity. *Annual Review of Public Health* 26:239-257.

Finkelstein, E.A., J.G. Trogdon, J.W. Cohen, and W. Dietz. 2009. Annual medical spending attributable to obesity: Payer- and service-specific estimates. *Health Affairs* 28(5):822-831.

Flegal, K.M., M.D. Carroll, C.L. Ogden, and L.R. Curtin. 2010. Prevalence and trends in obesity among US adults, 1999–2008. *Journal of the American Medical Association* 303(3):235-241.

Fox, K.R., and M. Hillsdon. 2007. Physical activity and obesity. *Obesity Reviews* 1(8):115-121.

French, S., M. Story, and R. Jeffery. 2001. Environmental influences on eating and physical activity. *Annual Review of Public Health* 22(1):309-335.

Girod, C.S., L.W. Mayne, S.A. Weltz, and S.K. Hart. 2014. *Milliman medical index.* Seattle: Milliman.

Goetzel, R.Z., and R.J. Ozminkowski. 2008. The health and cost benefits of work site health-promotion programs. *Annual Review of Public Health* 29:303-323.

Gordus, J.P., P. Jarley, and L.A. Feman. 1981. *Plant closings and economic dislocation.* Kalamazoo, MI: W.E. Upjohn Institute for Employment Research.

Groshen, E.L., S. Potter, and R.J. Sela. 2004. Economic restructuring in New York State. *Current Issues in Economics and Finance* 10(7):1-7.

Guh, D.P., W. Zhang, N. Bansback, Z. Amarsi, C.L. Birmingham, and A.H. Anis. 2009. The incidence of co-morbidities related to obesity and overweight: A systematic review and meta-analysis. *BMC Public Health* 9(1):1-20.

Harrington, D.M., T.V. Barreira, A.E. Staiano, and P.T. Katzmarzyk. 2014. The descriptive epidemiology of sitting among US adults, NHANES 2009/2010. *Journal of Science & Medicine in Sport* 17(4):371-375.

Hazlitt, H. 1979. *Economics in one lesson: The shortest and surest way to understand basic economics.* New York: Random House.

Hildebrandt, V.H., P.M. Bongers, J.J. Dul, F.H. van Dijk, and H.G. Kemper. 2000. The relationship between leisure time, physical activities and musculoskeletal symptoms and disability in worker populations. *International Archives of Occupational & Environmental Health* 73(8):507-518.

Hill, J.O., H.R. Wyatt, and J.C. Peters. 2012. Energy balance and obesity. *Circulation* 126:126-132.

Hill, J.O., H.R. Wyatt, G.W. Reed, and J.C. Peters. 2003. Obesity and the environment: Where do we go from here? *Science* 299(5608):853-855.

Jackson, A.S. 1994. Preemployment physical evaluation. *Exercise and Sport Science Reviews* 22:53-90.

———. 2006. Preemployment physical testing. In *Measurement theory and practice in kinesiology*, edited by T.M. Wood and W. Zhu, pp. 315-345. Champaign, IL: Human Kinetics.

Janowitz, M. 2010. *Social change and politics: 1920-1976*. New Brunswick, NJ: Transaction.

Joskow, P. 2010. Market imperfections versus regulatory imperfections. *CESifo DICE Report* 8(3):3-7.

Katzmarzyk, P.T., T.S. Church, C.L. Craig, and C. Bouchard. 2009. Sitting time and mortality from all causes, cardiovascular disease, and cancer. *Medicine and Science in Sports and Exercise* 41(5):998-1005.

Kenessey, Z. 1987. The primary, secondary, tertiary, and quaternary sectors of the economy. *Journal of the International Association for Research in Income and Wealth* 33(4):359-385.

Kirk, M.A., and R.E. Rhodes. 2011. Occupation correlates of adults' participation in leisure-time physical activity: A systematic review. *American Journal of Preventive Medicine* 40(4):476-485.

Kollmeyer, C. 2009. Explaining deindustrialization: How affluence, productivity growth, and globalization diminish manufacturing employment. *American Journal of Sociology* 114(6):1644-1677.

Kremers, S.P., F.F. Eves, and R.E. Andersen. 2012. Environmental changes to promote physical activity and healthy dietary behavior. *Journal of Environmental and Public Health* 2012:1-4.

Kruger, J.J. 2008. Productivity and structural change: A review of the literature. *Journal of Economic Surveys* 22(2):330–363.

Kuznets, S. 1973. Modern economic growth: Findings and reflections. *American Economic Review* 63(3):247-258.

Lakdawalla, D., and T. Philipson. 2009. The growth of obesity and technological change. *Economics and Human Biology* 7(3):283-293.

Loeppke, R., M. Taitel, D. Richling, T. Parry, R.C. Kessler, P. Hymel, and D. Konicki. 2007. Health and productivity as a business strategy. *Journal of Occupational and Environmental Medicine* 49(7):712-721.

Marteau, T., D. Ogilvie, M. Roland, M. Suhrcke, and M.P. Kelly. 2011. Judging nudging: Can nudging improve population health? *British Medical Journal* 342:263-265.

Masur, J.S., and E.A. Posner. 2012. Regulation, unemployment, and cost-benefit analysis. *Virginia Law Review* 98:579-634.

Matthews, C.E., K.Y. Chen, P.S. Freedson, M.S. Buchowski, B.M. Beech, R.R. Pate, and R.P. Trojano. 2008. Amount of time spent in sedentary behaviors in the United States, 2003–2004. *American Journal of Epidemiology* 167(7):875-881.

McLaughlin, P., and R. Greene. 2014. *The unintended consequences of federal regulatory accumulation*. Fairfax, VA: George Mason University.

McLaughlin, P., and R. Williams. 2014. *The consequences of regulatory accumulation and a proposed solution*. Fairfax, VA: George Mason University.

Morris, J.N., J.A. Heady, P.A.B. Raffle, C.G. Roberts, and J.W. Parks. 1953. Coronary heart-disease and physical activity of work. *Lancet* 265(6796):1111-1120.

Must, A., J. Spadano, E.H. Coakley, A.E. Field, G. Colditz, and W.H. Dietz. 1999. The disease burden associated with overweight and obesity. *JAMA* 282(16):1523-1529.

Ng, S.W., and B. Popkin. 2012. Time use of physical activity: A shift away from movement across the globe. *Obesity Reviews* 13(8):659-680.

Nyce, S., J. Grossmeier, D.R. Anderson, P.E. Terry, and B. Kelley. 2012. Association between changes in health risk status and changes in future health care costs: A multiemployer study. *Journal of Occupational and Environmental Medicine* 54(11):1364-1373.

Obama, B.H. 2011. Remarks by the President in the State of the Union address. Accessed August 6, 2014. www.whitehouse.gov/the-press-office/2011/01/25/remarks-president-state-union-address

Orbach, B. 2013. What is government failure? *Yale Journal on Regulation* 30:44-56.

Owen, N., E. Leslie, J. Salmon, and M.J. Fotheringham. 2000. Environmental determinants of physical activity and sedentary behavior. *Exercise and Sport Sciences Reviews* 28(4):153-158.

Palmer, K., W.E. Oates, and P.R. Portney. 1995. Tightening environmental standards: The benefit-cost or the no-cost paradigm? *Journal of Economic Perspectives* 9(4):119-132.

Palmer, K.T., R.A.F. Cox, and I. Brown I. 2007. *Fitness for work: The medical aspects*, 4th ed. Oxford, England: Oxford University Press.

Philipson, T.J., and R.A. Posner. 2003. The long-run growth in obesity as a function of technological change. *Perspectives in Biology and Medicine* 46(3):87-108.

Pilat, D., A. Cimper, K. Olsen, and C. Webb. 2006. The changing nature of manufacturing in OECD economies. *OECD Science, Technology and Industry Working Papers* 2006(9).

Porter, M. 1991. America's green strategy. *Scientific American* 264(4):168.

Porter, M., and C. van der Linde. 1995. Toward a new conception of the environment-competitiveness relationship. *Journal of Economic Perspectives* 9(4):97-118.

Pronk, N.P. 2015. Fitness of the US workforce. *Annual Review of Public Health* 36:131-149.

Pronk, N.P., and T.E. Kottke. 2009. Physical activity promotion as a strategic corporate priority to improve worker health and business performance. *Preventive Medicine* 49(4):316-321.

Pronk, N.P., B. Martinson, R.C. Kessler, A.L. Beck, G.E. Simon, and P. Wang. 2004. The association between work performance and physical activity, cardiorespiratory fitness, and obesity. *Journal of Occupational and Environmental Medicine* 46(1):19-25.

Rashid, M., D. Craig, C. Zimring, and M. Thitisawat. 2006. "Sedentary and fleeting activities and their spatial correlates in offices." Paper presented at proceedings of the 37th annual conference of the Environmental Design Research Association (EDRA), Atlanta, May 3-7.

Rashid, M., J. Wineman, and C. Zimring. 2009. Space, behavior, and environmental perception in open plan offices: A prospective study. *Environment and Planning B: Planning and Design* 36:432-449.

Rashid, M., K. Kampschroer, J. Wineman, and C. Zimring. 2006. Spatial layout and face-to-face interaction in offices—A study of the mechanisms of spatial effects on face-to-face interaction. *Environment and Planning B: Planning and Design* 33:825-844.

Rind, E., A. Jones, and H. Southall. 2014. How is post-industrial decline associated with the geography of physical activity? Evidence from the Health Survey for England. *Social Science & Medicine* 104:88-97.

Robinson, R. 1993. Cost-benefit analysis. *British Medical Journal* 307(6909):924-926.

Schinzinger, R. 1998. Ethics on the feedback loop. *Control Engineering Practices* 6(2):239-245.

Shephard, R.J. 1986. *Economic benefits of enhanced fitness.* Champaign, IL: Human Kinetics.

Sturm, R. 2005. Economics and physical activity: A research agenda. *American Journal of Preventive Medicine* 28(2):141-149.

Sunstein, C.R. 2002. *The cost-benefit state: The future of regulatory protection.* Chicago: American Bar Association.

Thaler, R.H., and C.R. Sunstein. 2008. *Nudge: Improving decisions about health, wealth, and happiness.* New York: Penguin.

Thompson, D., G. Oster, J. Brown, G. Nichols, and P. Elmer. 2001. Body mass index and future healthcare costs: A retrospective cohort study. *Obesity Research* 9(3):210-218.

Thornton, M., ed. 2011. *The Bastiat collection*, 2nd ed. Auburn, AL: Ludwig von Mises Institute.

Thorp, A.A., N. Owen, M. Neuhaus, and D.W. Dunstan. 2011. Sedentary behaviors and subsequent health outcomes in adults: A systematic review of longitudinal studies, 1996-2011. *American Journal of Preventive Medicine* 41(2):207-215.

Torbeyns, T., S. Bailey, and I. Bos. 2014. Active workstations to fight sedentary behavior. *Sports Medicine* 20:1-13.

Tudor-Locke, C., C. Leonardi, W.D. Johnson, and P.T. Katzmarzyk. 2011. Time spent in physical activity and sedentary behaviors on the working day: The American time use survey. Journal of Occupational and Environmental Medicine 53(12):1382-1387.

Ucci, M., S. Law, R. Andrews, A. Fisher, L. Smith, A. Sawye,r and A. Marmot. 2015. Indoor school environments, physical activity, sitting behaviour and pedagogy: a

scoping review. Building Research & Information, DOI: 10.1080/09613218.2015.1004275.

U.S. Department of Labor, Bureau of Labor Statistics. 2013. Economic news release. Accessed July 24, 2014. www.bls.gov/news.release/atus.t04.htm

van Amelsvoort, L.G., M.G. Spigt, G.M. Swaen, and I. Kant. 2006. Leisure time physical activity and sickness absenteeism; a prospective study. *Occupational Medicine* 56(3):210-212.

Wolfe, M. 1955. The concept of economic sectors. *Quarterly Journal of Economics* 69(3):402-420.

Chapter 7

Anderson, J.L., H.T. May, B.D. Horne, T.L. Bair, N.L. Hall, J.F. Carlquist, D.L. Lappé, and J.B. Muhlestein. 2010. Relation of vitamin D deficiency to cardiovascular risk factors, disease status, and incident events in a general healthcare population. *American Journal of Cardiology* 106:963-968.

Anderson, L.A., P.G. McTernan, A.H. Barnett, and S. Kumar. 2001. The effects of androgens and estrogens on preadipocyte proliferation in human adipose tissue: Influence of gender and site. *Journal of Clinical Endocrinology & Metabolism* 86:5045-5051.

Bell, N., R.N. Godsen, D.P. Henry, J. Shary, and S. Epstein. 1988. The effects of muscle-building exercise on vitamin D. *Journal of Bone and Mineral Research* 3:369-373.

Brock, K., R. Cant, L. Clemson, R.S. Mason, and D.R. Fraser. 2007. Effects of diet and exercise on plasma vitamin D (25(OH)D) levels in Vietnamese immigrant elderly in Sydney, Australia. *Journal of Steroid Biochemistry and Molecular Biology* 103:786-792.

Brock, K., W-Y. Huang, D.R. Fraser, L. Ke, M. Tseng, R. Stolzenberg-Solomon, U. Peters, et al. 2010. Low vitamin D status is associated with physical inactivity, obesity and low vitamin D intake in a large US sample of healthy middle-aged men and women. *Journal of Steroid Biochemistry and Molecular Biology* 121:462-466

Campos, P., A. Saguy, P. Ernsberger, E. Oliver, and G. Gaesser. 2006. The epidemiology of overweight and obesity: Public health crisis or moral panic? *International Journal of Epidemiology* 35:55-59.

Cannon, W.B. 1935. Stresses and strains of homeostasis. *American Journal of the Medical Sciences* 189:1-14.

Centers for Disease Control and Prevention. 2015. U.S. obesity trends: Trends by state 1985-2014. http://www.cdc.gov/obesity/data/prevalence-maps.html.

Clement, K., and D. Langin. 2007. Regulation of inflammation-related genes in human adipose tissue. *Journal of Internal Medicine* 262:422-430.

Conway, J.M., S.Z. Yanovski, N.A. Avila, and V.S. Hubbard. 1995. Visceral adipose tissue differences in black and white women. *American Journal of Clinical Nutrition* 61:765-771.

Cossrow, N., and B. Falkner. 2004. Race/ethnic issues in obesity and obesity-related comorbidities. *Journal of Clinical Endocrinology & Metabolism* 89:2590-2594.

Coutinho, T., K. Goel, D. Correa de Sa, C. Kragelund, A.M. Kanaya, M. Zeller, J-S. Park, et al. 2011. Central obesity and survival in subjects with coronary artery disease: A systematic review of the literature and collaborative analysis with individual subject data. *American Journal of Cardiology* 57:1877-1886.

Denison, F.C., K.A. Roberts, S.M. Barr, and J.E. Norman. 2010. Obesity, pregnancy, inflammation, and vascular function. *Reproduction* 140:373-385.

Deurenberg, P., M. Deurenberg-Yap, and S. Guricci. 2002. Asians are different from Caucasians and from each other in their body mass index/body fat per cent relationship. *Obesity Reviews* 3:141-146.

Donnelly, J.E., J.O. Hill, D.J. Jacobsen, J. Potteiger, D.K. Sullivan, S.L. Johnson, K. Heelan, et al. 2003. Effects of a 16-month randomized controlled exercise trial on body weight and composition in young, overweight men and women. *Archives of Internal Medicine* 163:1343-1350.

Fain, J.N. 2006. Release of interleukins and other inflammatory cytokines by human adipose tissue is enhanced in obesity and primarily due to the nonfat cells. *Vitamins & Hormones* 74:443-477.

Ferreira, I., M.B. Snijder, J.W.R. Twisk, W. Van Mechelen, H.C.G. Kemper, J.C. Seidell, and C.D.A. Stehouwer. 2004. Central fat mass versus peripheral fat and lean mass: Opposite (adverse versus favorable) associations with arterial stiffness? The Amsterdam growth and health longitudinal study. *Journal of Clinical Endocrinology & Metabolism* 89:2632-2639.

Flegal, K.M. 2006. Commentary: The epidemic of obesity—what's in a name? *International Journal of Epidemiology* 35:72-74.

Flegal, K.M., M.D. Carrol, C.L. Ogden, and L.P. Curtin. 2010. Prevalence and trends in obesity among US adults, 1999-2008. *JAMA* 303:235-241.

Fujioka, S., Y. Matsuzawa, K. Tokunaga, and S. Tarui. 1987. Contribution of intra-abdominal fat accumulation to the impairment of glucose and lipid metabolism in human obesity. *Metabolism* 36:54-59.

Garg, A. 2004. Regional adiposity and insulin resistance. *Journal of Clinical Endocrinology & Metabolism* 89:4206-4210.

Garland, C.F., and F.C. Garland. 1980. Do sunlight and vitamin D reduce the likelihood of colon cancer? *International Journal of Epidemiology* 9:227-231.

Goodpaster, B.H., S. Krishnaswami, T.B. Harris, A. Katsiaras, S.B. Kritchevsky, E.M. Simonsick, M. Nevitt, P. Holvoet, and A.B. Newman. 2005. Obesity, regional body fat distribution, and the metabolic syndrome in older men and women. *Archives of Internal Medicine* 165:777-783.

Gluckman, P., and M. Hanson. 2006. *Mismatch: Why our world no longer fits our bodies.* Oxford, England: Oxford University Press.

Grant, W.B., and C.F. Garland. 2004. A critical review of studies on vitamin D in relation to colorectal cancer. *Nutrition and Cancer* 48:115-123.

Hamadeh, M.J., M.C. Devries, and M.A. Tarnopolsky. 2005. Estrogen supplementation reduces whole body leucine and carbohydrate oxidation and increases lipid oxidation in men during endurance exercise. *Journal of Clinical Endocrinology & Metabolism* 90:3592-3599.

He, Q., M. Horlick, J. Thornton, J. Wang, R.N. Pierson Jr., S. Heshka, and D. Gallagher. 2004. Sex-specific fat distribution is not linear across pubertal groups in a multiethnic study. *Obesity Research* 12:725-733.

Hillman, L.S. 1990. Mineral and vitamin D adequacy in infants fed human milk or formula between 6 and 12 months of age. *Journal of Pediatrics* 117(2 Pt 2):S134-S142.

Holick, M.F., and T.C. Chen. 2008. Vitamin D deficiency: A worldwide problem with health consequences. *American Journal of Clinical Nutrition* 87(4):1080S-1086S.

Jenab, M., H.B. Bueno-de-Mesquita, P. Ferrari, F.J.B. van Duijnhoven, T. Norat, T. Pischon, E.H. Jansen, et al. 2010. Association between pre-diagnostic circulating vitamin D concentration and risk of colorectal cancer in European populations: A nested case-control study. *BMJ* 340:b5500.

Jensen, M.D. 2006. Is visceral fat involved in the pathogenesis of the metabolic syndrome? Human model. *Obesity* 14(Suppl. 1):20S-24S.

Karelis, A.D., D.H. St-Pierre, F. Conus, R. Rabasa-Lhoret, and E.T. Poehlman. 2004. Metabolic and body composition factors in subgroups of obesity: What do we know? *Journal of Clinical Endocrinology & Metabolism* 89:2569-2575.

Kershaw, E.E., and J.S. Flier. 2004. Adipose tissue as an endocrine organ. *Journal of Clinical Endocrinology & Metabolism* 89:2548-2556.

Kim, S., and B.M. Popkin. 2006. Current perspectives on obesity and health: Black and white, or shades of grey? *International Journal of Epidemiology* 35:69-71.

Kintscher, U., M. Hartge, K. Hess, A. Foryst-Ludwig, M. Clemenz, M. Wabitsch, P. Fischer-Posovszky, et al. 2008. T-lymphocyte infiltration in visceral adipose tissue. A primary event in adipose tissue inflammation and the development of obesity-mediated insulin resistance. *Arteriosclerosis, Thrombosis, and Vascular Biology* 28:1304-1310.

Kuk, J.L., S.J. Lee, S.B. Heymsfield, and R. Ross. 2005. Waist circumference and abdominal adipose tissue distribution: Influence of age and sex. *American Journal of Clinical Nutrition* 81:1330-1334.

Lamont, L.S. 2005. Gender differences in amino acid use during endurance exercise. *Nutrition Reviews* 63:419-422.

Lamont, L.S., A.J. McCullough, and S.C. Kalhan. 2001. Gender differences in leucine, but not lysine, kinetics. *Journal of Applied Physiology* 91:357-362.

Lemieux, S., D. Prud'homme, C. Bouchard, A. Tremblay, and J-P. Deprés. 1993. Sex differences in the relation of visceral adipose tissue accumulation to total body fatness. *American Journal of Clinical Nutrition* 58:463-467.

Llewellyn, D.J., I.A. Lang, K.M. Langa, G. Muniz-Terrera, C.L. Phillips, A. Cherubini, L. Ferrucci, and D. Melzer. 2010. Vitamin D and risk of cognitive decline in elderly persons. *Archives of Internal Medicine* 170:1135-1141.

Lumeng, C.N., J.B. DelProposto, D.J. Westcott, and A.R. Saltiel. 2008. Phenotypic switching of adipose tissue macrophages with obesity is generated by spatiotemporal differences in macrophage subtype. *Diabetes* 57:3239-3246.

Malik, V.S., Willett, W.C., and Hu, F.B. 2012. Global obesity: Trends, risk factors and policy implications. *Nature Reviews Endocrinology* 9:13-27.

McEwen, B.S. 1998. Stress, adaptation, and disease: Allostasis and allostatic load. *Annals of the New York Academy of Sciences* 840:33-44.

Mittendorfer, B. 2005. Sexual dimorphism in human lipid metabolism. *Journal of Nutrition* 135:681-686.

Mokha. J.S., S.R. Srinivasan, P. DasMahapatra, C. Fernandez, W. Chen, J. Xu, and G.S. Berenson. 2010. Utility of waist-to-height ratio in assessing the status of central obesity and related cardiometabolic risk profile among normal weight and overweight/obese children: The Bogalusa Heart Study. *BMC Pediatrics* 10:73.

Morris, D.L., K. Singer, and C.N. Lumeng. 2011. Adipose tissue macrophages: Phenotypic plasticity and diversity in lean and obese states. *Current Opinion in Clinical Nutrition & Metabolic Care* 14:341-346.

Nielsen, S., Z.K. Guo, J.B. Albu, S. Klein, P.C. O'Brien, and M.D. Jensen. 2003. Energy expenditure, sex, and endogenous fuel availability in humans. *Journal of Clinical Investigation* 111:981-988.

Nielsen, S., Z.K. Guo, M. Johnson, D.D. Hensrud, and M.D. Jensen. 2004. Splanchnic lipolysis in human obesity. *Journal of Clinical Investigation* 113:1582-1588.

Nishimura, S., I. Manabe, M. Nagasaki, K. Eto, H. Yamashita, M. Ohsugi, M. Otsu, et al. 2009. CD8+ effector T cells contribute to macrophage recruitment and adipose tissue inflammation in obesity. *Nature Medicine* 15:914-920.

Osei, K. 2010. 25-OH vitamin D: Is it the universal panacea for metabolic syndrome and type 2 diabetes? *Journal of Clinical Endocrinology & Metabolism* 95:4220-4222.

Park, Y-W., D.B. Allison, S.B. Heymsfield, and D. Gallagher. 2001. Larger amounts of visceral adipose tissue in Asian Americans. *Obesity Research* 9:381-387.

Pasquali, R., S. Cantobelli, F. Casimirri, M. Capelli, L. Bortoluzzi, R. Flamia, A.M.N. Labate, and L. Barbara. 1993. The hypothalamic-pituitary-adrenal axis in obese women with different patterns of body fat distribution. *Journal of Clinical Endocrinology & Metabolism* 77:341-346.

Pedersen, S.B., K. Kristensen, P.A. Hermann, J.A. Katzenellenbogen, and B. Richelsen. 2004. Estrogen controls lipolysis by up-regulating \ga\2A-adrenergic receptors directly in human adipose tissue through the estrogen receptor \ga\. Implications for the female fat distribution. *Journal of Clinical Endocrinology & Metabolism* 89:1869-1878.

Peters, A., U. Schweiger, L. Pellerin, C. Hubold, K.M. Oltmanns, M. Conrad, B. Schultes, J. Born, and H.L. Fehm. 2004. The selfish brain: Competition for energy resources. *Neuroscience & Biobehavioral Reviews* 28:144-178.

Power, M.L. 2004. Viability as opposed to stability: An evolutionary perspective on physiological regulation. In *Allostasis, homeostasis and the costs of adaptation*, edited by J. Schulkin, 343-364. Cambridge, England: Cambridge University Press.

Power, M.L., and J. Schulkin. 2009. *The evolution of obesity*. Baltimore: Johns Hopkins University Press.

Racette, S.B., J.M. Hagberg, E.M. Evans, J.O. Holloszy, and E.P. Weiss. 2006. Abdominal obesity is a stronger predictor of insulin resistance than fitness among 50-95 year olds. *Diabetes Care* 29:673-678.

Rask, E., B.R. Walker, S. Söderber, D.E.W. Livingstone, M. Eliasson, O. Johnson, R. Andrew, and T. Olsson. 2002. Tissue-specific changes in peripheral cortisol metabolism in obese women: Increased adipose 11\gb\-hydroxysteroid dehydrogenase type 1 activity. *Journal of Clinical Endocrinology & Metabolism* 87:3330-3336.

Rask, E., T. Olsson, S. Söderber, R. Andrew, D.E.W. Livingstone, O. Johnson, and B.R. Walker. 2001. Tissue-specific dysregulation of cortisol metabolism in human obesity. *Journal of Clinical Endocrinology & Metabolism* 86:1418-1421.

Rodríguez, G., M.P. Samper, J.L. Olivares, P. Ventura, L.A. Moreno, and J.M. Pérez-González. 2005. Skinfold measurements at birth: Sex and anthropometric influence. *Archives of Disease in Childhood—Fetal and Neonatal Edition* 90:F273-F275.

Rodriguez-Cuenca, S., M. Monjo, A.M. Proenza, and P. Roca. 2005. Depot differences in steroid receptor expression in adipose tissue: Possible role of the local steroid milieu. *American Journal of Physiology—Endocrinology and Metabolism* 288:E200-E207.

Ross, N. 1997. Effects of diet- and exercise-induced weight loss on visceral adipose tissue in men and women. *Sports Medicine* 24:55-64.

Roth, C.L., C. Elfers, M. Kratz, and A.N. Hoofnagle. 2011. Vitamin D deficiency in obese children and its relationship to insulin resistance and adipokines. *Journal of Obesity* Epub 2011 Dec 29. doi:10.1155/2011/495101.

Roth, J., J.S. Volek, M. Jacobson, J. Hickey, D.T. Stein, S. Klein, R. Feinman, G.J. Schwartz, and C.J. Segal-Isaacson. 2004. Paradigm shifts in obesity research and treatment: Roundtable discussion. *Obesity Research* 12:145S-148S.

Schleithoff, S.S., A. Zittermann, G. Tenderich, H.K. Berthold, P. Stehle, and R. Koerfer. 2006. Vitamin D supplementation improves cytokine profiles in patients with congestive heart failure: A double-blind, randomized, placebo-controlled trial. *American Journal of Clinical Nutrition* 83:754-759.

Schmidt-Nielsen, K. 1994. *Animal physiology: Adaptation and environment*. Cambridge, England: Cambridge University Press.

Schrauwen P., and M.K.C. Hesselink. 2004. Oxidative capacity, lipotoxicity, and mitochondrial damage in type 2 diabetes. *Diabetes* 53:1412-1417.

Schulkin, J. 2003. *Rethinking homeostasis: Allostatic regulation in physiology and pathophysiology.* Cambridge, England: MIT Press.

Seckl, J.R., and B.R. Walker. 2001. 11\gb\-hydroxysteroid dehydrogenase type 1: A tissue-specific amplifier of glucocorticoid action. *Endocrinology* 142:1371-1376.

Singh, R., J.N. Artaza, W.E. Taylor, M. Braga, X. Yuan, N.F. Gonzalez-Cadavid, and S. Bhasin. 2006. Testosterone inhibits adipogenic differentiation in 3T3-L1 cells: Nuclear translocation of androgen receptor complex with beta-catenin and T-cell factor 4 may bypass canonical Wnt signaling to down-regulate adipogenic transcription factors. *Endocrinology* 147:141-154.

Slawik, M., and A.J. Vidal-Puig. 2006. Lipotoxicity, overnutrition and energy metabolism in aging. *Ageing Research Reviews* 5:144-164.

Stewart, P.M., A. Boulton, S. Kumar, P.M.S. Clark, and C.H.L. Shakleton. 1999. Cortisol metabolism in human obesity: Impaired cortisone to cortisol conversion in subjects with central obesity. *Journal of Clinical Endocrinology & Metabolism* 84:1022-1027.

Stimson, R.H., J. Andersson, R. Andrew, D.N. Redhead, F. Karpe, P.C. Hayes, T. Olsson, and B.R. Walker. 2009. Cortisol release from adipose tissue by 11\gb\-hydroxysteroid dehydrogenase type 1 in humans. *Diabetes* 58:46-53.

Tchernof, A., A. Desmeules, C. Richard, P. Laberge, M. Daris, J. Mailloux, C. Rheaume, and P. Dupont. 2004. Ovarian hormone status and abdominal visceral adipose tissue metabolism. *Journal of Clinical Endocrinology & Metabolism* 89:3425-3430.

Tittelbach, T.J., D.M. Berman, B.J. Nicklas, A.S. Ryan, and A.P. Goldberg. 2004. Racial differences in adipocyte size and relationship to the metabolic syndrome in obese women. *Obesity Research* 12:990-998.

Tomlinson, J.W., J. Finney, B.A. Hughes, and P.M. Stewart. 2008. Reduced glucocorticoid production rate, decreased 5\ga\-reductase activity, and adipose tissue insulin sensitization after weight loss. *Diabetes* 57:1536-1543.

Tzotzas, T., F.G. Papadopoulou, K. Tziomalos, S. Karras, K. Gastaris, P. Perros, and G.E. Krassas. 2010. Rising serum 25 hydroxy-vitamin D levels after weight loss in obese women correlate with improvement in insulin resistance. *Journal of Clinical Endocrinology & Metabolism* 95:4251-4257.

Van Pelt, R.E., E.M. Evans, K.B. Schechtman, A.A. Ehsani, and W.M. Kohrt. 2002. Contributions of total and regional fat mass to risk for cardiovascular disease in older women. *American Journal of Physiology—Endocrinology and Metabolism* 282:E1023-E1028.

Van Pelt, R.E., Jankowski, C.M., Gozansky, W.S., Schwartz, R.S., & Kohrt, W.M. (2005). Lower-body adiposity and metabolic protection in postmenopausal women. *The Journal of Clinical Endocrinology & Metabolism,* 90(8), 4573-4578.

van Schoor, N.M., and P. Lips. 2011. Worldwide vitamin D status. *Best Practice & Research Clinical Endocrinology & Metabolism* 25:671-680.

Votruba, S.B., and M.D. Jensen. 2006. Sex-specific differences in leg fat uptake are revealed with a high-fat meal. *American Journal of Physiology—Endocrinology and Metabolism* 291:E1115-E1123.

Wake, D.J., M. Strand, E. Rask, J. Westerbacka, D.E. Livingstone, S. Soderberg, R. Andrew, H. Yki-Jarvinen, T. Olsson, and B.R. Walker. 2007. Intra-adipose sex steroid metabolism and body fat distribution in idiopathic human obesity. *Clinical Endocrinology* 66:440-446.

Weisberg, S.P., D. McCann, M. Desai, M. Rosenbaum, R.L. Leibel, and A.W. Ferrante Jr. 2003. Obesity is associated with macrophage accumulation in adipose tissue. *Journal of Clinical Investigation* 112:1796-1808.

Williams, C.M. 2004. Lipid metabolism in women. *Proceedings of the Nutrition Society* 63:153-160.

Wong, S.N.P., and P. Sicotte. 2007. Activity budget and ranging patterns of Colobus vellerosus in forest fragments in central Ghana. *Folia Primatologica* 78:245-254.

Woodhouse, L.J., N. Gupta, M. Bhasin, A.B. Singh, R. Ross, J. Phillips, and S. Bhasin. 2004. Dose-dependent effects of testosterone on regional adipose tissue distribution in healthy young men. *Journal of Clinical Endocrinology & Metabolism* 89:718-726.

Wortsman, J., L.Y. Matsuoka, T.C. Chen, Z. Lu, and M.F. Holick. 2000. Decreased bioavailability of vitamin D in obesity. *American Journal of Clinical Nutrition* 72:690-693.

Yajnik, C.S. 2004. Early life origins of insulin resistance and type 2 diabetes in India and other Asian countries. *Journal of Nutrition* 134:205-210.

Zhang, R., and D.P. Naughton. 2010. Vitamin D in health and disease: Current perspectives. *Nutrition Journal* 9:65.

Zittermann, A., S. Iodice, S. Pilz, W.B. Grant, V. Bagnardi, and S. Gandini. 2012. Vitamin D deficiency and mortality risk in the general population: A meta-analysis of prospective cohort studies. *American Journal of Clinical Nutrition* 95:91-100.

Chapter 8

Ainsworth, B.E., W.L. Haskell, S.D. Herrmann, N. Meckes, D.R. Bassett, C. Tudor-Locke, K.L. Greer, J. Vezina, M.C. Whitt-Glover, and A.S. Leon. 2011. Compendium of Physical Activities: A second update of codes and MET values. *Medicine and Science in Sports and Exercise* 43:1575-1581.

American Diabetes Association. 2013a. Standards of medical care in diabetes—2013. *Diabetes Care* 36(Suppl. 1):S11-S66.

———. 2013b. Economic costs of diabetes in the U.S. in 2012. *Diabetes Care* 36:1033-1046.

Aronson, D. 2003. Cross-linking of glycated collagen in the pathogenesis of arterial and myocardial stiffening of aging and diabetes. *Journal of Hypertension* 21:3-12.

Biswas, A, P.I. Oh, G.E. Faulkner, R.R. Bajaj, M.A. Silver, M.S. Mitchell, and D.A. Alter. 2015. Sedentary time and its association with risk for disease incidence, mortality, and hospitalization in adults: A systematic review and meta-analysis. *Annals of Internal Medicine* 162(2):123-132.

Bowman, S.A. 2006. Television-viewing characteristics of adults: Correlations to eating practices and overweight and health status. *Preventing Chronic Disease* 2006 Apr. www.cdc.gov/pcd/issues/2006/apr/05_0139.htm.

Boyle, J.P., T.J. Thompson, E.W. Gregg, L.E. Barker, and D.F. Williamson. 2010. Projection of the year 2050 burden of diabetes in the U.S. adult population: Dynamic modeling of incidence, mortality, and prediabetes prevalence. *Population Health Metrics* 8:29.

Caspersen, C.J. 1989. Physical activity epidemiology: Concepts, methods and applications to exercise science. *Exercise and Sport Sciences Reviews* 17:423-473.

Caspersen, C.J., K.E. Powell, and G.M. Christenson. 1985. Physical activity, exercise and physical fitness: Definitions and distinctions for health-related research. *Public Health Reports* 100:126-131.

Centers for Disease Control and Prevention. 2014. *National diabetes statistics report: Estimates of diabetes and its burden in the United States, 2014*. Atlanta: U.S. Department of Health and Human Services.

Church, T.S., D.M. Thomas, C. Tudor-Locke, P.T. Katzmarzyk, C.P. Earnest, R.Q. Rodarte, C.K. Martin, S.N. Blair, and C. Bouchard. 2011. Trends over 5 decades in U.S. occupation-related physical activity and their associations with obesity. *PLoS ONE* 6:e19657.

Clark, B.K., T. Sugiyama, G.N. Healy, J. Salmon, D.W. Dunstan, and N. Owen. 2009. Validity and reliability of measures of television viewing time and other nonoccupational sedentary behaviour of adults: A review. *Obesity Reviews* 10:7-16.

de Fronzo, RA., and D. Tripathy. 2009. Skeletal muscle insulin resistance is the primary defect in type 2 diabetes. *Diabetes Care* 32(Suppl. 2):S157-S163.

Dunstan, D.W., B.A. Kingwell, R. Larsen, G.N. Healy, E. Cerin, M.T. Hamilton, J.E. Shaw, D.A. Bertovic, P.Z. Zimmet, J.Salmon, and N. Owen. 2012. Breaking up prolonged sitting reduces postprandial glucose and insulin responses. *Diabetes Care* 35:976-983.

Dunstan, D.W., J. Salmon, G.N. Healy, J.E. Shaw, D. Jolley, P.Z. Zimmet, and N. Owen. 2007. Association of television viewing with fasting and 2-h postchallenge plasma glucose levels in adults without diagnosed diabetes. *Diabetes Care* 30:516-22.

Dunstan, D.W., J. Salmon, N. Owen, T. Armstrong, P.Z. Zimmet, T.A. Welborn, A.J. Cameron, T. Dwyer, D. Jolley, and J.E. Shaw. 2004. Physical activity and television viewing in relation to risk of undiagnosed abnormal glucose metabolism in adults. *Diabetes Care* 27:2603-2609.

———. 2005. Associations of TV viewing and physical activity with the metabolic syndrome in Australian adults. *Diabetologia* 48:2254-2261.

Engelgau, M.M., L.S. Geiss, J.B. Saaddine, J.P. Boyle, S.M. Benjamin, E.W. Gregg, E.F. Tierney, N. Rios-Burrows, A.H. Mokdad, E.S. Ford, G. Imperatore, and K.M. Narayan. 2004. The evolving diabetes burden in the United States. *Annals of Internal Medicine* 140:945-950.

Ford, E.S., and C.J. Caspersen. 2012. Sedentary behaviour and cardiovascular disease: A review of prospective studies. *International Journal of Epidemiology* 41:1338-53.

Ford, E.S., M.B. Schulze, J. Kroger, T. Pischon, M.M. Bergmann, and H. Boeing. 2010. Television watching and incident diabetes: Findings from the European Prospective Investigation into Cancer and Nutrition-Potsdam Study. *Journal of Diabetes* 2:23-27.

Geiss, L.S., L. Pan, B. Cadwell, E.W. Gregg, S.M. Benjamin, and M.M. Engelgau. 2006. Changes in incidence of diabetes in U.S. adults, 1997-2003. *American Journal of Preventive Medicine* 30:371-377.

Gu, K., C.C. Cowie, and M.I. Harris. 1998. Mortality in adults with and without diabetes in a national cohort of the U.S. population, 1971-1993. *Diabetes Care* 21:1138-1145.

Hamburg, N.M., C.J. McMackin, A.L. Huang, S.M. Shenouda, M.E. Widlansky, E. Schulz, N. Gokce, N.B. Ruderman, J.F. Keaney Jr., and J.A. Vita. 2007. Physical inactivity rapidly induces insulin resistance and microvascular dysfunction in healthy volunteers. *Arteriosclerosis, Thrombosis, and Vascular Biology* 27:2650-2656.

Healy, G.N., C.E. Matthews, D.W. Dunstan, E.A.H. Winkler, and N. Owen. 2011. Sedentary time and cardio-metabolic biomarkers in U.S. adults: NHANES 2003-06. *European Heart Journal* 32:590-597.

Healy, G.N., K. Wijndaele, D.W. Dunstan, J.E. Shaw, J. Salmon, P.Z. Zimmet, and N. Owen. 2008. Objectively measured sedentary time, physical activity, and metabolic risk: The Australian Diabetes, Obesity and Lifestyle Study (AusDiab). *Diabetes Care* 31:369-371.

Hill, A.B. 1965. President's address. The environment and disease: Association or causation? *Proceedings of the Royal Society of Medicine* 58:295-300.

Hu, F.B., M.F. Leitzmann, M.J. Stampfer, G.A. Colditz, W.C. Willett, and E.B. Rimm. 2001. Physical activity and television watching in relation to risk for type 2 diabetes mellitus in men. *Archives of Internal Medicine* 161:1542-1548.

Hu, F.B., T.Y. Li, G.A. Colditz, W.C. Willett, and J.E. Manson. 2003. Television watching and other sedentary behaviors in relation to risk of obesity and type 2 diabetes mellitus in women. *JAMA* 289:1785-1791.

Krishnan, S., L. Rosenberg, and J.R. Palmer. 2009. Physical activity and television watching in relation to risk of type 2 diabetes: The Black Women's Health Study. *American Journal of Epidemiology* 169:428-434.

Levine, J.A., N.L. Eberhardt, and M.D. Jensen. 1999. Role of nonexercise activity thermogenesis in resistance to fat gain in humans. *Science* 283:212-214.

Maher, C., T. Olds, E. Mire, and P.T. Katzmarzyk. 2014. Reconsidering the sedentary behaviour paradigm. *PLoS ONE* 9(1):e86403. doi:10.1371/journal.pone.0086403.

McKenzie, B., and M. Rapino. 2011. *Commuting in the United States: 2009. American Community Survey Reports No. ACS-15*. Washington, D.C.: U.S. Census Bureau.

McMurray, R.G., J. Soares, C.J. Caspersen, and T. McCurdy. 2014. Examining variations of resting metabolic rate of adults: A public health perspective. *Medicine and Science in Sports and Exercise* 46(7):1352-1358.

Mortensen, L.H., I.C. Siegler, J.C. Barefoot, M. Grønbæk, and T.I.A. Sørensen. 2006. Prospective associations between sedentary lifestyle and BMI in midlife. *Obesity* 14:1462-1471.

Narayan, K.M., J.P. Boyle, L.S. Geiss, J.B. Saaddine, and T.J. Thompson. 2006. Impact of recent increase in incidence on future diabetes burden: U.S., 2005-2050. *Diabetes Care* 29:2114-2116.

National Diabetes Education Program. 2012. *Are you at risk for type 2 diabetes?* www.niddk.nih.gov/health-information/health-communication-programs/ndep/ndep-health-topics/Documents/NDEP_Risk_test.pdf.

Nielsen Company. 2012. *State of the media: The Cross Platform Report Q2, 2012*. www.nielsen.com/us/en/reports/2012/state-of-the-media--cross-platform-report-q2-2012.html.

Noble, D., R. Mathur, T. Dent, C. Meads, and T. Greenhalgh. 2011. Risk models and scores for type 2 diabetes: Systematic review. *BMJ* 2011 Nov 28; 343:d7163. doi: 10.1136/bmj.d7163.

Powell, K.E., P.D. Thompson, C.J. Caspersen, and J.S. Kendrick. 1987. Physical activity and the incidence of coronary heart disease. *Annual Review of Public Health* 8:253-287.

Pulsford, R.M., E. Stamatakis, A.R. Britton, E.J. Brunner, and M.M. Hillsdon. 2013. Sitting behavior and obesity: Evidence from the Whitehall II Study. *American Journal of Preventive Medicine* 44(2):132-138.

Robinson, T.N. 1999. Reducing children's television viewing to prevent obesity: A randomized controlled trial. *JAMA* 282:1561-1567.

Rockette-Wagner, B., S. Edelstein, E.M. Venditti, D. Reddy, G.A. Bray, M.L. Carrion-Petersen, D. Dabelea, L.M. Delahanty, H. Florez, P.W. Franks, M.G. Montez, R. Rubin, and A.M. Kriska. 2015. The impact of lifestyle intervention on sedentary time in individuals at high risk of diabetes. *Diabetologia* 58(6):1198-1202.

Sedentary Behaviour Research Network. 2012. Letter to the Editor: Standardized use of the terms "sedentary" and "sedentary behaviours." *Applied Physiology: Nutrition Metabolism* 37:540-542.

Taylor, H.L., E.R. Buskirk, and R.D. Remington. 1973. Exercise in controlled trials of the prevention of coronary heart disease. *Federation Proceedings* 32:1623-1627.

Ulrich, P., and A. Cerami. 2001. Protein glycation, diabetes, and aging. *Recent Progress in Hormone Research* 56:1-21.

U.S. Department of Health and Human Services. 1996. *Physical activity and health: A report of the Surgeon General*. Atlanta: Author.

———. 2008. *2008 physical activity guidelines for Americans*. Washington, D.C.: Author. www.health.gov/paguidelines.

U.S. Public Health Service, Department of Health, Education, and Welfare. Smoking and Health. 1964. *Report of the Advisory Committee to the Surgeon General of the Public Health Service*. (DHEW publication no. (PHS) 1103). Washington, D.C.: Author.

Chapter 9

Aman, J., T.C. Skinner, C.E. de Beaufort, P.G. Swift, H.J. Aanstoot, and F. Cameron. 2009. Associations between physical activity, sedentary behavior, and glycemic control in a large cohort of adolescents with type 1 diabetes: The Hvidoere Study Group on Childhood Diabetes. *Pediatric Diabetes* 10(4):234-239.

Archer, E., and S.N. Blair. 2011. Physical activity and the prevention of cardiovascular disease: From evolution to epidemiology. *Progress in Cardiovascular Diseases* 53(6):387-396.

Archer, E., C.J. Lavie, S.M. McDonald, D.M. Thomas, J.R. Hébert, S.E. Taverno Ross, K.L. McIver, R.M. Malina, and S.N. Blair. 2013. Maternal inactivity: 45-year trends in mothers' use of time. *Mayo Clinic Proceedings* 88(12):1368-1377.

Archer, E., R.P. Shook, D.M. Thomas, T.S. Church, P.T. Katzmarzyk, J.R. Hebert, K.L. McIver, G.A. Hand, C.J. Lavie, and S.N. Blair. 2013. 45-year trends in women's use of time and household management energy expenditure. *PLoS One* 8(2):e56620.

Assmann, G., R. Carmena, P. Cullen, J.C. Fruchart, F. Jossa, B. Lewis, M. Mancini, and R. Paoletti. 1999. Coronary heart disease: Reducing the risk: A worldwide view. International Task Force for the Prevention of Coronary Heart Disease. *Circulation* 100(18):1930-1938.

Assmann, G., and A.M. Gotto Jr. 2004. HDL cholesterol and protective factors in atherosclerosis. *Circulation* 109(23 Suppl. 1):III8-14.

Australian Bureau of Statistics (ABS). 2008. *How Australians use their time*. Canberra: Author.

Ayer, J., and K. Steinbeck. 2010. Placing the cardiovascular risk of childhood obesity in perspective. *International Journal of Obesity* 34(1):4-5.

Beaglehole, R., R. Bonita, R. Horton, C. Adams, G. Alleyne, P. Asaria, V. Baugh, et al. 2011. Priority actions for the non-communicable disease crisis. *Lancet* 377(9775):1438-1447.

Beaglehole, R., S. Ebrahim, S. Reddy, J. Voute, S. Leeder, and Group Chronic Disease Action. 2007. Prevention of chronic diseases: A call to action. *Lancet* 370(9605):2152-2157.

Blair, S.N. 2009. Physical inactivity: The biggest public health problem of the 21st century. *British Journal of Sports Medicine* 43(1):1-2.

Blair, S.N., and S. Brodney. 1999. Effects of physical inactivity and obesity on morbidity and mortality: Current evidence and research issues. *Medicine & Science in Sports & Exercise* 31(11 Suppl.):S646-S662.

Blair, S.N., Y. Cheng, and J.S. Holder. 2001. Is physical activity or physical fitness more important in defining health benefits? *Medicine & Science in Sports & Exercise* 33(6 Suppl.):S379-S399; discussion S419-S420.

Blair, S.N., G. Davey Smith, I.M. Lee, K. Fox, M. Hillsdon, R.E. McKeown, W.L. Haskell, and M. Marmot. 2010. A tribute to Professor Jeremiah Morris: The man who invented the field of physical activity epidemiology. *Annals of Epidemiology* 20(9):651-660.

Blair, S.N., E. Horton, A.S. Leon, I.M. Lee, B.L. Drinkwater, R.K. Dishman, M. Mackey, and M.L. Kienholz. 1996a. Physical activity, nutrition, and chronic disease. *Medicine & Science in Sports & Exercise* 28(3):335-349.

Blair, S.N., J.B. Kampert, H.W. Kohl III, C.E. Barlow, C.A. Macera, R.S. Paffenbarger Jr., and L.W. Gibbons. 1996b. Influences of cardiorespiratory fitness and other precursors on cardiovascular disease and all-cause mortality in men and women. *JAMA* 276(3):205-210.

Blair, S.N., H.W. Kohl III, C.E. Barlow, R.S. Paffenbarger Jr., L.W. Gibbons, and C.A. Macera. 1995. Changes in physical fitness and all-cause mortality. A prospective study of healthy and unhealthy men. *JAMA* 273(14):1093-1098.

Blair, S.N., H.W. Kohl III, R.S. Paffenbarger Jr., D.G. Clark, K.H. Cooper, and L.W. Gibbons. 1989. Physical fitness and all-cause mortality: A prospective study of healthy men and women. *JAMA* 262(17):2395-2401.

Blair, S.N., and J.N. Morris. 2009. Healthy hearts—and the universal benefits of being physically active: Physical activity and health. *Annals of Epidemiology* 19(4):253-256.

Booth, F.W., M.J. Laye, and M.D. Roberts. 2011. Lifetime sedentary living accelerates some aspects of secondary aging. *Journal of Applied Physiology* 111(5):1497-1504.

Brunner, D., G. Manelis, M. Modan, and S. Levin. 1974. Physical activity at work and the incidence of myocardial infarction, angina pectoris and death due to ischemic heart disease. An epidemiological study in Israeli collective settlements (Kibbutzim). *Journal of Chronic Diseases* 27(4):217-233.

Burke, A., and G.A. FitzGerald. 2003. Oxidative stress and smoking-induced vascular injury. *Progress in Cardiovascular Diseases* 46(1):79-90.

Cecchini, M., F. Sassi, J.A. Lauer, Y.Y. Lee, V. Guajardo-Barron, and D. Chisholm. 2010. Tackling of unhealthy diets, physical inactivity, and obesity: Health effects and cost-effectiveness. *Lancet* 376(9754):1775-1784.

Charansonney, O.L. 2011. Physical activity and aging: A life-long story. *Discovery Medicine* 12(64):177-185.

Church, T.S., D.M. Thomas, C. Tudor-Locke, P.T. Katzmarzyk, C.P. Earnest, R.Q. Rodarte, C.K. Martin, S.N. Blair, and C. Bouchard. 2011. Trends over 5 decades in U.S. occupation-related physical activity and their associations with obesity. *PLoS One* 6(5):e19657.

Coccheri, S. 2007. Approaches to prevention of cardiovascular complications and events in diabetes mellitus. *Drugs* 67(7):997-1026.

Cooper, T.V., L.M. Klesges, M. Debon, R.C. Klesges, and M.L. Shelton. 2006. An assessment of obese and non obese girls' metabolic rate during television viewing, reading, and resting. *Eating Behaviors* 7(2):105-114.

Corbi, G., V. Conti, G. Russomanno, G. Rengo, P. Vitulli, A.L. Ciccarelli, A. Filippelli, and N. Ferrara. 2012. Is physical activity able to modify oxidative damage in cardiovascular aging? *Oxidative Medicine and Cellular Longevity* 2012:728547.

Davis, A.M., K.J. Bennett, C. Befort, and N. Nollen. 2011. Obesity and related health behaviors among urban and rural children in the United States: Data from the National Health and Nutrition Examination Survey 2003-2004 and 2005-2006. *Journal of Pediatric Psychology* 36(6):669-676.

Deanfield, J., A. Donald, C. Ferri, C. Giannattasio, J. Halcox, S. Halligan, A. Lerman, et al. 2005. Endothelial function and dysfunction. Part I: Methodological issues for assessment in the different vascular beds: a statement by the Working Group on Endothelin and Endothelial Factors of the European Society of Hypertension. *Journal of Hypertension* 23(1):7-17.

Di Angelantonio, E., P. Gao, L. Pennells, S. Kaptoge, M. Caslake, A. Thompson, A.S. Butterworth, et al. 2012. Lipid-related markers and cardiovascular disease prediction. *JAMA* 307(23):2499-2506.

Dunstan, D.W., E.L. Barr, G.N. Healy, J. Salmon, J.E. Shaw, B. Balkau, D.J. Magliano, A.J. Cameron, P.Z. Zimmet, and N. Owen. 2010. Television viewing time and mortality: The Australian Diabetes, Obesity and Lifestyle Study (AusDiab). *Circulation* 121(3):384-391.

Dwivedi, G., and S. Dwivedi. 2007. Sushruta—the clinician—Teacher par excellence. *Indian Journal of Chest Diseases and Allied Sciences* 49:243-244.

Earnest, C.P., E.G. Artero, X. Sui, D.C. Lee, T.S. Church, and S.N. Blair. 2013. Maximal estimated cardiorespiratory fitness, cardiometabolic risk factors, and metabolic syndrome in the Aerobics Center Longitudinal Study. *Mayo Clinic Proceedings* 88(3):259-270.

Evenson, K.R., W.D. Rosamond, J. Cai, A.V. Diez-Roux, and F.L. Brancati. 2002. Influence of retirement on leisure-time physical activity: The atherosclerosis risk in communities study. *American Journal of Epidemiology* 155(8):692-699.

Faulkner, R.A., and D.A. Bailey. 2007. Osteoporosis: A pediatric concern? *Medicine and Sport Science* 51:1-12.

Fletcher, G.F., G.J. Balady, S.N. Blair, J. Blumenthal, C. Caspersen, B. Chaitman, S. Epstein, et al. 1996. Statement on exercise: Benefits and recommendations for physical activity programs for all Americans: A statement for health professionals by the Committee on Exercise and Cardiac Rehabilitation of the Council on Clinical Cardiology, American Heart Association. *Circulation* 94(4):857-862.

Fletcher, G.F., S.N. Blair, J. Blumenthal, C. Caspersen, B. Chaitman, S. Epstein, H. Falls, E.S. Froelicher, V.F. Froelicher, and I.L. Pina. 1992. Statement on exercise. Benefits and recommendations for physical activity programs for all Americans. A statement for health professionals by the Committee on Exercise and Cardiac Rehabilitation of the Council on Clinical Cardiology, American Heart Association. *Circulation* 86(1):340-344.

Freedman, D.S., W.H. Dietz, S.R. Srinivasan, and G.S. Berenson. 1999. The relation of overweight to cardiovascular risk factors among children and adolescents: The Bogalusa Heart Study. *Pediatrics* 103(6 Pt 1):1175-1182.

Gidding, S.S., W. Bao, S.R. Srinivasan, and G.S. Berenson. 1995. Effects of secular trends in obesity on coronary risk factors in children: The Bogalusa Heart Study. *Journal of Pediatrics* 127(6):868-874.

Gidding, S.S., A.H. Lichtenstein, M.S. Faith, A. Karpyn, J.A. Mennella, B. Popkin, J. Rowe, L. Van Horn, and L. Whitsel. 2009. Implementing American Heart Association pediatric and adult nutrition guidelines: A scientific statement from the American Heart Association Nutrition Committee of the Council on Nutrition, Physical Activity and Metabolism, Council on Cardiovascular Disease in the Young, Council on Arteriosclerosis, Thrombosis and Vascular Biology, Council on Cardiovascular Nursing, Council on Epidemiology and Prevention, and Council for High Blood Pressure Research. *Circulation* 119(8):1161-1175.

Go, A.S., D. Mozaffarian, V.L. Roger, E.J. Benjamin, J.D. Berry, W.B. Borden, D.M. Bravata, et al. 2013. Executive summary: Heart disease and stroke statistics—2013 update: A report from the American Heart Association. *Circulation* 127(1):143-152.

Goldbourt, U., and H.N. Neufeld. 1986. Genetic aspects of arteriosclerosis. *Arteriosclerosis* 6(4):357-377.

Green, R.M., trans. 1951. *Galen's hygiene (De Sanitate Tuenda)*. Springfield, IL: Charles C. Thomas.

Grontved, A., and F.B. Hu. 2011. Television viewing and risk of type 2 diabetes, cardiovascular disease, and all-cause mortality: A meta-analysis. *JAMA* 305(23):2448-2455.

Gupta, R., and P. Deedwania. 2011. Interventions for cardiovascular disease prevention. *Cardiology Clinics* 29(1):15-34.

Guthrie, D. 1956. India's contribution to the history of medicine. *Nature* 178:1079-1134.

Guy, W.A. 1843. Contributions to a knowledge of the influence of employments upon health. *Journal of the Statistical Society of London* 6(3):197-211.

Halliwell, B. 2000. Lipid peroxidation, antioxidants and cardiovascular disease: How should we move forward? *Cardiovascular Research* 47(3):410-418.

Hamilton, M.T., D.G. Hamilton, and T.W. Zderic. 2007. Role of low energy expenditure and sitting in obesity, metabolic syndrome, type 2 diabetes, and cardiovascular disease. *Diabetes* 56(11):2655-2667.

Hedley, O.F. 1939. Five years' experience (1933-1937) with mortality from acute coronary occlusion in Philadelphia. Annals of Internal Medicine 13(4):598-611.

Heron, M., D.L. Hoyert, S.L. Murphy, J. Xu, K.D. Kochanek, and B. Tejada-Vera. 2009. Deaths: Final data for 2006. *National Vital Statistics Reports* 57(14):1-134.

Hippocrates. 1868. Hippocrates Collected Works I. In *Digital Hippocrates Collection*, edited by W.H.S. Jones. Cambridge, England: Harvard University Press.

Hu, G., J. Tuomilehto, K. Silventoinen, N.C. Barengo, M. Peltonen, and P. Jousilahti. 2005. The effects of physical activity and body mass index on cardiovascular, cancer and all-cause mortality among 47 212 middle-aged Finnish men and women. *International Journal of Obesity* 29(8):894-902.

Janz, K.F., J.D. Dawson, and L.T. Mahoney. 2000. Tracking physical fitness and physical activity from childhood to adolescence: The Muscatine study. *Medicine & Science in Sports & Exercise* 32(7):1250-1257.

Jensen, J., P.I. Rustad, A.J. Kolnes, and Y.C. Lai. 2011. The role of skeletal muscle glycogen breakdown for regulation of insulin sensitivity by exercise. *Frontiers in Physiology* 2:112.

Kahn, H.A. 1963. The relationship of reported coronary heart disease mortality to physical activity of work. *American Journal of Public Health Nations Health* 53:1058-1067.

Katzmarzyk, P.T., T.S. Church, C.L. Craig, and C. Bouchard. 2009. Sitting time and mortality from all causes, cardiovascular disease, and cancer. *Medicine & Science in Sports & Exercise* 41(5):998-1005.

Kavey, R.E., S.R. Daniels, R.M. Lauer, D.L. Atkins, L.L. Hayman, and K. Taubert. 2003. American Heart Association guidelines for primary prevention of atherosclerotic cardiovascular disease beginning in childhood. *Journal of Pediatrics* 142(4):368-372.

Klesges, R.C., M.L. Shelton, and L.M. Klesges. 1993. Effects of television on metabolic rate: Potential implications for childhood obesity. *Pediatrics* 91(2):281-286.

Kones, R. 2011. Primary prevention of coronary heart disease: Integration of new data, evolving views, revised goals, and role of rosuvastatin in management. A comprehensive survey. *Drug Design, Development and Therapy* 5:325-380.

Kushi, L.H., C. Doyle, M. McCullough, C.L. Rock, W. Demark-Wahnefried, E.V. Bandera, S. Gapstur, A.V. Patel, K. Andrews, and T. Gansler. 2012. American Cancer Society guidelines on nutrition and physical activity for cancer prevention: Reducing the risk of cancer with healthy food choices and physical activity. *CA: A Cancer Journal for Clinicians* 62(1):30-67.

Lagerros, Y.T., S.F. Hsieh, and C.C. Hsieh. 2004. Physical activity in adolescence and young adulthood and breast cancer risk: A quantitative review. European Journal of Cancer Prevention 13(1):5-12.

LaMonte, M.J., C.E. Barlow, R. Jurca, J.B. Kampert, T.S. Church, and S.N. Blair. 2005. Cardiorespiratory fitness is inversely associated with the incidence of metabolic syndrome: A prospective study of men and women. *Circulation* 112(4):505-512.

LaMonte, M.J., S.N. Blair, and T.S. Church. 2005. Physical activity and diabetes prevention. *Journal of Applied Physiology* 99(3):1205-1213.

Lavie, C.J., L.P. Cahalin, P. Chase, J. Myers, D. Bensimhon, M.A. Peberdy, E. Ashley, et al. 2013. Impact of cardiorespiratory fitness on the obesity paradox in patients with heart failure. *Mayo Clinic Proceedings* 88(3):251-258.

Lee, C.D., D.R. Jacobs Jr., A. Hankinson, C. Iribarren, and S. Sidney. 2009. Cardiorespiratory fitness and coronary artery calcification in young adults: The CARDIA Study. *Atherosclerosis* 203(1):263-268.

Lee, I.M., E.J. Shiroma, F. Lobelo, P. Puska, S.N. Blair, and P.T. Katzmarzyk. 2012. Effect of physical inactivity on major non-communicable diseases worldwide: An analysis of burden of disease and life expectancy. *Lancet* 380(9838):219-229.

Leung, F.P., L.M. Yung, I. Laher, X. Yao, Z.Y. Chen, and Y. Huang. 2008. Exercise, vascular wall and cardiovascular diseases: An update (Part 1). *Sports Medicine* 38(12):1009-1024.

Levine, J.A., L.M. Lanningham-Foster, S.K. McCrady, A.C. Krizan, L.R. Olson, P.H. Kane, M.D. Jensen, and M.M. Clark. 2005. Interindividual variation in posture allocation: Possible role in human obesity. *Science* 307(5709):584-586.

Lewington, S., F. Bragg, and R. Clarke. 2012. A review on metaanalysis of biomarkers: Promises and pitfalls. *Clinical Chemistry* 58(8):1192-1204.

Libby, P. 2000. Changing concepts of atherogenesis. *Journal of Internal Medicine* 247(3):349-358.

Lusis, A.J. 2000. Atherosclerosis. *Nature* 407(6801):233-241.

Lusis, A.J., A. Weinreb, and T.A. Drake. 1998. Risk factors for atherosclerosis. In *Textbook of Cardiovascular Medicine*, edited by E.J. Topol, pages 2389-2413. Philadelphia: Lippincott.

Macera, C.A., S.A. Ham, M.M. Yore, D.A. Jones, B.E. Ainsworth, C.D. Kimsey, and H.W. Kohl III. 2005. Prevalence of physical activity in the United States: Behavioral risk factor surveillance system, 2001. *Preventing Chronic Disease* 2(2):A17.

Martin, B.J., and T.J. Anderson. 2009. Risk prediction in cardiovascular disease: The prognostic significance of endothelial dysfunction. *Canadian Journal of Cardiology* 25(Suppl. A):15A-20A.

McDonald, N.C. 2007. Active transportation to school: Trends among U.S. schoolchildren, 1969-2001. *American Journal of Preventive Medicine* 32(6):509-516.

McDonogh, J.R., C.G. Hames, S.C. Stulb, and G.E. Garrison. 1965. Coronary heart disease among Negroes and Whites in Evans County, Georgia. *Journal of Chronic Diseases* 18:443-468.

McGill, H.C., Jr., C.A. McMahan, E.E. Herderick, A.W. Zieske, G.T. Malcom, R.E. Tracy, and J.P. Strong. 2002. Obesity accelerates the progression of coronary atherosclerosis in young men. *Circulation* 105(23):2712-2718.

Mendis, S., P. Puska, and B. Norrving. 2011. *Global atlas on cardiovascular disease prevention and control.* Geneva: World Health Organization.

Morris, J.N., J.A. Heady, P.A. Raffle, C.G. Roberts, and J.W. Parks. 1953. Coronary heart disease and physical activity of work. *Lancet* 265(6796):1111-1120; concl.

Nelson, M.C., P. Gordon-Larsen, L.S. Adair, and B.M. Popkin. 2005. Adolescent physical activity and sedentary behavior: Patterning and long-term maintenance. *American Journal of Preventive Medicine* 28(3):259-266.

Nielsen. 2011. State of the media: TV usage trends: Q3 and Q4 2010. www.nielsen.com/us/en/insights/reports/2011/state-of-the-media-tv-usage-trends-q3-and-q4-2010.html

Nieto, F.J. 1999. Cardiovascular disease and risk factor epidemiology: A look back at the epidemic of the 20th century. *American Journal of Public Health* 89(3):292-294.

Nikolaidis, M.G., A. Kyparos, C. Spanou, V. Paschalis, A.A. Theodorou, and I.S. Vrabas. 2012. Redox biology of exercise: An integrative and comparative consideration of some overlooked issues. *Journal of Experimental Biology* 215(Pt. 10):1615-1625.

Nikolopoulou, A., and N.P. Kadoglou. 2012. Obesity and metabolic syndrome as related to cardiovascular disease. *Expert Review of Cardiovascular Therapy* 10(7):933-939.

Nissinen, A., J. Pekkanen, A. Porath, S. Punsar, and M.J. Karvonen. 1989. Risk factors for cardiovascular disease among 55 to 74 year-old Finnish men: A 10-year follow-up. *Annals of Medicine* 21(3):239-240.

Nobili, V., A. Alisi, and M. Raponi. 2009. Pediatric non-alcoholic fatty liver disease: Preventive and therapeutic value of lifestyle intervention. *World Journal of Gastroenterology* 15(48):6017-6022.

Nordestgaard, B.G., M.J. Chapman, K. Ray, J. Boren, F. Andreotti, G.F. Watts, H. Ginsberg, et al. 2010. Lipoprotein(a) as a cardiovascular risk factor: Current status. *European Heart Journal* 31(23):2844-2853.

Norrving, B., and B. Kissela. 2013. The global burden of stroke and need for a continuum of care. *Neurology* 80(3 Suppl. 2):S5-S12.

Olsen, R.H., R. Krogh-Madsen, C. Thomsen, F.W. Booth, and B.K. Pedersen. 2008. Metabolic responses to reduced daily steps in healthy nonexercising men. *JAMA* 299(11):1261-1263.

Paffenbarger, R.S., and W.E. Hale. 1975. Work activity and coronary heart mortality. *New England Journal of Medicine* 292(11):545-550.

Pate, R.R., J.R. O'Neill, and F. Lobelo. 2008. The evolving definition of "sedentary". *Exercise and Sport Sciences Reviews* 36(4):173-178.

Piarulli, F., G. Sartore, and A. Lapolla. 2012. Glyco-oxidation and cardiovascular complications in type 2 diabetes: A clinical update. *Acta Diabetologica* Epub 2012 Jul 5. doi: 10.1007/s00592-012-0412-3.

Pillard, F., D. Laoudj-Chenivesse, G. Carnac, J. Mercier, J. Rami, D. Riviere, and Y. Rolland. 2011. Physical activity and sarcopenia. *Clinics in Geriatric Medicine* 27(3):449-470.

Roger, V.L., A.S. Go, D.M. Lloyd-Jones, E.J. Benjamin, J.D. Berry, W.B. Borden, D.M. Bravata, et al. 2012. Heart disease and stroke statistics—2012 update: A report from the American Heart Association. *Circulation* 125(1):e2-e220.

Rosenfeld, M.E. 1998. Inflammation, lipids, and free radicals: Lessons learned from the atherogenic process. *Seminars in Reproductive Endocrinology* 16(4):249-261.

Sallis, J.F., T.L. McKenzie, J.E. Alcaraz, B. Kolody, N. Faucette, and M.F. Hovell. 1997. The effects of a 2-year physical education program (SPARK) on physical activity and fitness in elementary school students. Sports, Play and Active Recreation for Kids. *American Journal of Public Health* 87(8):1328-1334.

Siri-Tarino, P.W., Q. Sun, F.B. Hu, and R.M. Krauss. 2010. Meta-analysis of prospective cohort studies evaluating the association of saturated fat with cardiovascular disease. *American Journal of Clinical Nutrition* 91(3):535-546.

Sisson, S.B., and S.T. Broyles. 2012. Social-ecological correlates of excessive TV viewing: Difference by race and sex. *Journal of Physical Activity & Health* 9(3):449-455.

Slattery, M.L., D.R. Jacobs, Jr., and M.Z. Nichaman. 1989. Leisure time physical activity and coronary heart disease death. The US Railroad Study. *Circulation* 79(2):304-311.

Smith, E. 1864. Report on the sanitary conditions of tailors in London. In *Report of the Medical Officer*, 416-430. London: The Privy Council.

Smith, S.C., A. Collins, R. Ferrari, D.R. Holmes, S. Logstrup, D.V. McGhie, J. Ralston, et al. 2012. Our time: A call to save preventable death from cardiovascular disease (heart disease and stroke). *European Heart Journal* 33(23):2910-2916.

Strong, J.P., G.T. Malcom, C.A. McMahan, R.E. Tracy, W.P. Newman III, E.E. Herderick, and J.F. Cornhill. 1999. Prevalence and extent of atherosclerosis in adolescents and young adults: Implications for prevention from the Pathobiological Determinants of Atherosclerosis in Youth Study. *JAMA* 281(8):727-735.

Sui, X., D.C. Lee, C.E. Matthews, S.A. Adams, J.R. Hebert, T.S. Church, C.D. Lee, and S.N. Blair. 2010. Influence of cardiorespiratory fitness on lung cancer mortality. *Medicine & Science in Sports & Exercise* 42(5):872-878.

Tabas, I., and C.K. Glass. 2013. Anti-inflammatory therapy in chronic disease: Challenges and opportunities. *Science* 339(6116):166-172.

Taveras, E.M., K.H. Hohman, S. Price, S.L. Gortmaker, and K. Sonneville. 2009. Televisions in the bedrooms of racial/ethnic minority children: How did they get there and how do we get them out? *Clinical Pediatrics* 48(7):715-719.

Thijssen, D.H., A.J. Maiorana, G. O'Driscoll, N.T. Cable, M.T. Hopman, and D.J. Green. 2010. Impact of inactivity and exercise on the vasculature in humans. *European Journal of Applied Physiology* 108(5):845-875.

Thorp, A.A., G.N. Healy, N. Owen, J. Salmon, K. Ball, J.E. Shaw, P.Z. Zimmet, and D.W. Dunstan. 2010. Deleterious associations of sitting time and television viewing time with cardiometabolic risk biomarkers: Australian Diabetes, Obesity and Lifestyle (AusDiab) study 2004-2005. *Diabetes Care* 33(2):327-334.

Thorp, A.A., N. Owen, M. Neuhaus, and D.W. Dunstan. 2011. Sedentary behaviors and subsequent health outcomes in adults: A systematic review of longitudinal studies, 1996-2011. *American Journal of Preventive Medicine* 41(2):207-215.

Thyfault, J.P., and R. Krogh-Madsen. 2011. Metabolic disruptions induced by reduced ambulatory activity in free living humans. *Journal of Applied Physiology* 111(4):1218-1224.

Touvier, M., S. Bertrais, H. Charreire, A.C. Vergnaud, S. Hercberg, and J.M. Oppert. 2010. Changes in leisure-time physical activity and sedentary behaviour at retirement: A prospective study in middle-aged French subjects. *International Journal of Behavioral Nutrition and Physical Activity* 7:14.

Truong, U.T., D.M. Maahs, and S.R. Daniels. 2012. Cardiovascular disease in children and adolescents with diabetes: Where are we, and where are we going? *Diabetes Technology & Therapeutics* 14(Suppl. 1):S11-S21.

Tucker, J.M., G.J. Welk, and N.K. Beyler. 2011. Physical activity in U.S.: Adults' compliance with the Physical Activity Guidelines for Americans. *American Journal of Preventive Medicine* 40(4):454-461.

Tuzcu, E.M., S.R. Kapadia, E. Tutar, K.M. Ziada, R.E. Hobbs, P.M. McCarthy, J.B. Young, and S.E. Nissen. 2001. High prevalence of coronary atherosclerosis in asymptomatic teenagers and young adults: Evidence from intravascular ultrasound. *Circulation* 103(22):2705-2710.

Vassalle, C., T. Simoncini, P. Chedraui, and F.R. Perez-Lopez. 2012. Why sex matters: The biological mechanisms of cardiovascular disease. *Gynecological Endocrinology* 28(9):746-751.

Vuori, I.M. 2001. Health benefits of physical activity with special reference to interaction with diet. *Public Health Nutrition* 4(2B):517-528.

Wai, F.K. 2004. On Hua Tuo's position in the history of Chinese medicine. *American Journal of Chinese Medicine* 32(2):313-320.

Warren, T.Y., V. Barry, S.P. Hooker, X. Sui, T.S. Church, and S.N. Blair. 2010. Sedentary behaviors increase risk of cardiovascular disease mortality in men. *Medicine & Science in Sports & Exercise* 42(5):879-885.

Wei, M., J.B. Kampert, C.E. Barlow, M.Z. Nichaman, L.W. Gibbons, R.S. Paffenbarger Jr., and S.N. Blair. 1999. Relationship between low cardiorespiratory fitness and mortality in normal-weight, overweight, and obese men. *JAMA* 282(16):1547-1553.

Weiss, C.O. 2011. Frailty and chronic diseases in older adults. *Clinics in Geriatric Medicine* 27(1):39-52.

Wile, D. 2007. Taijiquan and Taoism from religion to martial art and martial art to religion. *Journal of Asian Martial Arts* 16(4).

Xu, Y.J., P.S. Tappia, N.S. Neki, and N.S. Dhalla. 2014. Prevention of diabetes-induced cardiovascular complications upon treatment with antioxidants. *Heart Failure Reviews* 19(1):113-121.

Yung, L.M., I. Laher, X. Yao, Z.Y. Chen, Y. Huang, and F.P. Leung. 2009. Exercise, vascular wall and cardiovascular diseases: An update (part 2). *Sports Medicine* 39(1):45-63.

Chapter 10

Antuna-Puente, B., B. Feve, S. Fellahi, and J.-P. Bastard. 2008. Adipokines: The missing link between insulin resistance and obesity. *Diabetes and Metabolism* 34:2-11.

Arem, H., M.L. Irwin, Y. Zhou, L. Lu, H. Risch, and H. Yu. 2011. Physical activity and endometrial cancer in a population-based case-control study. *Cancer Causes & Control* 22(2):219-226.

Baan, R., Y. Grosse, K. Straif, B. Secretan, F. El Ghissassi, V. Bouvard, L. Benbrahim-Tallaa, et al. 2009. A review of human carcinogens—Part F: Chemical agents and related occupations. *Lancet Oncology* 10(12):1143-1144.

Bak, H., J. Christensen, B. Lykke Thomsen, A. Tjonneland, K. Overvad, S. Loft, and O. Raaschou-Nielsen. 2005. Physical activity and risk for lung cancer in a Danish cohort. *International Journal of Cancer* 116:439-445.

Balkau, B., L. Mhamdi, J.M. Oppert, J. Nolan, A. Golay, F. Porcellati, M. Laakso, and E. Ferrannini. 2008. Physical activity and insulin sensitivity: The RISC study. *Diabetes* 57:2613-2618.

Becker, S., L. Dossus, and R. Kaaks. 2009. Obesity related hyperinsulinaemia and hyperglycaemia and cancer development. *Archives of Physiology and Biochemistry* 115(2):86-96.

Belavy, D.L., M.J. Seibel, H.J. Roth, G. Armbrecht, J. Rittweger, and D. Felsenberg. 2012. The effects of bed rest and countermeasure exercise on the endocrine system in male adults—Evidence for immobilization induced reduction in sex hormone-binding globulin levels. *Journal of Endocrinological Investigation* 35(1):54-62.

Bey, L., N. Akunuri, P. Zhao, E.P. Hoffman, D.G. Hamilton, and M.T. Hamilton. 2003. Patterns of global gene expression in rat skeletal muscle during unloading and low-intensity ambulatory activity. *Physiological Genomics* 13:157-167.

Blanck, H.M., M.L. McCullough, A.V. Patel, C. Gillespie, E.E. Calle, V.E. Cokkinides, D.A. Galuska, L.K. Khan, and M.K. Serdula. 2007. Sedentary behavior, recreational physical activity, and 7-year weight gain among postmenopausal US women. *Obesity* 15(6):1578-1588.

Bouvard, V., R. Baan, K. Straif, Y. Grosse, B. Secretan, F. El Ghissassi, L. Benbrahim-Tallaa, et al. 2009. A review of

human carcinogens—Part B: Biological agents. *Lancet Oncology* 10(4):321-322.

Campbell, P.T., A.V. Patel, C. Newton, E. Jacobs, and S.M. Gapstur. 2013. Associations of recreational physical activity and leisure time spent sitting with colorectal cancer survival. *Journal of Clinical Oncology* 31(7):876-885.

Cohen, S., C.E. Matthews, P. Bradshaw, L. Lipworth, M.S. Buchowski, L.B. Signorello, and W.J. Blot. 2013. Sedentary behavior, physical activity, and likelihood of breast cancer among black and white women: A report from the Southern Community Cohort Study. *Cancer Prevention Research* 6(6):566-576.

Colbert, L.H., T.J. Hartman, N. Malila, P.J. Limburg, P. Pertinen, J. Virtamo, P.R. Taylore, and D. Albanes. 2001. Physical activity in relation to cancer of the colon and rectum in a cohort of male smokers. *Cancer Epidemiology Biomarkers & Prevention* 10:265-268.

Courneya, K.S., and C.M. Friedenreich, eds. 2011. *Physical activity and cancer.* Heidelberg, Germany: Springer-Verlag.

Coussens, L.M., and Z. Werb. 2002. Inflammation and cancer. *Nature* 420(6917):860-867.

Cust, A.E. 2011. Physical activity and gynecologic cancer prevention. In *Physical activity and cancer*, edited by K.S. Courneya and C.M. Friedenreich, 159-185. Berlin: Springer.

de Moura, M.B., L.S. dos Santos, and B. Van Houten. 2010. Mitochondrial dysfunction in neurodegenerative diseases and cancer. *Environmental and Molecular Mutagenesis* 51:391-405.

Dunstan, D.W., E.L.M. Barr, G.N. Healy, J. Salmon, J.E. Shaw, B. Balkau, D.J. Magliano, A.J. Cameron, P.Z. Zimmet, and N. Owen. 2010. Television viewing time and mortality: The Australian Diabetes, Obesity and Lifestyle Study (AusDiab). *Circulation* 121:384-391.

El Ghissassi, F., R. Baan, K. Straif, Y. Grosse, B. Secretan, V. Bouvard, L. Benbrahim-Tallaa, et al. 2009. A review of human carcinogens—Part D: Radiation. *Lancet Oncology* 10(8):751-752.

Ferlay, J., H.R. Shin, F. Bray, D. Forman, C. Mathers, and D.M. Parkin. 2010. GLOBOCAN 2008 v 1.2, Cancer Incidence, Mortality and Prevalence Worldwide. IARC CancerBase No. 10, International Agency for Research on Cancer.

Figueiredo, P.A., S.K. Powers, R.M. Ferreira, F. Amado, H.J. Appell, and J.A. Duarte. 2009. Impact of lifelong sedentary behavior in mitochondrial function of mice skeletal muscle. *Journals of Gerontology, Series A: Biological Sciences and Medical Sciences* 64A(9):927-939.

Forsythe, L.P., C.M. Alfano, S.M. George, A. McTiernan, K.B. Baumgartner, L. Bernstein, and R. Ballard-Barbash. 2013. Pain in long-term breast cancer survivors: The role of body mass index, physical activity, and sedentary behavior. *Breast Cancer Research and Treatment* 137(2):617-630.

Friberg, E., C.S. Mantzoros, and A. Wolk. 2006. Physical activity and risk of endometrial cancer: A population-based prospective cohort study. *Cancer Epidemiology Biomarkers & Prevention* 15(11):2136-2140.

Friedenreich, C.M., L.S. Cook, A.M. Magliocco, M.A. Duggan, and K.S. Courneya. 2010. Case-control study of lifetime of total physical activity and endometrial cancer risk. *Cancer Causes & Control* 21(7):1105-1116.

Friedenreich, C.M., T. Norat, K. Steindorf, M.C. Boutron-Ruault, T. Pischon, M. Mauir, F. Clavel-Chapelon, et al. 2006. Physical activity and risk of colon and rectal cancers: The European Prospective Investigation into Cancer and Nutrition. *Cancer Epidemiology Biomarkers & Prevention* 15(12):2398-2407.

Friedenreich, C.M., and M.R. Orenstein. 2002. Physical activity and cancer prevention: Etiologic evidence and biological mechanisms. *Journal of Nutrition* 132(11):3456S-3464S.

Fung, T.T., F.B. Hu, J. Yu, N.F. Chu, D. Spiegelman, G.H. Tofler, W.C. Willett, and E.B. Rimm. 2000. Leisure-time physical activity, television watching, and plasma biomarkers of obesity and cardiovascular disease risk. *American Journal of Epidemiology* 152(12):1171-1178.

George, S.M., C.M. Alfano, J. Groves, Z. Karabulut, K.L. Haman, B.A. Murphy, and C.E. Matthews. 2014. Objectively measured sedentary time is related to quality of life among cancer survivors. *Plos One* 9(2): e87937.

George, S.M., C.M. Alfano, A.W. Smith, M.L. Irwin, A. McTiernan, L. Bernstein, K.B. Baumgartner, and R. Ballard-Barbash. 2013. Sedentary behavior, health-related quality of life, and fatigue among breast cancer survivors. *Journal of Physical Activity and Health* 10(3):350-358.

George, S.M., M.L. Irwin, C.E. Matthews, S.T. Mayne, M.H. Gail, S.C. Moore, D. Albanes, et al. 2010. Beyond recreational physical activity: Examining occupational and household activity, transportation activity, and sedentary behavior in relation to postmenopausal breast cancer risk. *American Journal of Public Health* 100(11):2288-2295.

George, S.M., S.C. Moore, W. Chow, A. Schatzkin, A. Hollenbeck, and C.E. Matthews. 2011. A prospective analysis of prolonged sitting time and risk of renal cell carcinoma among 300,000 older adults. *Annals of Epidemiology* 21(10):787-790.

Grosse, Y., R. Baan, K. Straif, B. Secretan, F. El Ghissassi, V. Bouvard, L. Benbrahim-Tallaa, et al. 2009. A review of human carcinogens—Part A: Pharmaceuticals. *Lancet Oncology* 10(1):13-14.

Hamilton, M.T., D.G. Hamilton, and T.W. Zderic. 2007. Role of low energy expenditure and sitting in obesity, metabolic syndrome, type 2 diabetes, and cardiovascular disease. *Diabetes* 56(11):2655-2667.

Hawkes, A.L., B.M. Lynch, N. Owen, and J.F. Aitken. 2011. Lifestyle factors associated concurrently and prospectively with co-morbid cardiovascular disease in a population-based cohort of colorectal cancer survivors. *European Journal of Cancer* 47:267-276.

Healy, G.N., C.E. Matthews, D.W. Dunstan, E.A.H. Winkler, and N. Owen. 2011. Sedentary time and cardio-metabolic biomarkers in US adults: NHANES 2003-06. *European Heart Journal* 32(5):590-597.

Hildebrand, J.S., S.M. Gapstur, P.T. Campbell, M.M. Gaudet, and A.V. Patel. 2013. Recreational physical activity and leisure-time sitting in relation to postmenopausal breast cancer risk. *Cancer Epidemiology Biomarkers and Prevention* 22(10):1906-1912.

Howard, R.A., D.M. Freedman, Y. Park, A. Hollenbeck, A. Schatzkin, and M.F. Leitzmann. 2008. Physical activity, sedentary behavior, and the risk of colon and rectal cancer in the NIH-AARP Diet and Health Study. *Cancer Causes & Control* 19(9):939-953.

Hu, F.B., T.Y. Li, G.A. Colditz, W.C. Willett, and J.E. Manson. 2003. Television watching and other sedentary behaviors in relation to risk of obesity and type 2 diabetes mellitus in women. *JAMA* 289(14):1785-1791.

Johannsen, D.L., G.J. Welk, R.L. Sharp, and P.J. Flakoll. 2007. Differences in daily energy expenditure in lean and obese women: The role of posture allocation. *Obesity* 16(1):34-39.

Kaaks, R., and A. Lukanova. 2001. Energy balance and cancer: The role of insulin and insulin-like growth factor-I. *Proceedings of the Nutrition Society* 60(1):91-106.

Katzmarzyk, P.T., T.S. Church, C.L. Craig, and C. Bouchard. 2009. Sitting time and mortality from all causes, cardiovascular disease, and cancer. *Medicine and Science in Sports and Exercise* 41(5):998-1005.

Kendall, A., E.J. Folkerd, and M. Dowsett. 2007. Influences on circulating oestrogens in postmenopausal women: Relationship with breast cancer. *Journal of Steroid Biochemistry and Molecular Biology* 103:99-109.

Kershaw, E.E., and J.S. Flier. 2004. Adipose tissue as an endocrine organ. *Journal of Clinical Endocrinology & Metabolism* 89(6):2548-2556.

Kim, Y., L.R. Wilkens, S.Y. Park, M.T. Goodman, K.R. Monroe, and L.N. Kolonel. 2013. Association between various sedentary behaviours and all-cause, cardiovascular disease and cancer mortality: The Multiethnic Cohort Study. *International Journal of Epidemiology* 42(4):1040-1056.

Lacey, J., J. Deng, M. Dosemeci, Y.T. Gao, F.K. Mostofi, I.A. Sesterhenn, T. Xie, and A.W. Hsing. 2001. Prostate cancer, benign prostatic hyperplasia and physical activity in Shanghai, China. *International Journal of Epidemiology* 30:341-349.

Lahmann, P.H., C.M. Friedenreich, A.J. Schuit, S. Salvini, N.E. Allen, T.J. Key, K.T. Khaw, et al. 2007. Physical activity and breast cancer risk: The European Prospective Investigation into Cancer and Nutrition. *Cancer Epidemiology Biomarkers & Prevention* 16(1):36-42.

Lam, T.K., S.C. Moore, L.A. Brinton, L. Smith, A.R. Hollenbeck, G.L. Gierach, and N.D. Freedman. 2013. Anthropometric measures and physical activity and the risk of lung cancer in never-smokers: A prospective cohort study. *Plos One* 8(8):e70672.

Lee, Y.H., and R.E. Pratley. 2005. The evolving role of inflammation in obesity and the metabolic syndrome. *Current Diabetes Reports* 5:70-75.

Levi, F., C. Pasche, F. Lucchini, and C. La Vecchia. 1999. Occupational and leisure time physical activity and the risk of breast cancer. *European Journal of Cancer* 35(5):775-778.

Levine, J.A., L.M. Lanningham-Foster, S.K. McCrady, A.C. Krizan, L.R. Olson, P.H. Kane, M.D. Jensen, and M.M. Clark. 2005. Interindividual variation in posture allocation: Possible role in human obesity. *Science* 307(5709):584-586.

Lim, U., and M.A. Song. 2012. Dietary and lifestyle factors of DNA methylation. *Methods in Molecular Biology* 863:359-376.

Lowe, S.S., B. Danielson, C. Beaumont, S.M. Watanabe, V.E. Baracos, and K.S. Courneya. 2014. Correlates of objectively measured sedentary behavior in cancer patients with brain metastases: An application of the theory of planned behavior. *Psycho-Oncology* Epub 2014 Jul 29.

Lukanova, A., and R. Kaaks. 2005. Endogenous hormones and ovarian cancer: Epidemiology and current hypotheses. *Cancer Epidemiology Biomarkers & Prevention* 14(1):98-107.

Lynch, B.M. 2010. Sedentary behavior and cancer: A systematic review of the literature and proposed biological mechanisms. *Cancer Epidemiology Biomarkers & Prevention* 19(11):2691-2709.

Lynch, B.M., E. Cerin, N. Owen, A.L. Hawkes, and J.F. Aitken. 2011. Television viewing time of colorectal cancer survivors is associated prospectively with quality of life. *Cancer Causes & Control* 22(8):1111-1120.

Lynch, B.M., K.S. Courneya, and C.M. Friedenreich. 2013. A case-control study of lifetime occupational sitting and likelihood of breast cancer. *Cancer Causes & Control* 24(6):1257-1262.

Lynch, B.M., D.W. Dunstan, G.N. Healy, E. Winkler, E. Eakin, and N. Owen. 2010. Objectively measured physical activity and sedentary time of breast cancer survivors, and associations with adiposity: Findings from NHANES (2003-2006). *Cancer Causes & Control* 21:283-288.

Lynch, B.M., D.W. Dunstan, E. Winkler, G.N. Healy, E. Eakin, and N. Owen. 2011. Objectively assessed physical activity, sedentary time and waist circumference among prostate cancer survivors: Findings from the National Health and Nutrition Examination Survey (2003-2006). *European Journal of Cancer Care* 20:514-519.

Lynch, B.M., C.M. Friedenreich, K.A. Kopciuk, A.R. Hollenbeck, S.C. Moore, and C.E. Matthews. 2014. Sedentary behavior and prostate cancer risk in the NIH-AARP Diet and Health Study. *Cancer Epidemiology, Biomarkers & Prevention* 23(5):882-889.

Lynch, B.M., C.M. Friedenreich, E.A.H. Winkler, G.N. Healy, J.K. Vallance, E.G. Eakin, and N. Owen. 2011. Associations of objectively-assessed physical activity and sedentary time with biomarkers of breast cancer risk in postmenopausal women: Findings from NHANES (2003–2006). *Breast Cancer Research and Treatment* 130:183-194.

Mahabir, S., M.F. Leitzmann, P. Pietinen, D. Albanes, J. Virtamo, and P.R. Taylor. 2004. Physical activity and renal cell cancer risk in a cohort of male smokers. *International Journal of Cancer* 108:600-605.

Mathew, A., V. Gajalakshmi, R. Balakrishnan, V.C. Kanimozhi, P. Brennan, B.P. Binukumar, and P. Boffetta. 2009. Physical activity levels among urban and rural women in south India and the risk of breast cancer: A case-control study. *European Journal of Clinical Nutrition* 18(5):368-376.

Matthews, C.E., S.S. Cohen, J.H. Fowke, X. Han, Q. Xiao, M.S. Buchowski, M.K. Hargreaves, L.B. Signorello, and W.J. Blot. 2014. Physical activity, sedentary behavior, and cause-specific mortality in black and white adults in the southern community cohort study. *American Journal of Epidemiology* 180(4):394-405.

Matthews, C.E., S.M. George, S.C. Moore, H.R. Bowles, A. Blair, Y. Park, R.P. Troiano, A. Hollenbeck, and A. Schatzkin. 2012. Amount of time spent in sedentary behaviors and cause-specific mortality in US adults. *American Journal of Clinical Nutrition* 95:437-445.

McTiernan, A. 2008. Mechanisms linking physical activity with cancer. *Nature Reviews. Cancer* 8:205-211.

Moore, S.C., G.L. Gierach, A. Schatzkin, and C.E. Matthews. 2010. Physical activity, sedentary behaviours, and the prevention of endometrial cancer. *British Journal of Cancer* 103(7):933-938.

Nandeesha, H. 2009. Insulin: A novel agent in the pathogenesis of prostate cancer. *International Urology and Nephrology* 41(2):267-272.

Neilson, H.K., C.M. Friedenreich, N.T. Brockton, and R.C. Millikan. 2009. Physical activity and postmenopausal breast cancer: Proposed biologic mechanisms and areas for future research. *Cancer Epidemiology, Biomarkers & Prevention* 18(1):11-27.

Orsini, N., R. Bellocco, M. Bottai, M. Pagano, S.O. Andersson, J.E. Johansson, E. Giovannucci, and A. Wolk. 2009. A prospective study of lifetime physical activity and prostate cancer incidence and mortality. *British Journal of Cancer* 101(11):1932-1938.

Owen, N., G.N. Healy, C.E. Matthews, and D.W. Dunstan. 2010. Too much sitting: The population health science of sedentary behavior. *Exercise and Sport Sciences Reviews* 38(3):105-113.

Pan, S.Y., A.M. Ugnat, Y. Mao, and The Canadian Cancer Registries Research Group. 2005. Physical activity and the risk of ovarian cancer: A case-control study in Canada. *International Journal of Cancer* 117:300-307.

Patel, A.V., L. Bernstein, A. Deka, H.S. Feigelson, P.T. Campbell, S.M. Gapstur, G.A. Colditz, and M.J. Thun. 2010. Leisure time spent sitting in relation to total mortality in a prospective cohort of US adults. *American Journal of Epidemiology* 172(4):419-429.

Patel, A.V., H.S. Feigelson, J.T. Talbot, M.L. McCullough, C. Rodriguez, R.C. Patel, M.J. Thun, and E.E. Calle. 2008. The role of body weight in the relationship between physical activity and endometrial cancer: Results from a large cohort of US women. *International Journal of Cancer* 123(8):1877-1882.

Patel, A.V., C. Rodriguez, A.L. Pavluck, M.J. Thun, and E.E. Calle. 2006. Recreational physical activity and sedentary behavior in relation to ovarian cancer risk in a large cohort of US women. *American Journal of Epidemiology* 163(8):709-716.

Pou, K.M., J.M. Massaro, U. Hoffman, R.S. Vasan, P. Maurovich-Horvat, M.G. Larson, J.F. Keaney, et al. 2007. Visceral and subcutaneous adipose tissue volumes are cross-sectionally related to markers of inflammation and oxidative stress. The Framingham Heart Study. *Circulation* 116:1234-1241.

Proper, K.I., A.S. Singh, W. van Mechelen, and M.J.M. Chinapaw. 2011. Sedentary behaviors and health outcomes among adults: A systematic review of prospective studies. *American Journal of Preventive Medicine* 40(2):174-182.

Reeves, G.K., K. Pirie, V. Beral, J. Green, E. Spencer, and D. Bull. 2007. Cancer incidence and mortality in relation to body mass index in the Million Women Study: Cohort study. *British Medical Journal* 335(7630):1134-1139.

Renehan, A.G., M. Tyson, M. Egger, R.F. Heller, and M. Zwahlen. 2008. Body-mass index and incidence of cancer: A systematic review and meta-analysis of prospective observational studies. *Lancet* 371(9612):569-578.

Rogers, L.Q., S.J. Markwell, K.S. Courneya, E. McAuley, and S. Verhulst. 2011. Physical activity type and intensity among rural breast cancer survivors: Patterns and associations with fatigue and depressive symptoms. *Journal of Cancer Survivorship* 5(1):54-61.

Rosenberg, L., J.R. Palmer, T.N. Bethea, Y. Ban, K. Kipping-Ruane, and L.L. Adams-Campbell. 2014. A prospective study of physical activity and breast cancer incidence in African-American women. *Cancer Epidemiology, Biomarkers & Prevention* 23(11):2522-2531.

Schmidt, M.D., V.J. Cleland, R.J. Thomson, T. Dwyer, and A.J. Venn. 2008. A comparison of subjective and objective measures of physical activity and fitness in identifying associations with cardiometabolic risk factors. *Annals of Epidemiology* 18(5):378-386.

Secretan, B., K. Straif, R. Baan, Y. Grosse, F. El Ghissassi, V. Bouvard, L. Benbrahim-Tallaa, et al. 2009. A review of human carcinogens—Part E: Tobacco, areca nut, alcohol, coal smoke, and salted fish. *Lancet Oncology* 10(11):1033-1034.

Seguin, R., D.M. Buchner, J. Liu, M. Allison, T. Manini, C.Y. Wang, J.E. Manson, et al. 2014. Sedentary behavior and mortality in older women: The Women's Health Initiative. *American Journal of Preventive Medicine* 46(2):122-135.

Shenker, N.S., P.M. Ueland, S. Polidoro, K. van Veldhoven, F. Ricceri, R. Brown, J.M. Flanagan, and P. Vineis. 2013. DNA methylation as a long-term biomarker of exposure to tobacco smoke. *Epidemiology* 24(5):712-716.

Steindorf, K., C.M. Friedenreich, J. Linseisen, S. Rohrmann, A. Rundle, F. Veglia, P. Vineis, et al. 2006. Physical activity and lung cancer risk in the European Prospective Investigation into Cancer and Nutrition cohort. *International Journal of Cancer* 119:2389-2397.

Steindorf, K., B. Tobiasz-Adamczyk, T. Popiela, W. Jedrychowski, A. Penar, A. Matyja, and J. Wahrendorf. 2000. Combined risk assessment of physical activity and dietary habits on the development of colorectal cancer. A hospital-based case-control study in Poland. *European Journal of Cancer Prevention* 9:309-316.

Stolzenberg-Solomon, R., P. Pietinen, P.R. Taylor, J. Virtamo, and D. Albanes. 2002. A prospective study of medical conditions, anthropometry, physical activity, and pancreatic cancer in male smokers. *Cancer Causes & Control* 13:417-426.

Teras, L.R., S.M. Gapstur, W. Ryan Diver, B.M. Birmann, and A.V. Patel. 2012. Recreational physical activity, leisure sitting time and risk of non-Hodgkin lymphoid neoplasms in the American Cancer Society Cancer Prevention Study-II cohort. *International Journal of Cancer* 131(8):1912-1920.

Thorp, A.A., N. Owen, M. Neuhaus, and D.W. Dunstan. 2011. Sedentary behaviors and subsequent health outcomes in adults: A systematic review of longitudinal studies from 1996-2011. *American Journal of Preventive Medicine* 41(2):207-215.

Thune, I., T. Brenin, E. Lund, and M. Gaard. 1997. Physical activity and the risk of breast cancer. *The New England Journal of Medicine* 336(18):1269-1275.

Thune, I., and E. Lund. 1994. Physical activity and the risk of prostate and testicular cancer: A cohort study of 53,000 Norwegian men. *Cancer Causes & Control* 5:549-556.

———. 1996. Physical activity and risk of colorectal cancer in men and women. *British Journal of Cancer* 73:1134-1140.

———. 1997. The influence of physical activity on lung cancer risk: A prospective study of 81,516 men and women. *International Journal of Cancer* 70:57-62.

Tremblay, M.S., R.C. Colley, T.J. Saunders, G.N. Healy, and N. Owen. 2010. Physiological and health implications of a sedentary lifestyle. *Applied Physiology, Nutrition, and Metabolism* 35:725-740.

Trinh, L., R.C. Plotnikoff, R.E. Rhodes, S. North, and K.S. Courneya. 2013. Associations between sitting time and quality of life in a population-based sample of kidney cancer survivors. *Mental Health and Physical Activity* 6:16-23.

Tworoger, S.S., S.A. Missmer, A.H. Eliassen, R.L. Barbieri, M. Dowsett, and S.E. Hankinson. 2007. Physical activity and inactivity in relation to sex hormone, prolactin, and insulin-like growth factor concentrations in premenopausal women—Exercise and premenopausal hormones. *Cancer Causes & Control* 18(7):743-752.

Ukawa, S., A. Tamakoshi, K. Wakai, H. Noda, M. Ando, and H. Iso. 2013. Prospective cohort study on television viewing time and incidence of lung cancer: Findings from the Japan Collaborative Cohort Study. *Cancer Causes & Control* 24(8):1547-1553.

Vallance, J., T. Boyle, K.S. Courneya, and B. Lynch. 2014. Associations of objectively-assessed physical activity and sedentary time with health-related quality of life among colon cancer survivors. *Cancer* 120(18):2919-2926.

van Kruijsdijk, R.C.M., E. van der Wall, and F.L.J. Visseren. 2009. Obesity and cancer: The role of dysfunctional adipose tissue. *Cancer Epidemiology, Biomarkers & Prevention* 18(10):2569-2578.

Wijndaele, K., S. Brage, H. Besson, K.T. Khaw, S.J. Sharp, R. Luben, N.J. Wareham, and U. Ekelund. 2011. Television viewing time independently predicts all-cause and cardiovascular mortality: The EPIC Norfolk study. *International Journal of Epidemiology* 40(1):150-159.

Wijndaele, K., G.N. Healy, D.W. Dunstan, A.G. Barnett, J. Salmon, J.E. Shaw, P.Z. Zimmet, and N. Owen. 2010. Increased cardio-metabolic risk is associated with increased TV viewing time. *Medicine and Science in Sports and Exercise* 42(8):1511-1518.

Wijndaele, K., B.M. Lynch, N. Owen, D.W. Dunstan, S. Sharp, and J.F. Aitken. 2009. Television viewing time and weight gain in colorectal cancer survivors: A prospective population-based study. *Cancer Causes & Control* 20(8):1355-1362.

Wiseman, A.J., B.M. Lynch, A.J. Cameron, and D.W. Dunstan. 2014. Associations of change in television viewing time with biomarkers of postmenopausal breast cancer risk: The Australian Diabetes, Obesity and Lifestyle Study. *Cancer Causes & Control* 25(10):1309-1319.

World Cancer Research Fund and American Institute for Cancer Research. 2007. *Food, nutrition, and physical activity, and the prevention of cancer: A global perspective.* Washington D.C.: AICR.

Xiao, Q., H.P. Yang, N. Wentzensen, A. Hollenbeck, and C.E. Matthews. 2013. Physical activity in different periods of life, sedentary behavior, and the risk of ovarian cancer in the NIH-AARP diet and health study. *Cancer Epidemiology, Biomarkers & Prevention* 22(11):2000-2008.

Xue, F., and K.B. Michels. 2007. Diabetes, metabolic syndrome, and breast cancer: A review of the current evidence. *American Journal of Clinical Nutrition* 86(3):823S-835S.

Zhang, M., X. Xie, A.H. Lee, and C.W. Binns. 2004. Sedentary behaviours and epithelial ovarian cancer risk. *Cancer Causes & Control* 15(1):83-89.

Chapter 11

Ainsworth, B.E., W.L. Haskell, S.D. Herrmann, N. Meckes, D.R. Bassett Jr., C. Tudor-Locke, J.L. Greer, J. Vezina, M.C. Whitt-Glover, and A.S. Leon. 2011. 2011 compendium of physical activities: A second update of codes and MET values. *Medicine and Science in Sports and Exercise* 43(8):1575-1581.

Arendt-Nielsen, L., T. Graven-Nielsen, H. Svarrer, and P. Svensson. 1996. The influence of low back pain on muscle activity and coordination during gait: A clinical and experimental study. *Pain* 64(2):231-240.

Aultman, C.D., J.D.M. Drake, J.P. Callaghan, and S.M. McGill. 2004. The effect of static torsion on the compressive strength of the spine: An in vitro analysis using a porcine spine model. *Spine* 29(15):E304-E309.

Becker, A., H. Held, M. Redaelli, K. Strauch, J.F. Chenot, C. Leonhardt, S. Keller, et al. 2010. Low back pain in primary care: Costs of care and prediction of future health care utilization. *Spine* 35(18):1714-1720.

Berecki-Gisolf, J., F.J. Clay, A. Collie, and R.J. McClure. 2012. The impact of aging on work disability and return to work: Insights from workers' compensation claim records. *Journal of Occupational and Environmental Medicine / American College of Occupational and Environmental Medicine* 54(3):318-327.

Biering-Sørensen, F. 1984. Physical measurements as risk indicators for low-back trouble over a one-year period. *Spine* 9(2):106-119.

Bohannon, R.W. 2012. Measurement of sit-to-stand among older adults. *Topics in Geriatric Rehabilitation* 28(1):11-16.

Bone and Joint Decade. 2012. Musculoskeletal conditions: The second greatest cause of disability. http://bjdonline.org/2012/12/musculoskeletal-conditions-the-second-greatest-cause-of-disability-2.

Boscolo, M.S. 2013. "Optimization of inversion ankle taping: A Taguchi method based study." Dissertation, University of Illinois at Urbana-Champaign.

Burton, A.K., T.L. Symonds, E. Zinzen, K.M. Tillotson, D. Caboor, P. Van Roy, and J.P. Clarys. 1997. Is ergonomic intervention alone sufficient to limit musculoskeletal problems in nurses? *Occupational Medicine* 47(1):25-32.

Burton, A.K., K.M. Tillotson, T.L. Symonds, C. Burke, and T. Mathewson. 1996. Occupational risk factors for the first-onset and subsequent course of low back trouble. A study of serving police officers. *Spine* 21(22):2612-2620.

Cady, L.D., D.P. Bischoff, E.R. O'Connell, P.C. Thomas, and J.H. Allan. 1979. Strength and fitness and subsequent back injuries in firefighters. *Journal of Occupational Medicine: Official Publication of the Industrial Medical Association* 21(4):269-272.

Callaghan, J.P., and S.M. McGill. 2001. Intervertebral disc herniation: Studies on a porcine model exposed to highly repetitive flexion/extension motion with compressive force. *Clinical Biomechanics* 16(1):28-37.

Callaghan, J.P., A.E. Patla, and S.M. McGill. 1999. Low back three-dimensional joint forces, kinematics, and kinetics during walking. *Clinical Biomechanics* 14(3):203-216.

Chen, S.M., M.F. Liu, J. Cook, S. Bass, and S.K. Lo. 2009. Sedentary lifestyle as a risk factor for low back pain: A systematic review. *International Archives of Occupational and Environmental Health* 82(7):797-806.

Cholewicki, J., and S.M. McGill. 1996. Mechanical stability of the in vivo lumbar spine: Implications for injury and chronic low back pain. *Clinical Biomechanics* 11(1):1-15.

Chou, R. 2014. In the clinic: Low back pain. *Annals of Internal Medicine* 160(11):ITC6-ITC16.

Dagenais, S., J. Caro, and S. Haldeman. 2008. A systematic review of low back pain cost of illness studies in the United States and internationally. *The Spine Journal: Official Journal of the North American Spine Society* 8(1):8-20.

Debono, D.J., L.J. Hoeksema, and R.D. Hobbs. 2013. Caring for patients with chronic pain: Pearls and pitfalls. *JAOA: Journal of the American Osteopathic Association* 113(8):620-627.

Dunlop, D., J. Song, E. Arnston, P. Semanik, J. Lee, R. Chang, and J.M. Hootman. 2014. Sedentary time in U.S. older adults associated with disability in activities of daily living independent of physical activity. *Journal of Physical Activity and Health* Epub 2014 Feb 5. doi:10.1123/jpah.2013-0311.

Ehrlich, G.E. 2003. Low back pain. *Bulletin of the World Health Organization* 81(9):671-676.

Escamilla, R.F., C. Lewis, D. Bell, G. Bramblet, J. Daffron, S. Lambert, A. Pecson, R. Imamura, L. Paulos, and J.R. Andrews. 2010. Core muscle activation during Swiss ball and traditional abdominal exercises. *Journal of Orthopaedic and Sports Physical Therapy* 40(5):265-276.

Fanuele, J.C., W.A. Abdu, B. Hanscom, and J. N. Weinstein. 2002. Association between obesity and functional status in patients with spine disease. *Spine* 27(3):306-312.

File, T. 2013. *Computer and Internet use in the United States.* Washington, D.C.: U.S. Census Bureau. www.census.gov/prod/2013pubs/p20-569.pdf

Frymoyer, J.W., and W.L. Cats-Baril. 1991. An overview of the incidences and costs of low back pain. *Orthopedic Clinics of North America* 22(2):263-271.

Galli, M., M. Crivellini, F. Sibella, A. Montesano, P. Bertocco, and C. Parisio. 2000. Sit-to-stand movement analysis in obese subjects. *International Journal of Obesity and Related Metabolic Disorders: Journal of the International Association for the Study of Obesity* 24(11):1488-1492.

Gilkey, D. 2014. Ergonomics of the modern dynamic office [PowerPoint slides]. Colorado State University Online. May-December 2014.

Hamilton, M.T., G.N. Healy, D.W. Dunstan, T.W. Zderic, and N. Owen. 2008. Too little exercise and too much sitting: Inactivity physiology and the need for new recommendations on sedentary behavior. *Current Cardiovascular Risk Reports* 2(4):292-298.

Handrakis, J.P., K. Friel, F. Hoeffner, O. Akinkunle, V. Genova, E. Isakov, J. Mathew, and F. Vitulli. 2012. Key characteristics of low back pain and disability in college-aged adults: A pilot study. *Archives of Physical Medicine and Rehabilitation* 93(7):1217-1224.

Hendrick, P., S. Milosavljevic, L. Hale, D.A. Hurley, S.M. McDonough, P. Herbison, and G.D. Baxter. 2013. Does a patient's physical activity predict recovery from an episode of acute low back pain? A prospective cohort study. *BMC Musculoskeletal Disorders* 14:126.

Heuch, I., I. Heuch, K. Hagen, and J.A. Zwart. 2013. Body mass index as a risk factor for developing chronic low back pain: A follow-up in the Nord-Trøndelag Health Study. *Spine* 38(2):133-139.

Hootman, J.M. 2007. 'These old bones'—A growing public health problem. *Journal of Athletic Training* 42(3):325-326.

Hootman, J.M., C.A. Macera, B.E. Ainsworth, C.L. Addy, M. Martin, and S.N. Blair. 2002. Epidemiology of musculoskeletal injuries among sedentary and physically active adults. *Medicine and Science in Sports and Exercise* 34(5):838-844.

Hoozemans, M.J., L.L. Koppes, J.W. Twisk, and J.H. van Dieën. 2012. Lumbar bone mass predicts low back pain in males. *Spine* 37(18):1579-1585.

Howarth, S.J., D. Glisic, J.G.B. Lee, and T.A.C. Beach. 2013. Does prolonged seated deskwork alter the lumbar flexion relaxation phenomenon? *Journal of Electromyography and Kinesiology* 23(3):587-593.

Hoy, D., L. March, P. Brooks, F. Blyth, A. Woolf, C. Bain, G. Williams, et al. 2014. The global burden of low back pain: Estimates from the Global Burden of Disease 2010 Study. *Annals of the Rheumatic Diseases* 73(6):968-974.

Jackson, M., M. Solomonow, B. Zhou, R.V. Baratta, and M. Harris. 2001. Multifidus EMG and tension-relaxation recovery after prolonged static lumbar flexion. *Spine* 26(7):715-723.

Johnson, E.N., and J.S. Thomas. 2010. Effect of hamstring flexibility on hip and lumbar spine joint excursions during forward reaching tasks in individuals with and without low back pain. *Archives of Physical Medicine and Rehabilitation* 91(7):1140-1142.

Jones, L.D., H. Pandit, and C. Lavy. 2014. Back pain in the elderly: A review. *Maturitas.* doi:10.1016/j.maturitas.2014.05.004.

Koley, S., and N. Likhi. 2011. No relationship between low back pain and hamstring flexibility. *Anthropologist* 13(2):117-120.

Kubo, M., K.G. Holt, E. Saltzman, and R.C. Wagenaar. 2006. Changes in axial stiffness of the trunk as a function of walking speed. *Journal of Biomechanics* 39(4):750-757.

Kwon, B.K., D.M. Roffey, P.B. Bishop, S. Dagenais, and E.K. Wai. 2011. Systematic review: Occupational physical activity and low back pain. *Occupational Medicine (Oxford, England)* 61(8):541-548.

Leino, P.I. 1993. Does leisure time physical activity prevent low back disorders? A prospective study of metal industry employees. *Spine* 18(7):863-871.

Lis, A.M., K.M. Black, H. Korn, and M. Nordin. 2007. Association between sitting and occupational LBP. *European Spine Journal* 16(2):283-298.

Little, J.S., and P.S. Khalsa. 2005. Human lumbar spine creep during cyclic and static flexion: Creep rate, biomechanics, and facet joint capsule strain. *Annals of Biomedical Engineering* 33(3):391-401.

Luckhaupt, S.E., M.A. Cohen, J. Li, and G.M. Calvert. 2014. Prevalence of obesity among U.S. workers and associations with occupational factors. *American Journal of Preventive Medicine* 46(3):237-248.

Maetzel, A., and L. Li. 2002. The economic burden of low back pain: A review of studies published between 1996 and 2001. *Best Practice & Research Clinical Rheumatology* 16(1):23-30.

Manchikanti, L., V. Singh, S. Datta, S.P. Cohen, and J.A. Hirsch. 2009. Comprehensive review of epidemiology, scope, and impact of spinal pain. *Pain Physician* 12(4):E35-E70.

Manson, J.E., P.J. Skerrett, P. Greenland, and T.B. VanItallie. 2004. The escalating pandemics of obesity and sedentary lifestyle. A call to action for clinicians. *Archives of Internal Medicine* 164(3):249-258.

Matheson, L. 2003. The functional capacity evaluation. In *Disability evaluation*, 2nd ed., edited by S.L. Demeter and G.B.J. Andersson, Retrieved from: http://www.epicrehab.com/abstracts/ama-fce.pdf. Chicago: Mosby.

McCaffery, M., and C. Pasero. 1999. *Pain: Clinical manual for nursing practice,* 2nd ed. St. Louis: Mosby.

McGill, S.M. 1997. The biomechanics of low back injury: Implications on current practice in industry and the clinic. *Journal of Biomechanics* 30(5):465-475.

———. 1998. Low back exercises: Evidence for improving exercise regimens. *Physical Therapy* 78(7):754-765.

———. 2016. *Low back disorders: Evidence-based prevention and rehabilitation,* 3rd ed. Champaign, IL: Human Kinetics.

McGill, S.M., and S. Brown. 1992. Creep response of the lumbar spine to prolonged full flexion. *Clinical Biomechanics* 7(1):43-46.

McGill, S.M., S. Grenier, M. Bluhm, R. Preuss, S. Brown, and C. Russell. 2003. Previous history of LBP with work loss is related to lingering deficits in biomechanical, physiological, personal, psychosocial and motor control characteristics. *Ergonomics* 46(7):731-746.

McGill, S.M., M.T. Sharratt, and J.P. Seguin. 1995. Loads on spinal tissues during simultaneous lifting and ventilatory challenge. *Ergonomics* 38(9):1772-1792.

McQuade, K.J., J.A. Turner, and D.M. Buchner. 1988. Physical fitness and chronic low back pain. An analysis of the relationships among fitness, functional limitations, and depression. *Clinical Orthopaedics and Related Research* 233:198-204.

National Institute of Neurological Disorders and Stroke. 2015. Low back pain fact sheet. www.ninds.nih.gov/disorders/backpain/detail_backpain.htm

Ng, S.W., and B.M. Popkin. 2012. Time use and physical activity: A shift away from movement across the globe. *Obesity Reviews: An Official Journal of the International Association for the Study of Obesity* 13(8):659-80.

Nocera, J., T.W. Buford, T.M. Manini, K. Naugle, C. Leeuwenburgh, M. Pahor, M.G. Perri, and S.D. Anton. 2011. The impact of behavioral intervention on obesity mediated declines in mobility function: Implications for longevity. *Journal of Aging Research* 2011(October). doi:10.4061/2011/392510.

Nourbakhsh, M.R., and A.M. Arab. 2002. Relationship between mechanical factors and incidence of low back pain. *Journal of Orthopaedic & Sports Physical Therapy* 32(9):447-460.

Nutter, P. 1988. Aerobic exercise in the treatment and prevention of low back pain. *Occupational Medicine* 3(1):137-145.

O'Sullivan, K., P. O'Sullivan, L. O'Sullivan, and W. Dankaerts. 2012. What do physiotherapists consider to be the best sitting spinal posture? *Manual Therapy* 17(5):432-437.

O'Sullivan, P.B., A.J. Smith, D.J. Beales, and L.M. Straker. 2011. Association of biopsychosocial factors with degree of slump in sitting posture and self-report of back pain in adolescents: A cross-sectional study. *Physical Therapy* 91(4):470-483.

Owen, N., and A. Bauman. 1992. The descriptive epidemiology of a sedentary lifestyle in adult Australians. *International Journal of Epidemiology* 21(2):305-310.

Owen, N., P.B. Sparling, G.N. Healy, D.W. Dunstan, and C.E. Matthews. 2010. Sedentary behavior: Emerging evidence for a new health risk. *Mayo Clinic Proceedings* 85(12):1138-1141.

Pfile, K., M. Boiling, L. DiStefano, and A. Nguyen. 2014. The side plank as a measure of core stability is not associated with landing biomechanics. *Journal of Athletic Training* 49(3): S - 99.

Pinto, R.Z., P.H. Ferreira, A. Kongsted, M.L. Ferreira, C.G. Maher, and P. Kent. 2014. Self-reported moderate-to-vigorous leisure time physical activity predicts less pain and disability over 12 months in chronic and persistent low back pain. *European Journal of Pain (London, England),* Epub 2014 Feb 27. doi:10.1002/j.1532-2149.2014.00468.x.

Proper, K.I., A.S. Singh, W. Van Mechelen, and M.J.M. Chinapaw. 2011. Sedentary behaviors and health outcomes among adults: A systematic review of prospective studies. *American Journal of Preventive Medicine* 40(2):174-182.

Punnett, L., A. Prüss-Utün, D.I. Nelson, M.A. Fingerhut, J. Leigh, S.W. Tak, and S. Phillips. 2005. Estimating the global burden of low back pain attributable to combined occupational exposures. *American Journal of Industrial Medicine* 48(6):459-469.

Ramazzini, B. 2001. De morbis artificum diatriba [Diseases of workers]. *American Journal of Public Health* 91(9):1380-1382.

Ribeiro, D.C., D. Aldabe, J.H. Abbott, G. Sole, and S. Milosavljevic. 2012. Dose-response relationship between work-related cumulative postural exposure and low back pain: A systematic review. *The Annals of Occupational Hygiene* 56(6):684-696.

Roffey, D.M., E.K. Wai, P. Bishop, B.K. Kwon, and S. Dagenais. 2010. Causal assessment of occupational standing or walking and low back pain: Results of a systematic review. *The Spine Journal: Official Journal of the North American Spine Society* 10(3):262-272.

Salmon, J., M.S. Tremblay, S.J. Marshall, and C. Hume. 2011. Health risks, correlates, and interventions to reduce sedentary behavior in young people. *American Journal of Preventive Medicine* 41(2):197-206.

Steele, J., S. Bruce-Low, and D. Smith. 2014. A reappraisal of the deconditioning hypothesis in low back pain: Review of evidence from a triumvirate of research methods on specific lumbar extensor deconditioning. *Current Medical Research and Opinion* 30(5):865-911.

Stern, R.G. 2013. Ordering high-cost medical imaging: A right or a privilege? *The American Journal of Medicine* 126(11):939-940.

Stevenson, J.M., C.L. Weber, J.T. Smith, G.A. Dumas, and W.J. Albert. 2001. A longitudinal study of the development of low back pain in an industrial population. *Spine* 26(12):1370-1377.

Stewart, W.F., J.A. Ricci, E. Chee, D. Morganstein, and R. Lipton. 2003. Lost productive time and cost due to common pain conditions in the US workforce. *Journal of the American Medical Association* 290(18):2443-2454.

Strine, T.W., and J.M. Hootman. 2007. US national prevalence and correlates of low back and neck pain among adults. *Arthritis and Rheumatism* 57(4):656-665.

Tanaka, N., H.S. An, T.H. Lim, A. Fujiwara, C.H. Jeon, and V.M. Haughton. 2001. The relationship between disc degeneration and flexibility of the lumbar spine. *The Spine Journal* 1(1):47-56.

Taylor, J.B., A.P. Goode, S.Z. George, and C.E. Cook. 2014. Incidence and risk factors for first-time incident low back pain: A systematic review and meta-analysis. *The Spine Journal: Official Journal of the North American Spine Society* 14(10):2299-2319.

Tomlinson, D.J., R.M. Erskine, C.I. Morse, K. Winwood, and G.L. Onambélé-Pearson. 2014. Combined effects of body composition and ageing on joint torque, muscle activation and co-contraction in sedentary women. *Age* 36(3):9652.

Twomey, L., and J. Taylor. 1982. Flexion creep deformation and hysteresis in the lumbar vertebral column. *Spine* 7(2):116-122.

U.S. Department of Health and Human Services. 2008. *Physical Activity Guidelines for Americans*. www.health.gov/paguidelines.

U.S. Department of Labor. 2005. *Computer and Internet Use at Work Summary*. www.bls.gov./news.release/ciuaw.nr0.htm.

Videman, T., M. Nurminen, and J.D. Troup. 1990. 1990 Volvo award in clinical sciences. Lumbar spinal pathology in cadaveric material in relation to history of back pain, occupation, and physical loading. *Spine* 15(8):728-740.

Vincent, H.K., A.N. Seay, C. Montero, B.P. Conrad, R.W. Hurley, and K.R. Vincent. 2013. Functional pain severity and mobility in overweight older men and women with chronic low-back pain—Part I. *American Journal of Physical Medicine and Rehabilitation* 92(5):430-438.

Walsh, K., N. Varnes, C. Osmond, R. Styles, and D. Coggon. 1989. Occupational causes of low-back pain. *Scandinavian Journal of Work, Environment & Health* 15(1):54-59.

Chapter 12

Arnardottir, N.Y., A. Koster, D.R.V. Domelen, R.J. Brychta, P. Caserotti, G. Eiriksdottir, J.E. Sverrisdottir, et al. 2016. Association of change in brain structure to objectively measured physical activity and sedentary behavior in older adults: Age, Gene/Environment Susceptibility-Reykjavik Study. *Behavioural Brain Research* 296:118-124.

Balboa-Castillo, T., L.M. León-Muñoz, A. Graciani, F. Rodríguez-Artalejo, and P. Guallar-Castillón. 2011. Longitudinal association of physical activity and sedentary behavior during leisure time with health-related quality of life in community dwelling older adults. *Health and Quality of Life Outcomes* 9:47.

Ball, K., D.B. Berch, K.F. Helmers, J.B. Jobe, M.D. Leveck, M. Marsiske, J.N. Morris, et al. 2002. Effects of cognitive training interventions with older adults: A randomized controlled trial. *JAMA* 288(18):2271-2281.

Biddle, S.J.H., and M. Asare. 2011. Physical activity and mental health in children and adolescents: A review of reviews. *British Journal of Sports Medicine* 45(11):886-895.

Buschkuehl, M., S.M. Jaeggi, S. Hutchison, P. Perrig-Chiello, C. Däpp, M. Müller, F. Breil, H. Hoppeler, and W.J. Perrig. 2008. Impact of working memory training on memory performance in old-old adults. *Psychology and Aging* 23(4):743-753.

Capute, A.J., B.K. Shapiro, F.B. Palmer, A. Ross, and R.C. Wachtel. 1985. Cognitive-motor interactions: The relationship of infant gross motor attainment to IQ at 3 years. *Clinical Pediatrics* 24(12):671-675.

Christakis, D.A., F.J. Zimmerman, D.L. DiGiuseppe, and C.A. McCarty. 2004. Early television exposure and subsequent attentional problems in children. *Pediatrics* 113(4):708-713.

Clifford, A., A. Yesufu Udechuku, L. Edwards, S. Bandelow, and E. Hogervorst. 2009. Maintaining cognitive health in elderly women. *Aging Health* 5(5):655-670.

Colcombe, S., and A.F. Kramer. 2003. Fitness effects on the cognitive function of older adults: A meta-analytic study. *Psychological Science* 14(2):125-130.

Davies, C.A., C. Vandelanotte, M.J. Duncan, and J.G.Z. van Uffelen. 2012. Associations of physical activity and screen-time on health related quality of life in adults. *Preventive Medicine* 55(1):46-49.

Ekkekakis, P. 2013a. *The measurement of affect, mood, and emotion: A guide for health-behavioral research.* Cambridge, England: Cambridge University Press.

Ekkekakis, P., ed. 2013b. *Routledge handbook of physical activity and mental health.* London: Routledge.

Fox, K.R. 2000. The effects of exercise on self-perceptions and self-esteem. In *Physical activity and psychological well-being,* edited by S.J.H. Biddle, K.R. Fox, and S.H. Boutcher, 88-117. London: Routledge.

Gates, N., and M. Valenzuela. 2010. Cognitive exercise and its role in cognitive function in older adults. *Current Psychiatry Reports* 12(1):20-27.

Hamer, M., and Y. Chida. 2009. Physical activity and risk of neurodegenerative disease: A systematic review of prospective evidence. *Psychological Medicine* 39(1):3-11.

Hamer, M., and E. Stamatakis. 2014. Prospective study of sedentary behavior, risk of depression, and cognitive impairment. *Medicine and Science in Sports & Exercise* 46(4):718-723.

Hamer, M., E. Stamatakis, and G. Mishra. 2010. Television- and screen-based activity and mental well-being in adults. *American Journal of Preventive Medicine* 38(4):375-380. Henderson, M., N. Glozier, and K.H. Elliot. 2005. Long term sickness absence. *British Medical Journal* 330:802-803.

Hogervorst, E., A. Clifford, J. Stock, X. Xin, and S. Bandelow. 2012. Exercise to prevent cognitive decline and Alzheimer's disease: For whom, when, what, and (most importantly) how much? (Editorial). *Journal of Alzheimer's Disease & Parkinsonism* 2. doi: 10.4172/2161-0460.1000e117

Jefferis, B.J.M.H., C. Power, and C. Hertzman. 2002. Birth weight, childhood socioeconomic environment, and cognitive development in the 1958 British birth cohort study. *British Medical Journal* 325(7359):305-308.

Joseph, R.J., M. Alonso-Alonso, D.S. Bond, A. Pascual-Leone, and G.L. Blackburn. 2011. The neurocognitive connection between physical activity and eating behaviour. *Obesity Reviews* 12(10):800-812.

Ku, P-W., K.R. Fox, and L-J. Chen. 2015. Leisure-time physical activity, sedentary behaviors and subjective well-being in older adults: An eight-year longitudinal research. *Social Indicators Research* Epub 2015 June 12. doi: 10.1007/s11205-015-1005-7

LeBlanc, A.G., J.C. Spence, V. Carson, S.C. Gorber, C. Dillman, I. Janssen, M.E. Kho, J.A. Stearns, B.W. Timmons, and M.S. Tremblay. 2012. Systematic review of sedentary behaviour and health indicators in the early years (aged 0-4 years). *Applied Physiology, Nutrition & Metabolism* 37(4):753-772.

Lucas, M., R. Mekary, A. Pan, F. Mirzaei, E.J. O'Reilly, W.C. Willett, , K. Koenen, O.I. Okereke, and A. Ascherio. 2011. Relation between clinical depression risk and physical activity and time spent watching television in older women: A 10-year prospective follow-up study. *American Journal of Epidemiology* 174(9):1017-1027.

Mathers, C.D., and D. Loncar. 2006. Projections of global mortality and burden of disease from 2002 to 2030. *PLoS Med* 3(11):e442.

Moussavi, S., S. Chatterji, E. Verdes, A. Tandon, V. Patel, and B. Ustun. 2007. Depression, chronic diseases, and decrements in health: Results from the World Health Surveys. *Lancet* 370(9590):851-858.

Murray, C.J.L., and A.D. Lopez. 1997. Alternative projections of mortality and disability by cause 1990–2020: Global Burden of Disease Study. *Lancet* 349(9064):1498-1504.

Murray, G.K., J. Veijola, K. Moilanen, J. Miettunen, D.C. Glahn, T.D . Cannon, P.B. Jones, and M. Isohanni. 2006. Infant motor development is associated with adult cognitive categorisation in a longitudinal birth cohort study. *Journal of Child Psychology and Psychiatry* 47(1):25-29.

Mutrie, N. 2000. The relationship between physical activity and clinically defined depression. In *Physical activity and psychological well-being,* edited by S.J.H. Biddle, K.R. Fox, and S.H. Boutcher, 46-62. London: Routledge.

Newton, R.L., H. Han, T. Zderic, and M. Hamilton. 2013. The energy expenditure of sedentary behavior: A whole room calorimeter study. *PLoS ONE* 8(5):e63171.

Owen, A.M., A. Hampshire, J.A. Grahn, R. Stenton, S. Dajani, A.S. Burns, R.J. Howard, and C.G. Ballard. 2010. Putting brain training to the test. *Nature* 465(7299):775-778.

Papp, K.V., S.J. Walsh, and P.J. Snyder. 2009. Immediate and delayed effects of cognitive interventions in healthy elderly: A review of current literature and future directions. *Alzheimer's & Dementia* 5(1):50-60.

Pearson, N., and S.J.H. Biddle. 2011. Sedentary behaviour and dietary intake in children, adolescents and adults: A systematic review. *American Journal of Preventive Medicine* 41(2):178-188.

Primack, B.A., B. Swanier, A.M. Georgiopoulos, S.R Land, and M.J. Fine. 2009. Association between media use in adolescence and depression in young adulthood: A longitudinal study. *Archives of General Psychiatry* 66(2):181-188.

Rejeski, W.J., L.R. Brawley, and S.A. Shumaker. 1996. Physical activity and health-related quality of life. *Exercise and Sport Sciences Reviews* 24:71-108.

Rethorst, C.D., B.M. Wipfli, and D.M. Landers. 2009. The antidepressive effects of exercise: A meta-analysis of randomized trials. *Sports Medicine* 39(6):491-511.

Richards, M., R. Hardy, D. Kuh, and M.E.J. Wadsworth. 2001. Birth weight and cognitive function in the British 1946 birth cohort: Longitudinal population based study. *BMJ* 322(7280):199-203.

Sanchez-Villegas, A., I. Ara, F. Guillen-Grima, M. Bes-Rastrollo, J.J. Varo-Cenarruzabeitia, and M.A. Martinez-Gonzalez. 2008. Physical activity, sedentary index, and mental disorders in the SUN cohort study. *Medicine and Science in Sports & Exercise* 40(5):827-834.

Sedentary Behaviour Research Network. 2012. Letter to the editor: Standardized use of the terms "sedentary" and "sedentary behaviours". *Applied Physiology, Nutrition & Metabolism* 37(3):540-542.

Smith, E., P. Hay, L. Campbell, and J.N. Trollor. 2011. A review of the association between obesity and cognitive function across the lifespan: Implications for novel approaches to prevention and treatment. *Obesity Reviews* 12(9):740-755.

Smith, G.E., P. Housen, K. Yaffe, R. Ruff, R.F. Kennison, H.W. Mahncke, and E.M. Zelinski. 2009. A cognitive training program based on principles of brain plasticity: Results from the improvement in memory with plasticity-based adaptive cognitive training (IMPACT) study. *Journal of the American Geriatric Society* 57(4):594-603.

Spector, A., L. Thorgrimsen, B. Woods, L. Royan, S. Davies, M. Butterworth, and M. Orrell. 2003. Efficacy of an evidence-based cognitive stimulation therapy programme for people with dementia: Randomised controlled trial. *British Journal of Psychiatry* 183:248-254.

Spence, J.C., K.R. McGannon, and P. Poon. 2005. The effect of exercise on global self-esteem: A quantitative review. *Journal of Sport & Exercise Psychology* 27:311-334.

Stern, Y. 2002. What is cognitive reserve? Theory and research application of the reserve concept. *Journal of the International Neuropsychological Society* 8(3):448-460.

Suchert, V., R. Hanewinkel, and B. Isensee. 2015. Sedentary behavior and indicators of mental health in school-aged children and adolescents: A systematic review. *Preventive Medicine* 76:48-57.

Teychenne, M., K. Ball, and J. Salmon. 2008. Physical activity and likelihood of depression in adults: A review. *Preventive Medicine* 46(5):397-411.

———. 2010a. Physical activity, sedentary behavior and depression among disadvantaged women. *Health Education Research* 25(4):632-644.

———. 2010b. Sedentary behaviour and depression among adults: A review. *International Journal of Behavioural Medicine* 17(4):246-254.

Thorell, L.B., S. Lindqvist, S. Bergman Nutley, G. Bohlin, and T. Klingberg. 2009. Training and transfer effects of executive functions in preschool children. *Developmental Science* 12(1):106-113.

Thorp, A.A., N. Owen, M. Neuhaus, and D.W. Dunstan. 2011. Sedentary behaviors and subsequent health outcomes in adults: A systematic review of longitudinal studies, 1996-2011. *American Journal of Preventive Medicine* 41(2):207-215.

Tremblay, M., A. LeBlanc, M. Kho, T. Saunders, R. Larouche, R. Colley, G. Goldfield, and S.C. Gorber. 2011. Systematic review of sedentary behaviour and health indicators in school-aged children and youth. *International Journal of Behavioral Nutrition and Physical Activity* 8:98.

Uchida, S., and R. Kawashima. 2008. Reading and solving arithmetic problems improves cognitive functions of normal aged people: A randomized controlled study. *Age* 30(1):21-29.

Vallance, J.K., E.A.H. Winkler, P.A. Gardiner, G.N. Healy, B.M. Lynch, and N. Owen. 2011. Associations of objectively-assessed physical activity and sedentary time with depression: NHANES (2005-2006). *Preventive Medicine* 53(4-5):284-288.

van Uffelen, J.G.Z., J. Wong, J.Y. Chau, H.P. van der Ploeg, I. Riphagen, N.D. Gilson, N.W. Burton, et al. 2010. Occupational sitting and health risks: A systematic review. *American Journal of Preventive Medicine* 39(4):379-388.

Vance, D.E., V.G. Wadley, K.K. Ball, D.L. Roenker, and M. Rizzo. 2005. The effects of physical activity and sedentary behavior on cognitive health in older adults. *Journal of Aging and Physical Activity* 13(3):294-313.

Whalley, L.J., J.M. Starr, R. Athawes, D. Hunter, A. Pattie, and I.J. Deary. 2000. Childhood mental ability and dementia. *Neurology* 55(10):1455-1459.

Wilmot, E.G., C.L. Edwardson, F.A. Achana, M.J. Davies, T. Gorely, L.J. Gray, K. Khunti, T. Yates, and S.J.H. Biddle. 2012. Sedentary time in adults and the association with diabetes, cardiovascular disease and death: Systematic review and meta-analysis. *Diabetologia* 55(11):2895-2905.

Wilson, R., D.A. Bennett, D.W. Gilley, L.A. Beckett, L.L. Barnes, and D.A. Evans. 2000. Premorbid reading activity and patterns of cognitive decline in Alzheimer disease. *Archives of Neurology* 57(12):1718-1723.

Wipfli, B.M., C.D. Rethorst, and D.M. Landers. 2008. The anxiolytic effects of exercise: A meta-analysis of randomized trials and dose-response analysis. *Journal of Sport and Exercise Psychology* 30(4):392-410.

Woods, B., E. Aguirre, A.E. Spector, and M. Orrell. 2012. Cognitive stimulation to improve cognitive functioning in people with dementia. *Cochrane Database of Systematic Reviews* 2012 Feb 15. doi: 10.1002/14651858.CD005562.pub2

Zhai, L., Y. Zhang, and D. Zhang. 2015. Sedentary behaviour and the risk of depression: A meta-analysis. *British Journal of Sports Medicine* 49(11):705-709.

Zhao, E., M.J. Tranovich, and V.J. Wright. 2013. The role of mobility as a protective factor of cognitive functioning in aging adults: A review. *Sports Health: A Multidisciplinary Approach* 6(1):63-69.

Zimmerman, F.J., and D.A. Christakis. 2005. Children's television viewing and cognitive outcomes: A longitudinal analysis of national data. *Archives of Pediatric & Adolescent Medicine* 159(7):619-625.

Chapter 13

Ainsworth, B.E., C.J. Caspersen, C.E. Matthews, L.C. Masse, T. Baranowski, and W. Zhu. 2012. Recommendations to improve the accuracy of estimates of physical activity derived from self-report. *Journal of Physical Activity & Health* 9(Suppl. 1):S76-S84.

Ainsworth, B.E., W.L. Haskell, S.D. Herrmann, N. Meckes, D.R. Bassett Jr., C. Tudor-Locke, J.L. Greer, J. Vezina,

M.C. Whitt-Glover, and A.S. Leon. 2011. 2011 compendium of physical activities: A second update of codes and MET values. *Medicine and Science in Sports and Exercise* 43(8):1575-1581.

Arredondo, E.M., T. Mendelson, C. Holub, N. Espinoza, and S. Marshall. 2012. Cultural adaptation of physical activity self-report instruments. *Journal of Physical Activity & Health* 9(Suppl. 1):S37-S43.

Chastin, S.F.M., U. Schwarz, and D.A. Skelton. 2013. Development of a consensus taxonomy of sedentary behaviors (SIT): Report of Delphi Round 1. *PLoS One* 8(12):e82313.

Clark, B.K., A.A. Thorp, E.A. Winkler, P.A. Gardiner, G.N. Healy, N. Owen, and D.W. Dunstan. 2011. Validity of self-reported measures of workplace sitting time and breaks in sitting time. *Medicine and Science in Sports and Exercise* 43(10):1907-1912.

Clark, B.K., E. Winkler, G.N. Healy, P.G. Gardiner, D.W. Dunstan, N. Owen, and M.M. Reeves. 2013. Adults' past-day recall of sedentary time: Reliability, validity, and responsiveness. *Medicine and Science in Sports and Exercise* 45(6):1198-1207.

Craig, C.L., A.L. Marshall, M. Sjostrom, A.E. Bauman, M.L. Booth, B.E. Ainsworth, M. Pratt, et al. 2003. International Physical Activity Questionnaire: 12-country reliability and validity. *Medicine and Science in Sports and Exercise* 35(8):1381-1395.

Csizmadi, I., H.K. Neilson, K.A. Kopciuk, F. Khandwala, A. Liu, C.M. Friedenreich, Y. Yasui, et al. 2014. The Sedentary Time and Activity Reporting Questionnaire (STAR-Q): Reliability and validity against doubly labeled water and 7-day activity diaries. *American Journal of Epidemiology* 180(4):424-435.

DiPietro, L., C.J. Caspersen, A.M. Ostfeld, and E. R. Nadel. 1993. A survey for assessing physical activity among older adults. *Medicine & Science in Sports & Exercise* 25(5):628-642.

Gardiner, P.A., B.K. Clark, G.N. Healy, E.G. Eakin, E.A. Winkler, and N. Owen. 2011. Measuring older adults' sedentary time: Reliability, validity, and responsiveness. *Medicine and Science in Sports and Exercise* 43(11):2127-2133.

Hardy, L.L., M.L. Booth, and A.D. Okely. 2007. The reliability of the Adolescent Sedentary Activity Questionnaire (ASAQ). *Preventive Medicine* 45(1):71-74.

Healy, G.N., B.K. Clark, E.A. Winkler, P.A. Gardiner, W.J. Brown, and C.E. Matthews. 2011. Measurement of adults' sedentary time in population-based studies. *American Journal of Preventive Medicine* 41(2):216-227.

Hu, F.B., T.Y. Li, G.A. Colditz, W.C. Willett, and J.E. Manson. 2003. Television watching and other sedentary behaviors in relation to risk of obesity and type 2 diabetes mellitus in women. *JAMA* 289(14):1785-1791.

Lynch, B.M., C.M. Friedenreich, F. Khandwala, A. Liu, J. Nicholas, and I. Csizmadi. 2014. Development and testing of a past year measure of sedentary behavior: The SIT-Q. *BMC Public Health* 14:899.

Marshall, A.L., Y.D. Miller, N.W. Burton, and W.J. Brown. 2010. Measuring total and domain-specific sitting: A study of reliability and validity. *Medicine and Science in Sports and Exercise* 42(6):1094-1102.

Neilson, H.K., R. Ullman, P.J. Robson, C.M. Friedenreich, and I. Csizmadi. 2013. Cognitive testing of the STAR-Q: Insights in activity and sedentary time reporting. *Journal of Physical Activity & Health* 10(3):379-389.

Pate, R.R., R. Ross, M. Dowda, S.G. Trost, and J. Sirard. 2003. Validation of a 3-day physical activity recall instrument in female youth. *Pediatric Exercise Science* 15(3):257-265.

Pettee, K.K., S.A. Ham, C.A. Macera, and B.E. Ainsworth. 2009. The reliability of a survey question on television viewing and associations with health risk factors in US adults. *Obesity* 17(3):487-493.

Richardson, M.T., B.E. Ainsworth, H.C. Wu, D.R. Jacobs Jr., and A.S. Leon. 1995. Ability of the Atherosclerosis Risk in Communities (ARIC)/Baecke questionnaire to assess leisure-time physical activity. *International Journal of Epidemiology* 24(4):685-693.

Rivière, F., S. Aubert, A. Omorou, B.E. Ainsworth, and A. Vuillemin. 2015. "Content comparison of sedentary behavior questionnaires: A systematic review." Presentation at the Sedentary Behavior and Health Conference, Urbana Champaign, Illinois, October 15-17.

Rosenberg, D.E., F.C. Bull, A.L. Marshall, J.F. Sallis, and A.E. Bauman. 2008. Assessment of sedentary behavior with the International Physical Activity Questionnaire. *Journal of Physical Activity & Health* 5(Suppl. 1):S30-S44.

Rosenberg, D.E., G.J. Norman, N. Wagner, K. Patrick, K.J. Calfas, and J.F. Sallis. 2010. Reliability and validity of the Sedentary Behavior Questionnaire (SBQ) for adults. *Journal of Physical Activity & Health* 7(6):697-705.

Sallis, J.F., P.K. Strikmiller, D.W. Harsha, H.A. Feldman, S. Ehlinger, E.J. Stone, J. Williston, and S. Woods. 1996. Validation of interviewer- and self-administered physical activity checklists for fifth grade students. *Medicine and Science in Sports and Exercise* 28(7):840-851.

Schmitz, K.H., L. Harnack, J.E. Fulton, D.R. Jacobs Jr., S. Gao, L.A. Lytle, and P. Van Coevering. 2004. Reliability and validity of a brief questionnaire to assess television viewing and computer use by middle school children. *Journal of School Health* 74(9):370-377.

Thomas, J., J. Nelson, and S. Silverman. 2010. *Research methods in physical activity*, 6th ed. Champaign, IL: Human Kinetics.

U.S. Centers for Disease Control and Prevention. 2009. Behavioral Risk Factor Surveillance System. www.cdc.gov/brfss.

U.S. Centers for Disease Control and Prevention. 2014. Behavioral Risk Factor Surveillance System. www.cdc.gov/brfss.

U.S. Department of Commerce. 2010. 2010 Census Data. United States Census Bureau. www.census.gov

Wijndaele, K., D.E. Bourdeaudhuij, J.G. Godino, B.M. Lynch, S.J. Griffin, K. Westgate, and S. Brage. 2014. Reliability and validity of a domain-specific last 7-d sedentary time questionnaire. *Medicine and Science in Sports and Exercise* 46(6):1248-1260.

Yore, M.M., H.R. Bowles, B.E. Ainsworth, C.A. Macera, and H.W. Kohl. 2006. Single versus multiple item questions on occupational physical activity. *Journal of Physical Activity & Health* 3(1):1014.

Chapter 14

Allen, F.R., E. Ambikairajah, N.H. Lovell, and B.G. Celler. 2006. Classification of a known sequence of motions and postures from accelerometry data using adapted Gaussian mixture models. Physiological Measurement 27(10):935-951.

Arnardottir, N.Y., A. Koster, D.R. Van Domelen, R.J. Brychta, P. Caserotti, G. Eiriksdottir, J.E. Sverrisdottir, et al. 2012. Objective measurements of daily physical activity patterns and sedentary behaviour in older adults: Age, gene/environment susceptibility-Reykjavik Study. Age & Ageing 42(2):222-229.

Atkin, A.J., T. Gorely, S.A. Clemes, T. Yates, C. Edwardson, S. Brage, J. Salmon, S.J. Marshall, and S.J. Biddle. 2012. Methods of measurement in epidemiology: Sedentary behaviour. International Journal of Epidemiology 41(5):1460-1471.

Bankoski, A., T.B. Harris, J.J. McClain, R.J. Brychta, P. Caserotti, K.Y. Chen, D. Berrigan, R.P. Troiano, and A. Koster. 2011. Sedentary activity associated with metabolic syndrome independent of physical activity. Diabetes Care 34(2):497-503.

Barber, C., D. Evans, P.H. Fentem, and M.F. Wilson. 1973. A simple load transducer suitable for long-term recording of activity patterns in human subjects. Journal of Physiology 231(2):94P-95P.

Bassey, E.J., H.M. Dallosso, P.H. Fentem, J.M. Irving, and J.M. Patrick. 1987. Validation of a simple mechanical accelerometer (pedometer) for the estimation of walking activity. European Journal of Applied Physiology and Occupational Physiology 56(3):323-330.

Brody, S.I. 1992. The physician in aviation. Rhode Island Medical Society 75(8):391-395.

Broughton, R., J. Fleming, and J. Fleetham. 1996. Home assessment of sleep disorders by portable monitoring. Journal of Clinical Neurophysiology 13(4):272-284.

Bussmann, H.B., P.J. Reuvekamp, P.H. Veltink, W.L. Martens, and H.J. Stam. 1998. Validity and reliability of measurements obtained with an "activity monitor" in people with and without a transtibial amputation. Physical Therapy 78(9):989-998.

Butte, N.F., U. Ekelund, and K.R. Westerterp. 2012. Assessing physical activity using wearable monitors: Measures of physical activity. Medicine & Science in Sports & Exercise 44(1 Suppl. 1): S5-S12.

Butte, N.F., W.W. Wong, A.L. Adolph, M.R. Puyau, F.A. Vohra, and I.F. Zakeri. 2010. Validation of cross-sectional time series and multivariate adaptive regression splines models for the prediction of energy expenditure in children and adolescents using doubly labeled water. Journal of Nutrition 140(8):1516-1523.

Campbell, K.L., P.R. Crocker, and D.C. McKenzie. 2002. Field evaluation of energy expenditure in women using Tritrac accelerometers. Medicine & Science in Sports & Exercise 34(10):1667-1674.

Cauley, J.A., R.E. LaPorte, R.B. Sandler, M.M. Schramm, and A.M. Kriska. 1987. Comparison of methods to measure physical activity in postmenopausal women. American Journal of Clinical Nutrition 45(1):14-22.

Cavagna, G., F. Saibene, and R. Margaria. 1961. A three-directional accelerometer for analyzing body movements. Journal of Applied Physiology 16:191.

Chen, K.Y., S.A. Acra, K. Majchrzak, C.L. Donahue, L. Baker, L. Clemens, M. Sun, and M.S. Buchowski. 2003. Predicting energy expenditure of physical activity using hip- and wrist-worn accelerometers. Diabetes Technology & Therapeutics 5(6):1023-1033.

Chen, K.Y., and D.R. Bassett Jr. 2005. The technology of accelerometry-based activity monitors: Current and future. Medicine & Science in Sports & Exercise 37(11 Suppl):S490-S500.

Chen, K.Y., K.F. Janz, W. Zhu, and R.J. Brychta. 2012. Redefining the roles of sensors in objective physical activity monitoring. Medicine & Science in Sports & Exercise 44(1 Suppl. 1):S13-S23.

Chen, K.Y., and M. Sun. 1997. Improving energy expenditure estimation by using a triaxial accelerometer. Journal of Applied Physiology 83(6):2112-2122.

Choi, L., K.Y. Chen, S.A. Acra, and M.S. Buchowski. 2010. Distributed lag and spline modeling for predicting energy expenditure from accelerometry in youth. Journal of Applied Physiology 108(2):314-327.

Choi, L., Z. Liu, C.E. Matthews, and M.S. Buchowski. 2011. Validation of accelerometer wear and nonwear time classification algorithm. Medicine & Science in Sports & Exercise 43(2):357-364.

Cole, R.J., D.F. Kripke, W. Gruen, D.J. Mullaney, and J.C. Gillin. 1992. Automatic sleep/wake identification from wrist activity. Sleep 15(5):461-469.

Colley, R.C., D. Garriguet, I. Janssen, C.L. Craig, J. Clarke, and M.S. Tremblay. 2011. Physical activity of Canadian children and youth: Accelerometer results from the 2007 to 2009 Canadian Health Measures Survey. Health Reports 22(1):15-23.

Crouter, S.E., K.G. Clowers, and D.R. Bassett Jr. 2006. A novel method for using accelerometer data to predict energy expenditure. Journal of Applied Physiology 100(4):1324-1331.

Evenson, K.R., and J.W. Terry Jr. 2009. Assessment of differing definitions of accelerometer nonwear time. Research Quarterly for Exercise and Sport 80(2):355-362.

Giannakidou, D.M., A. Kambas, N. Ageloussis, I. Fatouros, C. Christoforidis, F. Venetsanou, I. Douroudos, and K. Taxildaris. 2012. The validity of two Omron pedometers during treadmill walking is speed dependent. European Journal of Applied Physiology 112(1):49-57.

Hart, T.L., J.J. McClain, and C. Tudor-Locke. 2011. Controlled and free-living evaluation of objective measures of sedentary and active behaviors. Journal of Physical Activity and Health 8(6):848-857.

Hoyt, R.W., J.J. Knapik, J.F. Lanza, B.H. Jones, and J.S. Staab. 1994. Ambulatory foot contact monitor to estimate metabolic cost of human locomotion. Journal of Applied Physiology 76(4):1818-1822.

Jackson, D.M., J.J. Reilly, L.A. Kelly, C. Montgomery, S. Grant, and J.Y. Paton. 2003. Objectively measured physical activity in a representative sample of 3- to 4-year-old children. Obesity Research 11(3):420-425.

Kiani, K., C.J. Snijders, and E.S. Gelsema. 1997. Computerized analysis of daily life motor activity for ambulatory monitoring. Technology and Health Care 5(4):307-318.

———. 1998. Recognition of daily life motor activity classes using an artificial neural network. Archives of Physical Medicine & Rehabilitation 79(2):147-154.

Klesges, R.C., L.M. Klesges, A.M. Swenson, and A.M. Pheley. 1985. A validation of two motion sensors in the prediction of child and adult physical activity levels. American Journal of Epidemiology 122(3):400-410.

Kozey-Keadle, S., A. Libertine, K. Lyden, J. Staudenmayer, and P.S. Freedson. 2011. Validation of wearable monitors for assessing sedentary behavior. Medicine & Science in Sports & Exercise 43(8):1561-1567.

Lanyon, L.E. 1971. Use of an accelerometer to determine support and swing phases of a limb during locomotion. American Journal of Veterinary Research 32(7):1099-1101.

Lau, H.Y., K.Y. Tong, and H. Zhu. 2009. Support vector machine for classification of walking conditions of persons after stroke with dropped foot. Human Movement Science 28(4):504-514.

Liu, S., R.X. Gao, and P.S. Freedson. 2012. Computational methods for estimating energy expenditure in human physical activities. Medicine & Science in Sports & Exercise 44(11):2138-2146.

Long, X., B. Yin, and R.M. Aarts. 2009. Single-accelerometer-based daily physical activity classification. Prococeedings of the Conference of the IEEE Engineering in Medicine and Biology Society 2009: 6107-6110.

MacCurdy, E. 1938. Leonardo Da Vinci. New York: Reynal & Hitchcock.

Mannini, A., and A.M. Sabatini. 2010. Machine learning methods for classifying human physical activity from on-body accelerometers. Sensors (Basel) 10(2):1154-1175.

Mathie, M.J., B.G. Celler, N.H. Lovell, and A.C. Coster. 2004. Classification of basic daily movements using a triaxial accelerometer. Medical & Biological Engineering & Computing 42(5):679-687.

Matthews, C.E., K.Y. Chen, P.S. Freedson, M.S. Buchowski, B.M. Beech, R.R. Pate, and R.P. Troiano. 2008. Amount of time spent in sedentary behaviors in the United States, 2003-2004. American Journal of Epidemiology 167(7):875-881.

Montoye, H.J., R. Washburn, S. Servais, A. Ertl, J.G. Webster, and F.J. Nagle. 1983. Estimation of energy expenditure by a portable accelerometer. Medicine & Science in Sports & Exercise 15(5):403-407.

Morris, J.R. 1972. Accelerometry in gait analysis. British Journal of Surgery 59(11):899.

———. 1973. Accelerometry—A technique for the measurement of human body movements. Journal of Biomechanics 6(6):729-736.

Mullaney, D.J., D.F. Kripke, and S. Messin. 1980. Wrist-actigraphic estimation of sleep time. Sleep 3(1):83-92.

Oliver, M., H.M. Badland, G.M. Schofield, and J. Shepherd. 2011. Identification of accelerometer nonwear time and sedentary behavior. Research Quarterly for Exercise and Sport 82(4):779-783.

Plasqui, G., A.G. Bonomi, and K.R. Westerterp. 2013. Daily physical activity assessment with accelerometers: New insights and validation studies. Obesity Reviews 14(6):451-462.

Plasqui, G., and K.R. Westerterp. 2007. Physical activity assessment with accelerometers: An evaluation against doubly labeled water. Obesity (Silver Spring) 15(10):2371-2379.

Pober, D.M., J. Staudenmayer, C. Raphael, and P.S. Freedson. 2006. Development of novel techniques to classify physical activity mode using accelerometers. Medicine & Science in Sports & Exercise 38(9):1626-1634.

Preece, S.J., J.Y. Goulermas, L.P. Kenney, D. Howard, K. Meijer, and R. Crompton. 2009. Activity identification using body-mounted sensors—A review of classification techniques. Physiological Measurement 30(4):R1-R33.

Puyau, M.R., A.L. Adolph, F.A. Vohra, and N.F. Butte. 2002. Validation and calibration of physical activity monitors in children. Obesity Research 10(3):150-157.

Puyau, M.R., A.L. Adolph, F.A. Vohra, I. Zakeri, and N.F. Butte. 2004. Prediction of activity energy expenditure using accelerometers in children. Medicine & Science in Sports & Exercise 36(9):1625-1631.

Rothney, M.P., M. Neumann, A. Beziat, and K.Y. Chen. 2007. An artificial neural network model of energy expenditure using nonintegrated acceleration signals. Journal of Applied Physiology 103(4):1419-1427.

Rowlands, A.V., T.S. Olds, M. Hillsdon, R. Pulsford, T.L. Hurst, R.G. Eston, S.R. Gomersall, K. Johnston, J. Lanford. 2014. Assessing sedentary behavior with the GENEActiv: introducing the sedentary sphere. Medicine & Science in Sports & Exercise 46(6): 1235-1247.

Rowlands, A.V., T. Yates, T.S. Olds, M. Davies, K. Khunti, C.L. Edwardson. 2016. Sedentary Sphere: Wrist-Worn Accelerometer-Brand Independent Posture Classification. Medicine & Science in Sports & Exercise 48(4): 748-754.

Ryan, C.G., P.M. Grant, W.W. Tigbe, and M.H. Granat. 2006. The validity and reliability of a novel activity monitor as a measure of walking. British Journal of Sports & Medicine 40(9):779-784.

Staudenmayer, J., D. Pober, S. Crouter, D. Bassett, and P. Freedson. 2009. An artificial neural network to estimate physical activity energy expenditure and identify physical activity type from an accelerometer. Journal of Applied Physiology 107(4):1300-1307.

Staudenmayer, J., W. Zhu, and D.J. Catellier. 2012. Statistical considerations in the analysis of accelerometry-based activity monitor data. Medicine & Science in Sports & Exercise 44(1 Suppl. 1):S61-S67.

Togowa, T., T. Tamura, and P.A. Oberg. 1998. Motion and force measurement. In Medical Instrumentation: Application and Design, edited by J.G. Webster, 183-200. New York: CRC Press.

Tracy, D.J., Z. Xu, L. Choi, S. Acra, K.Y. Chen, and M.S. Buchowski. 2014. Separating bedtime rest from activity using waist or wrist-worn accelerometers in youth. PLoS One 9(4):e92512.

Treuth, M.S., K. Schmitz, D.J. Catellier, R.G. McMurray, D.M. Murray, M.J. Almeida, S. Going, J.E. Norman, and R. Pate. 2004. Defining accelerometer thresholds for activity intensities in adolescent girls. Medicine & Science in Sports & Exercise 36(7):1259-1266.

Troiano, R.P., D. Berrigan, K.W. Dodd, L.C. Masse, T. Tilert, and M. McDowell. 2008. Physical activity in the United States measured by accelerometer. Medicine & Science in Sports & Exercise 40(1):181-188.

Troiano, R.P., J.J. McClain, R.J. Brychta, and K.Y. Chen. 2014. Evolution of accelerometer methods for physical activity research. British Journal of Sports Medicine 48(13):1019-1023.

Washburn, R., M.K. Chin, and H.J. Montoye. 1980. Accuracy of pedometer in walking and running. Research Quarterly for Exercise and Sport 51(4):695-702.

Webster, J.B., D.F. Kripke, S. Messin, D.J. Mullaney, and G. Wyborney. 1982. An activity-based sleep monitor system for ambulatory use. Sleep 5(4):389-399.

Weiss, A.R., N.L. Johnson, N.A. Berger, and S. Redline. 2010. Validity of activity-based devices to estimate sleep. Journal of Clinical Sleep Medicine 6(4):336-342.

Welk, G.J. 2002. Use of accelerometry-based activity monitors to assess physical activity. In Physical activity assessments for health-related research, edited by G.J. Welk, 125-141. Champaign, IL: Human Kinetics.

Welk, G.J., J. McClain, and B.E. Ainsworth. 2012. Protocols for evaluating equivalency of accelerometry-based activity monitors. Medicine & Science in Sports & Exercise 44(1 Suppl. 1):S39-S49.

Wong, T.C., J.G. Webster, H.J. Montoye, and R. Washburn. 1981. Portable accelerometer device for measuring human energy expenditure. IEEE Transactions on Biomedical Engineering 28(6):467-471.

Zakeri, I.F., A.L. Adolph, M.R. Puyau, F.A. Vohra, and N.F. Butte. 2010. Multivariate adaptive regression splines models for the prediction of energy expenditure in children and adolescents. Journal of Applied Physiology 108(1):128-136.

Chapter 15

Ainsworth, B.E., W.L. Haskell, S.D. Herrmann, N. Meckes, D.R. Bassett Jr., C. Tudor-Locke, J.L. Greer, J. Venzina, M.C. Whitt-Glover, and A.S. Leon. 2011. Compendium of physical activities: A second update of codes and MET values. *Medicine & Science in Sports & Exercise* 43(8):1575-1581.

Bassett, D., D. John, S.A. Conger, B.C. Rider, R.M. Passmore, and J.M. Clark. 2013. Detection of lying down, sitting, standing, and stepping using two activPAL monitors. *Medicine & Science in Sports & Exercise* 46(10): 2025-9.

Bey, L., and M. Hamilton. 2003. Supression of skeletal muscle lipoprotein lipase activity during physical inactivity: A molecular reason to maintain daily low-intensity activity. *The Journal of Physiology* 551(Pt 2):673-682.

Colbert, L., C. Matthews, T. Havighurst, K. Kim, and D. Schoeller. 2011. Comparative validity of physical activity measures in older adults. *Medicine & Science in Sports & Exercise* 43(5):867-876.

Drenowatz, C., and J. Eisenmann. 2011. Validation of the Sensewear armband at high intensity exercise. *European Journal of Applied Physiology* 111(5):833-837.

Dudley, P., D.R. Bassett, D. John, and S.E. Crouter. 2012. Validity of a multi-sensor armband for estimating energy expenditure during eighteen different activities. *Journal of Obesity and Weight Loss Therapy* 2(7):1-7.

Dunstan, D., E. Barr, G. Healy, J. Salmon, J.E. Shaw, B. Balkau, D.J. Magliano, A.J. Cameron, P.Z. Zimmet, and N. Owen. 2010. Television viewing time and mortality: The Australian Diabetes, Obesity and Lifestyle Study (AusDiab). *Circulation* 121(3):384-391.

Fruin, M.L., and J.W. Rankin. 2004. Validity of a multi-sensor armband in estimating rest and exercise energy expenditure. *Medicine & Science in Sports & Exercise* 36(6):1063-1069.

Hamilton, M., D. Hamilton, and T. Zderic. 2007. Role of low energy expenditure and sitting in obesity, metabolic syndrome, type 2 diabetes, and cardiovascular disease. *Diabetes* 56(11):2655-2667.

Haskell, W.L., M.C. Yee, A. Evans, and P. Irby. 1993. Simultaneous measurement of heart rate and body motion to quantitate physical activity. *Medicine & Science in Sports & Exercise* 25(1):109-115.

Helmerhorst, H., K. Wijndaele, S. Brage, N. Wareham, and U. Ekelund. 2009. Objectively measured sedentary time may predict insulin resistance independent of moderate- and vigorous-intensity physical activity. *Diabetes* 58(8):1776-1779.

Howard, B., S. Fraser, P. Sethi, E. Cerin, M.T. Hamilton, N. Owen, D.W. Dunstan, and B.A. Kingwell. 2013. Impact of hemostatic parameters of interrupting sitting with intermittent activity. *Medicine & Science in Sports Exercise* 45(7):1285-1291.

Jakicic, J.M., M. Marcus, K.I. Gallagher, C. Randall, E. Thomas, F.L. Goss, and R.J. Robertson. 2004. Evaluation of the SenseWear Pro Armband to assess energy expenditure during exercise. *Medicine & Science in Sports & Exercise* 36(5):897-904.

Janz, K.F. 2002. Use of heart rate monitors to assess physical activity. In *Physical activity assessments for health-related research,* edited by G.J. Welk, 143-161. Champaign, IL: Human Kinetics.

John, D., S. Liu, J. Sasaki, C.A. Howe, J. Staudenmayer, R.X. Gao, and P.S. Freedson. 2011. Calibrating a novel multi-sensor physical activity measurement system. *Physiological Measurement* 32(9):1473-1489.

John, D., D.L. Thompson, H. Raynor, K. Bielak, B. Rider, and D.R. Bassett. 2011. Treadmill workstations: A worksite physical activity intervention in overweight and obese office workers. *Journal of Physical Activity & Health* 8(8):1034-1043.

Katzmarzyk, P., T. Church, C. Craig, and C. Bouchard. 2000. Sitting time and mortality from all causes, cardiovascular disease, and cancer. *Medicine & Science in Sports & Exercise* 41(5):998-1005.

Katzmarzyk, P., and I. Lee. 2012. Sedentary behaviour and life expectancy in the USA: A cause-deleted life table analysis. *BMJ Open* 2(4): e000828.

King, G.A., N. Torres, C. Potter, T.J. Brooks, and K.J. Coleman. 2004. Comparison of activity monitors to estimate energy cost of treadmill exercise. *Medicine & Science in Sports & Exercise* 36(7):1244-1251.

Kozey-Keadle, S., A. Libertine, K. Lyden, J. Staudenmayer, and P. Freedson. 2011. Validation of wearable monitors for assessing sedentary behavior. *Medicine & Science in Sports & Exercise* 43(8):1561-1567.

Lyden, K., S.K. Keadle, J. Staudenmayer, and P. Freedson. 2012. Validity of two wearable monitors to estimate breaks from sedentary time. *Medicine & Science in Sports & Exercise* 44(11):2243-2252.

Morris, J., J. Heady, P. Raffle, C. Roberts, and J. Parks. 1953a. Coronary heart-disease and physical activity of work. *Lancet* 265(6795):1053-1057.

———. 1953b. Coronary heart disease and physical activity of work (conclusion). *Lancet* 265(6796):1111-1120.

Nag, P., S. Chintharia, S. Saiyed, and A. Nag. 1986. EMG analysis of sitting work postures in women. *Applied Ergonomics* 17(3):195-197.

Owen, N., G.N. Healy, B. Howard, and D.W. Dunstan. 2012. Too much sitting: Health risks of sedentary behaviour and opportunities for change. *Exercise & Sport Sciences Reviews* 38(3):105-113.

Owen, N., G. Healy, C. Matthews, and D. Dunstan. 2010. Too much sitting: The population health science of sedentary behavior. *Exercise & Sport Sciences Reviews* 38(3):105-113.

Paffenbarger, R.S., Jr., M.E. Laughlin, A.S. Gima, and R.A. Black. 1970. Work activity of longshoremen as related to death from coronary heart disease and stroke. *New England Journal of Medicine* 282(20):1109-1114.

Salmon, J., L. Arundell, C. Hume, H. Brown, K. Hesketh, D.W. Dunstan, R.M. Daly, et al. 2011. A cluster-randomized controlled trial to reduce sedentary behavior and promote physical activity and health of 8-9 year olds: The Transform Us! study. *BMC Public Health* 4(11):759.

Sedentary Behaviour Research Network. 2012. Standardised use of the terms "sedentary" and "sedentary behaviours". *Applied Physiology, Nutrition, and Metabolism* 37:540-542.

Soames, R., and J. Atha. 1981. The role of the antigravity musculature during quiet standing in man. *European Journal of Applied Physiology and Occupational Physiology* 47(2):159-167.

Steeves, J., D. Bassett, E. Fitzhugh, H. Raynor, and D. Thompson. 2012. Can sedentary behavior be made more active? A randomized pilot study of TV commercial stepping verus walking. *International Journal of Behavioral Nutrition and Physical Activity* 6(9):95.

Stephens, B., K. Granados, T. Zderic, M. Hamilton, and B. Braun. 2011. Effects of 1 day of inactivity on insulin action in healthy men and women: Interaction with energy intake. *Metabolism* 60(7):941-949.

Strath, S.J., D.R. Bassett, and D.L. Thompson. 2001. Simultaneous heart rate-motion sensor technique to estimate energy expenditure during lifestyle activities. *Medicine & Science in Sports & Exercise* 33(12):2118-2223.

Strath, S., D. Bassett, D. Thompson, and A. Swartz. 2002. Validity of the simultaneous heart rate-motion sensor technique for measuring energy expenditure. *Medicine & Science in Sports & Exercise* 34(5):888-894.

Suzuki, T., J. Hirata, K. Ohtsuki, and S. Watanabe. 2010. Electromyographic and haemodynamic activities in lumbar muscles during bicycle ergometer exercise and walking. *Electromyography and Clinical Neurophysiology* 50(5):213-218.

Tucker, S., L. Lanningham-Foster, J. Murphy, W.G. Thompson, A.J. Weymiller, C. Lohse, and J.A. Levine. 2011. Effects of a worksite physical activity intervention for hospital nurses who are working mothers. *American Association of Occupational Health Nurses Journal* 59(9):377-386.

Wadsworth, D., T. Howard, J. Hallam, and G. Blunt. 2005. A validation study of a continuous body-monitoring device: Assessing energy expenditure at rest and during exercise. *Medicine & Science in Sports & Exercise* 37(5):S24.

Warren, T., V. Barry, S. Hooker, X. Sui, T. Church, and S. Blair. 2010. Sedentary behaviors increase risk of cardiovascular disease mortality in men. *Medicine & Science in Sports & Exercise* 42(5):879-895.

Watanabe, S., A. Eguchi, K. Kobara, H. Ishida, and K. Otsuki. 2006. Electromyographic activity of selected trunk muscles during bicycle ergometer exercise and walking. *Electromyography and Clinical Neurophysiology* 46(5):311-315.

Welk, G., J. McClain, J. Eisenmann, and E. Wickel. 2007. Field validation of the MTI Actigraph and BodyMedia armband monitor using the IDEEA monitor. *Obesity* 15(4):918-928.

Zderic, T., and M. Hamilton. 2006. Physical inactivity amplifies the sensitivity of skeletal muscle to the lipid-induced downregulation of lipoprotein lipase activity. *Journal of Applied Physiology* 100(1):249-257.

Chapter 16

Abasolo, L., C. Lajas, L. Leon, L. Carmona, P. Macarron, G. Candelas, M. Blanco, and J.A. Jover. 2011. Prognostic factors for long-term work disability due to musculoskeletal disorders. *Rheumatology International* 32(2):3831-3839.

Albinali, F. 2013. "SPADES: Simplifying physical activity data collection." Paper presented at International Conference on Ambulatory Monitoring and Physical Activity Measurement, Amherst, Massachusetts, June 17-19.

Ancoli-Israel, S., R. Cole, C. Alessi, M. Chambers, W. Moorcroft, and C.P. Pollak. 2003. The role of actigraphy in the study of sleep and circadian rhythms. *Sleep* 26(3):342-392.

Azizyan, M., I. Constandache, and R.R. Choudhury. 2009. "SurroundSense: Mobile phone localization via ambience fingerprinting." Paper presented at the proceedings of the 15th annual International Conference on Mobile Computing and Networking, Beijing, China, Sept. 20-25.

Bankoski, A., T.B. Harris, J.J. McClain, R.J. Brychta, P. Caserotti, K.Y. Chen, D. Berrigan, R.P. Troiano, and A. Koster. 2011. Sedentary activity associated with metabolic syndrome independent of physical activity. *Diabetes Care* 34(2):497-503.

Barwais, F.A., T. Cuddihy, T. Washington, M.L. Tomson, and E. Brymer. 2013. Development and validation of a new self-report instrument for measuring sedentary behaviors and light-intensity physical activity in adults. *Journal of Physical Activity & Health* [Epub ahead of print].

Bloom, W.L., and M.F. Eidex. 1967. Inactivity as a major factor in adult obesity. *Metabolism* 16:679-684.

Brownson, R.C., T.K. Boehmer, and D.A. Luke. 2005. Declining rates of physical activity in the United States: What are the contributors? *Annual Review of Public Health* 26:421-443.

Chaput, J.-P., L. Klingenberg, and A. Sjodin. 2010. Do all sedentary activities lead to weight gain: Sleep does not. *Current Opinion in Clinical Nutrition & Metabolic Care* 13(6):601-607.

Chon, J., and H. Cha. 2011. Lifemap: A smartphone-based context provider for location-based services. *Pervasive Computing, IEEE* 10(2):58-67.

Dunstan, D.W., E.L. Barr, G.N. Healy, J. Salmon, J.E. Shaw, B. Balkau, D.J. Magliano, A.J. Cameron, P.Z. Zimmet, and N. Owen. 2010. Television viewing time and mortality: The Australian diabetes, obesity and lifestyle study (AusDiab). *Circulation* 121(3):384-391.

Eagle, N., and A. Pentland. 2004. *Social serendipity: Proximity sensing and cueing. MIT technical report.* http://vismod. media.mit.edu//tech-reports/TR-580. pdf

Fox, S., and M. Duggan. 2012. "Mobile Health 2012." *Pew Research Center.* www.pewinternet.org/2012/11/08/ mobile-health-2012

Healy, G.N., D.W. Dunstan, J. Salmon, E. Cerin, J.E. Shaw, P.Z. Zimmet, and N. Owen. 2007. Objectively measured light-intensity physical activity is independently associated with 2-h plasma glucose. *Diabetes Care* 30(6):1384-1389.

———. 2008. Breaks in sedentary time: Beneficial associations with metabolic risk. *Diabetes Care* 31(4):661-666.

Healy, G.N., D.W. Dunstan, J. Salmon, J.E. Shaw, P.Z. Zimmet, and N. Owen. 2008. Television time and continuous metabolic risk in physically active adults. *Medicine & Science in Sports & Exercise* 40(4):639-645.

Healy, G.N., E.G. Eakin, A.D. Lamontagne, N. Owen, E.A. Winkler, G. Wiesner, L. Gunning, et al. 2013. Reducing sitting time in office workers: Short-term efficacy of a multicomponent intervention. *Preventive Medicine* 57(1):43-48.

Hiden, H., S. Woodman, P. Watson, M. Catt, M. Trenell, and S. Zhang. 2013. Improving the scalability of movement monitoring workflows: An architecture for the integration of the Hadoop File System into e-Science Central. *Philosophical transactions Series A, Mathematical, physical, and engineering sciences* 371 (1983):20120085. doi:10.1098/rsta.2012.0085.

Huang, C.S., C.L. Lin, L.W. Ko, Y.K. Wang, J.W. Liang, and C.T. Lin. 2013. Automatic sleep stage classification GUI with a portable EEG device. In *HCI International 2013—-Posters' extended abstracts*, edited by C. Stephanidis, 613-617. New York: Springer.

Intille, S.S. 2007. Technological innovations enabling automatic, context-sensitive ecological momentary assessment. *The Science of Real-Time Data Capture. Self-Reports in Health Research*: 308-337.

Intille, S.S., K. Larson, J.S. Beaudin, J. Nawyn, E.M. Tapia, and P. Kaushik. 2005. "A living laboratory for the design and evaluation of ubiquitous computing technologies." Paper presented at Extended Abstracts on Human Factors in Computing Systems, Chicago, IL, April 2-7.

Intille, S.S., J. Lester, J.F. Sallis, and G. Duncan. 2012. New horizons in sensor development. *Medicine & Science in Sports & Exercise* 44(1 Suppl. 1):S24-S31.

John, D., S. Liu, J.E. Sasaki, C.A. Howe, J. Staudenmayer, R.X. Gao, and P.S. Freedson. 2011. Calibrating a novel multi-sensor physical activity measurement system. *Physiological Measurement* 32(9):1473-1489.

John, D., D.L. Thompson, H. Raynor, K. Bielak, B. Rider, and D.R. Bassett. 2011. Treadmill workstations: A worksite physical activity intervention in overweight and obese office workers. *Journal of Physical Activity & Health* 8(8):1034-1043.

Katzmarzyk, P.T., T.S. Church, C.L. Craig, and C. Bouchard. 2009. Sitting time and mortality from all causes, cardiovascular disease, and cancer. *Medicine & Science in Sports & Exercise* 41(5):998-1005.

Kerr, J., S.J. Marshall, S. Godbole, J. Chen, A. Legge, A.R. Doherty, P. Kelly, M. Oliver, H.M. Badland, and C. Foster. 2013. Using the SenseCam to improve classifications of sedentary behavior in free-living settings. *American Journal of Preventive Medicine* 44(3):290-296.

Kim, D.H., J. Hightower, R. Govindan, and D. Estrin. 2009. "Discovering semantically meaningful places from pervasive RF-beacons." Paper presented at the proceedings of the 11th International Conference on Ubiquitous Computing, Orlando, FL, Sept. 30- Oct. 3.

Kirchengast, S. 1998. Weight status of adult !Kung San and Kavango people from northern Namibia. *Annals of Human Biology* 25(6):541-551.

Koch, J., J. Wettach, E. Bloch, and K. Berns. 2007. "Indoor localisation of humans, objects, and mobile robots with RFID infrastructure." Paper presented at the proceedings of the 7th International Conference on Hybrid Intelligent Systems, Kaiserslautern, Germany, Sept. 17-19.

Kozey-Keadle, S., A. Libertine, K. Lyden, J. Staudenmayer, and P.S. Freedson. 2011. Validation of wearable monitors for assessing sedentary behavior. *Medicine & Science in Sports & Exercise* 43(8):1561-1567.

Kriska, A., and C. Caspersen. 1997. A collection of physical activity questionnaires for health-related research. *Medicine and Science in Sports and Exercise* 29(6):3-205.

Lyden, K., S.K. Keadle, J. Staudenmayer, and P.S. Freedson. 2014. A method to estimate free-living active and sedentary behavior from an accelerometer. *Medicine & Science in Sports & Exercise* 46(2):386-397.

Lyden, K., S.L. Kozey Keadle, J.W. Staudenmayer, and P.S. Freedson. 2012. Validity of two wearable monitors to estimate breaks from sedentary time. *Medicine & Science in Sports & Exercise* 44(11):2243-2252.

Makonin, S., and F. Popowich. 2011. An intelligent agent for determining home occupancy using power monitors and light sensors. In *Toward useful services for elderly and people with disabilities*, edited by B. Abdulrazak, S. Giroux, B. Bouchard, M. Mokhtari, and H. Pigot, 236-240. New York: Springer.

Mannini, A., S.S. Intille, M. Rosenberger, A.M. Sabatini, and W. Haskell. 2013. Activity recognition using a single accelerometer placed at the wrist or ankle. *Medicine & Science in Sports & Exercise* 45(11):2193-2203.

Marsiglia, M. 2009. "10 reasons we have daily 'stand up' meetings." *Atomic Object*. http://spin.atomicobject.com/2009/07/07/10-reasons-we-have-daily-stand-up-meetings

Matthews, C.E., K.Y. Chen, P.S. Freedson, M.S. Buchowski, B.M. Beech, R.R. Pate, and R.P. Troiano. 2008. Amount of time spent in sedentary behaviors in the United States, 2003-2004. *American Journal of Epidemiology* 167(7):875-881.

Matthews, C.E., S.K. Keadle, J. Sampson, K. Lyden, H.R. Bowles, S.C. Moore, A. Libertine, P.S. Freedson, and J.H. Fowke. 2013. Validation of a previous-day recall measure of active and sedentary behaviors. *Medicine & Science in Sports & Exercise* 45(8):1629-1638.

Mayagoitia, R.E., A.V. Nene, and P.H. Veltink. 2002. Accelerometer and rate gyroscope measurement of kinematics: An inexpensive alternative to optical motion analysis systems. *Journal of Biomechanics* 35(4):537-542.

Mun, M., D. Estrin, J. Burke, and M. Hansen. 2008. "Parsimonious mobility classification using GSM and wifi traces." Paper presented at the proceedings of the 5th workshop on Embedded Networked Sensors, Sydney, Australia, June 2-3.

Nam, Y., S. Rho, and C. Lee. 2013. Physical activity recognition using multiple sensors embedded in a wearable device. *ACM Transactions on Embedded Computing Systems (TECS)* 12(2):26.

Nielsen Company. 2013. "Mobile majority: U.S. smartphone ownership tops 60%." www.nielsen.com/us/en/newswire/2013/mobile-majority--u-s--smartphone-ownership-tops-60-.html

Owen, N., T. Sugiyama, E.E. Eakin, P.A. Gardiner, M.S. Tremblay, and J.F. Sallis. 2011. Adults' sedentary behavior determinants and interventions. *American Journal of Preventive Medicine* 41(2):189-196.

Peng, W., J.H. Lin, and J. Crouse. 2011. Is playing exergames really exercising? A meta-analysis of energy expenditure in active video games. *Cyberpsychology, Behavior, and Social Networking* 14(11):681-688.

Peng, Y., C.Y. Lin, and M.T. Sun. 2006. "A distributed multimodality sensor system for home-used sleep condition inference and monitoring." Paper presented at the 1st Transdisciplinary Conference on Distributed Diagnosis and Home Healthcare, Arlington, VA, April 2-4.

Pollak, C.P., W.W. Tryon, H. Nagaraja, and R. Dzwonczyk. 2001. How accurately does wrist actigraphy identify the states of sleep and wakefulness? *Sleep* 24(8):957-965.

Shiffman, S., A.A. Stone, and M.R. Hufford. 2008. Ecological momentary assessment. *Annual Review of Clinical Psychology* 4:1-32.

Smith, D., L. Ma, and N. Ryan. 2006. Acoustic environment as an indicator of social and physical context. *Personal and Ubiquitous Computing* 10(4):241-254.

Stratton, G., R. Murphy, M. Rosenberg, P. Fergus, and A. Attwood. 2012. "Creating intelligent environments to monitor and manipulate physical activity and sedentary behavior in public health and clinical settings." Paper presented at the International Conference on Communications (ICC), Ottawa, Canada, June 10-15.

Tapia, E.M., S.S. Intille, W. Haskell, K. Larson, J. Wright, A. King, and R. Friedman. 2007. "Real-time recognition of physical activities and their intensities using wireless accelerometers and a heart rate monitor." Paper prented at the 11th IEEE International Symposium on Wearable Computers. Boston, MA, Oct. 11-13.

Tapia, E.M., S.S. Intille, and K. Larson. 2007. Portable wireless sensors for object usage sensing in the home: Challenges and practicalities. In Ambient Intelligence, edited by S. Bernt, A.K. Dey, H. Gellersen, D. Boris, M.

Tscheligi, R. Wichert, E. Aarts, and A. Buchmann. 19-37. New York: Springer.

Thiagarajan, A., J. Biagioni, T. Gerlich, and J. Eriksson. 2010. "Cooperative transit tracking using smart-phones." Paper presented at the proceedings of the 8th ACM Conference on Embedded Networked Sensor Systems, Zurich, Switzerland, Nov. 3-5.

Troiano, R., and J. McClain. 2012. "Objective measures of physical activity, sleep, and strength in U.S. National Health and Nutrition Examination Survey (NHANES) 2011-2014." Paper presented at the International Conference on Diet and Activity Methods, Rome, Italy, May 14-17.

UK Biobank. n.d. Activity Monitor. Accessed July 20,2013. www.ukbiobank.ac.uk/physical-activity-monitor

Van Dantzig, S., G. Geleijnse, and A.T. van Halteren. 2011. Toward a persuasive mobile application to reduce sedentary behavior. *Personal and Ubiquitous Computing* 1-10.

Chapter 17

Aitchison, J. 1981. A new approach to null correlations of proportions. *Mathematical Geology* 13(2):175-189.

———. 1982. The statistical analysis of compositional data (with discussion). *Journal of the Royal Statistical Society, Series B (Statistical Methodology)* 44(2):139-177.

———. 1983. Principal component analysis of compositional data. *Biometrika* 70(1):57-65.

———. 1984. The statistical analysis of geochemical compositions. *Mathematical Geology* 16(6):531-564.

———. 1986. *The statistical analysis of compositional data, monographs on statistics and applied probability.* Caldwell, NJ: The Blackburn Press.

———. 2004. *The statistical analysis of compositional data.* Caldwell, NJ: The Blackburn Press.

Aitchison, J., C. Barcelo-Vidal, and V. Pawlowsky-Glahn. 2002. Some comments on compositional data analysis in archaeometry, in particular the fallacies in Tangri and Wright's dismissal of log ratio analysis. *Archaeometry* 44:295-304.

Billheimer, D., P. Guttorp, and W. Fagan. 2001. Statistical interpretation of species composition. *Journal of the American Statistical Association* 96:1205-1214.

Bolger, N., and J-P. Laurenceau. 2013. Intensive longitudinal methods: An introduction to diary and experience sampling research. New York: Guilford.

Breton, M., and B. Kovatchev. 2008. Analysis, modeling, and simulation of the accuracy of continuous glucose sensors. *Journal of Diabetes Science and Technology* 2(5):853-862.

Buccianti, A., G. Mateu-Figueras, and V. Pawlowsky-Glahn, eds. 2006. *Compositional data analysis in the geosciences: From theory to practice.* London: Geological Society of London.

Cain, K.L., J.F. Sallis, T.L. Conway, D. Van Dyck, and L. Calhoon. 2013. Using accelerometers in youth physical activity studies: A review of methods. *Journal of Physical Activity and Health* 10(3):437-450.

Cattell, R.B. 1952. The three basic factor-analytic research designs—their interrelations and derivatives. *Psychological Bulletin* 49(5):499-520.

———. 1988. The data box: Its ordering of total resources in terms of possible relational systems. In *Handbook of multivariate experimental psychology*, 2nd ed., edited by J.R. Nesselroade and R.B. Cattell, pp. 69-130.

Chayes, F. 1960. On correlation between variables of constant sum. *Journal of Geophysical Research* 65:4185-4193.

Clarke, W.L., D. Cox, L.A. Gonder-Frederick, W. Carter, and S.L. Pohl. 1987. Evaluating clinical accuracy of systems for self-monitoring of blood glucose. *Diabetes Care* 10(5):622-628.

Cohen, J. 1994. The earth is round (p < .05). *American Psychologist* 49:997-1003.

Dunstan, D.W., G.N. Healy, T. Sugiyama, and N. Owen. 2010. 'Too much sitting' and metabolic risk—Has modern technology caught up with us? *European Endocrinology* 6:19-23.

Engle, R., and M. Watson. 1981. A one-factor multivariate time series model of metropolitan wage rates. *Journal of American Statistical Association* 76:774-781.

Gilliam, L.K., and I.B. Hirsch. 2009. Practical aspects of real-time continuous glucose monitoring. *Diabetes Technology & Therapeutics* 11(Suppl.1):75-82.

Healy, G., D. Dunstan, J. Salmon, E. Cerin, J. Shaw, P. Zimmet, and N. Owen. 2008. Breaks in sedentary time: Beneficial associations with metabolic risk. *Diabetes Care* 31(4):661-666.

Healy, G.N., C.E. Matthews, D.W. Dunstan, E.A.H. Winkler, and N. Owen. 2011. Sedentary time and cardio-metabolic biomarkers in US adults: NHANES 2003-06. *European Heart Journal* 32(5):590-597.

Kane, M. 1994. Validating the performance standards associated with passing scores. *Review of Educational Research* 64:425-461.

———. 2001. So much remains the same: Conception and status of validation in setting standards. In *Setting performance standards: Concepts, methods, and perspectives*, edited by G. Cizek, pp. 53-88. Mahwah, NJ: Lawrence Erlbaum.

Owen, N., G.N. Healy, C.E. Matthews, and D.W. Dunstan. 2010. Too much sitting: The population health science of sedentary behavior. *Exercise and Sport Sciences Reviews* 38(3):105-109.

Pate, R.R., J.R. O'Neill, and F. Lobelo. 2008. The evolving definition of "sedentary". *Exercise and Sport Sciences Reviews* 36(4):173-178.

Pawlowsky-Glahn, V., and A. Buccianti, eds. 2011. *Compositional data analysis: Theory and applications.* Hoboken, NJ: Wiley

Pawlowsky-Glahn, V., and J.J. Egozcue. 2001. Geometric approach to statistical analysis on the simplex. *Sto-*

chastic Environmental Research and Risk Assessment (SERRA) 15:384-398.

Pawlowsky-Glahn, V., J.J. Egozcue, and R. Tolosana-Delgado. 2015. *Modelling and analysis of compositional data (Statistics in practice).* Hoboken, NJ: Wiley.

Pearson, K. 1897. Mathematical contributions to the theory of evolution—On a form of spurious correlation which may arise when indices are used in the measurement of organs. *Proceedings of the Royal Society of London* 60:489-498.

Ram, N., and K.J. Grimm. 2015. Growth curve modeling and longitudinal factor analysis. *Handbook of Child Psychology and Development Science* 1:1-31.

Raudenbush, S.W., and A.S. Bryk. 2002. *Hierarchical linear models: Applications and data analysis methods,* 2nd ed. Newbury Park, CA: Sage.

Rice, M.J., and D.B. Coursin. 2012. Continuous measurement of glucose: Facts and challenges. *Anesthesiology* 116(1):199-204.

van den Boogaart, K.G., and R. Tolosana-Delgado. 2013. *Analyzing compositional data with R.* New York: Springer.

Wentholt, I.M., J.B. Hoekstra, and J.H. DeVries. 2006. A critical appraisal of the continuous glucose-error grid analysis. *Diabetes Care* 29(8):1805-1811.

Zhu, W. 1997. A multi-level analysis of school factors associated with health-related fitness. *Research Quarterly for Exercise and Sport* 68:124-135.

———. 2012. Sadly, the earth is still round ($p < 0.05$). *Journal of Sport and Health Science* 1:9-11.

———. 2013. Science and art of setting performance standards and cutoff scores in kinesiology. *Research Quarterly for Exercise and Sport* 84(4):456-468.

Zhu, W., and S.J. Erbaugh. 1997. Assessing changes in swimming skills using the hierarchical linear model. *Measurement in Physical Education and Exercise Science* 1:179-201.

Zhu, W., M.T. Mahar, G.J. Welk, S.B. Going, and K.J. Cureton. 2011. Approaches for development of criterion-referenced standards in health-related youth fitness tests. American Journal of Preventive Medicine 41(4 Suppl. 2):68-76.

Chapter 18

Academy of Nutrition and Dietetics. 2006. Childhood overweight evidence analysis project. Available at: http://andevidencelibrary.com/topic.cfm?cat=3013&auth=1 Accessed on June 03, 2013 from http://andevidencelibrary.com/topic.cfm?cat=3013&auth=1

American Academy of Pediatrics. 2001. Children, adolescents, and television. Pediatrics 107(2):423-426.

Aminian, S., and E.A. Hinckson. 2012. Examining the validity of the ActivPAL monitor in measuring posture and ambulatory movement in children. International Journal of Behavioral Nutrition and Physical Activity 9:119.

Andersen, R.E., C.J. Crespo, S.J. Bartlett, L.J. Cheskin, and M. Pratt. 1998. Relationship of physical activity and television watching with body weight and level of fatness among children: Results from the Third National Health and Nutrition Examination Survey. JAMA 279(12):938-942.

Atkin, A.J., U. Ekelund, N.C. Moller, K. Froberg, L.B. Sardinha, L.B. Andersen, and S. Brage. 2013. Sedentary time in children: Influence of accelerometer processing on health relations. Medicine & Science in Sports & Exercise 45(6):1097-1104.

Babey, S.H., T.A. Hastert, and J. Wolstein. 2013. Adolescent sedentary behaviors: Correlates differ for television viewing and computer use. Journal of Adolescent Health 52(1):70-76.

Bailey, D.P., L.M. Boddy, L.A. Savory, S.J. Denton, and C.J. Kerr. 2013. Choice of activity-intensity classification thresholds impacts upon accelerometer-assessed physical activity-health relationships in children. PLOS ONE 8(2):e57101.

Biddle, S.J., T. Gorely, S.J. Marshall, I. Murdey, and N. Cameron. 2004. Physical activity and sedentary behaviours in youth: Issues and controversies. Journal of the Royal Society for the Promotion of Health 124(1):29-33.

Biddle, S.J.H., T. Gorely, and S.J. Marshall. 2009. Is television viewing a suitable marker of sedentary behavior in young people? Annals of Behavioral Medicine 38(2):147-153.

Biddle, S.J., S.J. Marshall, T. Gorely, and N. Cameron. 2009. Temporal and environmental patterns of sedentary and active behaviors during adolescents' leisure time. International Journal of Behavioral Medicine 16(3):278-286.

Boone-Heinonen, J., P. Gordon-Larsen, and L.S. Adair. 2008. Obesogenic clusters: Multidimensional adolescent obesity-related behaviors in the U.S. Annals of Behavioral Medicine 36(3):217-230.

Bowles, H.R. 2012. Measurement of active and sedentary behaviors: Closing the gaps in self-report methods. Journal of Physical Activity & Health 9:S1-S4.

Brodersen, N.H., A. Steptoe, D.R. Boniface, and J. Wardle. 2007. Trends in physical activity and sedentary behaviour in adolescence: Ethnic and socioeconomic differences. British Journal of Sports & Medicine 41(3):140-144.

Byun, W., J. Liu, and R.R. Pate. 2013. Association between objectively measured sedentary behavior and body mass index in preschool children. International Journal of Obesity 37(7):961-965.

Celis-Morales, C.A., F. Perez-Bravo, L. Ibanez, C. Salas, M.E. Bailey, and J.M. Gill. 2012. Objective vs. self-reported physical activity and sedentary time: Effects of measurement method on relationships with risk biomarkers. PLOS ONE 7(5):e36345.

Chaput, J.P., M. Lambert, M.E. Mathieu, M.S. Tremblay, J. O'Loughlin, and A. Tremblay. 2012. Physical activity vs. sedentary time: Independent associations with adiposity in children. Pediatric Obesity 7(3):251-258.

Chinapaw, M.J.M., M. Yildirim, T.M. Altenburg, A.S. Singh, E. Kovacs, D. Molnar, and J. Brug. 2012. Objective and self-rated sedentary time and indicators of metabolic health in Dutch and Hungarian 10-12 year olds: The ENERGY-Project. PLOS ONE 7(5):e36657.

Clark, B.K., E. Winkler, G.N. Healy, P.G. Gardiner, D.W. Dunstan, N. Owen, and M.M. Reeves. 2013. Adults' past-day recall of sedentary time: Reliability, validity, and responsiveness. Medicine & Science in Sports & Exercise 45(6):1198-1207.

Cliff, D.P., A.D. Okely, T.L. Burrows, R.A. Jones, P.J. Morgan, C.E. Collins, and L.A. Baur. 2013. Objectively measured sedentary behavior, physical activity, and plasma lipids in overweight and obese children. Obesity 21(2):382-385.

Colley, R.C., D. Garriguet, I. Janssen, S.L. Wong, T.J. Saunders, V. Carson, and M.S. Tremblay. 2013. The association between accelerometer-measured patterns of sedentary time and health risk in children and youth: Results from the Canadian Health Measures Survey. BMC Public Health 13:200.

Dall, P.M., P.R. McCrorie, M.H. Granat, and B.W. Stansfield. 2013. Step accumulation per minute epoch is not the same as cadence for free-living adults. Medicine & Science in Sports & Exercise 45(10):1995-2001.

Davies, G., J.J. Reilly, A.J. McGowan, P.M. Dall, M.H. Granat, and J.Y. Paton. 2012. Validity, practical utility, and reliability of the activPAL in preschool children. Medicine & Science in Sports & Exercise 44(4):761-768.

Delmas, C., C. Platat, B. Schweitzer, A. Wagner, M. Oujaa, and C. Simon. 2007. Association between television in bedroom and adiposity throughout adolescence. Obesity (Silver Spring) 15(10):2495-2503.

DeMattia, L., L. Lemont, and L. Meurer. 2007. Do interventions to limit sedentary behaviours change behaviour and reduce childhood obesity? A critical review of the literature. Obesity Reviews 8(1):69-81.

Denton, S.J., M.I. Trenell, T. Plotz, L.A. Savory, D.P. Bailey, and C.J. Kerr. 2013. Cardiorespiratory fitness is associated with hard and light intensity physical activity but not time spent sedentary in 10-14 year old schoolchildren: The HAPPY Study. PLOS ONE 8(4):e61073.

Dietz, W.H., and S.L. Gortmaker. 1985. Do we fatten our children at the television set? Obesity and television viewing in children and adolescents. Pediatrics 75(5):807-812.

Dolinsky, D.H., R.J. Brouwer, K.R. Evenson, A.M. Siega-Riz, and T. Ostbye. 2011. Correlates of sedentary time and physical activity among preschool-aged children. Preventing Chronic Disease 8(6):A131.

Dunstan, D.W., B. Howard, G.N. Healy, and N. Owen. 2012. Too much sitting—A health hazard. Diabetes Research and Clinical Practice 97(3):368-376.

Eaton, D.K., L. Kann, S. Kinchen, S. Shanklin, K.H. Flint, J. Hawkins, W.A. Harris, et al. 2012. Youth risk behavior surveillance—United States, 2011. MMWR Surveillance Summaries 61(4):1-162.

Ekelund, U., S. Brage, K. Froberg, M. Harro, S.A. Anderssen, L.B. Sardinha, C. Riddoch, and L.B. Andersen. 2006. TV viewing and physical activity are independently associated with metabolic risk in children: The European Youth Heart Study. PLOS Medicine 3(12):e488.

Ekelund, U., J. Luan, L.B. Sherar, D.W. Esliger, P. Griew, and A. Cooper. 2012. Moderate to vigorous physical activity and sedentary time and cardiometabolic risk factors in children and adolescents. JAMA 307(7):704-712.

Evenson, K.R., D.J. Catellier, K. Gill, K.S. Ondrak, and R.G. McMurray. 2008. Calibration of two objective measures of physical activity for children. Journal of Sports Sciences 26(14):1557-1565.

Fairclough, S.J., L.M. Boddy, A.F. Hackett, and G. Stratton. 2009. Associations between children's socioeconomic status, weight status, and sex, with screen-based sedentary behaviours and sport participation. International Journal of Pediatric Obesity 4(4):299-305.

Fakhouri, T.H.I., J.P. Hughes, D.J. Brody, B.K. Kit, and C.L. Ogden. 2013. Physical activity and screen-time viewing among elementary school-aged children in the United States from 2009 to 2010. JAMA Pediatrics 167(3):223-229.

Feldman, D.E., T. Barnett, I. Shrier, M. Rossignol, and L. Abenhaim. 2003. Is physical activity differentially associated with different types of sedentary pursuits? Archives of Pediatrics and Adolescent Medicine 157(8):797-802.

Fischer, C., M. Yildirim, J. Salmon, and M.J.M. Chinapaw. 2012. Comparing different accelerometer cut-points for sedentary time in children. Pediatric Exercise Science 24(2):220-228.

Foley, L., R. Maddison, T. Olds, and K. Ridley. 2012. Self-report use-of-time tools for the assessment of physical activity and sedentary behaviour in young people: Systematic review. Obesity Review 13(8):711-722.

Fuller-Tyszkiewicz, M., H. Skouteris, L.L. Hardy, and C. Halse. 2012. The associations between TV viewing, food intake, and BMI. A prospective analysis of data from the Longitudinal Study of Australian Children. Appetite 59(3):945-948.

Fulton, J.E., X. Wang, M.M. Yore, S.A. Carlson, D.A. Galuska, and C.J. Caspersen. 2009. Television viewing, computer use, and BMI among U.S. children and adolescents. Journal of Physical Activity and Health 6(Suppl. 1): S28-S35.

Gortmaker, S.L., A. Must, A.M. Sobol, K. Peterson, G.A. Colditz, and W.H. Dietz. 1996. Television viewing as a cause of increasing obesity among children in the United States, 1986-1990. Archives of Pediatrics & Adolescent Medicine 150(4):356-362.

Guinhouya, C.B., S. Soubrier, C. Vilhelm, P. Ravaux, M. Lemdani, A. Durocher, and H. Hubert. 2007. Physical activity and sedentary lifestyle in children as time-limited functions: Usefulness of the principal component analysis method. Behavioral Research Methods 39(3):682-688.

Hardy, L.L., T.A. Dobbine, E.A. Denney-Wilson, A.D. Okely, and M.L. Booth. 2009. Sedentariness, small-screen recreation, and fitness in youth. American Journal of Preventative Medicine 36(2):120-125.

Hardy, L.L., T.A. Dobbins, E.A. Denney-Wilson, A.D. Okely, and M.L. Booth. 2006. Descriptive epidemiology of small screen recreation among Australian adolescents. Journal of Paediatrics and Child Health 42(11):709-714.

Hardy, L.L., A.P. Hills, A. Timperio, D. Cliff, D. Lubans, P.J. Morgan, B.J. Taylor, and H. Brown. 2013. A hitchhiker's guide to assessing sedentary behaviour among young people: Deciding what method to use. Journal of Science and Medicine in Sport 16(1):28-35.

Hart, T.L., B.E. Ainsworth, and C. Tudor-Locke. 2011. Objective and subjective measures of sedentary behavior and physical activity. Medicine and Science in Sports and Exercise 43(3):449-456.

Healy, G.N., D.W. Dunstan, J. Salmon, J.E. Shaw, P.Z. Zimmet, and N. Owen. 2008. Television time and continuous metabolic risk in physically active adults. Medicine & Science in Sports & Exercise 40(4):639-645.

Herman, K.M., C.M. Sabiston, M.E. Mathieu, A. Tremblay, and G. Paradis. 2014. Sedentary behavior in a cohort of 8- to 10-year-old children at elevated risk of obesity. Preventative Medicine 60:115-120.

Hesketh, K.R., A.M. McMinn, U. Ekelund, S.J. Sharp, P.J. Collings, N.C. Harvey, K.M. Godfrey, H.M. Inskip, C. Cooper, and E.M. van Sluijs. 2014. Objectively measured physical activity in four-year-old British children: A cross-sectional analysis of activity patterns segmented across the day. International Journal of Behavioral Nutrition and Physical Activity 11:1.

Hinkley, T., J. Salmon, A.D. Okely, and S.G. Trost. 2010. Correlates of sedentary behaviours in preschool children: A review. International Journal of Behavioral Nutrition and Physical Activity 7:66.

Hislop, J.F., C. Bulley, T.H. Mercer, and J.J. Reilly. 2012. Comparison of accelerometry cut points for physical activity and sedentary behavior in preschool children: A validation study. Pediatric Exercise Science 24(4):563-576.

Hsu, Y.W., B.R. Belcher, E.E. Ventura, C.E. Byrd-Williams, M.J. Weigensberg, J.N. Davis, A.D. McClain, M.I. Goran, and D. Spruijt-Metz. 2011. Physical activity, sedentary behavior, and the metabolic syndrome in minority youth. Medicine & Science in Sports and Exercise 43(12):2307-2313.

Iannotti, R.J., and J. Wang. 2013. Trends in physical activity, sedentary behavior, diet, and BMI among US adolescents, 2001-2009. Pediatrics 132(4):606-614.

Jago, R., A. Page, K. Froberg, L.B. Sardinha, L. Klasson-Heggebo, and L.B. Andersen. 2008. Screen-viewing and the home TV environment: The European Youth Heart Study. Preventative Medicine 47(5):525-529.

Janz, K.F., T.L. Burns, and S.M. Levy. 2005. Tracking of activity and sedentary behaviors in childhood: The Iowa Bone Development Study. American Journal of Preventative Medicine 29(3):171-178.

Johnson, R., G. Welk, P.F. Saint-Maurice, and M. Ihmels. 2012. Parenting styles and home obesogenic environments. International Journal of Environmental Research and Public Health 9(4):1411-1426.

Kamath, C.C., K.S. Vickers, A. Ehrlich, L. McGovern, J. Johnson, V. Singhal, R. Paulo, A. Hettinger, P.J. Erwin, and V.M. Montori. 2008. Clinical review: Behavioral interventions to prevent childhood obesity: A systematic review and metaanalyses of randomized trials. Journal of Clinical Endocrinology & Metabolism 93(12):4606-4615.

Kim, Y., J.M. Lee, B.P. Peters, G.A. Gaesser, and G.J. Welk. 2014. Examination of different accelerometer cut-points for assessing sedentary behaviors in children. PLOS ONE 9(4):e90630.

King, A.C., K.N. Parkinson, A.J. Adamson, L. Murray, H. Besson, J.J. Reilly, L. Basterfield, and Gateshead Millennium Study Core Team. 2011. Correlates of objectively measured physical activity and sedentary behaviour in English children. European Journal of Public Health 21(4):424-431.

Kriska, A., L. Delahanty, S. Edelstein, N. Amodei, J. Chadwick, K. Copeland, B. Galvin, M. Haymond, M. Kelsey, C. Lassiter, and E. Mayer-Davis. 2013. Sedentary behavior and physical activity in youth with recent onset of type 2 diabetes. Pediatrics 131(3): e850-e856.

Kwon, S., T.L. Burns, S.M. Levy, and K.F. Janz. 2013. Which contributes more to childhood adiposity—High levels of sedentarism or low levels of moderate-through-vigorous physical activity? The Iowa Bone Development Study. Journal of Pediatrics 162(6):1169-1174.

Leung, M.M., A. Agaronov, K. Grytsenko, and M.C. Yeh. 2012. Intervening to reduce sedentary behaviors and childhood obesity among school-age youth: A systematic review of randomized trials. Journal of Obesity 2012:685430.

Li, S., M.S. Treuth, and Y. Wang. 2010. How active are American adolescents and have they become less active? Obesity Reviews 11(12):847-862.

Liao, Y., J. Liao, C.P. Durand, and G.F. Dunton. 2014. Which type of sedentary behaviour intervention is more effective at reducing body mass index in children? A meta-analytic review. Obesity Reviews 15(3):159-168.

Lowry, R., S.M. Lee, J.E. Fulton, Z. Demissie, and L. Kann. 2013. Obesity and other correlates of physical activity and sedentary behaviors among US high school students. Journal of Obesity 2013:276318.

Lubans, D.R., K. Hesketh, D.P. Cliff, L.M. Barnett, J. Salmon, J. Dollman, P.J. Morgan, A.P. Hills, and L.L. Hardy. 2011. A systematic review of the validity and reliability of sedentary behaviour measures used with children and adolescents. Obesity Reviews 12(10):781-799.

Marshall, S.J., S.J. Biddle, T. Gorely, N. Cameron, and I. Murdey. 2004. Relationships between media use, body fatness and physical activity in children and youth: A meta-analysis. International Journal of Obesity and Related Metabolic Disorders 28(10):1238-1246.

Marshall, S.J., S.J.H. Biddle, J.F. Sallis, T.L. McKenzie, and T.L. Conway. 2002. Clustering of sedentary behaviors and physical activity among youth: A cross-national study. Pediatric Exercise Science 14(4):401-417.

Martinez-Gomez, D., J.C. Eisenmann, G.N. Healy, S. Gomez-Martinez, L.E. Diaz, D.W. Dunstan, O.L. Veiga, and A. Marcos. 2012. Sedentary behaviors and emerging cardiometabolic biomarkers in adolescents. Journal of Pediatrics 160(1):104-110.e2.

Matthews, C.E., K.Y. Chen, P.S. Freedson, M.S. Buchowski, B.M. Beech, R.R. Pate, and R.P. Troiano. 2008. Amount of time spent in sedentary behaviors in the United States, 2003-2004. American Journal of Epidemiology 167(7):875-881.

Matthews, C.E., S.C. Moore, S.M. George, J. Sampson, and H.R. Bowles. 2012. Improving self-reports of active and sedentary behaviors in large epidemiologic studies. Exercise and Sports Sciences Reviews 40(3):118-126.

Mitchell, J.A., C. Mattocks, A.R. Ness, S.D. Leary, R.R. Pate, M. Dowda, S.N. Blair, and C. Riddoch. 2009. Sedentary behavior and obesity in a large cohort of children. Obesity (Silver Spring) 17(8):1596-1602.

Mitchell, J.A., R.R. Pate, M.W. Beets, and P.R. Nader. 2013. Time spent in sedentary behavior and changes in childhood BMI: A longitudinal study from ages 9 to 15 years. International Journal of Obesity 37(1):54-60.

Mitchell, J.A., R.R. Pate, and S.N. Blair. 2012. Screen-based sedentary behavior and cardiorespiratory fitness from age 11 to 13. Medicine & Science in Sports & Exercise 44(7):1302-1309.

Mitchell, J.A., R.R. Pate, M. Dowda, C. Mattocks, C. Riddoch, A.R. Ness, and S.N. Blair. 2012. A prospective study of sedentary behavior in a large cohort of youth. Medicine & Science in Sports & Exercise 44(6):1081-1087.

Must, A., L.G. Bandini, D.J. Tybor, S.M. Phillips, E.N. Naumova, and W.H. Dietz. 2007. Activity, inactivity, and screen time in relation to weight and fatness over adolescence in girls. Obesity (Silver Spring) 15(7):1774-1781.

Must, A., and D.J. Tybor. 2005. Physical activity and sedentary behavior: A review of longitudinal studies of weight and adiposity in youth. International Journal of Obesity 29(Suppl. 2):S84-S96.

Nelson, M.C., D. Neumark-Stzainer, P.J. Hannan, J.R. Sirard, and M. Story. 2006. Longitudinal and secular trends in physical activity and sedentary behavior during adolescence. Pediatrics 118(6):e1627-e1634.

Nilsson, A., L.B. Andersen, Y. Ommundsen, K. Froberg, L.B. Sardinha, K. Piehl-Aulin, and U. Ekelund. 2009. Correlates of objectively assessed physical activity and sedentary time in children: A cross-sectional study (The European Youth Heart Study). BMC Public Health 9:322.

Nilsson, A., S.A. Anderssen, L.B. Andersen, K. Froberg, C. Riddoch, L.B. Sardinha, and U. Ekelund. 2009. Between- and within-day variability in physical activity and inactivity in 9-and 15-year-old European children. Scandinavian Journal of Medicine & Science in Sports 19(1):10-18.

Olds, T.S., K.E. Ferrar, N.K. Schranz, and C.A. Maher. 2011. Obese adolescents are less active than their normal-weight peers, but wherein lies the difference? Journal of Adolescent Health 48(2):189-195.

Olds, T.S., C.A. Maher, K. Ridley, and D.M. Kittel. 2010. Descriptive epidemiology of screen and non-screen sedentary time in adolescents: A cross sectional study.

International Journal of Behavioral Nutrition and Physical Activity 7:92.

Olshansky, S.J., D.J. Passaro, R.C. Hershow, J. Layden, B.A. Carnes, J. Brody, L. Hayflick, R.N. Butler, D.B. Allison, and D.S. Ludwig. 2005. A potential decline in life expectancy in the United States in the 21st century. New England Journal of Medicine 352(11):1138-1145.

Ortega, F.B., K. Konstabel, E. Pasquali, J.R. Ruiz, A. Hurtig-Wennlof, J. Maestu, M. Lof, et al. 2013. Objectively measured physical activity and sedentary time during childhood, adolescence and young adulthood: A cohort study. PLOS ONE 8(4):e60871.

Owen, N., G.N. Healy, C.E. Matthews, and D.W. Dunstan. 2010. Too much sitting: The population health science of sedentary behavior. Exercise and Sport Sciences Reviews 38(3):105-113.

Pate, R.R., J.A. Mitchell, W. Byun, and M. Dowda. 2011. Sedentary behaviour in youth. British Journal of Sports Medicine 45(11):906-913.

Pate, R.R., J. Stevens, C. Pratt, J.F. Sallis, K.H. Schmitz, L.S. Webber, G. Welk, and D.R. Young. 2006. Objectively measured physical activity in sixth-grade girls. Archives of Pediatric and Adolescent Medicine 160(12):1262-1268.

Pearson, N., and S.J. Biddle. 2011. Sedentary behavior and dietary intake in children, adolescents, and adults. A systematic review. American Journal of Preventative Medicine 41(2):178-188.

Pearson, N., R.E. Braithwaite, S.J. Biddle, E.M. van Sluijs, and A.J. Atkin. 2014. Associations between sedentary behaviour and physical activity in children and adolescents: A meta-analysis. Obesity Reviews 15(8):666-675.

Puyau, M.R., A.L. Adolph, F.A. Vohra, and N.F. Butte. 2002. Validation and calibration of physical activity monitors in children. Obesity Research 10(3):150-157.

Reilly, J.J., J. Coyle, L. Kelly, G. Burke, S. Grant, and J.Y. Paton. 2003. An objective method for measurement of sedentary behavior in 3- to 4-year olds. Obesity Research 11(10):1155-1158.

Robinson, T.N. 1999. Reducing children's television viewing to prevent obesity: A randomized controlled trial. JAMA 282(16):1561-1567.

Rowlands, A.V. 2009. Methodological approaches for investigating the biological basis for physical activity in children. Pediatric Exercise Science 21(3):273-278.

Ruiz, J.R., F.B. Ortega, D. Martinez-Gomez, I. Labayen, L.A. Moreno, I. De Bourdeaudhuij, Y. Manios, et al. 2011. Objectively measured physical activity and sedentary time in European adolescents: The HELENA study. American Journal of Epidemiology 174(2):173-184.

Rusby, J.C., E. Westling, R. Crowley, and J.M. Light. 2013. Psychosocial correlates of physical and sedentary activities of early adolescent youth. Health Education & Behavior 41(1):42-51.

Saint-Maurice, P.F., Y. Kim, G.J. Welk, and G.A. Gaesser. 2015. Kids are not little adults: What MET threshold captures sedentary behavior in children? European Journal of Applied Physiology 116(1):29-38.

Sallis, J.F., N. Owen, and M.J. Fotheringham. 2000. Behavioral epidemiology: A systematic framework to classify phases of research on health promotion and disease prevention. Annals of Behavioral Medicine 22(4):294-298.

Saunders, T.J., J.P. Chaput, and M.S. Treblay. 2014. Sedentary behaviour as an emerging risk factor for cardiometabolic diseases in children and youth. Canadian Journal of Diabetes 38(1): 53-61.

Sellers, C.E., P.M. Grant, C.G. Ryan, C. O'Kane, K. Raw, and D. Conn. 2012. Take a walk in the park? A crossover pilot trial comparing brisk walking in two different environments: Park and urban. Preventive Medicine 55(5):438-443.

Sisson, S.B., T.S. Church, C.K. Martin, C. Tudor-Locke, S.R. Smith, C. Bouchard, C.P. Earnest, T. Rankinen, R.L. Newton, and P.T. Katzmarzyk. 2009. Profiles of sedentary behavior in children and adolescents: The US National Health and Nutrition Examination Survey, 2001-2006. International Journal of Pediatric Obesisty 4(4):353-359.

Stamatakis, E., N. Coobms, R. Jago, A. Gama, I. Mourão, H. Nogueira, V. Rosado, and C. Padez. 2013. Type-specific screen time associations with cardiovascular risk markers in children. American Journal of Preventive Medicine 44(5): 481-488.

Steele, R.M., E.M. van Sluijs, S.J. Sharp, J.R. Landsbaugh, U. Ekelund, and S.J. Griffin. 2010. An investigation of patterns of children's sedentary and vigorous physical activity throughout the week. International Journal of Behavioral Nutrition and Physical Activity 7:88.

Steeves, J.A., D.L. Thompson, D.R. Bassett, E.C. Fitzhugh, and H.A. Raynor. 2012. A review of different behavior modification strategies designed to reduce sedentary screen behaviors in children. Journal of Obesity 2012:379215.

Sternfeld, B., and L. Goldman-Rosas. 2012. A systematic approach to selecting an appropriate measure of self-reported physical activity or sedentary behavior. Journal of Physical Activity and Health 9(Suppl. 1):S19-S28.

Stone, M.R., A.V. Rowlands, and R.G. Eston. 2009. Relationships between accelerometer-assessed physical activity and health in children: Impact of the activity-intensity classification method. Journal of Sports Science and Medicine 8(1):136-143.

Straker, L., A. Smith, B. Hands, T. Olds, and R. Abbott. 2013. Screen-based media use clusters are related to other activity behaviours and health indicators in adolescents. BMC Public Health 13:1174.

Tanaka, C., J.J. Reilly, and W.Y. Huang. 2014. Longitudinal changes in objectively measured sedentary behaviour and their relationship with adiposity in children and adolescents: Systematic review and evidence appraisal. Obesity Reviews 15(10):791-803.

Tremblay, M.S., A.G. LeBlanc, M.E. Kho, T.J. Saunders, R. Larouche, R.C. Colley, G. Goldfield, and S. Connor Gorber. 2011. Systematic review of sedentary behaviour

and health indicators in school-aged children and youth. International Journal of Behavioral Nutrition and Physical Activity 8:98.

Treuth, M.S., C.D. Baggett, C.A. Pratt, S.B. Going, J.P. Elder, E.Y. Charneco, and L.S. Webber. 2009. A longitudinal study of sedentary behavior and overweight in adolescent girls. Obesity 17(5):1003-1008.

Treuth, M.S., K. Schmitz, D.J. Catellier, R.G. McMurray, D.M. Murray, M.J. Almeida, S. Going, J.E. Norman, and R. Pate. 2004. Defining accelerometer thresholds for activity intensities in adolescent girls. Medicine & Science in Sports & Exercise 36(7):1259-1266.

Trilk, J.L., R.R. Pate, K.A. Pfeiffer, M. Dowda, C.L. Addy, K.M. Ribisl, D. Neumark-Sztainer, and L.A. Lytle. 2012. A cluster analysis of physical activity and sedentary behavior patterns in middle school girls. Journal of Adolescent Health 51(3):292-298.

Troiano, R.P., D. Berrigan, K.W. Dodd, L.C. Masse, T. Tilert, and M. McDowell. 2008. Physical activity in the United States measured by accelerometer. Medicine & Science in Sports & Exercise 40(1):181-188.

Troiano, R.P., K.K. Pettee Gabriel, G.J. Welk, N. Owen, and B. Sternfeld. 2012. Reported physical activity and sedentary behavior: Why do you ask? Journal of Physical Activity and Health 9(Suppl. 1):S68-S75.

Trost, S.G., B.S. Fees, S.J. Haar, A.D. Murray, and L.K. Crowe. 2012. Identification and validity of accelerometer cut-points for toddlers. Obesity 20(11):2317-2319.

Trost, S.G., P.D. Loprinzi, R. Moore, and K.A. Pfeiffer. 2011. Comparison of accelerometer cut points for predicting activity intensity in youth. Medicine & Science in Sports & Exercise 43(7):1360-1368.

Tudor-Locke, C., W.D. Johnson, and P.T. Katzmarzyk. 2011. U.S. population profile of time-stamped accelerometer outputs: Impact of wear time. Journal of Physical Activity & Health 8(5):693-698.

Van Cauwenberghe, E., R.A. Jones, T. Hinkley, D. Crawford, and A.D. Okely. 2012. Patterns of physical activity and sedentary behaviour in preschool children. International Journal of Behavioral Nutrition and Physical Activity 9:138.

Van Cauwenberghe, E., L. Wooller, L. Mackay, G. Cardon, and M. Oliver. 2012. Comparison of Actical and activPAL measures of sedentary behaviour in preschool children. Journal of Science and Medicine in Sport 15(6):526-531.

Van Der Horst, K., M.J. Paw, J.W. Twisk, and W.Van Mechelen. 2007. A brief review on correlates of physical activity and sedentariness in youth. Medicine & Science in Sports Exercise 39(8):1241-1250.

van Grieken, A., N.P. Ezendam, W.D. Paulis, J.C. van der Wouden, and H. Raat. 2012. Primary prevention of overweight in children and adolescents: A meta-analysis of the effectiveness of interventions aiming to decrease sedentary behaviour. International Journal of Behavioral Nutrition and Physical Activity 9:61.

van Sluijs, E.M.F., A. Page, Y. Ommundsen, and S.J. Griffin. 2010. Behavioural and social correlates of sedentary time in young people. British Journal of Sports Medicine 44(10):747-755.

Welk, Greg. 2002. Physical activity assessments for health-related research. Champaign, IL: Human Kinetics.

Whitt-Glover, M.C., W.C. Taylor, M.F. Floyd, M.M. Yore, A.K. Yancey, and C.E. Matthews. 2009. Disparities in physical activity and sedentary behaviors among US children and adolescents: Prevalence, correlates, and intervention implications. Journal of Public Health Policy 30(Suppl. 1):S309-S334.

Winkler, E.A.H., P.A. Gardiner, B.K. Clark, C.E. Matthews, N. Owen, and G.N. Healy. 2012. Identifying sedentary time using automated estimates of accelerometer wear time. British Journal of Sports Medicine 46(6):436-442.

Zabinski, M.F., G.J. Norman, J.F. Sallis, K.J. Calfas, and K. Patrick. 2007. Patterns of sedentary behavior among adolescents. Health Psychology 26(1):113-120.

Chapter 19

Allman-Farinelli, M.A., T. Chey, D. Merom, and A.E. Bauman. 2010. Occupational risk of overweight and obesity: An analysis of the Australian Health Survey. Journal of Occupational Medicine and Toxicology 5:14.

Au, N., and B. Hollingsworth. 2011. Employment patterns and changes in body weight among young women. Preventive Medicine 52(5):310-316.

Ball, K., W. Brown, and D. Crawford. 2002. Who does not gain weight? Prevalence and predictors of weight maintenance in young women. International Journal of Obesity 26(12):1570-1578.

Bassett, D.R., P.R. Schneider, and G.E. Huntington. 2004. Physical activity in an Old Order Amish community. Medicine & Science in Sports & Exercise 36(1):79-85.

Brown, W.J., A.E. Bauman, and N. Owen. 2009. Stand up, sit down, keep moving: Turning circles in physical activity research? British Journal of Sports Medicine 43(2):86-88.

Brown, W.J., Y.D. Miller, and R. Miller. 2003. Sitting time and work patterns as indicators of overweight and obesity in Australian adults. International Journal of Obesity 27(11):1340-1346.

Brown, H.E., G.C. Ryde, N.D. Gilson, N.W. Burton, and W.J. Brown. 2013. Objectively measured sedentary behaviour and physical activity in office employees: Relationships with presenteeism. Journal of Occupational and Environmental Medicine 55(8):945-953.

Brown, W.J., L. Williams, J.H. Ford, K. Ball, and A.J. Dobson. 2005. Identifying the energy gap: Magnitude and determinants of 5-year weight gain in mid-age women. Obesity Research 13(8):1431-1441.

Chapman, L.S. 2005. Presenteeism and its role in worksite health promotion. American Journal of Health Promotion 19(4):1-8.

Chau, J.Y., H.P. van der Ploeg, D. Merom, T. Chey, and A.E. Bauman. 2012. Cross-sectional associations between occupational and leisure-time sitting, physical activity and obesity in working adults. Preventative Medicine 54(3-4):195-200.

Chau, J.Y., H.P. van der Ploeg, J.G.Z. van Uffelen, J. Wong, I. Riphagen, G.N. Healy, N.D. Gilson, et al. 2010. Are workplace interventions to reduce sitting effective? A systemic review. Preventive Medicine 51(5):352-356.

Church, T.S., D.M. Thomas, C. Tudor-Locke, P.T. Katzmarzyk, C.P. Earnest, R.Q. Rodarte, C.K. Martin, S.N. Blair, and C. Bouchard. 2011. Trends over 5 decades in U.S. occupation-related physical activity and their associations with obesity. PLoS ONE 6(5):e19657.

de Cocker, K., M.J. Duncan, C. Short, J.G. van Uffelen, and C. Vandelanotte. 2014. Understanding occupational sitting: Prevalence, correlates and moderating effects in Australian employees. Preventive Medicine 67:288-294.

Duncan, M.J., H.M. Badland, and W.K. Mummery. 2010. Physical activity level by occupational category in non-metropolitan Australian adults. Journal of Physical Activity and Health 7(6):718-723.

Dunstan, D.W., B.A. Kingwell, R. Larsen, G.N. Healy, E. Cerin, M.T. Hamilton, J.E. Shaw, et al. 2012. Breaking up prolonged sitting reduces postprandial glucose and insulin responses. Diabetes Care 35(5):976-983.

Ekelund, U., Steene-Johannessen, J., Brown, W.J., Fagerland, M.W., Owen, N., Powell, K.E., ... & Lee, I. M. (2016). Physical activity attenuates the detrimental association of sitting time with mortality: A harmonised meta-analysis of data from more than one million men and women. The Lancet.

Gilson, N.D., T.G. Pavey, C. Vandelanotte, M.J. Duncan, S.R. Gomersall, S.G. Trost, and W.J. Brown. 2015. Chronic disease risks and use of a smartphone application during a physical activity and dietary intervention in Australian truck drivers. Australian and New Zealand Journal of Public Health, Epub ahead of print, 2015 Dec 29. doi: 10.1111/1753-6405.12501

Hallman, D.M., N. Gupta, S.E. Mathiassen, and A. Holtermann. 2015. Association between objectively measured sitting time and neck-shoulder pain among blue-collar workers. International Archives of Occupational Environment and Health 88(8):1031-1042.

Healy, G.N., D.W. Dunstan, J. Salmon, E. Cerin, J.E. Shaw, P.Z. Zimmet, and N. Owen. 2008. Breaks in sedentary time: Beneficial associations with metabolic risk. Diabetes Care 31(4):661-666.

Hu, F.B., T.Y. Li, G.A. Colditz, W.C. Willett, and J.E. Manson. 2003. Television watching and other sedentary behaviors in relation to risk of obesity and type 2 diabetes mellitus in women. Journal of the American Medical Association 289(14):1785-1791.

Jans, M.P., K.I. Proper, and V.H. Hildebrandt. 2007. Sedentary behavior in Dutch workers: Differences between occupations and business sectors. American Journal of Preventative Medicine 33(6):450-454.

Lis, A.M., K.M. Black, H. Korn, and M. Nordin. 2007. Association between sitting and occupational LBP. European Spine Journal 16(2):283-298.

Lyden, K., S.L. Kozey-Keadle, J.W. Staudenmayer, and P.S. Freedson. 2012.Validity of two wearable monitors to estimate breaks from sedentary time. *Medicine & Science in Sports & Exercise* 44(11):2243-2252.

McCrady, S.K., and J.A. Levine. 2009. Sedentariness at work: How much do we really sit? *Obesity* 17(11):2103-2105.

Miller, R., and W. Brown. 2004. Steps and sitting in a working population. *International Journal of Behavioral Medicine* 11(4):219-224.

Mummery, W.K., G.M. Schofield, R. Steele, E.G. Eakin, and W.J. Brown. 2005. Occupational sitting time and overweight and obesity in Australian workers. *American Journal of Preventative Medicine* 29(2):91-97.

Ng, S.W., and B.M. Popkin. 2012. Time use and physical activity: A shift away from movement across the globe. *Obesity Reviews* 13(8):659-680.

Paffenbarger R.S., S.N. Blair, and I.M. Lee. 2001. A history of physical activity, cardiovascular health and longevity: The scientific contributions of Jeremy N Morris, DSc, DPH, FRCP. *International Journal of Epidemiology* 30(5):1184-1192.

Parry, S., and L. Straker. 2013. The contribution of office work to sedentary behaviour associated risk. *BMC Public Health* 13:296.

Roffey, D.M., E.K. Wai, P. Bishop, B.K. Kwon, and S. Dagenias. 2010. Causal assessment of occupational sitting and low back pain: Results of a systemic review. *The Spine Journal* 10(3):252-261.

Rütten, A., and K. Abu-Omar. 2004. Prevalence of physical activity in the European Union. *Sozial-und Präventivmedzin* 49(4):281-289.

Ryan, C.G., P.M. Dall, M.H. Granat, and P.M. Grant. 2011. Sitting patterns at work: Objective measurement of adherence to current recommendations. *Ergonomics* 54(6):531-538.

Ryde, G.C., N.D. Gilson, A. Suppini, and W.J. Brown. 2012. Validation of a novel, objective measure of occupational sitting. *Journal of Occupational Health* 54:383-386.

Ryde, G., H.E. Brown, N.D. Gilson, and W.J. Brown. 2014. Are we chained to our desks? Describing desk based sitting using a novel measure of occupational sitting. *Journal of Physical Activity and Health* 11(7):1318-1323.

Steele, R., and K. Mummery. 2003. Occupational physical activity across occupational categories. *Journal of Science and Medicine in Sport* 6(4):398-407.

Steeves, J.A., C. Tudor-Locke, R.A. Murphy, G.A. King, E.C. Fitzhugh, and T.B. Harris. 2015. Classification of occupational activity categories using accelerometry: NHANES 2003-2004. *International Journal of Behavioral Nutrition and Physical Activity* 12(1):89.

Thorp, A.A., G.N. Healy, E. Winkler, B.K. Clark, P.A. Gardiner, N. Owen, and D.W. Dunstan. 2012. Prolonged sedentary time and physical activity in workplace and non-work contexts: A cross-sectional study of office, customer service and call centre employees. *International Journal of Behavioral Nutrition and Physical Activity* 9:128-137.

Toomingas, A., M. Forsman, S.E. Mathiassen, M. Heiden, and T. Nilsson. 2012. Variation between seated and standing/walking postures among male and female call centre operators. *BMC Public Health* 12:154.

Varela-Mato, V., T. Yates, S.J. Biddle, and S. Clemes. 2015. Time spent sitting during and outside working hours in bus drivers: A pilot study. *Preventive Medicine Reports* 3:36-39.

van Uffelen, J.G.Z., M.J. Watson, A.J. Dobson, and W.J. Brown. 2010. Sitting time is associated with weight but not with weight gain in mid-aged Australian women. *Obesity* 18(9):1788-1794.

van Uffelen J.G.Z., J. Wong, J.Y. Chau, H.P. van der Ploeg, I. Riphagen, N.D. Gilson, N.W. Burton, et al. 2010. Associations between occupational sitting and health risks: A systematic review. *American Journal of Preventative Medicine* 39(4):379-388.

Wane, S.L. 2012. "Young women and weight gain: What is the role of patterns of physical activity and sedentary behaviour?" PhD diss., The University of Queensland, Australia.

Wong, J.Y., N.D. Gilson, R.A. Bush, and W.J. Brown. 2014. Patterns and perceptions of physical activity and sedentary time in male transport drivers working in regional Australia. *Australian and New Zealand Journal of Public Health* 38(4):314-320.

Chapter 20

Aggarwal, B., M. Liao, A. Christian, and L. Mosca. 2009. Influence of caregiving on lifestyle and psychosocial risk factors among family members of patients hospitalized with cardiovascular disease. Journal of General Internal Medicine 24(1):93-98.

American College of Sports Medicine. 2013. About Exercise is Medicine. Exercise is Medicine. http://exerciseismedicine.org/about.htm

Ashburner, J.M., J.A. Cauley, P. Cawthon, K.E. Ensrud, M.C. Hochberg, and L. Fredman. 2011. Self-ratings of health and change in walking speed over 2 years: Results from the Caregiver-Study of Osteoporotic Fractures. American Journal of Epidemiology 173(8): 882-889.

Atienza, A.A., B.W. Hesse, T.B. Baker, D.B. Abrams, B.K. Rimer, R.T. Croyle, and L.N. Volckmann. 2007. Critical issues in eHealth research. American Journal of Preventive Medicine 32(5 Suppl.):S71-S74.

Balboa-Castillo, T., L.M. Leon-Munoz, A. Graciani, F. Rodriguez-Artalejo, and P. Guallar-Castillon. 2011. Longitudinal association of physical activity and sedentary behavior during leisure time with health-related quality of life in community-dwelling older adults. Health and Quality of Life Outcomes 9:47.

Barnes, P.M., and C.A. Schoenborn. 2012. Trends in adults receiving a recommendation for exercise or other physical activity from a physician or other health professional. NCHS Data Brief 86:1-8.

Bowerman, J. 2006. Designing the primary health care centre of the future: A community experience. International Journal of Health Care Quality Assurance Incorporating Leadership in Health Services 19(6-7):xvi-xxiii.

Bowman, S.A. 2006. Television-viewing characteristics of adults: Correlations to eating practices and overweight and health status. Preventing Chronic Disease 3(2):A38.

Brown, C.J., D.T. Redden, K.L. Flood, and R.M. Allman. 2009. The underrecognized epidemic of low mobility during hospitalization of older adults. Journal of the American Geriatrics Society 57(9):1660-1665.

Buckley, J., G. Tucker, G. Hugo, G. Wittert, R.J. Adams, and D.H. Wilson. 2013. The Australian baby boomer population-factors influencing changes to health-related quality of life over time. Journal of Aging and Health 25(1):29-55.

Buman, M.P., S.J. Winter, J.L. Sheats, E.B. Hekler, J.J. Otten, L.A. Grieco, and A.C. King. 2013. The Stanford healthy neighborhood discovery tool: A computerized tool to assess active living environments. American Journal of Preventive Medicine 44(4):e41-e47.

Burton, N.W., M. Haynes, J.G. van Uffelen, W.J. Brown, and G. Turrell. 2012. Mid-aged adults' sitting time in three contexts. American Journal of Preventive Medicine 42(4):363-373.

Centers for Disease Control and Prevention. 2012. Falls among older adults: An overview. www.cdc.gov/home-andrecreationalsafety/falls/adultfalls.html

Chastin, S.F., E. Ferriolli, N.A. Stephens, K.C. Fearon, and C. Greig. 2012. Relationship between sedentary behaviour, physical activity, muscle quality and body composition in healthy older adults. Age and Ageing 41(1):111-114.

Chen, B., K.E. Covinsky, I. Stijacic Cenzer, N. Adler, and B.A. Williams. 2012. Subjective social status and functional decline in older adults. Journal of General Internal Medicine 27(6):693-699.

Clark, B.K., T. Sugiyama, G.N. Healy, J. Salmon, D.W. Dunstan, and N. Owen. 2009. Validity and reliability of measures of television viewing time and other non-occupational sedentary behaviour of adults: A review. Obesity Reviews 10(1):7-16.

Covinsky, K.E., R.M. Palmer, R.H. Fortinsky, S.R. Counsell, A.L. Stewart, D. Kresevic, C.J. Burant, and C.S. Landefeld. 2003. Loss of independence in activities of daily living in older adults hospitalized with medical illnesses: Increased vulnerability with age. Journal of the American Geriatrics Society 51(4):451-458.

Covinsky, K.E., E. Pierluissi, and C.B. Johnston. 2011. Hospitalization-associated disability: "She was probably able to ambulate, but I'm not sure". Journal of the American Medical Association 306(16):1782-1793.

De Greef, K., B. Deforche, C. Tudor-Locke, and I. De Bourdeaudhuij. 2010. A cognitive-behavioural pedometer-based group intervention on physical activity and sedentary behaviour in individuals with type 2 diabetes. Health Education Research 25(5):724-736.

De Greef, K.P., B.I. Deforche, J.B. Ruige, J.J. Bouckaert, C.E. Tudor-Locke, J.M. Kaufman, and I.M. De Bourdeaudhuij. 2011. The effects of a pedometer-based behavioral modification program with telephone support on physical activity and sedentary behavior in type 2 diabetes patients. Patient Education and Counseling 84(2):275-279.

Depp, C.A., D.A. Schkade, W.K. Thompson, and D.V. Jeste. 2010. Age, affective experience, and television use. American Journal of Preventive Medicine 39(2):173-178.

Ding, D., T. Sugiyama, E. Winkler, E. Cerin, K. Wijndaele, and N. Owen. 2012. Correlates of change in adults' television viewing time: A four-year follow-up study. Medicine and Science in Sports and Exercise 44(7):1287-1292.

Dogra, S., and L. Stathokostas. 2012. Sedentary behavior and physical activity are independent predictors of successful aging in middle-aged and older adults. Journal of Aging Research 2012:190654.

Egger, G. 2007. Personal carbon trading: A potential "stealth intervention" for obesity reduction? Medical Journal of Australia 187(3):185-187.

Evenson, K.R., D.M. Buchner, and K.B. Morland. 2012. Objective measurement of physical activity and sedentary behavior among US adults aged 60 years or older. Preventing Chronic Disease 9:E26.

Evenson, K.R., W.D. Rosamond, J. Cai, A.V. Diez-Roux, F.L. Brancati, and Atherosclerosis Risk in Communities Study Investigators. 2002. Influence of retirement on leisure-time physical activity: The Atherosclerosis Risk in Communities Study. American Journal of Epidemiology 155(8):692-699.

Fitzsimons, C.F., A. Kirk, G. Baker, F. Michie, C. Kane, and N. Mutrie. 2013. Using an individualised consultation and activPAL feedback to reduce sedentary time in older Scottish adults: Results of a feasibility and pilot study. Preventive Medicine 57(5):718-720.

Foley, D.J., M.V. Vitiello, D.L. Bliwise, S. Ancoli-Israel, A.A. Monjan, and J.K. Walsh. 2007. Frequent napping is associated with excessive daytime sleepiness, depression, pain, and nocturia in older adults: Findings from the National Sleep Foundation '2003 Sleep in America' Poll. American Journal of Geriatric Psychiatry 15(4):344-350.

Fried, L.P., M.C. Carlson, M. Freedman, K.D. Frick, T.A. Glass, J. Hill, S. McGill, et al. 2004. A social model for health promotion for an aging population: Initial evidence on the Experience Corps model. Journal of Urban Health 81(1):64-78.

Gardiner, P.A., E.G. Eakin, G.N. Healy, and N. Owen. 2011. Feasibility of reducing older adults' sedentary time. American Journal of Preventive Medicine 41(2):174-177.

Gardiner, P.A., G.N. Healy, E.G. Eakin, B.K. Clark, D.W. Dunstan, J.E. Shaw, P.Z. Zimmet, and N. Owen. 2011. Associations between television viewing time and overall sitting time with the metabolic syndrome in older men and women: The Australian Diabetes, Obesity and Lifestyle Study. Journal of the American Geriatrics Society 59(5):788-796.

Gennuso, K.P., R.E. Gangnon, C.E. Matthews, K.M. Thraen-Borowski, and L.H. Colbert. 2013. Sedentary behavior, physical activity, and markers of health in older adults. Medicine and Science in Sports and Exercise 45(8):1493-1500.

Hawkes, A.L., S. Gollschewski, B.M. Lynch, and S. Chambers. 2009. A telephone-delivered lifestyle intervention for colorectal cancer survivors 'Can Change': A pilot study. Psycho-Oncology 18(4):449-455.

Hawkley, L.C., R.A. Thisted, and J.T. Cacioppo. 2009. Loneliness predicts reduced physical activity: Cross-sectional and longitudinal analyses. Health Psychology 28(3):354-363.

Healy, G.N., D.W. Dunstan, J. Salmon, E. Cerin, J.E. Shaw, P.Z. Zimmet, and N. Owen. 2008. Breaks in sedentary time: Beneficial associations with metabolic risk. Diabetes Care 31(4):661-666.

Irvine, A.B., V.A. Gelatt, J.R. Seeley, P. Macfarlane, and J.M. Gau. 2013. Web-based intervention to promote physical activity by sedentary older adults: Randomized controlled trial. Journal of Medical Internet Research 15(2):e19.

Kempen, G.I., J.C. van Haastregt, K.J. McKee, K. Delbaere, and G.A. Zijlstra. 2009. Socio-demographic, health-related and psychosocial correlates of fear of falling and avoidance of activity in community-living older persons who avoid activity due to fear of falling. BMC Public Health 9:170.

Kesse-Guyot, E., H. Charreire, V.A. Andreeva, M. Touvier, S. Hercberg, P. Galan, and J.M. Oppert. 2012. Cross-sectional and longitudinal associations of different sedentary behaviors with cognitive performance in older adults. PLoS One 7(10):e47831.

Kikuchi, H., S. Inoue, T. Sugiyama, N. Owen, K. Oka, and T. Shimomitsu. 2013. Correlates of prolonged television viewing time in older Japanese men and women. BMC Public Health 13:213.

King, A.C., D.K. Ahn, B.M. Oliveira, A.A. Atienza, C.M. Castro, and C.D. Gardner. 2008. Promoting physical activity through hand-held computer technology. American Journal of Preventive Medicine 34(2):138-142.

King, A.C., T.W. Bickmore, M.I. Campero, L.A. Pruitt, and J.L. Yin. 2013. Employing 'virtual advisors' in preventive care for underserved Latino communities: Results from the COMPASS Study. Journal of Health Communication 18(12):1449-1464.

King, A.C., R. Friedman, B. Marcus, C. Castro, M. Napolitano, D. Ahn, and L. Baker. 2007. Ongoing physical activity advice by humans versus computers: The Community Health Advice by Telephone (CHAT) Trial. Health Psychology 26(6):718-727.

King, A.C., J.H. Goldberg, J. Salmon, N. Owen, D. Dunstan, D. Weber, C. Doyle, and T.N. Robinson. 2010. Identifying subgroups of US adults at risk for prolonged television viewing to inform program development. American Journal of Preventive Medicine 38(1):17-26.

King, A.C., and J.M. Guralnik. 2010. Maximizing the potential of an aging population. Journal of the American Medical Association 304(17):1944-1945.

King, A.C., E.B. Hekler, L.A. Grieco, S.J. Winter, M.P. Buman, B. Banerjee, J. Cirimele, T.N. Robinson, E. Mezias, and F. Chen. 2012. "Mobile phone applications to promote physical activity increases: Preliminary results from the MILES Pilot Study." Paper presented at 33rd annual meeting and scientific sessions of the Society of Behavioral Medicine. New Orleans, LA, April 11-14.

King, A.C., and D.E. King. 2010. Physical activity for an aging population. Public Health Nutrition 32(2):56-81.

Kortebein, P., T.B. Symons, A. Ferrando, D. Paddon-Jones, O. Ronsen, E. Protas, S. Conger, J. Lombeida, R. Wolfe, and W.J. Evans. 2008. Functional impact of 10 days of bed rest in healthy older adults. The Journals of Gerontology Series A: Biological Sciences and Medical Sciences 63(10):1076-1081.

Kozo, J., J.F. Sallis, T.L. Conway, J. Kerr, K. Cain, B.E. Saelens, L.D. Frank, and N. Owen. 2012. Sedentary behaviors of adults in relation to neighborhood walkability and income. Health Psychology 31(6):704-713.

Lee, R.E., and A.C. King. 2003. Discretionary time among older adults: How do physical activity promotion interventions affect sedentary and active behaviors? Annals of Behavioral Medicine 25(2):112-129.

Lu, Z., S.D. Rodiek, M.M. Shepley, and M. Duffy. 2011. Influences of physical environment on corridor walking among assisted living residents: Findings from focus group discussions. Journal of Applied Gerontology 30(4):463-484.

Matthews, C.E., K.Y. Chen, P.S. Freedson, M.S. Buchowski, B.M. Beech, R.R. Pate, and R.P. Troiano. 2008. Amount of time spent in sedentary behaviors in the United States, 2003-2004. American Journal of Epidemiology 167(7):875-881.

McBeth, J., B.I. Nicholl, L. Cordingley, K.A. Davies, and G J. Macfarlane. 2010. Chronic widespread pain predicts physical inactivity: Results from the prospective EPIFUND Study. European Journal of Pain 14(9):972-979.

National Center on Senior Transportation. n.d. Transportation options for older adults: Choices for mobility independence. Washington, D.C.: National Center on Senior Transportation.

National Collaborating Centre for Nursing and Supportive Care. 2004. Clinical practice guideline for the assessment and prevention of falls in older people. London: Royal College of Nursing.

Owen, N., T. Sugiyama, E.E. Eakin, P.A. Gardiner, M.S. Tremblay, and J.F. Sallis. 2011. Adults' sedentary behavior determinants and interventions. American Journal of Preventive Medicine 41(2):189-196.

Perissinotto, C.M., I. Stijacic Cenzer, and K.E. Covinsky. 2012. Loneliness in older persons: A predictor of functional decline and death. Archives of Internal Medicine 172(14):1078-1083.

Physical Activity Guidelines Advisory Committee. 2008. Physical activity guidelines advisory committee report, 2008. Washington, D.C.: U.S. Department of Health and Human Services.

Rhodes, R.E., R.S. Mark, and C.P. Temmel. 2012. Adult sedentary behavior: A systematic review. American Journal of Preventive Medicine 42(3):e3-e28.

Robinson, T.N. 2010. Save the world, prevent obesity: Piggybacking on existing social and ideological movements. Obesity 18(Suppl. 1):S17-S22.

———. 2012. Solution-oriented policy research: Using research to drive obesity prevention and control policies. Archives of Pediatrics and Adolescent Medicine 166(2):189-190.

Sari, N. 2010. A short walk a day shortens the hospital stay: Physical activity and the demand for hospital services for older adults. Canadian Journal of Public Health 101(5):385-389.

Seguin, R., M. Lamonte, L. Tinker, J. Liu, N. Woods, Y.L. Michael, C. Bushnell, and A.Z. Lacroix. 2012. Sedentary behavior and physical function decline in older women: Findings from the Women's Health Initiative. Journal of Aging Research 2012:271589.

Senior Mobility Initiative. 2013. Mobility ambassadors. www.seniormobility.org/ambassadors.html

Shankar, A., A. McMunn, J. Banks, and A. Steptoe. 2011. Loneliness, social isolation, and behavioral and biological health indicators in older adults. Health Psychology 30(4):377-385.

Sofi, F., D. Valecchi, D. Bacci, R. Abbate, G.F. Gensini, A. Casini, and C. Macchi. 2011. Physical activity and risk of cognitive decline: A meta-analysis of prospective studies. Journal of Internal Medicine 269(1):107-117.

Stamatakis, E., M. Davis, A. Stathi, and M. Hamer. 2012. Associations between multiple indicators of objectively-measured and self-reported sedentary behaviour and cardiometabolic risk in older adults. Preventive Medicine 54(1):82-87.

Steeves, J.A., D.R. Bassett, E.C. Fitzhugh, H.A. Raynor, and D.L. Thompson. 2012. Can sedentary behavior be made more active? A randomized pilot study of TV commercial stepping versus walking. International Journal of Behavioral Nutrition and Physical Activity 9:95.

Strong, L.L., L.R. Reitzel, D.W. Wetter, and L.H. McNeill. 2013. Associations of perceived neighborhood physical and social environments with physical activity and television viewing in African-American men and women. American Journal of Health Promotion 27(6):401-409.

Thibaud, M., F. Bloch, C. Tournoux-Facon, C. Breque, A.S. Rigaud, B. Dugue, and G. Kemoun. 2012. Impact of physical activity and sedentary behaviour on fall risks in older adults: A systematic review and meta-analysis of observational studies. European Review of Aging and Physical Activity 9(1):5-15.

Thorp, A.A., N. Owen, M. Neuhaus, and D.W. Dunstan. 2011. Sedentary behaviors and subsequent health outcomes in adults: A systematic review of longitudinal studies, 1996-2011. American Journal of Preventive Medicine 41(2):207-215.

Tremblay, M.S., R.C. Colley, T.J. Saunders, G.N. Healy, and N. Owen. 2010. Physiological and health implications of a sedentary lifestyle. Applied Physiology, Nutrition, and Metabolism 35(6):725-740.

U.S. Department of Health and Human Services. 2008. 2008 physical activity guidelines for Americans. Washington, D.C.: U.S. Department of Health and Human Services.

———. 2013. Healthy People 2020: Physical Activity. Office of Disease Prevention and Health Promotion. https://www.healthypeople.gov/2020/topics-objectives/topic/physical-activity.

U.S. Department of Labor, Bureau of Labor Statistics. 2015. Volunteering in the United States, 2015. Accessed December 9, 2016. www.bls.gov/news.release/volun.nr0.htm

Van Dyck, D., E. Cerin, T.L. Conway, I. De Bourdeaudhuij, N. Owen, J. Kerr, G. Cardon, L.D. Frank, B.E. Saelens, and J.F. Sallis. 2012. Perceived neighborhood environmental attributes associated with adults' transport-related walking and cycling: Findings from the USA, Australia and Belgium. International Journal of Behavioral Nutrition and Physical Activity 9:70.

Verghese, J., R.B. Lipton, M.J. Katz, C.B. Hall, C.A. Derby, G. Kuslansky, A.F. Ambrose, M. Sliwinski, and H. Buschke. 2003. Leisure activities and the risk of dementia in the elderly. New England Journal of Medicine 348(25):2508-2516.

Wang, C., and L. Bai. 2012. Sarcopenia in the elderly: Basic and clinical issues. Geriatrics and Gerontology International 12(3):388-396.

Wang, H.X., A. Karp, B. Winblad, and L. Fratiglioni. 2002. Late-life engagement in social and leisure activities is associated with a decreased risk of dementia: A longitudinal study from the Kungsholmen Project. American Journal of Epidemiology 155(12):1081-1087.

Wen, C.P., and X. Wu. 2012. Stressing harms of physical inactivity to promote exercise. Lancet 380(9838):192-193.

Weuve, J., J.H. Kang, J E. Manson, M.M. Breteler, J.H. Ware, and F. Grodstein. 2004. Physical activity, including walking, and cognitive function in older women. Journal of the American Medical Association 292(12):1454-1461.

Wilkie, R., A. Tajar, and J. McBeth. 2013. The onset of widespread musculoskeletal pain is associated with a decrease in healthy ageing in older people: A population-based prospective study. PLoS One 8(3):e59858.

Xu, L., C.Q. Jiang, T.H. Lam, W.S. Zhang, G.N. Thomas, and K.K. Cheng. 2011. Dose-response relation between physical activity and cognitive function: Guangzhou Biobank Cohort Study. Annals of Epidemiology 21(11):857-863.

Zickuhr, K., and M. Madden. 2012. Older adults and Internet use. Washington, D.C.: Pew Research Center.

Chapter 21

Adegoke, B.O., and A.L. Oyeyemi. 2011. Physical inactivity in Nigerian young adults: Prevalence and socio-demographic correlates. Journal of Physical Activity & Health 8(8):1135-1142.

Ainsworth, B.E., S. Wilcox, W.W. Thompson, D.L. Richter, and K.A. Henderson. 2003. Personal, social, and physical environmental correlates of physical activity in African-American women in South Carolina. American Journal of Preventive Medicine 25(3 Suppl. 1):23-29.

Airhihenbuwa, C.O. 1995. Health and culture: Beyond the Western paradigm. Thousand Oaks, CA: Sage.

Airhihenbuwa, C.O., S. Kumanyika, T.D. Agurs, and A. Lowe. 1995. Perceptions and beliefs about exercise, rest, and health among African-Americans. American Journal of Health Promotion 9(6):426-429.

Airhihenbuwa, C.O., S.K. Kumanyika, T.R. TenHave, and C.B. Morssink. 2000. Cultural identity and health lifestyles among African Americans: A new direction for health intervention research? Ethnicity & Disease 10(2):148-164.

Allison, M.A., N.E. Jensky, S.J. Marshall, A.G. Bertoni, and M. Cushman. 2012. Sedentary behavior and adiposity-associated inflammation: The Multi-Ethnic Study of Atherosclerosis. American Journal of Preventive Medicine 42(1):8-13.

Babey, S.H., T.A. Hastert, and J. Wolstein. 2013. Adolescent sedentary behaviors: Correlates differ for television viewing and computer use. Journal of Adolescent Health 52(1):70-76.

Barr-Anderson, D.J., J.A. Fulkerson, M. Smyth, J.H. Himes, P.J. Hannan, B. Holy Rock, and M. Story. 2011. Associations of American Indian children's screen-time behavior with parental television behavior, parental perceptions of children's screen time, and media-related resources in the home. Preventing Chronic Disease 8(5):A105.

Barr-Anderson, D.J., and S.B. Sisson. 2012. Media use and sedentary behavior in adolescents: What do we know, what has been done, and where do we go? Adolescent Medicine: State of the Art Reviews 23(3):511-528.

Boslaugh, S.E., D.A. Luke, R.C. Brownson, K.S. Naleid, and M.W. Kreuter. 2004. Perceptions of neighborhood environment for physical activity: Is it "who you are" or "where you live"? Journal of Urban Health 81(4):671-681.

Boyington, J.E., L. Carter-Edwards, M. Piehl, J. Hutson, D. Langdon, and S. McManus. 2008. Cultural attitudes toward weight, diet, and physical activity among overweight African American girls. Preventing Chronic Disease 5(2):A36.

Buchowski, M.S., S.S. Cohen, C.E. Matthews, D.G. Schlundt, L.B. Signorello, M.K. Hargreaves, and W.J. Blot. 2010. Physical activity and obesity gap between black and white women in the southeastern U.S. American Journal of Preventive Medicine 39(2): 140-147.

Byun, W., M. Dowda, and R.R. Pate. 2011. Correlates of objectively measured sedentary behavior in US preschool children. Pediatrics 128(5):937-945.

Byun, W., X. Sui, J.R. Hebert, T.S. Church, I.M. Lee, C.E. Matthews, and S.N. Blair. 2011. Cardiorespiratory fitness and risk of prostate cancer: Findings from the Aerobics Center Longitudinal Study. Cancer Epidemiology 35(1):59-65.

Casagrande, S.S., M.C. Whitt-Glover, K.J. Lancaster, A.M. Odoms-Young, and T.L. Gary. 2009. Built environment and health behaviors among African Americans: A systematic review. American Journal of Preventive Medicine 36(2):174-181.

Centers for Disease Control and Prevention. 2010a. 1988-2008 No leisure-time physical activity trend chart. https://stacks.cdc.gov/view/cdc/33752/cdc_33752_DS2.txt

———. 2010b. U.S. physical activity estimates, 2001—national average: Recommended physical activity; by race. http://apps.nccd.cdc.gov/PASurveillance/DemoCompareResultV.asp?State=1&Cat=4&Year=2001&CI=on&Go=GO

———. 2010c. U.S. physical activity estimates, 2008–national average: Recommended physical activity; by race. http://apps.nccd.cdc.gov/PASurveillance/DemoCompareResultV.asp?Year=2008&State=1&Cat=4&CI=on#result

Chang, M.W., S. Nitzke, E. Guilford, C.H. Adair, and D.L. Hazard. 2008. Motivators and barriers to healthful eating and physical activity among low-income overweight and obese mothers. Journal of the American Dietetic Association 108(6):1023-1028.

Cong, Z., D. Feng, Y. Liu, and M.C. Esperat. 2012. Sedentary behaviors among Hispanic children: Influences of parental support in a school intervention program. American Journal of Health Promotion 26(5):270-280.

Evenson, K.R., D.M. Buchner, and K.B. Morland. 2012. Objective measurement of physical activity and sedentary behavior among US adults aged 60 years or older. Preventing Chronic Disease 9(11).

Evenson, K.R., M.K. Moos, K. Carrier, and A.M. Siega-Riz. 2009. Perceived barriers to physical activity among pregnant women. Maternal and Child Health Journal 13(3):364-375.

Ewing, R., T. Schmid, R. Killingsworth, A. Zlot, and S. Raudenbush. 2003. Relationship between urban sprawl and physical activity, obesity, and morbidity. American Journal of Health Promotion 18(1):47-57.

Eyler, A.A., E. Baker, L. Cromer, A.C. King, R.C. Brownson, and R.J. Donatelle. 1998. Physical activity and minority women: A qualitative study. Health Education & Behavior 25(5):640-652.

Fitzgibbon, M.L., M.R. Stolley, A.R. Dyer, L. VanHorn, and K. KauferChristoffel. 2002. A community-based obesity prevention program for minority children: Rationale and study design for Hip-Hop to Health Jr. Preventive Medicine 34(2):289-297.

Fitzgibbon, M.L., M.R. Stolley, L.A. Schiffer, C.L. Braunschweig, S.L. Gomez, L. Van Horn, and A.R. Dyer. 2011. Hip-Hop to Health Jr. Obesity prevention effectiveness trial: Postintervention results. Obesity 19(5):994-1003.

Fitzgibbon, M.L., M.R. Stolley, L. Schiffer, L. Van Horn, K. KauferChristoffel, and A. Dyer. 2005. Two-year follow-up results for Hip-Hop to Health Jr.: A randomized controlled trial for overweight prevention in preschool minority children. Journal of Pediatrics 146(5):618-625.

———. 2006. Hip-Hop to Health Jr. for Latino preschool children. Obesity 14(9):1616-1625.

Gordon-Larsen, P., P. Griffiths, M.E. Bentley, D.S. Ward, K. Kelsey, K. Shields, and A. Ammerman. 2004. Barriers to physical activity: Qualitative data on caregiver-daughter perceptions and practices. American Journal of Preventive Medicine 27(3):218-223.

Gordon-Larsen, P., M.C. Nelson, P. Page, and B.M. Popkin. 2006. Inequality in the built environment underlies key health disparities in physical activity and obesity. Pediatrics 117(2):417-424.

Gortmaker, S.L., L.W. Cheung, K.E. Peterson, G. Chomitz, J.H. Cradle, H. Dart, M.K. Fox, et al. 1999. Impact of a school-based interdisciplinary intervention on diet and physical activity among urban primary school children: Eat well and keep moving. Archives of Pediatrics and Adolescent Medicine 153(9):975-983.

Grow, H.M., B.E. Saelens, J. Kerr, N.H. Durant, G.J. Norman, and J.F. Sallis. 2008. Where are youth active? Roles of proximity, active transport, and built environment. Medicine and Science in Sports and Exercise 40(12):2071-2079.

Hanson, M.D., and E. Chen. 2007. Socioeconomic status, race, and body mass index: The mediating role of physical activity and sedentary behaviors during adolescence. Journal of Pediatric Psychology 32(3):250-259.

Henderson, K.A., and B.E. Ainsworth. 2000a. Enablers and constraints to walking for older African American and American Indian women: The Cultural Activity Participation Study. Research Quarterly for Exercise and Sport 71(4):313-321.

———. 2000b. Sociocultural perspectives on physical activity in the lives of older African American and American Indian women: A cross cultural activity participation study. Women Health 31(1):1-20.

———. 2000c. The connections between social support and women's physical activity involvement: The Cultural Activity Participation Study. Women's Sport and Physical Activity Journal 9(2):27-53.

———. 2001. Research leisure and physical activity with women of color: Issues and emerging questions. Leisure Sciences 23:21-34.

———. 2003. A synthesis of perceptions about physical activity among older African American and American Indian women. American Journal of Public Health 93(2):313-317.

Hsu, Y.W., B.R. Belcher, E.E. Ventura, C.E. Byrd-Williams, M.J. Weigensberg, J.N. Davis, A.D. McClain, M.I. Goran, and D. Spruijt-Metz. 2011. Physical activity, sedentary behavior, and the metabolic syndrome in minority youth. Medicine and Science in Sports and Exercise 43(12):2307-2313.

Katzmarzyk, P.T., T.S. Church, C.L. Craig, and C. Bouchard. 2009. Sitting time and mortality from all causes, cardiovascular disease, and cancer. Medicine and Science in Sports and Exercise 41(5):998-1005.

King, A.C., C. Castro, S. Wilcox, A.A. Eyler, J.F. Sallis, and R.C. Brownson. 2000. Personal and environmental factors associated with physical inactivity among different racial-ethnic groups of U.S. middle-aged and older-aged women. Health Psychology 19(4):354-364.

Lee, R.E., S.K. Mama, and H.J. Adamus-Leach. 2012. Neighborhood street scale elements, sedentary time and cardiometabolic risk factors in inactive ethnic minority women. PLoS One 7(12):e51081.

Mathews, A.E., S.B. Laditka, J.N. Laditka, S. Wilcox, S.J. Corwin, R. Liu, D.B. Friedman, R. Hunter, W. Tseng, and R.G. Logsdon. 2010. Older adults' perceived physical activity enablers and barriers: A multicultural perspective. Journal of Aging and Physical Activity 18(2):119-140.

Matthews, C.E., K.Y. Chen, P.S. Freedson, M.S. Buchowski, B.M. Beech, R.R. Pate, and R.P. Troiano. 2008. Amount of time spent in sedentary behaviors in the United States, 2003-2004. American Journal of Epidemiology 167(7):875-881.

McDonald, N.C. 2008. The effect of objectively measured crime on walking in minority adults. American Journal of Health Promotion 22(6):433-436.

Miller K.H., C. Ziegler, R. Greenberg, P.D. Patel, and M.B. Carter 2012. Why physicians should share PDA/smartphone findings with their patients: A brief report. Journal of Health Communication 17(Suppl. 1):54-61.

Moore, J.B., S.B. Jilcott, K.A. Shores, K.R. Evenson, R.C. Brownson, and L.F. Novick. 2010. A qualitative examination of perceived barriers and facilitators of physical activity for urban and rural youth. Health Education Research 25(2):355-367.

Moore, L.V., A.V. Diez Roux, K.R. Evenson, A.P. McGinn, and S.J. Brines. 2008. Availability of recreational resources in minority and low socioeconomic status areas. American Journal of Preventive Medicine 34(1):16-22.

National Center for Health Statistics, U.S. Department of Health and Human Services. 2016. Health, United States, 2015: With special feature on racial and ethnic health disparities. Hyattsville, MD.

Norman, G.J., B.A. Schmid, J.F. Sallis, K.J. Calfas, and K. Patrick. 2005. Psychosocial and environmental correlates of adolescent sedentary behaviors. Pediatrics 116(4):908-916.

Parra-Medina, D., S. Wilcox, J. Salinas, C. Addy, E. Fore, M. Poston, and D.K. Wilson. 2011. Results of the Heart Healthy and Ethnically Relevant Lifestyle trial: A cardiovascular risk reduction intervention for African American women attending community health centers. American Journal of Public Health 101(10):1914-1921.

Powell, L.M., S. Slater, and F.J. Chaloupka. 2004. The relationship between community physical activity settings and race, ethnicity and socioeconomic status. Evidence-Based Preventive Medicine 1(2):135-144.

Rees, R., J. Kavanagh, A. Harden, J. Shepherd, G. Brunton, S. Oliver, and A. Oakley. 2006. Young people and physical activity: A systematic review matching their views to effective interventions. Health Education Research 21(6):806-825.

Robinson, T.N., J.D. Killen, H.C. Kraemer, D.M. Wilson, D.M. Matheson, W.L. Haskell, L.A. Pruitt, et al. 2003. Dance and reducing television viewing to prevent weight gain in African-American girls: The Stanford GEMS pilot study. Ethnicity & Disease 13(1 Suppl. 1):S65-S77.

Rosenberg, D., D. Ding, J.F. Sallis, J. Kerr, G.J. Norman, N. Durant, S.K. Harris, and B.E. Saelens. 2009. Neighborhood Environment Walkability Scale for Youth (NEWS-Y): Reliability and relationship with physical activity. Preventive Medicine 49(2-3):213-218.

Sander, A.P., J. Wilson, N. Izzo, S.A. Mountford, and K.W. Hayes. 2012. Factors that affect decisions about physical activity and exercise in survivors of breast cancer: A qualitative study. Physical Therapy 92(4):525-536.

Sanderson, B.K., H.R. Foushee, V. Bittner, C.E. Cornell, V. Stalker, S. Shelton, and L. Pulley. 2003. Personal, social, and physical environmental correlates of physical activity in rural African-American women in Alabama. American Journal of Preventive Medicine 25(3 Suppl. 1):30-37.

Shuval, K., T. Leonard, J. Murdoch, M.O. Caughy, H.W. Kohl III, and C.S. Skinner. 2013. Sedentary behaviors and obesity in a low-income, ethnic-minority population. Journal of Physical Activity & Health 10(1):132-136.

Sidney, S., B. Sternfeld, W.L. Haskell, D.R. Jacobs Jr., M.A. Chesney, and S.B. Hulley. 1996. Television viewing and cardiovascular risk factors in young adults: The CARDIA study. Annals of Epidemiology 6(2):154-159.

Singh, G.K., S.M. Yu, M. Siahpush, and M.D. Kogan. 2008. High levels of physical inactivity and sedentary behaviors among US immigrant children and adolescents. Archives of Pediatrics and Adolescent Medicine 162(8):756-763.

Stathi, A., H. Gilbert, K.R. Fox, J. Coulson, M. Davis, and J.L. Thompson. 2012. Determinants of neighborhood activity of adults age 70 and over: A mixed-methods study. Journal of Aging and Physical Activity 20(2):148-170.

Thorp, A.A., N. Owen, M. Neuhaus, and D.W. Dunstan. 2011. Sedentary behaviors and subsequent health outcomes in adults: A systematic review of longitudinal studies, 1996-2011. American Journal of Preventive Medicine 41(2):207-215.

Troiano, R.P., D. Berrigan, K.W. Dodd, L.C. Masse, T. Tilert, and M. McDowell. 2008. Physical activity in the United States measured by accelerometer. Medicine and Science in Sports and Exercise 40(1):181-188.

Trowbridge, M.J., and N.C. McDonald. 2008. Urban sprawl and miles driven daily by teenagers in the United States. American Journal of Preventive Medicine 34(3):202-206.

U.S. Census Bureau. 2014. 2014 American community survey 1-year estimates. American Fact Finder. http://factfinder.census.gov/faces/tableservices/jsf/pages/productview.xhtml?pid=ACS_14_SPL_K200201&prodType=table

U.S. Department of Health and Human Services. 1996. Physical activity and health: A report of the Surgeon General. Hyattsville, MD: Author.

———. 2001. The Surgeon General's call to action to prevent and decrease overweight and obesity, 2001. Rockville, MD: Author.

Weintraub, D.L., E.C. Tirumalai, K.F. Haydel, M. Fujimoto, J.E. Fulton, and T.N. Robinson. 2008. Team sports for overweight children: The Stanford Sports to Prevent Obesity Randomized Trial (SPORT). Archives of Pediatrics and Adolescent Medicine 162(3):232-237.

Whitt-Glover, M.C., G. Bennett, and J.F. Sallis. 2013. Introduction to the Active Living Research Supplement: Disparities in environments and policies that support active living. Annals of Behavioral Medicine 45(Suppl. 1):S1-S5.

Whitt-Glover, M.C., W.C. Taylor, M.F. Floyd, M.M. Yore, A.K. Yancey, and C.E. Matthews. 2009. Disparities in physical activity and sedentary behaviors among U.S. children and adolescents: Prevalence, correlates, and intervention implications. Journal of Public Health Policy 30(Suppl. 1):S309-S334.

Wolch, J., J.P. Wilson, and J. Fehrenbach. 2005. Parks and parks funding in Los Angeles: An equity mapping analysis. Urban Geography 26(1):4-35.

Wolin, K.Y., L.A. Colangelo, B.C. Chiu, B. Ainsworth, R. Chatterton, and S.M. Gapstur. 2007. Associations of physical activity, sedentary time, and insulin with percent breast density in Hispanic women. Journal of Women's Health 16(7):1004-1011.

Chapter 22

Bandura, A. 1969. *Principles of behavior modification*. New York: Holt, Rinehart, & Winston.

———. 1977. Self-efficacy: Toward a unifying theory of behavioral change. *Psychological Review* 84(2):191.

———. 1982. Self-efficacy mechanism in human agency. *American Psychologist* 37(2):122.

———. 1986. *Social foundations of thought and action: A social cognitive theory*. Englewood Cliffs, NJ: Prentice-Hall.

———. 1997. *Self-efficacy: The exercise of control*. New York: Freeman.

Bickel, W.K. and R.E. Vuchinich, eds. 2000. *Reframing health behavior change with behavioral economics*. Mahwah, NJ: Erlbaum

Booth, S.L., J.F. Sallis, C. Ritenbaugh, J.O. Hill, L.L. Birch, L.D. Frank, K. Glanz, et al. 2001. Environmental and societal factors affect food choice and physical activity: Rationale, influences, and leverage points. *Nutrition Reviews* 59(3):S21-S36.

Cohen, D.A., R.A. Scribner, and T.A. Farley. 2000. A structural model of health behavior: A pragmatic approach to explain and influence health behaviors at the population level. *Preventive Medicine* 30(2):146-154.

Craig, C.L., E.V. Lambert, H.W. Kohl III, S. Inoue, J.R. Alkandari, G. Leetongin, S. Kahlmeier, and the Lancet Physical Activity Series Working Group. 2012. The pandemic of physical inactivity: Global action for public health. *Lancet* 380(9838):294-305.

DiClemente, C.C., and J.O. Prochaska. 1982. Self-change and therapy change of smoking behavior: A comparison of processes of change in cessation and maintenance. *Addictive Behaviors* 7(2):133-142.

Dunstan, D.W., B.A. Kingwell, R. Larsen, G.N. Healy, E. Cerin, M.T. Hamilton, J.E. Shaw, et al. 2012. Breaking up prolonged sitting reduces postprandial glucose and insulin responses. *Diabetes Care* 35(5):976-983.

Fishbein, M. 1967. *Readings in attitude theory and measurement.* New York: Wiley.

Fishbein, M., and I. Ajzen 1975. *Belief, attitude, intention, and behavior: An introduction to theory and research.* Reading, MA: Addison-Wesley.

Fisher, E.B. 2008. The importance of context in understanding behavior and promoting health. *Annals of Behavioral Medicine* 35(1):3-18.

Freud, S. 1969. *The question of lay analysis: Conversations with an impartial person.* New York: W.W. Norton & Company.

Glanz, K., B.K. Rimer, and K. Viswanath. 2008. *Health behavior and health education: Theory, research, and practice.* New York: John Wiley & Sons.

Green, L.W., and M.W. Kreuter 1991. *Health education planning.* Palo Alto, CA: Mayfield.

Hagger, M.S., N.L. Chatzisarantis, and S.J.H. Biddle. 2002. A meta-analytic review of the theories of reasoned action and planned behavior in physical activity: Predictive validity and the contribution of additional variables. *Journal of Sport & Exercise Psychology* 24(1):3-32.

Hochbaum, G.M. 1958. *Public participation in medical screening programs: A socio-psychological study.* Washington, D.C.: Division of Special Health Services, U.S. Public Health Service.

Hollis, J.F., M.R. Polen, E.P. Whitlock, E. Lichtenstein, J.P. Mullooly, W.F. Velicer, and C.A. Redding. 2005. Teen reach: Outcomes from a randomized, controlled trial of a tobacco reduction program for teens seen in primary medical care. *Pediatrics* 115(4):981-989.

Hovell, M.F., D.R. Wahlgren, and C.A. Gehrman. 2002. The behavioral ecological model. In *Emerging theories in health promotion practice and research. Strategies for improving public health*, edited by R.J. DiClemente, 347-385. San Francisco: Jossey-Bass.

Humpel, N., N. Owen, and E. Leslie. 2002. Environmental factors associated with adults' participation in physical activity: A review. *American Journal of Preventive Medicine* 22(3):188-199.

Kohl, A., W. Rief, and J.A. Glombiewski. 2012. How effective are acceptance strategies? A meta-analytic review of experimental results. *Journal of Behavior Therapy and Experimental Psychiatry* 43(4):988-1001.

Lewin, K. 1939. Field theory and experiment in social psychology: Concepts and methods. *American Journal of Sociology* 44:868-896.

Marshall, S.J., S.J. Biddle, I. Murdey, T. Gorely, and N. Cameron. 2003. But what are you doing now? Ecological momentary assessment of sedentary behavior among youth. *Medicine & Science in Sports & Exercise* 35(5):S180.

Matthews, C.E., S.M. George, S.C. Moore, H.R. Bowles, A. Blair, Y. Park, R.P. Troiano, A. Hollenbeck, and A. Schatzkin. 2012. Amount of time spent in sedentary behaviors and cause-specific mortality in US adults. *The American Journal of Clinical Nutrition* 95(2):437-445.

McKenzie, T.L., and D. Cohen. 2011. Introduction to SOPARC and the science of systematic observation. *Research Quarterly for Exercise and Sport* 82(1):A5-A5.

McLeroy, K.R., D. Bibeau, A. Steckler, and K. Glanz. 1988. An ecological perspective on health promotion programs. *Health Education & Behavior* 15(4):351-377.

Prochaska, J.O., S. Butterworth, C.A. Redding, V. Burden, N. Perrin, M. Leo, M. Flaherty-Robb, and J.M. Prochaska. 2008. Initial efficacy of MI, TTM tailoring and HRI's with multiple behaviors for employee health promotion. *Preventive Medicine* 46(3):226-231.

Richard, L., L. Potvin, N. Kischuk, H. Prlic, and L.W. Green. 1996. Assessment of the integration of the ecological approach in health promotion programs. *American Journal of Health Promotion* 10(4):318-328.

Rogers, C.R. 1951. *Client-centered therapy: Its current practice, implications and theory.* Boston: Houghton Mifflin.

Rosenstock, I.M., V.J. Strecher, and M.H. Becker. 1988. Social learning theory and the health belief model. *Health Education Quarterly* 15(2):175-183.

Russell, B. 1950. Logical positivism. *Revue Internationale de Philosophie* 4(11):3-19.

Saelens, B.E., J.F. Sallis, and L.D. Frank. 2003. Environmental correlates of walking and cycling: Findings from the transportation, urban design, and planning literatures. *Annals of Behavioral Medicine* 25(2):80-91.

Sallis, J.F., T.L. McKenzie, T.L. Conway, J.P. Elder, J.J. Prochaska, M. Brown, M.M. Zive, S.J. Marshall, and J.E. Alcaraz. 2003. Environmental interventions for eating and physical activity: A randomized controlled trial in middle schools. *American Journal of Preventive Medicine* 24(3):209-217.

Sallis, J.F., and N. Owen 1999. *Physical activity & behavioral medicine.* Thousand Oaks, CA: Sage.

Sallis, J.F., N. Owen, and E. Fisher. 2008. Ecological models of health behavior. *Health Behavior and Health Education: Theory, Research, and Practice* 4:465-486.

Sallis, J.F., J.J. Prochaska, and W.C. Taylor. 2000. A review of correlates of physical activity of children and adolescents. *Medicine & Science in Sports & Exercise* 32(5):963-975.

Schunk, D.H. 1987. Peer models and children's behavioral change. *Review of Educational Research* 57(2):149-174.

Skinner, B.F. 1938. *The behavior of organisms: An experimental analysis.* New York: Appleton-Century-Crofts.

———. 1972. *Beyond freedom and dignity.* New York: Springer.

Smedley, B., and S. Syme 2001. Promoting health: Intervention strategies from social and behavioral research. *American Journal of Health Promotion* 15:149-166.

Stamps, J.A., V.V. Krishnan, and M.L. Reid 2005. Search costs and habitat selection by dispersers. *Ecology* 86:510-518.

Stevens, J., D.M. Murray, D.J. Catellier, P.J. Hannan, L.A. Lytle, J.P. Elder, D.R. Young, D.G. Simons-Morton, and L.S. Webber. 2005. Design of the trial of activity in adolescent girls (TAAG). *Contemporary Clinical Trials* 26(2):223-233.

Stokols, D. 1992. Establishing and maintaining healthy environments: Toward a social ecology of health promotion. *American Psychologist* 47(1):6.

Thorndike, E.L. 1911. *Animal intelligence: Experimental studies.* New York: Macmillan.

Tolman, E.C. 1932. *Purposive behavior in animals and men.* Berkeley, CA: University of California Press.

United States Department of Health and Human Services. 2000. *Healthy people 2010.* Washington D.C.: Author.

World Health Organization. 1986. *Ottawa charter for health promotion.* Geneva: Author.

Watson, J.B. 1913. Psychology as the behaviorist views it. *Psychological Review* 20(2):158.

———. 1925. *Behaviorism.* New Brunswick, NJ: Transaction Books.

Wittgenstein, L. 1922. *Tractatus Logico-Philosophicus,* translated by C.K. Ogden. London: Kegan Paul, Trench, & Trubner.

Chapter 23

Barnett, A., E. Cerin, and T. Baranowski. 2011. Active video games for youth: A systematic review. *Journal of Physical Activity and Health* 8(5):724-737.

Bauman, A.E., R.S. Reis, J.F. Sallis, J.C. Wells, R.J.F. Loos, and B.W. Martin. 2012. Correlates of physical activity: Why are some people physically active and others not? *Lancet* 380:258-271.

Beers, E., J.N. Roemmich, L.H. Epstein, and P.J. Horvath. 2008. Increasing passive energy expenditure during clerical work. *European Journal of Applied Physiology* 103(3):353-360.

Blake, J.J., M.E. Benden, and M.L. Wendel. 2012. Using stand/sit workstations in classrooms: Lessons learned from a pilot study in Texas. *Journal of Public Health Management and Practice* 18(5):412-415.

Cardon, G., D. De Clercq, I. De Bourdeaudhuij, and D. Breithecker. 2004. Sitting habits in elementary school children: A traditional versus a "moving school". *Patient Education and Counseling* 54(2):133-142.

Clemes, S.A., S.E. Barber, D.D. Bingham, N.D. Ridgers, E. Fletcher, N. Pearson, J. Salmon, and D.W. Dunstan. 2015. Reducing children's classroom sitting time using sit-to-stand desks: Findings from pilot studies in UK and Australian primary schools. *Journal of Public Health,* Epub ahead of print, 2015 Jun 14. http://jpubhealth. oxfordjournals.org/content/early/2015/06/14/pubmed. fdv084.short

De Decker, E., M. De Craemer, I. De Bourdeaudhuij, K. Wijndaele, K. Duvinage, B. Koletzko, E. Grammatikaki, et al. 2012. Influencing factors of screen time in preschool children: An exploration of parents' perceptions through focus groups in six European countries. *Obesity Reviews* 13(Suppl. 1):75-84.

Epstein, L.H., J.N. Roemmich, J.L. Robinson, R.A. Paluch, D.D. Winiewicz, J.H. Fuerch, and T.N. Robinson. 2008. A randomized trial of the effects of reducing television viewing and computer use on body mass index in young children. *Archives of Pediatric and Adolescent Medicine* 162(3):239-245.

Evans, R.E., H.O. Fawole, S. Sheriff, P.M. Dall, P.M. Grant, and C.G. Ryan. 2012. Point-of-choice prompts to reduce sitting time at work: A randomized trial. *American Journal of Preventive Medicine* 43(3):293-297.

Faith, M.S., N. Berman, M. Heo, A. Pietrobelli, D. Gallagher, L.H. Epstein, M.T. Eiden, and D.B. Allison. 2001. Effects of contingent television on physical activity and television viewing in obese children. *Pediatrics* 107(5):1043-1048.

Giles-Corti, B., F. Bull, M. Knuiman, G. McCormack, K. Van Niel, A. Timperio, H. Christian, S. Foster, M. Divitini, N. Middleton, and B. Boruff. 2013. The influence of urban design on neighbourhood walking following residential relocation: Longitudinal results from the RESIDE study. *Social Science & Medicine* 77(11):20-30.

Gilson, N.D., A. Suppini, G.C. Ryde, H.E. Brown, and W.J. Brown. 2012. Does the use of standing "hot" desks change sedentary work time in an open plan office? *Preventive Medicine* 54(1):65-67.

Goldfield, G.S., R. Mallory, T. Parker, T. Cunningham, C. Legg, A. Lumb, K. Parker, D. Prud'homme, I. Gaboury, and K.B. Adamo. 2006. Effects of open-loop feedback on physical activity and television viewing in overweight and obese children: A randomized, controlled trial. *Pediatrics* 118(1):157-166.

Handy, S. 2005. Smart growth and the transportation-land use connection: What does the research tell us? *International Regional Science Review* 28(2):146-167.

Healy, G.N., E.G. Eakin, A.D. Lamontagne, N. Owen, E.A. Winkler, G. Wiesner, L. Gunning, et al. 2013. Reducing sitting time in office workers: Short-term efficacy of a multicomponent intervention. *Preventive Medicine* 57(1):43-48.

Hinckson, E.A., S. Aminian, E. Ikeda, T. Stewart, M. Oliver, S. Duncan, and G. Schofield. 2013. Acceptability of standing workstations in elementary school: A pilot study. *Preventive Medicine* 56(1):82-85.

Ingram, D.K. 2000. Age-related decline in physical activity: Generalization to nonhumans. *Medicine and Science in Sports and Exercise* 32(9):1623-1629.

Kerr, J., D.E. Rosenberg, A. Nathan, R. Millstein, J. Carlson, K. Crist, K. Wasilenko, et al. 2012. Applying the ecological model of behavior change to a physical activity trial in retirement communities: Description of the study protocol. *Contemporary Clinical Trials* 33(6):1180-1188.

Kibbe, D.L., J. Hackett, M. Hurley, A. McFarland, K.G. Schubert, A. Schultz, and S. Harris. 2011. Ten years of TAKE 10! Integrating physical activity with academic concepts in elementary school classrooms. *Preventive Medicine* 52(Suppl. 1):43-50.

Kozo, J., J.F. Sallis, T.L. Conway, J. Kerr, K. Cain, B.E. Saelens, L.D. Frank, and N. Owen. 2012. Sedentary behaviors of adults in relation to neighborhood walkability and income. *Health Psychology* 31(6):704-713.

Lanningham-Foster, L., T.B. Jensen, R.C. Foster, B. Redmond, B. Walker, D. Heinz, and J. Levine. 2006. Energy expenditure of sedentary screen time compared with active screen time for children. *Pediatrics* 118(6):1831-1835.

Lazarovici, L. 2012. Exercise breaks reduce injuries, stress and sick days. *Instant Recess*. www.toniyancey.com/IR_About_Case_Studies.html

Maloney, A.E., T.C. Bethea, K.S. Kelsey, J.T. Marks, S. Paez, A.M. Rosenberg, D.J. Catellier, R.M. Hamer, and L. Sikich. 2008. A pilot of a video game (DDR) to promote physical activity and decrease sedentary screen time. *Obesity* 16(9):2074-2080.

McWilliams, C., S.C. Ball, S.E. Benjamin, D. Hales, A. Vaughn, and D.S. Ward. 2009. Best-practice guidelines for physical activity at child care. *Pediatrics* 124(6):1650-1659.

Ni Mhurchu, C., V. Roberts, R. Maddison, E. Dorey, Y. Jiang, A. Jull, and S. Tin. 2009. Effect of electronic time monitors on children's television watching: Pilot trial of a home-based intervention. *Preventive Medicine* 49(5):413-417.

Owen, N., G.N. Healy, C.E. Matthews, and D.W. Dunstan. 2010. Too much sitting: The population health science of sedentary behaviors. *Exercise and Sport Science Reviews* 38:105-113.

Owen, N., T. Sugiyama, E.E. Eakin, P.A. Gardiner, M.S. Tremblay, and J.F. Sallis. 2011. Adults' sedentary behavior: Determinants and interventions. *American Journal of Preventive Medicine* 41:189-196.

Pucher, J., J. Dill, and S. Handy. 2010. Infrastructure, programs, and policies to increase bicycling: An international review. *Preventive Medicine* 50(Suppl. 1):106-125.

Robinson T.N. 1999. Reducing children's television viewing to prevent obesity: A randomized controlled trial. *Journal of the American Medical Association* 282(16):1561-1567.

Sallis, J.F., M.F. Floyd, D.A. Rodriguez, and B.E. Saelens. 2012. The role of built environments in physical activity, obesity, and CVD. *Circulation* 125:729-737.

Sallis, J.F., N. Owen, and E.B. Fisher. 2008. Ecological models of health behavior. In *Health behavior and health education: Theory, research, and practice*, 4th ed., edited by K. Glanz, B.K. Rimer, and K. Viswanath, 465-486. San Francisco: Jossey-Bass.

Sallis, J.F., M. Story, and D. Lou. 2009. Study designs and analytic strategies for environmental and policy research on obesity, physical activity, and diet: Recommendations from a meeting of experts. *American Journal of Preventive Medicine* 36(2 Suppl. 2):S72-S77.

Singh, A., L. Uijtdewilligen, J.W.R. Twisk, W. van Mechelen, and M.J.M. Chinapaw. 2012. Physical activity and performance at school: A systematic review of the literature including a methodological quality assessment. *Archives of Pediatric & Adolescent Medicine* 166(1):49-55.

Sugiyama, T., J. Salmon, D.W. Dunstan, A.E. Bauman, and N. Owen. 2007. Neighborhood walkability and TV viewing time among Australian adults. *American Journal of Preventive Medicine* 33:444-449.

Van Dyck, D., G. Cardon, B. Deforche, N. Owen, J.F. Sallis, and I. De Bourdeaudhuij. 2010. Neighborhood walkability and sedentary time in Belgian adults. *American Journal of Preventive Medicine* 39:25-32.

Chapter 24

Alkhajah, T.A., M.M. Reeves, E.G. Eakin, E.A. Winkler, N. Owen, and G.N. Healy. 2012. Sit-stand workstations: A pilot intervention to reduce office sitting time. *American Journal of Preventive Medicine* 43:298-303.

Balci, R., and F. Aghazadeh. 2003. The effect of work-rest schedules and type of task on the discomfort and performance of VDT users. *Ergonomics* 46:455-465.

Barr-Anderson, D.J., M. AuYong, M.C. Whitt-Glover, B.A. Glenn, and A.K. Yancey. 2011. Integration of short bouts of physical activity into organizational routine: A systematic review of the literature. *American Journal of Preventive Medicine* 40:76-93.

Berry, L.L., A.M. Mirabito, and W.B. Baun. 2011. What's the hard return on employee wellness programs? *Harvard Business Review* 89:20-21.

Brown, H.E., N.D. Gilson, N.W. Burton, and W.J. Brown. 2011. Does physical activity impact on presenteeism and other indicators of workplace well-being? *Sports Medicine* 41:249-262.

Cancelliere, C., J.D. Cassidy, C. Ammendolia, and P. Cote. 2011. Are workplace health promotion programs effective at improving presenteeism in workers? A systematic review and best evidence synthesis of the literature. *BMC Public Health* 11:395.

Carnethon, M., L.P. Whitsel, B.A. Franklin, P. Kris-Etherton, R. Milani, C.A. Pratt, and G.R. Wagner. 2009. Worksite wellness programs for cardiovascular disease prevention: A policy statement from the American Heart Association. *Circulation* 120:1725-1741.

Chapman, L.S. 2004. Expert opinions on "best practices" in worksite health promotion. *American Journal of Health Promotion* 18:1-6.

Chau, J.Y., H.P. van der Ploeg, J.G.Z. van Uffelen, J. Wong, I. Riphagen, G.N. Healy, N.D. Gilson, et al. 2010. Are workplace interventions to reduce sitting effective? A systematic review. *Preventive Medicine* 51:352-356.

Church, T.S., D.M. Thomas, C. Tudor-Locke, P.T. Katzmarzyk, C.P. Earnest, R.Q. Rodarte, C.K. Martin, S.N. Blair, and C. Bouchard. 2011. Trends over 5 decades in U.S. occupation-related physical activity and their associations with obesity. *PLoS ONE* 6(5):e19657.

Dishman, R.K., D.M. DeJoy, M.G. Wilson, and R.J. Vandenberg. 2009. Move to improve: A randomized workplace trial to increase physical activity. *American Journal of Preventive Medicine* 36:133-141.

Evans, R.E., H.O. Fawole, S.A. Sheriff, P.M. Dall, M. Grant, and C.G. Ryan. 2012. Point-of-choice prompts to reduce sitting time at work: A randomized trial. *American Journal of Preventive Medicine* 43:293-297.

Galinsky, T., N.G. Swanson, S.L. Sauter, R. Dunkin, J. Hurrell, and L. Schleifer. 2007. Supplementary breaks and stretching exercises for data entry operators: A follow-up field study. *American Journal of Industrial Medicine* 50:519-527.

Galinsky, T., N. Swanson, S.L. Sauter, J. Hurrell, and L. Schleifer. 2000. A field study of supplementary rest breaks for data-entry operators. *Ergonomics* 43:622-638.

Gardiner, P.A., E.G. Eakin, G.N. Healy, and N. Owen. 2011. Feasibility of reducing older adults' sedentary time. *American Journal of Preventive Medicine* 41:174-177.

Gilson, N.D., A. Suppini, G.C. Ryde, H.E. Brown, and W.J. Brown. 2012. Does the use of standing 'hot' desks change sedentary work time in an open plan office? *Preventive Medicine* 54:65-67.

Goetzel, R.Z., X. Pei, M.J. Tabrizi, R.M. Henke, N. Kowlessar, C.F. Nelson, and R.D. Metz. 2012. Ten modifiable health risk factors are linked to more than one-fifth of employer-employee health care spending. *Health Affairs* 31:2474-2484.

Goetzel, R.Z., and N.P. Pronk. 2010. Worksite health promotion: How much do we really know about what works? *American Journal of Preventive Medicine* 38(2 Suppl.):S223-S225.

Goetzel, R.Z., D. Shechter, R.J. Ozminkowski, P.F. Marmet, M.J. Tabrizi, and E.C. Roemer. 2007. Promising practices in employer health and productivity management efforts: Findings from a benchmarking study. *Journal of Occupational and Environmental Medicine* 49:111-130.

Healy, G.N., D.W. Dunstan, J. Salmon, E. Cerin, J.E. Shaw, P.Z. Zimmet, and N. Owen. 2008. Breaks in sedentary time: Beneficial associations with metabolic risk. *Diabetes Care* 31:661-666.

John, D., D. Bassett, D. Thompson, J. Fairbrother, and D. Baldwin. 2009. Effect of using a treadmill workstation on performance of simulated office work tasks. *Journal of Physical Activity and Health* 6:617-624.

John, D., D.L. Thompson, H. Raynor, K. Bielak, B. Rider, and D.R. Bassett. 2011. Treadmill workstations: A worksite physical activity intervention in overweight and obese office workers. *Journal of Physical Activity and Health* 8:1034-1043.

Kosteas, V.D. 2013. *The effect of exercise on earnings: Evidence from the NLSY.* Paper from Cleveland State University. http://academic.csuohio.edu/kosteas_b/Exercise%20 and%20Earnings.pdf

Kozey-Keadle, S., A. Libertine, J. Staudenmayer, and P. Freedson. 2012. The feasibility of reducing and measuring sedentary time among overweight, non-exercising office workers. *Journal of Obesity* 2012:282303.

Langley, G.J., R. Moen, K.M. Nolan, T.W. Nolan, C.L. Norman, and L.P. Provost. 2009. *The improvement guide: A practical approach to enhancing organizational performance,* 2nd ed. San Francisco: Jossey-Bass.

McLean, L., M. Tingley, R.N. Scott, and J. Rickards. 2001. Computer terminal work and the benefit of microbreaks. *Applied Ergonomics* 32:225-237.

Morris, J.N., P.A. Heady, C.G. Raffle, and J.W. Parks. 1953. Coronary heart disease and physical activity of work. *Lancet* 2:1053-1057.

Mummery, W.K., G.M. Schofield, R. Steele, E.G. Eakin, and W.J. Brown. 2005. Occupational sitting time and overweight and obesity in Australian workers. *American Journal of Preventive Medicine* 29:91-97.

National Institute for Occupational Safety and Health (NIOSH). 2008. *Essential elements of effective workplace programs and policies for improving worker health and well-being.* Atlanta: Author. www.cdc.gov/niosh/docs/2010-140/pdfs/2010-140.pdf

Nicoll, G., and C. Zimring. 2009. Effect of innovative building design on physical activity. *Journal of Public Health Policy* 30(Suppl. 1):S111-S123.

O'Donnell, M.P., ed. 2002. *Health promotion in the workplace,* 3rd ed. Florence, KY: Delmar Thomson Learning.

Owen, N., G.N. Healy, C.E. Matthews, and D.W. Dunstan. 2010. Too much sitting: The population health science of sedentary behavior. *Exercise and Sports Science Reviews* 38:105-113.

Panter, J., C. Desousa, and D. Ogilvie. 2013. Incorporating walking or cycling into car journeys to and from work: The role of individual, workplace, and environmental characteristics. *Journal of Obesity* 56(3-4):211-217.

Physical Activity Guidelines Advisory Committee. 2008. *Physical Activity Guidelines Advisory Committee Report.* Washington, D.C.: Department of Health and Human Services.

Pronk, N.P. 2009a. Physical activity promotion in business and industry: Evidence, context, and recommendations for a national plan. *Journal of Physical Activity and Health* 6(Suppl. 2):S220-S235.

———. 2009b. *ACSM's worksite health handbook: A guide to building healthy and productive companies*, 2nd ed. Champaign, IL: Human Kinetics.

———. 2010. The problem with too much sitting: A workplace conundrum. *ACSM's Health & Fitness Journal* 15:41-43.

———. 2011. A global approach. *ACSM's Health & Fitness Journal* 15:48-50.

Pronk, N.P., and R.Z. Goetzel. 2010. The practical use of evidence: Practice and research connected. *American Journal of Preventive Medicine* 38(2 Suppl.):S229-S231.

Pronk, N.P., M.J. Goodman, P.J. O'Connor, and B.C. Martinson. 1999. Relationship between modifiable health risks and short-term health care costs. *JAMA* 282:2235-2239.

Pronk, N.P., A.S. Katz, M. Lowry, and J.R. Payfer. 2012. Reducing occupational sitting time and improving worker health: The Take-a-Stand Project, 2011. *Preventing Chronic Disease* 9:E154.

Pronk, N.P., and T.E. Kottke. 2009. Physical activity promotion as a strategic corporate priority to improve worker health and business performance. *Preventive Medicine* 49:316-321.

Pronk, S.J., N.P. Pronk, A. Sisco, D.S. Ingalls, and C. Ochoa. 1995. Impact of a daily 10-minute strength and flexibility program in a manufacturing plant. *American Journal of Health Promotion* 9:175-178.

Pronk, N.P., A.W. Tan, and P.J. O'Connor. 1999. Obesity, fitness, willingness to communicate and health care costs. *Medicine and Science in Sports and Exercise* 31:1535-1543.

Proper, K.I., B.J. Staal, V.H. Hildebrandt, A.J. van der Beek, and W. van Mechelen. 2002. Effectiveness of physical activity programs at worksites with respect to work-related outcomes. *Scandinavian Journal of Work and Environmental Health* 28:75-84.

Ramazzini, B [trans. by W.C. Wright]. 1713/1940. *Diseases of workers (Latin)*. Chicago: University of Chicago Press.

Robertson, M.M., V.M. Ciriello, and A.M. Garabet. 2013. Office ergonomics training and a sit-stand workstation: Effects on musculoskeletal and visual symptoms and performance of office workers. *Applied Ergonomics* 44:73-85.

Roelofs, A., and L. Straker. 2002. The experience of musculoskeletal discomfort amongst bank tellers who just sit, just stand, or sit and stand at work. *Ergonomics Journal of South Africa* 14:11-29.

Soler, R.E., K.D. Leeks, S. Razi, D.P. Hopkins, M. Griffith, A. Aten, S.K. Chattopadhyay, et al. 2010. A systematic review of selected interventions for worksite health promotion: The assessment of health risks with feedback. *American Journal of Preventive Medicine* 38(2 Suppl.):S237-S262.

Soler, R.E., K.D. Leeks, L.R. Buchanan, R.C. Brownson, G.W. Heath, D.H. Hopkins, and the Task Force on Community Preventive Services. 2010. Point-of-decision prompts to increase stair use: A systematic review update. *American Journal of Preventive Medicine* 38(2 Suppl.):S292-S300.

Sparling, P.B. 2010. Worksite health promotion: Principles, resources, and challenges. *Preventing Chronic Disease* 7:A25.

Straker, L.M. 1998. An overview of occupational injury/disease statistics in Australia. *Ergonomics Australia* 12:11-16.

Thompson, W.G., R.C. Foster, D.S. Eide, and J.A. Levine. 2008. Feasibility of a walking workstation to increase daily walking. *British Journal of Sports Medicine* 42:225-228.

Thorp, A.A., G.N. Healy, E. Winkler, B.K. Clark, P.A. Gardiner, N. Owen, and D.W. Dunstan. 2012. Prolonged sedentary time and physical activity in workplace and non-work contexts: A cross-sectional study of office, customer service and call centre employees. *International Journal of Behavioral Nutrition and Physical Activity* 9:128.

Tudor-Locke, C., C. Leonardi, W.D. Johnson, and P.T. Katzmarzyk. 2011. Time spent in physical activity and sedentary behaviors on the working day: The American time use survey. *Journal of Occupational and Environmental Medicine* 53:1382-1387.

Van Domelen, D.R., A. Koster, P. Caserotti, R.J. Brychta, K.Y. Chen, J.J. McClain, R.P. Troiano, D. Berrigan, and T.B. Harris. 2011. Employment and physical activity in the U.S. *American Journal of Preventive Medicine* 41:136-145.

Yancey, A.K., L.B. Lewis, J.J. Guinyard, D.C. Sloane, L.M. Nascimento, L. Galloway-Gilliam, A.L. Diamant, and W.J. McCarthy. 2006. Putting promotion into practice: The African Americans building a legacy of health organizational wellness program. *Health Promotion Practice* 7(3 Suppl.):233S-246S.

Chapter 25

Anand, S.S., A.D. Davis, R. Ahmed, R. Jacobs, C. Xie, A. Hill, J. Sowden, et al. 2007. A family-based intervention to promote healthy lifestyles in an aboriginal community in Canada. *Canadian Journal of Public Health* 98:447-452.

Biddle, S.J.H., S. O'Connell, and R.E. Braithwaite, 2011. Sedentary behaviour interventions in young people: A meta-analysis. *British Journal of Sports Medicine* 45:937-942.

Campbell, K.J., and K.D. Hesketh. 2007. Strategies which aim to positively impact on weight, physical activity, diet and sedentary behaviours in children from zero to five years. A systematic review of the literature. *Obesity Reviews* 8:327-338.

Chau, J.Y., H. van der Ploeg, J.G.Z. van Uffelen, J. Wong, I. Riphagen, G.N. Healy, N.D. Gilson, et al. 2010. Are workplace interventions to reduce sitting effective? A systematic review. *Preventive Medicine* 51(5):352-356.

Cong, Z., D. Feng, Y. Liu, and M.C. Esperat. 2012. Sedentary behaviors among Hispanic children: Influences of parental support in a school intervention program. *American Journal of Health Promotion* 26:270-280.

Cui, Z., S. Shah, L. Yan, Y. Pan, A. Gao, X. Shi, Y. Wu, and M.J. Dibley. 2012. Effect of a school-based peer education intervention on physical activity and sedentary behaviour in Chinese adolescents: A pilot study. *BMJ Open* 2:e000721.

De Cocker, K.A., I.M. De Bourdeaudhuij, W.J. Brown, and G.M. Cardon. 2008. The effect of a pedometer-based physical activity intervention on sitting time. *Preventive Medicine* 47:179-181.

de Silva-Sanigorski, A., D. Elea, C. Bell, P. Kremer, L. Carpenter, M. Nichols, M. Smith, S. Sharp, R. Boak, and B. Swinburn. 2011. Obesity prevention in the family day care setting: Impact of the romp & chomp intervention on opportunities for children's physical activity and healthy eating. *Child: Care, Health and Development* 37:385-393.

DeMattia, L., L. Lemont, and L. Meurer. 2007. Do interventions to limit sedentary behaviours change behaviour and reduce childhood obesity? A critical review of the literature. *Obesity Reviews* 8:69-81.

Dennison, B.A., T.J. Russo, P.A. Burdick, and P.L. Jenkins. 2004. An intervention to reduce television viewing by preschool children. *Archives of Pediatrics & Adolescent Medicine* 158:170-176.

Faith, M.S., N. Berman, M. Heo, A. Pietrobelli, D. Gallagher, L.H. Epstein, M.T. Eiden, and D.B. Allison. 2001. Effects of contingent television on physical activity and television viewing in obese children. *Pediatrics* 107:1043-1048.

Fitzsimons, C., G. Baker, S. Gray, M. Nimmo, N. Mutrie, and The Scottish Physical Activity Research Collaboration. 2012. Does physical activity counselling enhance the effects of a pedometer-based intervention over the long-term: 12-month findings from the Walking for Wellbeing in the west study. *BMC Public Health* 12:206.

Ford, B.S., T.E. McDonald, A.S. Owens, and T.N. Robinson. 2002. Primary care interventions to reduce television viewing in African-American children. *American Journal of Preventive Medicine* 22:106-109.

Foster, G.D., S. Sherman, K.E. Borradaile, K.M. Grundy, S.S. Vander Veur, J. Nachmani, A. Karpyn, S. Kumanyika, and J. Shults. 2008. A policy-based school intervention to prevent overweight and obesity. *Pediatrics* 121:e794-e802.

French, S.A., A.F. Gerlach, N.R. Mitchell, P.J. Hannan, and E.M. Welsh. 2011. Household obesity prevention: Take action—A group-randomized trial. *Obesity* 19:2082-2088.

Goldfinger, J.Z., G. Arniella, J. Wylie-Rosett, and C.R. Horowitz. 2008. Project HEAL: Peer education leads to weight loss in Harlem. *Journal of Health Care for the Poor and Underserved* 19:180-192.

Gortmaker, S.L., K. Peterson, J. Wiecha, A.M. Sobol, S. Dixit, M.K. Fox, and N. Laird. 1999. Reducing obesity via a school-based interdisciplinary intervention among youth: Planet health. *Archives of Pediatrics & Adolescent Medicine* 153:409-418.

Jones, D., D. Hoelscher, S. Kelder, A. Hergenroeder, and S. Sharma. 2008. Increasing physical activity and decreasing sedentary activity in adolescent girls—The Incorporating More Physical Activity and Calcium in Teens (IMPACT) study. *International Journal of Behavioral Nutrition and Physical Activity* 5:42.

Kahn, E.B., L.T. Ramsey, R.C. Brownson, G.W. Heath, E.H. Howze, K.E. Powell, E.J. Stone, M.W. Rajab, and P. Corso.

2002. The effectiveness of interventions to increase physical activity: A systematic review. *American Journal of Preventive Medicine* 22:73-107.

Kamath, C.C., K.S. Vickers, A. Ehrlich, L. McGovern, J. Johnson, V. Singhal, R. Paulo, A. Hettinger, P.J. Erwin, and V.M. Montori. 2008. Behavioral interventions to prevent childhood obesity: A systematic review and metaanalyses of randomized trials. *Journal of Clinical Endocrinology & Metabolism* 93:4606-4615.

Leung, M.M., A. Agaronov, K. Grytsenko, and M.C. Yeh. 2012. Intervening to reduce sedentary behaviors and childhood obesity among school-age youth: A systematic review of randomized trials. *Journal of Obesity* 2012:685430.

Milat, A.J., L. King, A.E. Bauman, and S. Redman. 2013. The concept of scalability: Increasing the scale and potential adoption of health promotion interventions into policy and practice. *Health Promotion International* 28(3):285-298.

Muller, M.J., I. Asbeck, M. Mast, and K. Langnase. 2001. Prevention of obesity—More than an intention. Concept and first results of the Kiel Obesity Prevention Study (KOPS). *International Journal of Obesity* 25:S66-S74.

Nguyen, B., V.A. Shrewsbury, J. O'Connor, K.S. Steinbeck, A. Lee, A.J. Hill, S. Shah, M.R. Kohn, S. Torvaldsen, and L.A. Bauer. 2012. Twelve-month outcomes of the Loozit randomized controlled trial: A community-based healthy lifestyle program for overweight and obese adolescents. *Archives of Pediatrics & Adolescent Medicine* 166:170-177.

O'Hara, B.J., P. Phongsavan, L. King, E. Develin, A.J. Milat, D. Eggins, E. King, J. Smith, and A.E. Bauman. 2014. Translational formative evaluation: Critical in up-scaling public health programmes. *Health Promotion International* 29(1):38-46.

Otten, J.J., K.E. Jones, B. Littenberg, and J. Harvey-Berino. 2009. Effects of television viewing reduction on energy intake and expenditure in overweight and obese adults: A randomized controlled trial. *Archives of Internal Medicine* 169:2109-2115.

Owen, N., T. Sugiyama, E.E. Eakin, P.A. Gardiner, M.S. Tremblay, and J.F. Sallis. 2011. Adults' sedentary behavior: Determinants and interventions. *American Journal of Preventive Medicine* 41:189-196.

Plachta-Danielzik, S., B. Landsberg, D. Lange, J. Seiberl, and M.J. Müller. 2011. Eight-year follow-up of school-based intervention on childhood overweight—The Kiel Obesity Prevention Study. *Obesity Facts* 4:35-43.

Plachta-Danielzik, S., S. Pust, I. Asbeck, M. Czerwinski-Mast, K. Langnäse, C. Fischer, A. Bosy-Westphal, P. Kriwy, and M.J. Müller. 2007. Four-year follow-up of school-based intervention on overweight children: The KOPS study. *Obesity* 15:3159-3169.

Robinson, T.N. 1999. Reducing children's television viewing to prevent obesity: A randomized controlled trial. *JAMA* 282:1561-1567.

Rogers, E.M. 2002. Diffusion of preventive innovations. *Addictive Behaviors* 27:989-993.

Sacher, P.M., M. Kolotourou, P.M. Chadwick, T.J. Cole, M.S. Lawson, A. Lucas, and A. Singhal. 2010. Randomized controlled trial of the MEND program: A family-based community intervention for childhood obesity. *Obesity* 18:S62-S68.

Salmon, J., K. Ball, C. Hume, M. Booth, and D. Crawford. 2008. Outcomes of a group-randomized trial to prevent excess weight gain, reduce screen behaviours and promote physical activity in 10-year-old children: Switch-Play. *International Journal of Obesity* 32:601-612.

Salmon, J., M.S. Tremblay, S.J. Marshall, and C. Hume. 2011. Health risks, correlates, and interventions to reduce sedentary behavior in young people. *American Journal of Preventive Medicine* 41:197-206.

Sepulveda, M.J., C. Lu, S. Sill, J.M. Young, and D.W. Edington. 2010. An observational study of an employer intervention for children's healthy weight behaviors. *Pediatrics* 126:e1153-1160.

Shrewsbury, V., B. Nguyen, J. O'Connor, K. Steinbeck, A. Lee, A. Hill, S. Shah, M. Kohn, S. Torvaldsen, and L. Baur. 2011. Short-term outcomes of community-based adolescent weight management: The Loozit(R) Study. *BMC Pediatrics* 11:13.

Simon, C., A. Wagner, C. DiVita, E. Rauscher, C. Klein-Platat, D. Arveiler, B. Schweitzer, and E. Triby. 2004. Intervention centred on adolescents' physical activity and sedentary behaviour (ICAPS): Concept and 6-month results. *International Journal of Obesity and Related Metabolic Disorders* 28(Suppl. 3):S96-S103.

Stahl, C.E., J.W. Necheles, J.H. Mayefsky, L.K. Wright, and K.M. Rankin. 2011. 5-4-3-2-1 go! Coordinating pediatric resident education and community health promotion to address the obesity epidemic in children and youth. *Clinical Pediatrics* 50:215-224.

Wahi, G., P.C. Parkin, J. Beyene, E.M. Uleryk, and C.S. Birken. 2011. Effectiveness of interventions aimed at reducing screen time in children: A systematic review and meta-analysis of randomized controlled trials. *Archives of Pediatrics and Adolescent Medicine* 165:979-986.

Wen, L.M., L.A. Baur, J.M. Simpson, C. Rissel, K. Wardle, and V.M. Flood. 2012. Effectiveness of home based early intervention on children's BMI at age 2: Randomised controlled trial. *BMJ* 344:e3732.

Chapter 26

American College of Sports Medicine (ACSM). 1978. Position statement on the recommended quantity and quality of exercise for developing and maintaining fitness in healthy adults. *Medicine and Science in Sports and Exercise* 10:vii-x.

Andersson, B.J., and R. Ortengren. 1974. Myoelectric back muscle activity during sitting. *Scandinavian Journal of Rehabilitative Medicine* 3(Suppl.):73-90.

Åstrand, P.O. 1992. Physical activity and fitness. *The American Journal of Clinical Nutrition* 55:1231S-1236S.

Bagatell, N., G. Mirigliani, C. Patterson, Y. Reyes, and L. Test. 2010. Effectiveness of therapy ball chairs on classroom participation in children with autism spectrum disorders. *American Journal of Occupational Therapy* 64:895-903.

Baute, K.J. 2008. An examination of the lower limb musculature involvement while using a stability ball as a chair at a workstation while performing a reaching task. Master's thesis, Indiana University, Bloomington.

Bherer, L., A.F. Kramer, M.S. Peterson, S. Colcombe, K. Erickson, and E. Becic. 2005. Training effects on dual-task performance: Are there age-related differences in plasticity of attentional control? *Psychology and Aging* 20:695.

Callaghan, J.P., and S.M. McGill. 2001. Low back joint loading and kinematics during standing and unsupported sitting. *Ergonomics* 44:280-294.

Cooper, K.H. 2013. *Aerobics program for total well-being: Exercise, diet, and emotional balance.* New York: Random House.

Dean, C., R. Shepherd, and R. Adams. 1999. Sitting balance I: Trunk–arm coordination and the contribution of the lower limbs during self-paced reaching in sitting. *Gait & Posture* 10:135-146.

Dunn, W., C. Brown, and A. McGuigan. 1994. The ecology of human performance: A framework for considering the effect of context. *American Journal of Occupational Therapy* 48:595-607.

Ekblom-Bak, E., M.-L. Hellénius, and B. Ekblom. 2010. Are we facing a new paradigm of inactivity physiology? *British Journal of Sports Medicine* 44:834-835.

Erickson, K.I., S.J. Colcombe, R. Wadhwa, L. Bherer, M.S. Peterson, P.E. Scalf, J.S. Kim, M. Alvarado, and A.F. Kramer. 2007. Training-induced functional activation changes in dual-task processing: An FMRI study. *Cerebral Cortex* 17:192-204.

Fedewa, A.L., and H.E. Erwin. 2011. Stability balls and students with attention and hyperactivity concerns: Implications for on-task and in-seat behavior. *American Journal of Occupational Therapy* 65:393-399.

Grandjean, E., W. Hünting, and M. Pidermann. 1983. VDT workstation design: Preferred settings and their effects. *Human Factors: The Journal of the Human Factors and Ergonomics Society* 25:161-175.

Gregory, D.E., N.M. Dunk, and J.P. Callaghan. 2006. Stability ball versus office chair: Comparison of muscle activation and lumbar spine posture during prolonged sitting. *Human Factors: The Journal of the Human Factors and Ergonomics Society* 48:142-153.

Hamilton, M.T., D.G. Hamilton, and T.W. Zderic. 2007. Role of low energy expenditure and sitting in obesity, metabolic syndrome, type 2 diabetes, and cardiovascular disease. *Diabetes* 56:2655-2667.

Hill, K., H. Kaplan, K. Hawkes, and A.M. Hurtado. 1985. Men's time allocation to subsistence work among the Ache of eastern Paraguay. *Human Ecology* 13:29-47.

Hodges, P.W. 2001. Changes in motor planning of feedforward postural responses of the trunk muscles in low back pain. Experimental Brain Research 141:261-266.

Hodges, P.W., G.L. Moseley, A. Gabrielsson, and S.C. Gandevia. 2003. Experimental muscle pain changes feedforward postural responses of the trunk muscles. Experimental Brain Research 151:262-271.

Hodges, P.W., and C.A. Richardson. 1997. Relationship between limb movement speed and associated contraction of the trunk muscles. Ergonomics 40:1220-1230.

Illi, U. 1994. Balls instead of chairs in the classroom. Swiss Journal of Physical Education 6:37-39.

Katzmarzyk, P.T., T.S. Church, C.L. Craig, and C. Bouchard. 2009. Sitting time and mortality from all causes, cardiovascular disease, and cancer. Medicine & Science in Sports & Exercise 41:998-1005.

Kingma, I., and J.H. van Dieën. 2009. Static and dynamic postural loadings during computer work in females: Sitting on an office chair versus sitting on an exercise ball. Applied Ergonomics 40:199-205.

Kramer, A.F., J.F. Larish, and D.L. Strayer. 1995. Training for attentional control in dual task settings: A comparison of young and old adults. Journal of Experimental Psychology: Applied 1:50-76.

Krämer, J. 1973. Biomechanics of the lumbar locomotion segment. Fortschritte der Medizin 91:863.

Kroemer, K.H.E., and E. Grandjean. 2005. Fitting the task to the human: A textbook of occupational ergonomics. Boca Raton, FL: CRC Press.

Kroemer, K., H. Kroemer, and K.E. Kroemer-Elbert. 2001. Ergonomics: How to design for ease and efficiency. Upper Saddle River, NJ: Prentice Hall.

Kumar, S. 1990. Cumulative load as a risk factor for back pain. Spine 15:1311-1316.

———, ed. 1999. Biomechanics in ergonomics. Boca Raton, FL: CRC Press.

———. 2001. Theories of musculoskeletal injury causation. Ergonomics 44:17-47.

Li, K.Z.H., E. Roudaia, M. Lussier, L. Bherer, A. Leroux, and P.A. McKinley. 2010. Benefits of cognitive dual-task training on balance performance in healthy older adults. The Journals of Gerontology Series A: Biological Sciences and Medical Sciences 65:1344-1352.

Lundberg, U. 2002. Psychophysiology of work: Stress, gender, endocrine response, and work related upper extremity disorders. American Journal of Industrial Medicine 41:383-392.

Lundervold, A.J. 1951. Electromyographic investigations of position and manner of working in typewriting. Acta Physiologica Scandinavica 24(Suppl.):1.

———. 1958. Electromyographic investigations during typewriting. Ergonomics 1:226-233.

Magnusson, M., and M.H. Pope. 1996. Body height changes with hyperextension. Clinical Biomechanics 11:236-238.

Magnusson, M.L., and M.H. Pope. 1998. A review of the biomechanics and epidemiology of working postures. Journal of Sound and Vibration 215:965-976.

Malina, R.M., and B.B. Little. 2008. Physical activity: The present in the context of the past. American Journal of Human Biology 20:373-391.

Marks, C.R.C., K.E. Hylland, and J. Terrell. 2012. Stability ball sitting versus chair sitting during sub-maximal arm ergometry. International Journal of Exercise Science 5:3.

McGill, S.M., N.S. Kavcic, and E. Harvey. 2006. Sitting on a chair or an exercise ball: Various perspectives to guide decision making. Clinical Biomechanics 21:353-360.

Merritt, L.G., and C.M. Merritt. 2007. The gym ball as a chair for the back pain patient: A two case report. Journal of the Canadian Chiropractic Association 51:50.

Miller, L.J., M.E. Anzalone, S.J. Lane, S.A. Cermak, and E.T. Osten. 2007. Concept evolution in sensory integration: A proposed nosology for diagnosis. American Journal of Occupational Therapy 61:135-140.

Miller, L.J., and S.J. Lane. 2000. Toward a consensus in terminology in sensory integration theory and practice: Part 1: Taxonomy of neurophysiological processes. Sensory Integration Special Interest Section Quarterly 23:1-4.

Morgan, W.P., ed. 2013. Physical activity and mental health. Washington, D.C.: Taylor & Francis.

O'Sullivan, P., W. Dankaerts, A. Burnett, L. Straker, G. Bargon, N. Moloney, M. Perry, and S. Tsang. 2006. Lumbopelvic kinematics and trunk muscle activity during sitting on stable and unstable surfaces. Journal of Orthopaedic and Sports Physical Therapy 36:19.

Pellecchia, G.L. 2005. Dual-task training reduces impact of cognitive task on postural sway. Journal of Motor Behavior 37:239-246.

Pesce, C. 2012. Shifting the focus from quantitative to qualitative exercise characteristics in exercise and cognition research. Journal of Sport & Exercise Psychology 34:766-786.

Schilling, D.L., and I.S. Schwartz. 2004. Alternative seating for young children with autism spectrum disorder: Effects on classroom behavior. Journal of Autism and Developmental Disorders 34:423-432.

Schilling, D.L., K. Washington, F.F. Billingsley, and J. Deitz. 2003. Classroom seating for children with attention deficit hyperactivity disorder: Therapy balls versus chairs. American Journal of Occupational Therapy 57:534-541.

Silsupadol, P., A. Shumway-Cook, V. Lugade, P. van Donkelaar, L. Chou, U. Mayr, and M.H. Woollacott. 2009. Effects of single-task versus dual-task training on balance performance in older adults: A double-blind, randomized controlled trial. Archives of Physical Medicine and Rehabilitation 90:381.

Urquhart, D.M., P.W. Hodges, T.J. Allen, and I.H. Story. 2005. Abdominal musclerecruitment during a range of voluntary exercises. Manual Therapy 10:144-153.

Vieira, E.R., and S. Kumar. 2004. Working postures: A literature review. Journal of Occupational Rehabilitation 14:143-159.

Westgaard, R.H., and J. Winkel. 2011. Occupational musculoskeletal and mental health: Significance of rationalization and opportunities to create sustainable production systems—A systematic review. Applied Ergonomics 42:261-296.

Witt, D., and R. Talbot. 1998. Let's get our kids on the ball. Advance for Physical Therapists, 27-28.

Yogev-Seligmann, G., J.M. Hausdorff, and N. Giladi. 2008. The role of executive function and attention in gait. Movement Disorders 23:329-342.

Chapter 27

Adams, J.S. 1961. Reduction of cognitive dissonance by seeking consonant information. Journal of Abnormal and Social Psychology 62:74-78.

Adorno, T.W., E. Frenkel-Brunswik, D.J. Levinson, and R.N. Sanford. 1950. The authoritarian personality. Oxford, England: Harpers.

Ajzen, I., and T.J. Madden. 1986. Prediction of goal-directed behavior: Attitudes, intentions, and perceived behavioral control. Journal of Experimental Social Psychology 22(5):453-474.

Albarracín, D. 2002. Cognition in persuasion: An analysis of information processing in response to persuasive communications. In Advances in experimental social psychology, vol. 34, edited by M.P. Zanna, 61-132. San Diego: Academic Press.

Albarracín, D., B.T. Johnson, M. Fishbein, and P.A. Muellerleile. 2001. Theories of reasoned action and planned behavior as models of condom use: A meta-analysis. Psychological Bulletin 127:142-161.

Albarracín, D., and A.L. Mitchell. 2004. The role of defensive confidence in preference for proattitudinal information: How believing that one is strong can sometimes be a defensive weakness. Personality and Social Psychology Bulletin 30:1565-1584.

Albarracín, D., M.P. Zanna, B.T. Johnson, and G.T. Kumkale. 2005. Attitudes: Introduction and scope. Mahwah, NJ: Lawrence Erlbaum.

Altemeyer B. 1981. Right-wing authoritarianism. Winnipeg, MB: University of Manitoba Press.

———. 1998. The other 'authoritarian personality'. Advances in Experimental Social Psychology 30:47-91.

Anderson-Bill, E.S., R.A. Winett, and J.R. Wojcik. 2011. Social cognitive determinants of nutrition and physical activity among web-health users enrolling in an online intervention: The influence of social support, self-efficacy, outcome expectations, and self-regulation. Journal of Medical Internet Research 13(1):e28.

Baker, L., T.H. Wagner, S. Singer, and M. Bundorf. 2003. Use of the internet and e-mail for health care information. Journal of the American Medical Association 289:2401-2406.

Bandura, A. 1986. Social foundations of thought and action: A social cognitive theory. Englewood Cliffs, NJ: Prentice-Hall.

———. 1989. Human agency in social cognitive theory. American Psychologist 44:1175-1184.

———. 1994. Social cognitive theory of mass communication. In Media effects: Advances in theory and research, edited by J. Bryant and D. Zillman, 61-90. Hillsdale, NJ: Lawrence Erlbaum.

Baranowski, T., R. Buday, D.I. Thompson, and J. Baranowski. 2008. Playing for real: Video games and stories for health-related behavior change. American Journal of Preventive Medicine 34:74-82.

Bardram, J.E., M. Frost, K. Szántó, and G. Marcu. 2012. The MONARCA self-assessment system: A persuasive personal monitoring system for bipolar patients. Proceedings of the 2nd ACM SIGHIT International Health Informatics Symposium 2012:21-30.

Bartholomew, L.K., M.M. Sockrider, S.L. Abramson, P.R. Swank, D.I. Czyzewski, S.R. Tortolero, C.M. Markham, M.E. Fernandez, R. Shegog, and S. Tyrrell. 2006. Partners in school asthma management: Evaluation of a self-management program for children with asthma. Journal of School Health 76:283-290.

Beauvois, J., and R. Joule. 1996. A radical dissonance theory. Philadelphia: Taylor and Francis.

Berger, J., and K. Milkman. 2010. "Social transmission, emotion, and the virality of online content." Research paper, The Wharton School, University of Philadelphia. http://robingandhi.com/wp-content/uploads/2011/11/Social-Transmission-Emotion-and-the-Virality-of-Online-Content-Wharton.pdf

———. 2012. What makes online content viral? Journal of Marketing Research 49:192-205.

Berkowitz, L. 1965. Cognitive dissonance and communication preferences. Human Relations 18:361-372.

Betsch, T., S. Haberstroh, A. Glöckner, T. Haar, and K. Fiedler., 2001. The effects of routine strength on adaptation and information search in recurrent decision making. Organizational Behavior and Human Decision Processes 84(1):23-53.

Biddiss, E., and J. Irwin. 2010. Active video games to promote physical activity in children and youth: A systematic review. Archives of Pediatrics and Adolescent Medicine 164(7):664-672.

Bielik, P., M. Tomlein, P. Krátky, Š. Mitrík, M. Barla, and M. Bieliková. 2012. "Move2Play: An innovative approach to encouraging people to be more physically active." Paper presented at the proceedings of the 2nd ACM SIGHIT International Health Informatics Symposium, Miami, FL, January 28-30.

Blanchard, C.G., T.L. Albrecht, J.C. Ruckdeschel, C.H. Grant, and R.M. Hemmick. 1995. The role of social support in adaptation to cancer and to survival. *Journal of Psychosocial Oncology* 13(1-2):75-95.

Bosak, K.A.S. 2007. "An internet physical activity intervention to reduce coronary heart disease risk in the metabolic syndrome population." PhD diss., University of Nebraska Medical Center. PsycINFO (AAI3289621).

Brechan, I. 2002. "Selective exposure and selective attention: The moderating effect of confidence in attitudes and the knowledge basis for these attitudes." M.S. thesis, University of Florida, Gainesville, FL.

Brehm, J.W., and A.R. Cohen. 1962. *Explorations in cognitive dissonance.* Hoboken, NJ: John Wiley and Sons.

Brodbeck, M. 1956. The role of small groups in mediating the effects of propaganda. *Journal of Abnormal and Social Psychology* 52(2):166-170.

Broder, A., M. Fontoura, V. Josifovski, and L. Riedel. 2007. "A semantic approach to contextual advertising." Paper presented at the proceedings of the 30th annual International ACM SIGIR conference on research and development information retrieval, New York, July 23-27.

Brown, R., H. Sugarman, and A. Burstin. 2009. Use of the Nintendo Wii fit for the treatment of balance problems in an elderly patient with stroke: A case report. *International Journal of Rehabilitation Research* 32:S109-S110.

Brown, S.J., D.A. Lieberman, B.A. Gemeny, Y.C. Fan, D.M. Wilson, and D.J. Pasta. 1997. Educational video game for juvenile diabetes: Results of a controlled trial. *Informatics for Health and Social Care* 22(1):77-89.

Burke, M., R. Kraut, and D. Williams. 2010. "Social use of computer-mediated communication by adults on the autism spectrum." Paper presented at the proceedings of the 2010 ACM conference on computer supported cooperative work, Savannah, GA, February 6-10.

Canon, L.K. 1964. Self-confidence and selective exposure to information. In *Conflict, decision, and dissonance*, edited by L. Festinger, 83-95. Stanford, CA: Stanford University Press.

Cappella, J., H. Kim, and D. Albarracín. 2015. Selection and transmission processes for information in the emerging media environment: Psychological motives and message characteristics. *Media Psychology* 18(3):396-424.

Carr, L.J. 2009. "Short and long-term efficacy of an internet-delivered physical activity behavior change program on physical activity and cardiometabolic disease risk factors in sedentary, overweight adults." PhD diss., University of Wyoming. PsycINFO (AAI3340668).

Carr, L.J., R.T. Bartee, C. Dorozynski, J.F. Broomfield, M.L. Smith, and D.T. Smith. 2008. Internet-delivered behavior change program increases physical activity and improves cardiometabolic disease risk factors in sedentary adults: Results of a randomized controlled trial. *Preventive Medicine: An International Journal Devoted to Practice and Theory* 46(5):431-438.

Carr, L.J., S.I. Dunsiger, B. Lewis, J.T. Ciccolo, S. Hartman, B. Bock, G. Dominick, and B.H. Marcus. 2013. Randomized controlled trial testing: An Internet physical activity intervention for sedentary adults. *Health Psychology* 32(3):328-336.

Carter, O.B.J., R. Donovan, and G. Jalleh. 2011. Using viral e-mails to distribute tobacco control advertisements: An experimental investigation. *Journal of Health Communication* 16(7):698-707.

Cavallo, D.N. 2013. "Using online social network technology to increase social support for physical activity: The internet support for healthy associations promoting exercise (INSHAPE) study." PhD diss., University of North Carolina, Chapel Hill. PsycINFO (AAI3526113).

Chaiken, S., A. Liberman, and A.H. Eagly. 1989. Heuristic and systematic information processing within and beyond the persuasion context. In *Unintended thought*, edited by J.S. Uleman and J.A. Bargh, 212-252. New York: Guilford Press.

Chaiken, S., W. Wood, and A.H. Eagly. 1996. *Principles of persuasion.* New York: Guilford Press.

Chretien, K.C., J. Azar, and T. Kind. 2011. Physicians on Twitter. *JAMA* 305(6):566-568.

Chung, D.S., and S. Kim. 2008. Blogging activity among cancer patients and their companions: Uses, gratifications, and predictors of outcomes. *Journal of the American Society for Information Science and Technology* 59(2):297-306.

Consolvo, S., K. Everitt, I. Smith, and J.A. Landay. 2006. "Design requirements for technologies that encourage physical activity." Paper presented at the proceedings of the 2006 SIGCHI conference on human factors in computing systems, Paris, April 24-27.

Cooperberg, J. 2014. "Food for thought: A parental internet-based intervention to treat childhood obesity in preschool-aged children." PhD diss., Washington University, St Louis. PsycINFO (AAI3559780).

Coulson, N.S. 2005. Receiving social support online: An analysis of a computer-mediated support group for individuals living with irritable bowel syndrome. *CyberPsychology and Behavior* 8(6):580-584.

Cullen, K.W., D. Thompson, C. Boushey, K. Konzelmann, and T.A. Chen. 2013. Evaluation of a web-based program promoting healthy eating and physical activity for adolescents: Teen Choice: Food and Fitness. *Health Education Research* 28(4):704-714.

Darke, P.R., and S. Chaiken. 2005. The pursuit of self-interest: Self-interest bias in attitude judgment and persuasion. *Journal of Personality and Social Psychology* 89(6):864-883.

Davies, E.B., R. Morriss, and C. Glazebrook. 2014. Computer-delivered and web-based interventions to improve depression, anxiety, and psychological well-being of university students: A systematic review and meta-analysis. *Journal of Medical Internet Research* 16(5):e130

Davis, M.A., A.L. Quittner, C.M. Stack, and M.C. Yang. 2004. Controlled evaluation of the STARBRIGHT CD-ROM program for children and adolescents with cystic fibrosis. *Journal of Pediatric Psychology* 29(4):259-267.

Davis, J.C., E. Verhagen, S. Bryan, T. Liu-Ambrose, J. Borland, D. Buchner, M.R.C. Hendricks, et al. 2014. Consensus statement from the first Economics of Physical Inactivity Consensus (EPIC) Conference (Vancouver). *British Journal of Sports Medicine* 48:947-951.

De Bourdeaudhuij, I., L. Maes, S. De Henauw, T. De Vriendt, L.A. Moreno, M. Kersting, K. Sarri, et al. 2010. Evaluation of a computer-tailored physical activity intervention in adolescents in six European countries: The Activ-O-Meter in the HELENA intervention study. *Journal of Adolescent Health* 46(5):458-466.

De la Torre-Díez, I., F.J. Díaz-Pernas, and M. Antón-Rodríguez. 2012. A content analysis of chronic diseases social groups on Facebook and Twitter. *Telemedicine and e-Health* 18(6):404-408.

De Oliveira, R., and N. Oliver. 2008. "TripleBeat: Enhancing exercise performance with persuasion." Paper presented at the proceedings of the 10th international conference on Human computer interaction with mobile devices and services, New York, September 2-5.

Deterding, S., D. Dixon, R. Khaled, and L. Nacke. 2011. "From game design elements to gamefulness: Defining gamification." Paper presented at the proceedings of the 15th international academic MindTrek conference, Tampere, Finland, 28-30 September. Dunton, G.F., and T.P. Robertson. 2008. A tailored internet-plus-email intervention for increasing physical activity among ethnically-diverse women. *Preventive Medicine: An International Journal Devoted to Practice and Theory* 47(6):605-611.

Eagly, A.H., and S. Chaiken. 1993. *The psychology of attitudes*. Orlando, FL: Harcourt Brace Jovanovich College.

Eagly, A.H., S. Chen, S. Chaiken, and K. Shaw-Barnes. 1999. The impact of attitudes on memory: An affair to remember. *Psychological Bulletin* 125(1):64-89.

Earl, A., D. Albarracín, M.R. Durantini, J.B. Gunnoe, J. Leeper, and J.H. Levitt. 2009. Participation in counseling programs: High-risk participants are reluctant to accept HIV-prevention counseling. *Journal of Consulting and Clinical Psychology* 77(4):668-679.

Eckler, P., and P. Bolls. 2011. Spreading the virus: Emotional tone of viral advertising and its effect on forwarding intentions and attitudes. *Journal of Interactive Advertising* 11(2):1-11.

Farnham, S., L. Cheng, L. Stone, M. Zaner-Godsey, C. Hibbeln, K. Syrjala, A.M. Clark, and J. Abrams. 2002. "HutchWorld: Clinical study of computer-mediated social support for cancer patients and their caregivers." Paper presented at the proceedings of the 2002 SIGCHI conference on human factors in computing systems, New York, April 20-25.

Feather, N.T. 1962. Cigarette smoking and lung cancer: A study of cognitive dissonance. *Australian Journal of Psychology* 14(1):55-64.

Felfernig, A., M. Jeran, G. Ninaus, F. Reinfrank, and S. Reiterer. 2013. Toward the next generation of recommender systems: Applications and research challenges. *Multimedia Services in Intelligent Environments* 24:81-98.

Festinger, L. 1957. *A theory of cognitive dissonance*. Stanford, CA: Stanford University Press.

———. 1964. *Conflict, decision, and dissonance*. Stanford, CA: Stanford University Press.

Fishbein, M., and I. Ajzen. 1975. *Belief, attitude, intention, and behavior: An introduction to theory and research*. Reading, MA: Addison-Wesley.

Fisher, J.D., and W.A. Fisher. 1992. Changing AIDS-risk behavior. *Psychological Bulletin* 111(3):455-474.

Floyd, D.L., S. Prentice-Dunn, and R.W. Rogers. 2000. A meta-analysis of research on protection motivation theory. *Journal of Applied Social Psychology* 30:407-429.

Fogel, J., S.M. Albert, F. Schnabel, B.A. Ditkoff, and A.I. Neugut. 2002. Use of the Internet by women with breast cancer. *Journal of Medical Internet Research* 4(2):e9.

Fox, S. and M. Duggan. 2013. Health Online 2013. *Pew Internet and American Life Project*. http://pewinternet.org/Reports/2013/Health-online.aspx

Franklin, P.D., P.F. Rosenbaum, M.P. Carey, and M.F. Roizen. 2006. Using sequential email messages to promote health behaviors: Evidence of feasibility and reach in a worksite sample. *Journal of Medical Internet Research* 8(1):e3.

Freedman, J.L. 1965. Confidence, utility, and selective exposure: A partial replication. *Journal of Personality and Social Psychology* 2(5):778-780.

Freedman, J.L., and D.O. Sears. 1965. Selective exposure. In *Advances in experimental social psychology*, vol. 2, edited by L. Berkowitz, 57-97. New York: Academic Press.

Frey, D. 1986. Recent research on selective exposure to information. In *Advances in experimental social psychology*, vol. 19, edited by L. Berkowitz, 41-80. New York: Academic Press.

Frey, D., and M. Rosch. 1984. Information seeking after decisions: The roles of novelty of information and decision reversibility. *Personality and Social Psychology Bulletin* 10(1):91-98.

Gao, Y., and R. Mandryk. 2012. "The acute cognitive benefits of casual exergame play." Paper presented at the proceedings of the 2012 ACM annual conference on human factors in computing systems, Austin, TX, May 5-10.

Glasgow, R.E., D. Kurz, D. King, J.M. Dickman, A.J. Faber, E. Halterman, T. Wooley, et al. 2010. Outcomes of minimal and moderate support versions of an Internet-based diabetes self-management support program. *Journal of General Internal Medicine* 25(12):1315-1322.

Gow, R.W., S.E. Trace, and S.E. Mazzeo. 2010. Preventing weight gain in first year college students: An online intervention to prevent the "freshman fifteen." *Eating Behaviors* 11(1):33-39.

Grimes, A., V. Kantroo, and R.E. Grinter. 2010. "Let's play! Mobile health games for adults." Paper presented at the proceedings of the 12th ACM international conference on ubiquitous computing, Copenhagen, Denmark, September 26-29.

Hammer, S., J. Kim, and E. André. 2010. "MED-StyleR: METABO diabetes-lifestyle recommender." Paper presented at the proceedings of the 4th ACM conference on recommender systems, Barcelona, Spain, September 26-30.

Hart, W., D. Albarracín, A.H. Eagly, I. Brechan, M.J. Lindberg, and L. Merrill. 2009. Feeling validated versus being correct: A meta-analysis of selective exposure to information. Psychological Bulletin 135(4):555-588.

Hatchett, A.G. 2009. "Evaluation of a social cognitive theory based intervention to enhance the physical activity of patients recovering from breast cancer." PhD diss.,The University of Mississippi. PsycINFO (AAI3361173).

Heider, F. 1958. *The psychology of interpersonal relations.* New York: John Wiley and Sons.

Herndon, C.A., M. Decambre, and P.H. McKenna. 2001. Interactive computer games for treatment of pelvic floor dysfunction. *Journal of Urology* 166(5):1893-1898.

Hibbard, J.H., and E. Peters. 2003. Supporting informed consumer health care decisions: Data presentation approaches that facilitate the use of information in choice. *Annual Review of Public Health* 24(1):413-433.

Hillsdon, M., C. Foster, and M. Thorogood. 2005. Interventions for promoting physical activity. *Cochrane Database of Systematic Reviews* 2005 Jan 25(1):CD003180.

Heaivilin, N., B. Gerbert, J.E. Page, and J.L. Gibbs, 2011. Public health surveillance of dental pain via Twitter. *Journal of Dental Research* 90(9):1047-1051.

Hoff, T., M. Mishel, and I. Rowe. 2008. Using new media to make HIV personal. *Cases in Public Health Communication and Marketing* 2:190-197.

Hoffman, H.G., A. Garcia-Palacios, D.R. Patterson, M. Jensen, T. Furness III, and W.F. Ammons Jr. 2001. The effectiveness of virtual reality for dental pain control: A case study. *CyberPsychology and Behavior* 4(4):527-535.

Huang, S.J., W.C. Hung, M. Chang, and J. Chang. 2009. The effect of an Internet-based, stage-matched message intervention on young Taiwanese women's physical activity. *Journal of Health Communication* 14(3):210-227.

Hwang, K.O., A.J. Ottenbacher, A.P. Green, M.R. Cannon-Diehl, O. Richardson, E.V. Bernstam, and E.J. Thomas. 2010. Social support in an Internet weight loss community. *International Journal of Medical Informatics* 79(1):5-13.

Irvine, A.B., V.A. Gelatt, J.R. Seeley, P. Macfarlane, and J.M. Gau. 2013. Web-based intervention to promote physical activity by sedentary older adults: Randomized controlled trial. *Journal of Medical Internet Research* 15(2):18-33.

Jafarinaimi, N., J. Forlizzi, A. Hurst, and J. Zimmerman. 2005. "Breakaway: An ambient display designed to change human behavior." Paper presented at the CHI'05 extended abstracts on human factors in computing systems, Portland, OR, April 2-7.

Jamison-Powell, S., C. Linehan, L. Daley, A. Garbett, and S. Lawson. 2012. "I can't get no sleep: Discussing #insomnia on Twitter." Paper presented at the proceedings of the 2012 ACM annual conference on human factors in computing systems, Austin, TX, May 5-10.

Janz, N.K., and M.H. Becker. 1984. The health belief model: A decade later. *Health Education Quarterly* 11(1):1-47.

Joachims, T., L.A. Granka, B. Pan, H. Hembrooke, and G. Gay. 2005. Accurately interpreting clickthrough data as implicit feedback. *SIGIR* August:154-161

Johnson, B.T., and A.H. Eagly. 1989. Effects of involvement on persuasion: A meta-analysis. *Psychological Bulletin* 106(2):290-314.

Jonas, E., and D. Frey. 2003. Information search and presentation in advisor-client interaction. *Organizational Behavior and Human Decision Processes* 91(2):154-168.

Kahn, E.B., L.T. Ramsey, R.C. Brownson, G.W. Heath, E.H. Howze, K.E. Powell, E.J. Stone, M.W. Rajab, and P. Corso. 2002. The effectiveness of interventions to increase physical activity: A systematic review. *American Journal of Preventive Medicine* 22:73-106.

Kang, M., S.J. Marshall, T.V. Barreira, and J.O. Lee. 2009. Effect of pedometer-based physical activity interventions: A meta-analysis. *Research Quarterly for Exercise and Sport* 80(3):648-655.

Kassin, S.M., and D.J. Hochreich. 1977. Instructional set: A neglected variable in attribution research? *Personality and Social Psychology Bulletin* 3(4):620-623.

Kato, P.M., S.W. Cole, A.S. Bradlyn, and B.H. Pollock. 2008. A video game improves behavioral outcomes in adolescents and young adults with cancer: A randomized trial. *Pediatrics* 122(2):e305-e317.

Katz, D. 1960. The functional approach to the study of attitudes. *Public Opinion Quarterly* 24(2):163-204.

Kelders, S.M., J.E.W.C. Van Gemert-Pijnen, A. Werkman, N. Nijland, and E.R. Seydel. 2011. Effectiveness of a web-based intervention aimed at healthy dietary and physical activity behavior: A randomized controlled trial about users and usage. *Journal of Medical Internet Research* 13(2):3-18.

Kiesler, C.A. 1971. *The psychology of commitment.* New York: Academic Press.

Kim, H.S., S. Lee, J.N. Cappella, L. Vera, and S. Emery. 2013. Content characteristics driving the diffusion of antismoking messages: Implications for cancer prevention in the emerging public communication environment. *Journal of the National Cancer Institute Monographs* 2013(47):182-187.

Kim, S., J.A. Kientz, S.N. Patel, and G.D. Abowd. 2008. "Are you sleeping? Sharing portrayed sleeping status within a social network." Paper presented at the proceedings of the 2008 ACM conference on computer support cooperative work, San Diego, November 8-12.

Klemm, P., D. Bunnell, M. Cullen, R. Soneji, P. Gibbons, and A. Holecek. 2003. Online cancer support groups: A review of the research literature. *Computers Informatics Nursing* 21(3):136-142.

Kosma, M., B.J. Cardinal, and J.A. McCubbin. 2005. A pilot study of a web-based physical activity motivational program for adults with physical disabilities. *Disability and Rehabilitation: An International, Multidisciplinary Journal* 27(23):1435-1442.

Krebs, D. 1975. Empathy and altruism. *Journal of Personality and Social Psychology* 32(6):1134-1146.

Kruglanski, A.W., and T. Freund. 1983. The freezing and unfreezing of lay-inferences: Effects on impressional primacy, ethnic stereotyping, and numerical anchoring. *Journal of Experimental Social Psychology* 19(5):448-468.

Kunda, Z. 1990. The case for motivated reasoning. *Psychological Bulletin* 108(3):480-498.

Lasker, J.N., E.D. Sogolow, and R.R. Sharim. 2005. The role of an online community for people with a rare disease: Content analysis of messages posted on a primary biliary cirrhosis mailing list. *Journal of Medical Internet Research* 7(1):e10.

Lau, E.Y., P.W.C. Lau, P.K. Chung, L.B. Ransdell, and E. Archer. 2012. Evaluation of an Internet–short message service–based intervention for promoting physical activity in Hong Kong Chinese adolescent school children: A pilot study. *Cyberpsychology, Behavior, and Social Networking* 15(8):425-434.

Lee, I.M., E.J. Shiroma, F. Lobelo, P. Puska, S.N. Blair, P.T. Katzmarzyk, and Lancet Physical Activity Working Group. 2012. Effect of physical inactivity on major non-communicable diseases worldwide: An analysis of burden of disease and life expectancy. *Lancet* 380:219-229.

Lee, M.K., S. Kiesler, and J. Forlizzi. 2011. "Mining behavioral economics to design persuasive technology for healthy choices." Paper presented at the proceedings of the 2011 SIGCHI conference on human factors in computing systems, Vancouver, Canada, May 7-12.

Leung, F.L.E. 2011. "The efficacy of an Internet-based behavioural intervention for physical activity promotion among university students." PhD diss., The Chinese University of Hong Kong. PsycINFO (AAI3514520).

Liebreich, T., R.C. Plotnikoff, K.S. Courneya, and N. Boulé. 2009. Diabetes NetPLAY: A physical activity website and linked email counselling randomized intervention for individuals with type 2 diabetes. *International Journal of Behavioral Nutrition and Physical Activity* 6:18.

Lin, C.T., L. Wittevrongel, L. Moore, B.L. Beaty, and S.E. Ross. 2005. An Internet-based patient-provider communication system: Randomized controlled trial. *Journal of Medical Internet Research* 7(4):347.

Lin, J.J., L. Mamykina, S. Lindtner, G. Delajoux, and H.B. Strub. 2006. Fish'n'Steps: Encouraging physical activity with an interactive computer game. Paper presented at the proceedings of the 2006 *International Conference on Ubiquitous Computing*, Orange County, CA, September 17-21.Berlin: Springer.

Liu, L.S., J. Huh, T. Neogi, K. Inkpen, and W. Pratt. 2013. "Health vlogger-viewer interaction in chronic illness management." Paper presented at the proceedings of the 2013 SIGCHI conference on human factors in computing systems, Paris, France, April 27-May 2.

Liu, T.Y. 2009. Learning to rank for information retrieval. *Foundations and Trends in Information Retrieval* 3(3):225-331.

Lubans, D.R., P.J. Morgan, R. Callister, and C.E. Collins. 2009. Effects of integrating pedometers, parental materials, and e-mail support within an extracurricular school sport intervention. *Journal of Adolescent Health* 44(2):176-183.

Lundgren, S.R., and R. Prislin. 1998. Motivated cognitive processing and attitude change. *Personality and Social Psychology Bulletin* 24(7):715-726.

Maher, C.A., M.T. Williams, T. Olds, and A.E. Lane. 2010. An internet-based physical activity intervention for adolescents with cerebral palsy: A randomized controlled trial. *Developmental Medicine and Child Neurology* 52(5):448-455.

Mailey, E.L., T.R. Wójcicki, R.W. Motl, L. Hu, D.R. Strauser, K.D. Collins, and E. McAuley. 2010. Internet-delivered physical activity intervention for college students with mental health disorders: A randomized pilot trial. *Psychology, Health and Medicine* 15(6):646-659.

Maitland, J., and M. Chalmers. 2011. "Designing for peer involvement in weight management." Paper presented at the proceedings of the 2011 SIGCHI conference on human factors in computing systems. Vancouver, Canada, May 7-12.

Maitland, J., S. Sherwood, L. Barkhuus, I. Anderson, M. Hall, B. Brown, M. Chalmers, and H. Muller. 2006. "Increasing the awareness of daily activity levels with pervasive computing." Paper presented at the pervasive health conference and workshops. Innsbruck, Austria, November November 29-December 1.

Mamykina, L., E. Mynatt, P. Davidson, and D. Greenblatt. 2008. "MAHI: Investigation of social scaffolding for reflective thinking in diabetes management." Paper presented at the proceedings of the 2008 SIGCHI conference on human factors in computing systems, Florence, Italy, April 5-10.

Mankoff, J., G. Hsieh, H.C. Hung, S. Lee, and E. Nitao. 2002. Using low-cost sensing to support nutritional awareness. Paper presented at the proceedings of the 2002 *International Conference on Ubiquitous Computing*, Goteborg, Sweden, Setemper 29- October 1.

Marks, J.T., M.K. Campbell, D.S. Ward, K.M. Ribisl, B.M. Wildemuth, and M.J. Symons. 2006. A comparison of web and print media for physical activity promotion among adolescent girls. *Journal of Adolescent Health* 39(1):96-104.

Marshall, A.L., E.R. Leslie, A.E. Bauman, B.H. Marcus, and N. Owen. 2003. Print versus website physical activity programs. *American Journal of Preventive Medicine* 25(2):88-94.

Matthews, M., G. Doherty, J. Sharry, and C. Fitzpatrick. 2008. Mobile phone mood charting for adolescents. *British Journal of Guidance and Counselling* 36(2):113-129.

Micucci, J.A. 1972. "Self-esteem and preference for consonant information." M.S. thesis, Cornell University, Ithaca, NY.

Miller, R.S. 1987. Empathic embarrassment: Situational and personal determinants of reactions to the embarrassment of another. *Journal of Personality and Social Psychology* 53(6):1061-1069.

Mo, P.K., and N.S. Coulson. 2008. Exploring the communication of social support within virtual communities: A content analysis of messages posted to an online HIV/AIDS support group. *CyberPsychology and Behavior* 11(3):371-374.

Morgan, P.J., D.R. Lubans, C.E. Collins, J.M. Warren, and R. Callister. 2009. The SHED-IT randomized controlled trial: Evaluation of an internet-based weight-loss program for men. *Obesity* 17(11):2025-2032.

Napolitano, M.A., M. Fotheringham, D. Tate, C. Sciamanna, E. Leslie, N. Owen, A. Bauman, and B. Marcus. 2003. Evaluation of an Internet-based physical activity intervention: A preliminary investigation. *Annals of Behavioral Medicine* 25(2):92-99.

Neiger, B.L., R. Thackeray, S.A. Van Wagenen, C.L. Hanson, J.H. West, M.D. Barnes, and M.C. Fagen. 2012. Use of social media in health promotion purposes, key performance indicators, and evaluation metrics. *Health Promotion Practice* 13(2):159-164.

Newman, M.W., D. Lauterbach, S.A. Munson, P. Resnick, and M.E. Morris. 2011. "It's not that I don't have problems, I'm just not putting them on Facebook: Challenges and opportunities in using online social networks for health." Paper presented at the proceedings of the ACM 2011 conference on computer supported cooperative work, Hangzhou, China, March 19-23.

Norton, M.I., B. Monin, J. Cooper, and M.A. Hogg. 2003. Vicarious dissonance: Attitude change from the inconsistency of others. *Journal of Personality and Social Psychology* 85(1):47-62.

Object Frontier [blog]. 2013. 10 examples of gamification to influence employee behavior. http://info.objectfrontier.com/blog/bid/316541/10-Examples-of-Gamification-to-Influence-Employee-Behavior

Oenema, A., J. Brug, A. Dijkstra, I. de Weerdt, and H. de Vries. 2008. Efficacy and use of an internet-delivered computer-tailored lifestyle intervention, targeting saturated fat intake, physical activity and smoking cessation: A randomized controlled trial. *Annals of Behavioral Medicine* 35(2):125-135.

Olson, J.M., and J. Stone. 2005. The influence of behavior on attitudes. In *The handbook of attitudes*, edited by D. Albarracín, B.T. Johnson, and M.P. Zanna, 223-272. Mahwah, NJ: Lawrence Erlbaum Associates.

O'Reilly, D., K. Gaebel, F. Xie, J.E. Tarride, and R. Goeree. 2011. Health economic evaluations help inform payers of the best use of scarce health care resources. *International Journal of Circumpolar Health* 70:417-427.

Orji, R., J. Vassileva, and R.L. Mandryk. 2013. LunchTime: A slow-casual game for long-term dietary behavior change. *Personal and Ubiquitous Computing* 17(6):1211-1221.

Pan, B., H. Hembrooke, T. Joachims, L. Lorigo, G. Gay, and L.A. Granka. 2007. In Google we trust: Users' decisions on rank, position, and relevance. *Journal of Computer-Mediated Communication* 12(3):801-823.

Pekmezi, D.W., D.M. Williams, S. Dunsiger, E.G. Jennings, B.A. Lewis, J.M. Jakicic, and B.H. Marcus. 2010. Feasibility of using computer-tailored and Internet-based interventions to promote physical activity in underserved populations. *Telemedicine and e-Health* 16(4):498-503.

Peng, W., J.H. Lin, and J. Crouse. 2011. Is playing exergames really exercising? A meta-analysis of energy expenditure in active video games. *Cyberpsychology, Behavior, and Social Networking* 14(11):681-688.

Pettee, G.K.K., J.R. Morrow Jr., and A.L. Woolsey. 2012. Framework for physical activity as a complex and multidimensional behavior. *Journal of Physical Activity and Health* 9(Suppl. 1):S11-S18.

Petty, R.E., and J.T. Cacioppo. 1986. The elaboration likelihood model of persuasion. In *Advances in experimental social psychology*, edited by L. Berkowitz, 1-24. New York: Academic Press.

Poole, E.S., A.D. Miller, Y. Xu, E. Eiriksdottir, R. Catrambone, and E.D. Mynatt. 2011. "The place for ubiquitous computing in schools: Lessons learned from a school-based intervention for youth physical activity." Paper presented at the proceedings of the 13th international conference on ubiquitous computing, Beijing, China, September 17-21.

Preece, J. 1998. Empathic communities: Reaching out across the Web. *Interactions* 5(2):32-43.

Prislin, R., and W. Wood. 2005. Social influence in attitudes and attitude change. In *The handbook of attitudes*, edited by D. Albarracín, B.T. Johnson, and M.P. Zanna, 671-706. Mahwah, NJ: Lawrence Erlbaum.

Prochaska, J.J., C. Pechmann, R. Kim, and J.M. Leonhardt. 2012. Twitter = quitter? An analysis of Twitter quit smoking social networks. *Tobacco Control* 21(4):447-449.

Purpura, S., V. Schwanda, K. Williams, W. Stubler, and P. Sengers. 2011. "Fit4life: The design of a persuasive technology promoting healthy behavior and ideal weight." Paper presented at the proceedings of the 2011 SIGCHI conference on human factors in computing systems, Vancouver, Canada, May 7-12.

Ressler, P.K., Y.S. Bradshaw, L. Gualtieri, and K.K.H. Chui. 2012. Communicating the experience of chronic pain and illness through blogging. *Journal of Medical Internet Research* 14(5):e143.

Ricci, F., L. Rokach, B. Shapira, and P.B. Kantor. 2011. *Recommender systems handbook*. New York: Springer.

Richardson, C.R., L.R. Buis, A.W. Janney, D.E. Goodrich, A. Sen, M.L. Hess, K.S. Mehari, L.A. Fortlage, P.J. Resnick, B.J. Zikmund-Fisher, V.J. Strecher, and J.D. Piette. 2010. An online community improves adherence in an internet-mediated walking program. Part 1: Results of a randomized controlled trial. Journal of Medical Internet Research12(4):e71.

Robroek, S.J.W., S. Polinder, F.J. Bredt, and A. Burdorf. 2012. Cost-effectiveness of a long-term Internet-delivered worksite health promotion programme on physical activity and nutrition: A cluster randomized controlled trial. *Health Education Research* 27(3):399-410.

Rodgers, S., and Q. Chen. 2005. Internet community group participation: Psychosocial benefits for women with breast cancer. *Journal of Computer Mediated Communication* 10(4).

Rogers, R.W. 1975. A protection motivation theory of fear appeals and attitude change. *Journal of Psychology* 91:93-114.

Rosenstock, I.M. 1974. Historical origins of the health belief model. *Health Education & Behavior* 2(4):328-335.

Rosenstock, I.M., V.J. Strecher, and M.H. Becker. 1994. The health belief model and HIV risk behavior change. In *Preventing AIDS: Theories and methods of behavioral interventions.* New York: Plenum Press.

Rothman, A.J., and M.T. Kiviniemi. 1999. Treating people with information: An analysis and review of approaches to communicating health risk information. *JNCI Monographs* 1999(25):44-51.

Salem, D.A., G.A. Bogat, and C. Reid. 1997. Mutual help goes online. *Journal of Community Psychology* 25(2):189-207.

Scanfeld, D., V. Scanfeld, and E.L. Larson. 2010. Dissemination of health information through social networks: Twitter and antibiotics. *American Journal of Infection Control* 38(3):182-188.

Schlenker, B.R. 1980. *Impression management: The self-concept, social identity, and interpersonal relations.* Monterey, CA: Brooks/Cole.

Schwinn, T.M., S. Schinke, L. Fang, and S. Kandasamy. 2014. A web-based, health promotion program for adolescent girls and their mothers who reside in public housing. *Addictive Behaviors* 39(4):757-760.

Sears, D.W., and J.L. Freedman. 1965. Effects of expected familiarity with arguments upon opinion change and selective exposure. *Journal of Personality and Social Psychology* 2(3):420-426.

Shen, X., B. Tan, and C.X. Zhai. 2005. "Implicit user modeling for personalized search." Paper presented at the proceedings of the 14th ACM international conference on information and knowledge management, Bremen, Germany, October 31 - November 05.

Sillence, E., P. Briggs, P. Harris, and L. Fishwick. 2006. "Changes in online health usage over the last 5 years." Paper presented at the proceedings of the 2006 SIGCHI conference on human factors in computing systems, Montreal, Canada, April 24-27.

———. 2007. How do patients evaluate and make use of online health information? *Social Science and Medicine* 64(9):1853-1862.

Skår, S., F.F. Sniehotta, G.J. Molloy, A. Prestwich, and V. Araújo-Soares. 2011. Do brief online planning inter-ventions increase physical activity amongst university students? A randomised controlled trial. *Psychology and Health* 26(4):399-417.

Skeels, M.M., K.T. Unruh, C. Powell, and W. Pratt. 2010. "Catalyzing social support for breast cancer patients." Paper presented at the proceedings of the 2010 SIGCHI conference on human factors in computing systems, Atlanta, April 10-15.

Slootmaker, S.M., M.J.M. Chinapaw, A.J. Schuit, J.C. Seidell, and W. Van Mechelen. 2009. Feasibility and effectiveness of online physical activity advice based on a personal activity monitor: Randomized controlled trial. *Journal of Medical Internet Research* 11(3):1-13.

Spittaels, H., I. De Bourdeaudhuij, and C. Vandelanotte. 2007. Evaluation of a website-delivered computer-tailored intervention for increasing physical activity in the general population. *Preventive Medicine: An International Journal Devoted to Practice and Theory* 44(3):209-217.

Staiano, A.E., and S.L. Calvert. 2011. Exergames for physical education courses: Physical, social, and cognitive benefits. *Child Development Perspectives* 5(2):93-98.

Steele, R.M., W.K. Mummery, and T. Dwyer. 2007a. Examination of program exposure across intervention delivery modes: Face to face versus Internet. International Journal of Behavioral Nutrition and Physical Activity 2007(4):7.

———. 2007b. Using the internet to promote physical activity: A randomized trial of intervention delivery modes. *Journal of Physical Activity and Health* 4(3):245-260.

Sullivan, S.J., A.G. Schneiders, C.W. Cheang, E. Kitto, H. Lee, J. Redhead, S. Ward, O.H. Ahmed, and P.R. McCrory. 2012. 'What's happening?' A content analysis of concussion-related traffic on Twitter. *British Journal of Sports Medicine* 46(4):258-263.

Tetlock, P.E., and J.I. Kim. 1987. Accountability and judgment processes in a personality prediction task. *Journal of Personality and Social Psychology* 52(4):700-709.

Tetlock, P.E., and A.S. Manstead. 1985. Impression management versus intrapsychic explanations in social psychology: A useful dichotomy? *Psychological Review* 92(1):59-77.

Thayer, S. 1969. Confidence and postjudgment exposure to consonant and dissonant information in a free-choice situation. *Journal of Social Psychology* 77(1):113-120.

Thomas, R., J. Cahill, and L. Santilli. 1997. Using an interactive computer game to increase skill and self-efficacy regarding safer sex negotiation: Field test results. *Health Education and Behavior* 24(1):71-86.

Thorson, E.A. 2008. Changing patterns of news consumption and participation: News recommendation engines. *Information, Communication and Society* 11(4):473-489.

Unnithan, V.B., W. Houser, and B. Fernhall. 2006. Evaluation of the energy cost of playing a dance simulation video game in overweight and non-overweight children and adolescents. *International Journal of Sports Medicine* 27(10):804-809.

Valle, C.G., D.F. Tate, D.K. Mayer, M. Allicock, and J. Cai. 2012. A randomized trial of a Facebook-based physical activity intervention for young adult cancer survivors. *American Journal of Cardiology* 109:1754.

van Genugten, L., P. van Empelen, B. Boon, G. Borsboom, T. Visscher, and A. Oenema. 2012. Results from an online computer-tailored weight management intervention for overweight adults: Randomized controlled trial. *Journal of Medical Internet Research* 14(2):100-114.

van Wier, M.F., J.C. Dekkers, I.J.M. Hendriksen, M.W. Heymans, G.A.M. Ariëns, N.P. Pronk, T. Smid, and W. van Mechelen. 2011. Effectiveness of phone and e-mail lifestyle counseling for long term weight control among overweight employees. *Journal of Occupational and Environmental Medicine* 53(6):680-686.

Wadsworth, D. 2006. "Evaluation of a social cognitive theory based e-mail intervention to increase physical activity of college females." PhD diss., University of Mississippi. PsycINFO (AAI3190576).

Wagner, J., G. Geleijnse, and A. van Halteren. 2011. "Guidance and support for healthy food preparation in an augmented kitchen." Paper presented at the proceedings of the 2011 workshop on context-awareness in retrieval and recommendation, Palo Alto, CA, February 13.

Wang, H., X. He, M.W. Chang, Y. Song, R.W. White, and W. Chu. 2013. "Personalized ranking model adaptation for web search." Paper presented at the proceedings of the 36th international ACM SIGIR conference on research and development in information retrieval, Dublin, July 28 - August 01.

Wanner, M., E. Martin-Diener, C. Braun-Fahrländer, G. Bauer, and B.W. Martin. 2009. Effectiveness of Active-Online, an individually tailored physical activity intervention, in a real-life setting: Randomized controlled trial. *Journal of Medical Internet Research* 11(3):1-14.

Webber, K.H., D.F. Tate, and J.M. Bowling. 2008. A randomized comparison of two motivationally enhanced internet behavioral weight loss programs. *Behaviour Research and Therapy* 46(9):1090-1095.

White, M., and S.M. Dorman. 2001. Receiving social support online: Implications for health education. *Health Education Research* 16(6):693-707.

White, R.W. 2013. "Beliefs and biases in web search." Paper presented at the proceedings of the 36th international ACM SIGIR conference on research and development in information retrieval, Dublin, July 28 - August 01.

White, R.W., and E. Horvitz. 2009a. "Experiences with web search on medical concerns and self-diagnosis." Paper presented at the proceedings of the 2009 AMIA annual symposium, San Francisco, November 14-18.

————. 2009b. Cyberchondria: Studies of the escalation of medical concerns in web search. *ACM Transactions on Information Systems* 27(4):23.

————. 2013. From health search to health care: Explorations of intention and utilization via query logs and user surveys. *Journal of the American Medical Informatics Association* 21(1):49-55.

Whittemore, R., S. Jeon, and M. Grey. 2013. An internet obesity prevention program for adolescents. *Journal of Adolescent Health* 52(4):439-447.

Wicks, P., M. Massagli, J. Frost, C. Brownstein, S. Okun, T. Vaughan, R. Bradley, and J. Heywood. 2010. Sharing health data for better outcomes on PatientsLikeMe. *Journal of Medical Internet Research* 12(2):e19.

Wilkinson, N., R.P. Ang, and D.H. Goh. 2008. Online video game therapy for mental health concerns: A review. *International Journal of Social Psychiatry* 54(4):370-382.

Winett, R.A., E.S. Anderson, J.R. Wojcik, S.G. Winett, and T. Bowden. 2007. Guide to health: Nutrition and physical activity outcomes of a group-randomized trial of an internet-based intervention in churches. *Annals of Behavioral Medicine* 33(3):251-261.

Wyer, R.S., Jr., and D. Albarracín. 2005. *Belief formation, organization, and change: Cognitive and motivational influences.* Mahwah, NJ: Lawrence Erlbaum.

Zanna, M.P., and J.K. Rempel. 1988. Attitudes: A new look at an old concept. In *The social psychology of knowledge,* edited by D. Bar-Tal and A.W. Kruglanski, 283-301. New York: Cambridge University Press.

Zhai, C.X. 2008. *Statistical language models for information retrieval (Synthesis lectures series on human language technologies).* San Rafael, CA: Morgan and Claypool.

Ziebland, S., and S. Wyke. 2012. Health and illness in a connected world: How might sharing experiences on the internet affect people's health? *Milbank Quarterly* 90:219-249.

INDEX

ABOUT THE EDITORS

Weimo Zhu is a professor in the Department of Kinesiology and Community Health at the University of Illinois at Urbana-Champaign, USA. An internationally known scholar in Kines-metrics (Measurement and Evaluation in Kinesiology), Dr. Zhu's primary research interests are in the study and application of new measurement theories and statistical models and methods to the field of kinesiology, especially in youth physical fitness, the impact of body-mind exercises on health, and physical activity and inactivity and public health. He has published more than 100 SCI/SSCI journal articles and his research has been funded by external grants, including NIH and RWJF. He is the editor-in-chief of the *Research Quarterly for Exercise and Sport*, one of the most respected research journals in Kinesiology with a long, rich history, and he was an associate editor of the *Journal of Physical Activity and Health* and *Frontiers in Physiology*. He is an active fellow of the US National Academy of Kinesiology, the American College of Sports Medicine, and the Research Consortium of SHAPE America. He was a member of the Scientific Board of the President's Council on Physical Fitness and Sports from 2005 to 2008, and he was appointed as a panel member of the Institute of Medicine of the US National Academies' committee on "Fitness Measures and Health Outcomes in Youth" in 2011. Dr. Zhu has served on the FITNESSGRAM/ACTIVITYGRAM Advisory Committee since 2002.

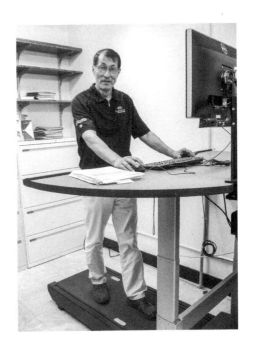

Photo by Anna Flanagan, courtesy of UIUC.

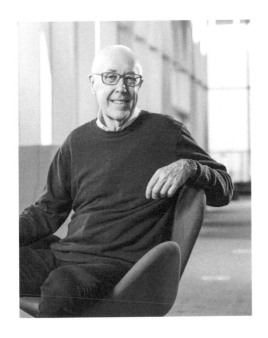

Neville Owen is a National Health and Medical Research Council of Australia Senior Principal Research Fellow, Head of the Behavioural Epidemiology Laboratory at the Baker Heart & Diabetes Institute, and Distinguished Professor of Health Sciences at Swinburne University, in Melbourne, Australia. He has appointments as an adjunct professor in Medicine at Monash University, Population and Global Health at the University of Melbourne, and Public Health at the University of Queensland. His research aims to identify how environmental and policy initiatives may be used to prevent type 2 diabetes, cardiovascular disease, and cancer. His early studies were in tobacco control and behavior change for smoking cessation and exercise. His research now focuses on changing the environmental determinants of physical activity and sedentary behavior. This is through mechanistically focused laboratory experiments, epidemiologic observational studies, real-world intervention trials, and improving the health of urban populations through influencing the built environment to increase physical activity.

Photo courtesy of Swinburne University of Technology. Image: Eamon Gallagher.

CONTRIBUTORS

Barbara E. Ainsworth,
Arizona State University
(Tempe, AZ, United States)

Dolores Albarracin,
University of Illinois at Urbana-Champaign
(Urbana, IL, United States)

Edward Archer,
EnduringFX
(Columbia, SC, United States)

Enrique G. Artero,
University of Almería
(Almería, Spain)

Jorge A. Banda,
Stanford University School of Medicine
(Stanford, CA, United States)

Stephan Bandelow,
Loughborough University
(Loughborough, UK)

David Bassett,
University of Tennessee
(Knoxville, TN, United States)

Adrian Bauman,
University of Sydney
(Sydney, Australia)

Kelly J. Baute,
A Splendid Earth Wellness, LLC
(Seymour, IN, United States)

Audrey Bergouignan,
Baker IDI Heart and Diabetes Institute
(Melbourne, Australia)

Stuart J.H. Biddle,
Victoria University
(Melbourne, Australia)

Steven N. Blair,
retired, University of South Carolina
(Columbia, SC, United States)

Marco S. Boscolo,
California State University
(Sacramento, CA, United States)

Wendy J. Brown,
University of Queensland
(Brisbane, Australia)

Jordan A. Carlson,
Children's Mercy Hospital
(San Diego, CA, United States)

Carl J. Caspersen,
retired, Centers for Disease Control and Prevention
(Atlanta, GA, United States)

Tyrone G. Ceaser,
Gramercy Research Group
(Winston-Salem, NC, United States)

Josephine Y. Chau,
University of Sydney
(Sydney, Australia)

Kong Y. Chen,
National Institutes of Health
(Bethesda, MD, United States)

Galen Cranz,
University of California
(Berkeley, CA, United States)

David W. Dunstan,
Baker IDI Heart and Diabetes Institute
(Melbourne, Australia)

John P. Elder,
San Diego State University
(San Diego, CA, United States)

Alberto Flórez Pregonero,
Pontificia Universidad Javeriana
(Bogotá, Colombia)

Christine M. Friedenreich,
Alberta Health Services
(Calgary, AB, Canada)

Kenneth A. Glover,
CSX Transportation
(Jacksonville, FL, United States)

Bethany J. Howard,
Baker IDI Heart and Diabetes Institute
(Melbourne, Australia)

Stephen Intille,
Northeastern University
(Boston, MA, United States)

Dinesh John,
Northeastern University
(Boston, MA, United States)

Youngwon Kim,
University of Cambridge
(Cambridge, England)

Abby C. King,
Stanford University School of Medicine
(Stanford, CA, United States)

Bronwyn A. Kingwell,
Baker IDI Heart and Diabetes Institute
(Melbourne, Australia)

Vera Liao,
University of Illinois at Urbana-Champaign
(Urbana, IL, United States)

Brigid M. Lynch,
Cancer Council Victoria
(Melbourne, Australia)

Kevin O. Moran,
Northwestern University
(Evanston, IL, United States)

Michael L. Power,
Smithsonian Conservation Biology Institute
(Washington, DC, United States)

Nicolaas P. Pronk,
HealthPartners Institute
(Bloomington, MN, United States) and
Harvard School of Public Health
(Boston, MA, United States)

Fabien Rivière,
University of Lorraine
(Vandoeuvre-lès-Nancy, France)

Thomas N. Robinson,
Stanford University School of Medicine and
Lucile Packard Children's Hospital
(Stanford, CA, United States)

James F. Sallis,
University of California
(San Diego, CA, United States)

John B. Shea,
Indiana University
(Bloomington, IN, United States)

G. Darlene Thomas,
retired, Centers for Disease Control and Prevention
(Atlanta, GA, United States)

Richard P. Troiano,
National Institutes of Health
(Bethesda, MD, United States)

Joan Vernikos,
Third Age, LLC
(Culpeper, VA, United States)

Gregory J. Welk,
Iowa State University
(Ames, IA, United States)

Melicia C. Whitt-Glover,
Gramercy Research Group
(Greensboro/Winston-Salem, NC, United States)

Sandra J. Winter,
Stanford University School of Medicine
(Stanford, CA, United States)

Jessica Yi,
University of Illinois at Urbana-Champaign
(Urbana, IL, United States)

ChengXiang Zhai,
University of Illinois at Urbana-Champaign
(Urbana, IL, United States)

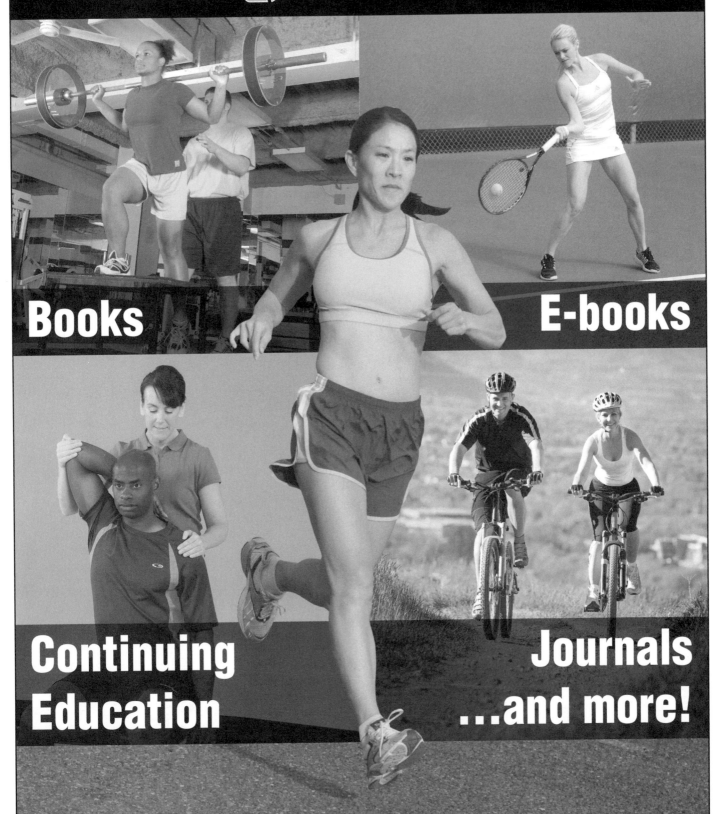
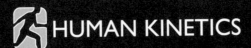